ATLAS OF
Roentgenographic positions and standard radiologic procedures

Volume three

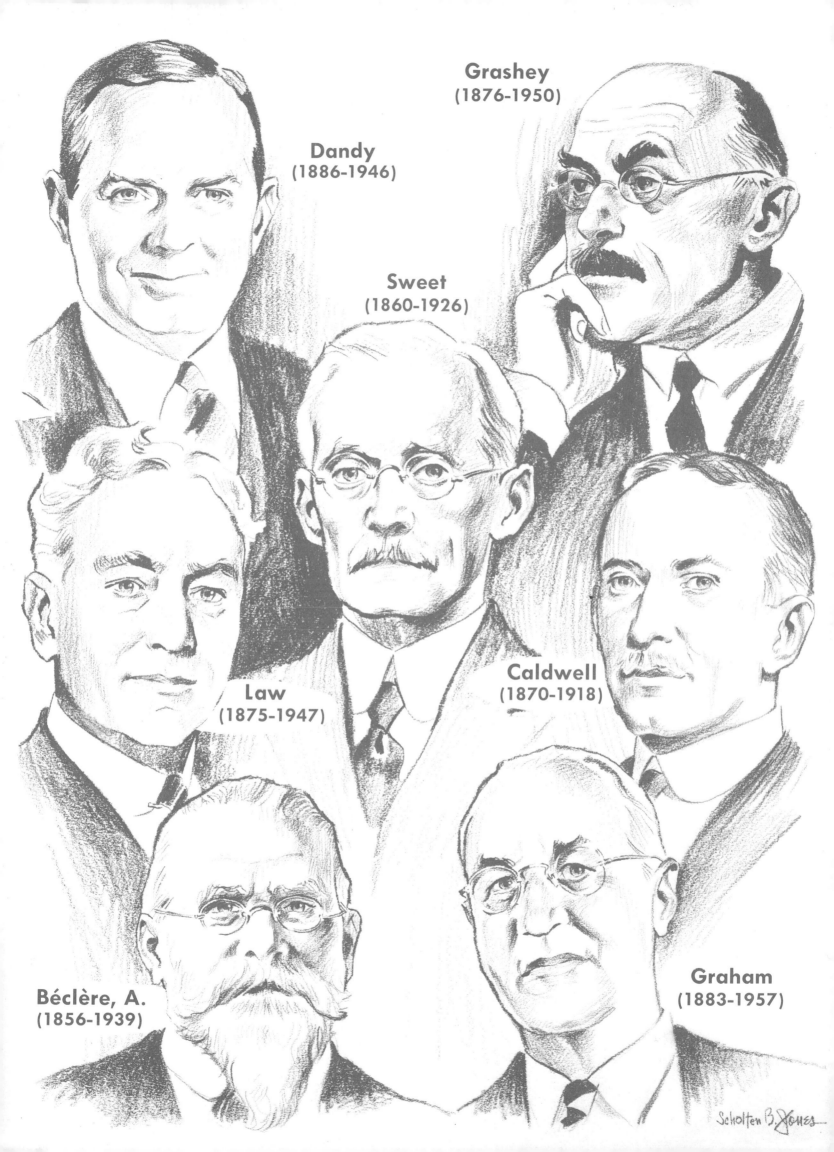

Grashey
(1876-1950)

Dandy
(1886-1946)

Sweet
(1860-1926)

Law
(1875-1947)

Caldwell
(1870-1918)

Béclère, A.
(1856-1939)

Graham
(1883-1957)

Scholten B. Jones

ATLAS OF
Roentgenographic positions and standard radiologic procedures

Vinita Merrill

WITH CONTRIBUTIONS BY

David L. Benninghoff, M.D.
Carl R. Bogardus, Jr., M.D.
Barbara M. Curcio, R.T.
John P. Dorst, M.D.
Joseph W. Kaplan, Jr., R.T.
Richard G. Lester, M.D.
William J. Setlak, N.M.T.(A.R.R.T.), B.S.
William H. Shehadi, M.D., F.A.C.R.
Roy D. Strand, M.D.
Donald L. Sucher
Carole A. Sullivan, R.T.

Volume three of three volumes

FOURTH EDITION

The C. V. Mosby Company

Saint Louis   1975

FOURTH EDITION

Copyright © 1975 by The C. V. Mosby Company

All rights reserved. No part of this book may be reproduced in any manner without written permission of the publisher.

Previous editions copyrighted 1949, 1959, 1967

Printed in the United States of America
Distributed in Great Britain by Henry Kimpton, London

Library of Congress Cataloging in Publication Data

Merrill, Vinita, 1905-
    Atlas of roentgenographic positions and standard radiologic procedures.

    Includes bibliographies and index.
    1. Radiography, Medical—Positioning—Atlases.
I. Title. II. Title: Roentgenographic positions and standard radiologic procedures. [DNLM: 1. Technology, Radiology—Atlases. WN17 M571a]
RC78.4.M47   616.07′572   75-1144
ISBN 0-8016-3412-1

TS/U/B 9 8 7 6 5 4 3 2 1

Contents

Volume three

ATLAS OF
Roentgenographic positions and standard radiologic procedures

Volume three

Anatomy and positioning of the anterior part of the neck

SOFT PALATE, PHARYNX, LARYNX, AND THYROID GLAND

Anterior part of the neck

The neck occupies the region between the skull and the thorax, its upper limit being defined by an imaginary line extending from the inferior border of the symphysis menti to the external occipital protuberance, and its lower limit being defined by a line extending from the suprasternal notch to the superior border of the first thoracic vertebra. For radiographic purposes, the neck is divided into posterior and anterior portions in accordance with the tissue composition and function of the contained structures. The several procedures that are required to demonstrate the osseous structures occupying the posterior division of the neck are described in the discussion on the cervical vertebrae. The portions of the central nervous system and of the circulatory system passing through the neck are described under the respective headings. The portion of the neck lying in front of the vertebrae is composed largely of soft tissues, the upper part of the respiratory and digestive systems being the principal structures and the ones under consideration in this discussion. The thyroid and parathyroid glands, and the larger part of the submaxillary glands, are also located in the anterior portion of the neck.

The *thyroid gland* consists of two lateral lobes connected together at their lower thirds by a narrow median portion called the isthmus. The lobes are approximately 2 inches in length, 1¼ inches in width, and ¾ inch thick. The gland lies at the front and sides of the upper part of the trachea, its lobes reaching from the lower third of the thyroid cartilage to the level of the first thoracic vertebra. While the thyroid gland is normally suprasternal in position, occasionally it presents a retrosternal extension into the upper aperture of the thorax. The *parathyroid glands* are small ovoid bodies and are normally four in number—two on each side. They are situated, one above the other, on the posterior part of the adjacent lobe of the thyroid gland.

The *pharynx*, serving as a passage for both air and food, is common to the respiratory and digestive systems. The pharynx is a musculomembranous, tubular structure situated in front of the vertebrae and behind the nose, the mouth, and the larynx. It is approximately 5 inches in length, extending from the undersurface of the body of the sphenoid bone and the basilar part of the occipital bone downward to the level of the disk between the sixth and seventh cervical vertebrae, where it becomes continuous with the esophagus. The pharyngeal cavity is subdivided into nasal, oral, and laryngeal portions. The nasopharynx lies above the soft palate, the upper part of which forms its floor, and communicates with the nasal fossae anteriorly and with the eustachian tubes laterally. On the roof and posterior wall of the nasopharynx, between the orifices of the eustachian tubes, the mucosa contains a mass of lymphadenoid tissue known as the *pharyngeal tonsil*, or *adenoids*. Hypertrophy of this tissue interferes with nasal breathing and is common in children. This condition is well demonstrated in a lateral projection of the nasopharynx. The oropharynx is the portion extending from the soft palate to the level of the hyoid bone; it communicates with the mouth through the faucial isthmus and has the *palatine tonsils*, which are located on its lateral walls between the two palatine, or faucial, arches. The base, or root, of the tongue forms the anterior wall of the oropharynx. The laryngeal pharynx, or hypopharynx, lies behind the larynx, its anterior wall being formed by the back of the larynx, and communicates with it by means of the upper laryngeal aperture. The air-containing nasal and oral pharynges are well visualized in lateral projections, except during the act of phonation, when the soft palate contracts and tends to obscure the nasal pharynx. An opaque medium is required for the demonstration of the lumen of the laryngeal pharynx, though it can be distended with air during the Valsalva maneuver.

The *larynx* is the organ of voice and, serving as the air passage between the pharynx and the trachea, it is also one of the divisions of the respiratory system.

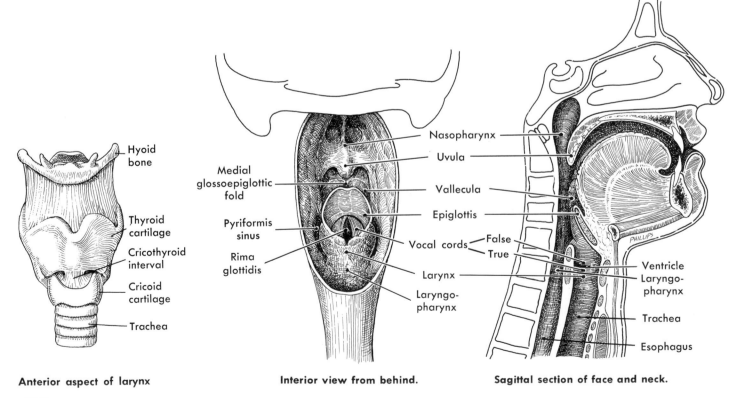

Anterior aspect of larynx

Interior view from behind.

Sagittal section of face and neck.

The larynx is a movable, tubular structure, is broader above than below, and is approximately 1½ inches in length. It is situated below the root of the tongue and in front of the laryngeal pharynx, where, suspended from the hyoid bone, it extends from the level of the superior margin of the fourth cervical vertebra to its junction with the trachea at the level of the inferior margin of the sixth cervical vertebra. The framework of the larynx is composed of nine cartilages—three single (epiglottis, thyroid, cricoid) and three paired (arytenoid, corniculate, cuneiform). These cartilages are connected together with ligaments, are moved by muscles, and are clothed in mucous membrane that is drawn into folds over certain of these structures. The thin, leaf-shaped epiglottis is situated behind the root of the tongue and the hyoid bone and above the laryngeal entrance. The thyroid cartilage, the largest of the group, forms the laryngeal prominence, or "Adam's apple." The lower border of the cricoid cartilage, the second largest of the group, is connected to the first ring of the trachea. The space between the ventral aspect of the thyroid and cricoid cartilages, called the *cricothyroid interval*, is the site of entry in percutaneous transtracheal bronchography.

The inlet of the larynx is oblique, slanting from above downward and backward. A pouchlike fossa, called the *pyriform recess* or *sinus* of the hypopharynx, is located on each side of the larynx and external to its orifice. The pyriform sinuses are well shown on frontal projections when insufflated with air (Valsalva maneuver) and when filled with an opaque medium.

The anterior surface of the free upper part of the epiglottis is attached to the root of the tongue by a median and two lateral folds of mucous membrane that bound two depressions called the *epiglottic valleculae*. The median glossoepiglottic fold extends between the front of the epiglottis and the base of the tongue. The lateral glosso-epiglottic folds extend lateralward and forward from the margin of the epiglottis to the junction of the side walls of the pharynx and the tongue. It has been stated that the epiglottis and valleculae serve as a trap to prevent leakage into the throat between acts of swallowing.

The entrance of the larynx is guarded above and in front by the epiglottis, and laterally and posteriorly by folds of mucous membrane called the aryepiglottic and interarytenoid folds. These folds extend around the margin of the laryngeal orifice from their junction with the epiglottis, and they function as a sphincter during deglutition (swallowing).

The laryngeal cavity is subdivided into three compartments by two pairs of mucosal folds which, extending anteroposteriorly, project from its lateral walls. The upper pair of folds, separated from each other by a median interval called the *vestibular slit*, or *rima vestibuli*, are the ventricular folds, or false vocal cords. The space above them is called the *laryngeal vestibule*. The lower pair of folds are separated from each other by a median fissure called the *rima glottidis*, and they are known as the *vocal folds*, or *true vocal cords*. The vocal cords and the rima glottidis comprise the vocal apparatus of the larynx and are collectively referred to as the *glottis*. The middle compartment, the space between the upper and lower mucosal folds, expands into a space on each side called the *laryngeal ventricle*. The lower space or compartment is continuous with the cavity of the trachea. The position and contour of the laryngeal structures vary considerably during speech and during deglutition.

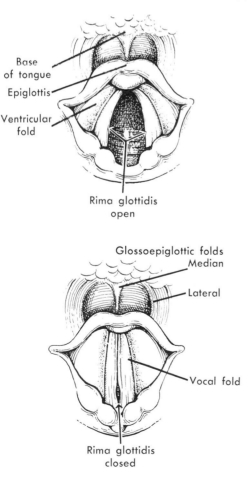

Base of tongue
Epiglottis
Ventricular fold
Rima glottidis open

Glossoepiglottic folds
Median
Lateral
Vocal fold
Rima glottidis closed

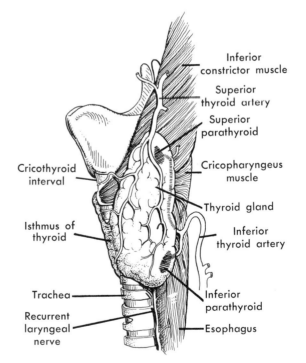

Inferior constrictor muscle
Superior thyroid artery
Superior parathyroid
Cricopharyngeus muscle
Thyroid gland
Inferior thyroid artery
Inferior parathyroid
Esophagus
Cricothyroid interval
Isthmus of thyroid
Trachea
Recurrent laryngeal nerve

597

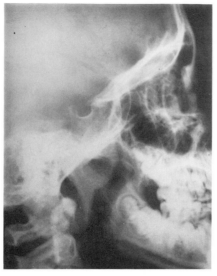

Hypertrophy of pharyngeal tonsil.

Radiograph and diagnostic information courtesy Dr. Judah Zizmor.

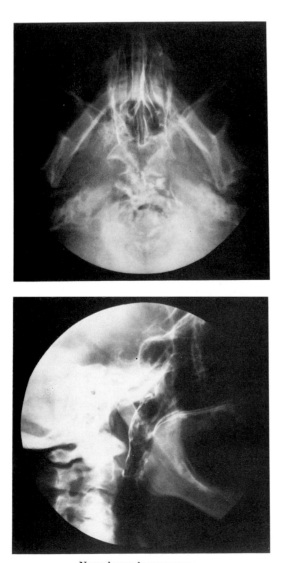

Normal nasopharyngograms.

Radiographs and diagnostic information courtesy Dr. M. J. Wisenberg.

ANTERIOR PART OF THE NECK
Soft palate, pharynx, and larynx
Methods of examination

The throat structures may be examined without or with an opaque medium; the method employed depends upon the abnormality being investigated.

PALATOGRAPHY

Bloch and Quantrill[1] investigate suspected tumors of the soft palate by a positive contrast technique. The patient is seated laterally before a vertical head unit with the nasopharynx centered to the film. For the first palatogram the patient is required to swallow a small amount of a thick, creamy barium sulfate mixture to coat the inferior surface of the soft palate and the uvula. A second lateral projection is obtained after the injection of 0.5 ml. of the creamy barium mixture into each nasal cavity to coat the upper surface of the soft palate and the posterior wall of the nasopharynx.

Morgan and associates[2] described a method of evaluating abnormalities of chewing and swallowing in children. These examiners record the chewing and swallowing function with cineradiography as the child chews barium-impregnated chocolate fudge, the recipe for which they include in their paper.

Cleft palate studies are taken with the patient seated laterally erect and are centered to the nasopharynx. The exposures are made during phonation to demonstrate the range of movement of the soft palate and the position of the tongue during each of the following sounds:[3,4] "d-a-h," "m-m-m," "s-s-s," and "e-e-e."

NASOPHARYNGOGRAPHY

Hypertrophy of the pharyngeal tonsil, or adenoids, is clearly delineated in a direct lateral projection centered to the nasopharynx (¾ inch directly forward from the external auditory meatus). To ensure filling the nasopharynx with air, the film must be exposed during the intake of a deep breath *through the nose*. Mouth breathing moves the soft palate backward to near approximation with the posterior wall of the nasopharynx, and thus causes the air intake to bypass the nasopharynx as it is directed downward into the larynx.

Positive contrast nasopharyngography is performed to assess the extent of nasopharyngeal tumors. Some examiners recommend an iodized oil for this examination.[5] Others prefer finely ground barium sulfate, either mixed in paste form[6] or applied dry with a pressure blower.[7]

[1]Bloch, S., and Quantrill, J. R.: The radiology of nasopharyngeal tumors, including positive contrast nasopharyngography, S. Afr. Med. J. **42**:1030-1036, 1968.

[2]Morgan, J. A., Gyepes, M. T., Jones, M. H., and Disilets, D. T.: Barium-impregnated chocolate fudge for the study of chewing mechanism in children, Radiology **94**:432-433, 1970.

[3]Randall, P., O'Hara, A. E., and Bakes, F. P.: A simple roentgen examination for the study of soft palate function in patients with poor speech, Plast. Reconstr. Surg. **21**:345-356, 1958.

[4]O'Hara, A. E.: Roentgen evaluation of patients with cleft palate, Radiol. Clin. N. Amer. **1**:1-11, 1963.

[5]Johnson, T. H., Green, A. E., and Rice, E. N.: Nasopharyngography: its technic and uses, Radiology **88**:1166-1169, 1967.

[6]Khoo, F. Y., Chia, K. B., and Nalpon, J.: A new technique of contrast examination of the nasopharynx with cinefluorography and roentgenography, Amer. J. Roentgen. **99**:238-248, 1967.

[7]Chittinand, S., Patheja, S. S., and Wisenberg, M. J.: Barium nasopharyngography, Radiology **98**:387-390, 1971.

Preliminary filming commonly consists of a submentovertical projection of the skull and an erect lateral projection centered to the nasopharynx (¾ inch directly forward from the external auditory meatus). When an iodized oil or a barium paste is used, the patient is placed on the examining table in the supine position after local anesthetization. The shoulders are elevated to flex the neck enough to permit the orbitomeatal line to be adjusted at an angle of 40 to 45 degrees to the horizontal. The head is kept in this position throughout the examination. Both before and after the instillation of the contrast medium into the nasal cavities, the basal views are obtained with the central ray directed midway between the mandibular angles at an angle of 15 to 20 degrees toward the head. Lateral views are obtained by cross-table projections centered to the nasopharynx. On completion of this phase of the examination, the patient is requested to sit up and blow his nose. This act evacuates most of the contrast medium, and the remainder will be swallowed. It is reported that none of the contrast medium is aspirated because the swallowing mechanism is triggered before the contrast medium reaches the larynx. Additional studies in the erect position are then made as directed by the examining radiologist.

Chittinand and associates[7] described an opaque contrast nasopharyngographic procedure wherein the patient is not required to keep his neck in the uncomfortable flexed position for the entire examination. These examiners have the patient seated before a vertical head unit or Potter-Bucky diaphragm. Preliminary lateral and submentovertical films are obtained. The authors state that topical anesthetization is not required for their method of examination. Using a standard spray bottle, they spray each nasal cavity with water as a wetting agent, after which they spray Micropaque powder through each nostril with a powder blower connected to a pressure unit. Two basal projections, one at rest and one during a modified Valsalva maneuver, and a lateral projection are then taken. Any of the medium not expelled when the patient blows his nose is swallowed. The authors state that immediate chest films reveal no barium in the lungs and that 24-hour follow-up films reveal complete clearing of the nasopharynx.

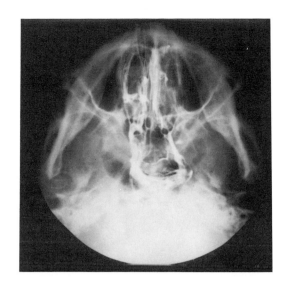

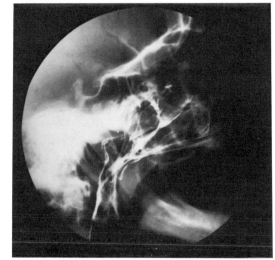

Right ninth nerve signs. There is asymmetry of the nasopharynx with flattening on the right and irregularity demonstrated on the basal view. The lateral view shows a mass in the posterior aspect of the nasopharynx with an umbilication.

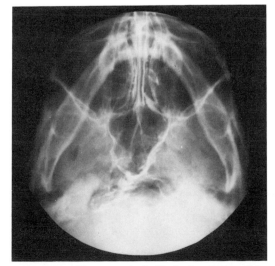

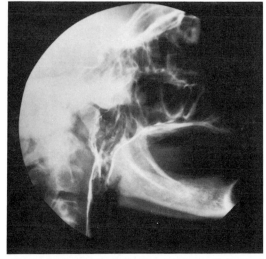

Two views of a 69-year-old woman who had had a long history of decreased hearing on the left side and left facial paresthesia. The nasopharynx is asymmetrical with blunting of the fossa of Rosenmuller and poor definition of the torus tubarius. There is a soft tissue density in the nasopharynx posteriorly. On the lateral view a shallow niche is seen at the C1 level, which may represent an ulcer.

Above radiographs and diagnostic information courtesy Dr. M. J. Wisenberg.

599

ANTERIOR PART OF THE NECK

Soft palate, pharynx, and larynx
Methods of examination—cont'd

PHARYNGOGRAPHY

Opaque studies of the pharynx are made with an ingestible contrast medium, usually with a thick, creamy mixture of equal parts, by volume, of water and barium sulfate. This examination is frequently carried out under radioscopy with spot-film studies only, these and/or conventional projections being made during deglutition.

Deglutition. The act of swallowing is performed by the rapid and highly coordinated action of many muscles. The student is referred to the papers listed in the bibliography for a detailed description of deglutition. The following are points of importance in radiography of the pharynx and upper esophagus:

1. The mid-area of the tongue becomes depressed to collect the mass, or bolus, of material to be swallowed.

2. The base of the tongue forms a central groove to accommodate the bolus and then moves upward and backward along the roof of the mouth to propel the bolus through the faucial isthmus into the pharynx.

3. Simultaneously with the backward thrust of the tongue, the larynx moves forward and upward under the root of the tongue, the sphincteric folds nearly closing the laryngeal orifice.

4. The epiglottis divides the passing bolus and drains the two portions laterally into the pyriform sinuses as it lowers over the laryngeal entrance.

The bolus is projected into the pharynx at the height of the forward movement of the larynx. The student has only to swallow a few times to study the process of deglu-tition and to understand the need to synchronize a rapid exposure with the peak of the act.

The shortest exposure time possible must be utilized for studies made during deglutition. The patient is asked to hold the barium sulfate bolus in his mouth until signaled and then to swallow the bolus *in one movement.* He is asked to refrain from swallowing again if a mucosal study is to be attempted. The mucosal study is taken during the modified Valsalva maneuver for double-contrast delineation.

Gunson method

Gunson[1] made an excellent and practical suggestion for synchronizing the exposure with the height of the swallowing act in deglutition studies of the pharynx and upper esophagus. Gunson's method consists of tying a dark-colored shoestring (metal tips removed) snugly around the patient's throat above the thyroid cartilage. The forward and upward travel of the larynx is then shown by the elevation of the shoestring as the thyroid cartilage moves forward and, immediately thereafter, by the displacement of the shoestring as the cartilage passes upward.

It is desirable to have the exposure coincide with the peak of the *forward* movement of the larynx, the instant at which the bolus of contrast material is projected into the pharynx, but as stated by Templeton and Kredel,[2] the action is so rapid that satisfactory filling is usually obtained if the exposure is made as soon as the forward movement is noted.

[1]Gunson, Edward F.: Radiography of the pharynx and upper esophagus, shoestring method, Xray Techn. **33**:1-8, 1961.
[2]Templeton, F. E., and Kredel, R. A.: The cricopharyngeal sphincter, Laryngoscope **53**:1-12, 1943.

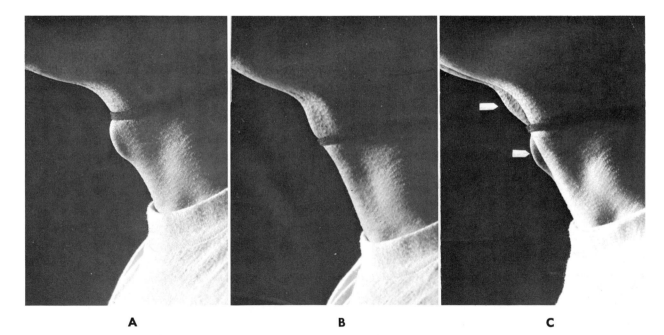

| A | B | C |

A, Ordinary dark shoelace has been tied snugly around the patient's neck above the Adam's apple. **B,** Exposure was made at peak of upward and forward movement of larynx during swallowing. At this moment pharynx is completely filled with barium, representing the ideal instant for making x-ray exposure. **C,** Double-exposure photograph emphasizing movement of the Adam's apple during swallowing. Note extent of anterior as well as upward excursion.

Photographs and legends courtesy Edward F. Gunson.

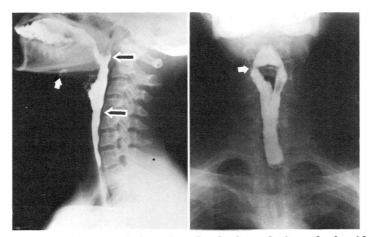

Both exposures are made at the peak of laryngeal elevation. In the lateral view, the hyoid bone (arrow) is almost at the level of the mandible. The pharynx (between the large arrows) is completely distended with barium. In the anteroposterior projection, the epiglottis divides the bolus into two streams, filling the pyriform sinuses below. Barium can also be seen entering the upper esophagus.

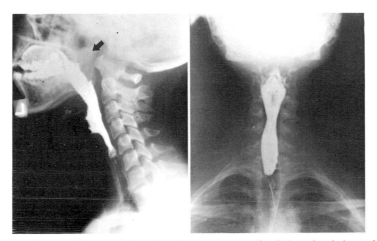

Examples of the type of radiographs readily made by the shoestring method for obtaining views of the swallowing mechanism. Note that the lateral view provides a clear view of the pharynx and esophagus as well as the mouth, the soft palate (arrow), the soft tissues of the neck, and the cervical vertebrae, all important in disorders of the swallowing function. The anteroposterior view also provides a record of the lung apices and the upper mediastinum, in addition to the pharynx and the esophagus.

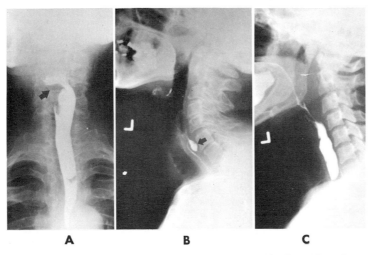

A   **B**   **C**

Anteroposterior view of the pharynx and upper esophagus with barium. The head has been turned to the right, with resultant asymmetric filling of the pharynx. **A,** The bolus is passing through the left pyriform sinus, leaving the right side unfilled (arrow). **B,** Lateral view after barium, showing a diverticulum. **C,** The lateral view made slightly late, with optimal filling of the upper esophagus.

Pharyngograms and legends courtesy Edward F. Gunson.

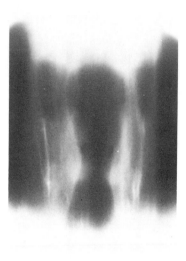

Linear tomogram during inspiration.

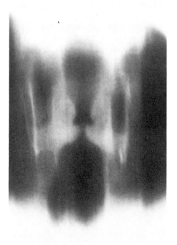

Linear tomogram during phonation of "e-e-e."

ANTERIOR PART OF THE NECK
Soft palate, pharynx, and larynx
Methods of examination—cont'd
LARYNGOPHARYNGOGRAPHY

Plain film studies, or more correctly, negative contrast studies, of the air-containing laryngopharyngeal structures are made in both frontal and lateral directions, the latter in the erect position with a soft tissue technique (10 kilovolts less than for the cervical spine). Frontal studies are made with the patient in either the supine or the seated erect position, with the head extended enough to prevent superimposition of the mandibular shadow on that of the larynx.

A Potter-Bucky technique is usually employed for the frontal projections. Thornbury and Latourette[1] and Zizmor[2] recommend the use of a high kilovoltage–heavy filtration technique for frontal studies of the larynx. The former examiners use a nongrid technique with a 3 mm. brass filter and, with Parspeed screens, the following exposure factors: 150 kvp., 300 milliamperes, 1/20 to 1/30 second, and a 40-inch focal film distance. Zizmor uses a grid technique with 2 mm. of aluminum and, with Parspeed screens, the following exposure factors: 150 kvp., 100 milliamperes, ¼ second, and a 40-inch focal film distance. The high kilovolt–heavy filtration technique greatly diminishes the image of the underlying cervical spine, giving near tomographic delineation of the larynx.

Negative contrast studies of the laryngopharyngeal structures provide considerable information concerning any alteration in the normal anatomy and function of these organs. Both negative and positive contrast studies are made during the following respiratory and stress maneuvers, with the patient in the frontal position:

1. *Quiet inspiration* to test abduction of the vocal cords. The resultant radiograph should show the cords open (abducted), with an uninterrupted column of air extending from the laryngeal vestibule downward into the trachea.

2. *Normal (expiratory) phonation* to test adduction of the vocal cords. The patient is instructed to take a deep breath and then, as he slowly exhales, to phonate either

[1]Thornbury, J. R., and Latourette, H. B.: Comparison study of laryngography techniques: 150 kvp plain roentgenography vs positive contrast roentgenography, Amer. J. Roentgen. **99**:555-561, 1967.
[2]Zizmor, Judah: Personal communication.

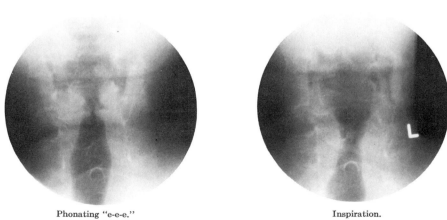

Phonating "e-e-e."   Inspiration.

This pair of radiographs was made with high-filtration technique.

All radiographs courtesy Dr. Judah Zizmor.

a high pitched "e-e-e" or a low pitched "a-a-h." The resultant radiograph should show the closed (adducted) vocal cords just above the break in the air column at the closed rima glottidis.

Phonation is normally performed during expiration. This test is now generally referred to as *normal* or *expiratory* phonation to distinguish it from the following test.

3. Powers and associates[1] introduced the use of *inspiratory phonation* (also called reverse phonation and aspirate or aspirant maneuver) for the demonstration of the laryngeal ventricle. The patient is instructed to exhale completely and then, as he slowly inhales, to make a harsh, stridulous sound with the phonation of "e" or other high-pitched sound. This test adducts the vocal cords, moves them downward, and balloons the ventricle for clear delineation.

4. *True Valsalva maneuver* to show complete closure of the glottis. This maneuver tests the elasticity and functional integrity of the glottis.

For the true Valsalva maneuver, ask the patient to take a deep breath and, while holding the breath in, to bear down as if trying to move his bowels (there is no delicate way to describe this maneuver to the patient). This act forces the breath against the closed glottis, and it increases both intrathoracic and intra-abdominal pressure.

5. *Modified Valsalva maneuver* to test the elasticity of the hypopharynx and the pyriform sinuses. The resultant radiograph should show the glottis closed and the hypopharynx and pyriform sinuses distended with air.

For the modified Valsalva maneuver, ask the patient to pinch his nostrils together with the thumb and forefinger of one hand and, with his mouth closed, to make and sustain a slight effort to blow his nose. Another way is to have the patient blow his cheeks outward against the closed nostrils and mouth as if he were blowing into a horn or balloon.

Each maneuver to be employed must be carefully explained and demonstrated just prior to its use, and the patient then required to perform the maneuver one or more times until he is able to perform it correctly.

[1]Powers, W. E., Holtz, S., and Ogura, J.: Contrast examination of the larynx and pharynx: inspiratory phonation, Amer. J. Roentgen. 92:40-42, 1964.

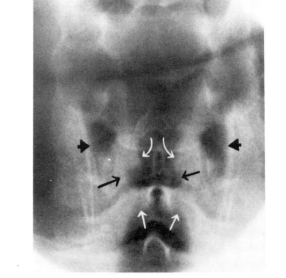

Inspiratory phonation showing the laryngeal ventricle (horizontal black arrows), the false vocal cords (curved white arrows), the true vocal cords (straight white arrows) and the pyriform sinuses (black arrow heads).

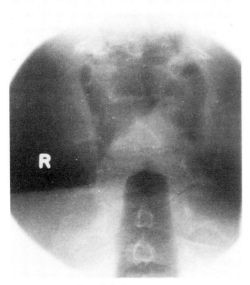

True Valsalva maneuver.

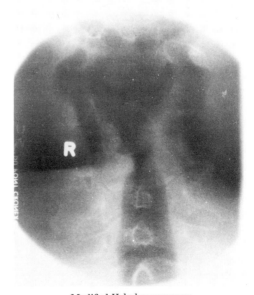

Modified Valsalva maneuver.

Above radiographs courtesy Dr. Judah Zizmor.

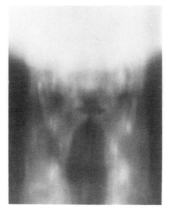

Linear tomogram during phonation of "e-e-e."

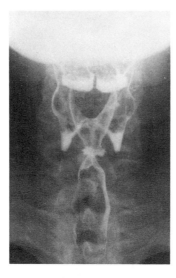

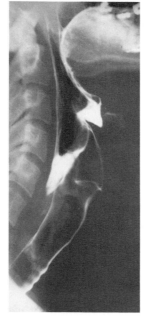

Normal laryngograms.

Above radiographs and clinical information courtesy Dr. Judah Zizmor.

ANTERIOR PART OF THE NECK
Soft palate, pharynx, and larynx
Methods of examination—cont'd
LARYNGOPHARYNGOGRAPHY—cont'd
Tomolaryngography

Tomographic studies of the laryngopharyngeal structures, either before or after the introduction of a radiopaque contrast medium, are made in the frontal plane. One set is usually made during quiet inspiration and one during normal (expiratory) phonation, but the stress maneuvers are used as indicated. The rapid-travel linear sweep is generally considered to be the method of choice for these studies, and the exposures are made during the first half of a wide arc (40 to 50 degrees) to prevent overlap streaking by the facial bones and teeth.

Positive contrast laryngopharyngography

Positive contrast examinations of the larynx and hypopharynx are usually performed to determine the exact site, size, and extent of tumor masses of these structures. The examination is carried out under radioscopy with the use of spot-films and/or cineradiographic recordings.

An iodized oil, in conjunction with the examination procedure described by Powers and associates,[1] is the medium most commonly used, although other radiopaque media are employed (see bibliography). In this procedure atropine sulfate and, when indicated, a mild sedative are administered 45 to 60 minutes prior to the examination. Atropine is used to dry the mucous membranes (1) for more immediate contact of the topical anesthetic and (2) for better and more uniform adherence of the contrast medium.

After satisfactory preliminary films, and with the patient seated erect, the radiologist sprays the laryngopharyngeal structures with a topical anesthetic to inhibit the gag, cough and deglutition reflexes. He then examines the patient radioscopically, gives him explicit instructions on each of the test maneuvers to be used, and cautions him to avoid coughing and swallowing after the introduction of the radiopaque medium.

[1]Powers, W. E., McGee, H. H., and Seaman, W. B.: Contrast examination of the larynx and pharynx, Radiology **68**:169-178, 1957.

Positive contrast laryngopharyngography—cont'd

A syringe loaded with the specified amount of iodized oil is attached to a curved metal cannula for the administration of the medium. With the patient seated erect, the radiologist slowly drips the iodized oil over the back of the tongue or directly into the larynx, coating all structures of the larynx and hypopharynx. The patient is then again examined radioscopically, and spot films are exposed at the height of each of the various test maneuvers. Some examiners obtain cineradiographic recordings with a continuous catheter drip of thin barium or iodized oil into the larynx.

• • •

Conventional films, the high kilovoltage–selective filtration method, tomography, positive contrast laryngography and cineradiography are the present radiographic methods for the study of the larynx.

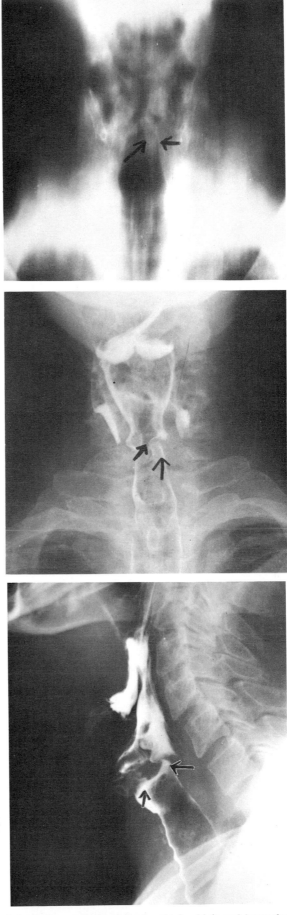

Rounded soft tissue mass involving two-thirds of left cord hangs down into subglottic larynx. On lateral view this is best demonstrated with the Valsalva maneuver.

Radiographs and diagnostic information courtesy Dr. Judah Zizmor.

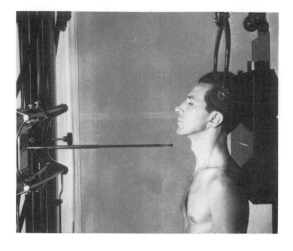

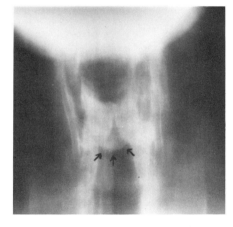

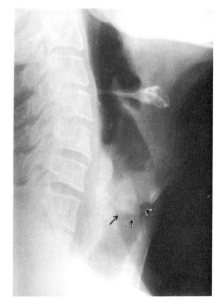

Polypoid mass of right false cord hanging into subglottic larynx.
Radiographs and diagnostic information courtesy Dr. Judah Zizmor.

PHARYNX AND LARYNX
Anteroposterior projection
Posteroanterior view

Radiographic studies of the pharyngolaryngeal structures are made during breathing, phonation, stress maneuvers, and swallowing. In order to minimize the incidence of motion, the shortest possible exposure time must be used in these examinations. For the purpose of obtaining better contrast on the anteroposterior projections, the studies in this plane may be made with a stationary or with a high-speed movable grid where high-capacity apparatus is available; otherwise, a nongrid technique must be employed.

Film: $8'' \times 10''$ or $10'' \times 12''$ lengthwise.

Position of patient

Except for tomographic studies, the patient is placed in the erect position, seated or standing, whenever possible.

Position of part

Center the median sagittal plane of the body to the midline of the cassette stand or Potter-Bucky diaphragm. Ask the patient to sit or stand straight; in the latter position, the weight of the body must be equally distributed on the feet. Adjust the patient's shoulders to lie in the same transverse plane to prevent rotation of the head and neck, with resultant obliquity of the throat structures.

Center the film at the level of, or just below, the laryngeal prominence. Extend the patient's head only enough to prevent the mandibular shadow from obscuring the laryngeal area. Immobilize the head with a head clamp or other suitable means.

Central ray

Direct the central ray perpendicularly to the laryngeal prominence.

Filming in the frontal plane

Preliminary films, both anteroposterior and lateral, are made during the inspiratory phase of quiet nasal breathing to ensure filling the throat passages with air. The optimum time for the exposure is easily determined by watching the breathing movements of the chest; the exposure should be made just before the chest comes to rest at the end of one of its inspiratory expansions.

PHARYNX AND LARYNX
Anteroposterior position
Posteroanterior view
Filming in the frontal plane—cont'd

Further studies of the pharynx and larynx (the procedure or procedures to be employed usually determined radioscopically) may be made at the following times:

1. During the Valsalva and/or the modified Valsalva stress maneuvers (page 603).

2. At the height of the act of swallowing a bolus of 1 tablespoon of creamy barium sulfate mixture. After practicing with one or more swallows of water, the patient is asked to hold the barium sulfate bolus in his mouth until signaled, and then to swallow it *in one movement.* He is asked to refrain from swallowing again if a double-contrast study is to be attempted.

3. During the modified Valsalva maneuver immediately after the barium swallow for double-contrast delineation of the pyriform sinuses.

4. During phonation and/or with the larynx in the rest position following its opacification with an iodinated contrast medium.

Tomographic studies of the larynx are made during the phonation of a high-pitched "e-e-e." Following these tomographic studies of the larynx, one or more sectional studies may be made at the selected level or levels with the larynx at rest.

Even when the patient has been instructed in the performance of these maneuvers during the radioscopic examination, the newness of the maneuver necessitates that he be reinstructed in each maneuver just prior to its use in the filming procedure.

NOTE: For an adequate demonstration of tumor masses in the neck, place the patient in the seated position and rotate the body so that the mass is tangent to the film. Direct the central ray horizontally to the inner border of the mass.

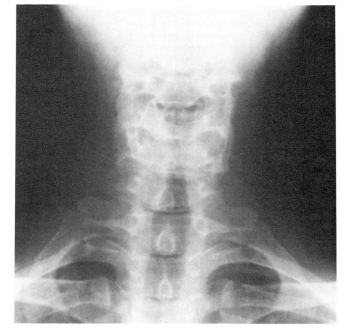

Quiet breathing.

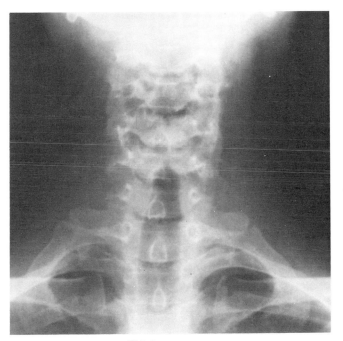

Valsalva maneuver.

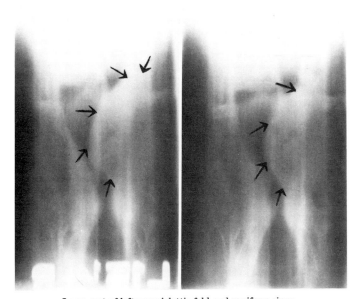

Large cyst of left aryepiglottic fold and pyriform sinus.

Radiographs and clinical information courtesy Dr. Judah Zizmor.

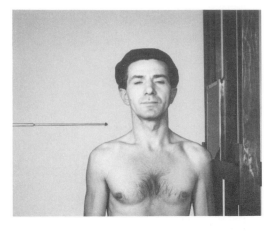

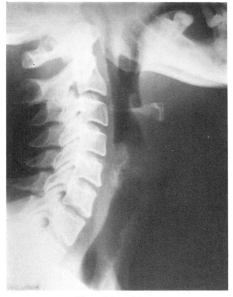

Normal breathing.

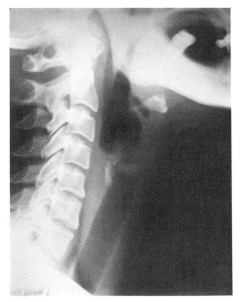

Phonating "e-e-e."

SOFT PALATE, PHARYNX, AND LARYNX
Lateral position

All other exposure factors remaining the same, lateral studies of the laryngopharyngeal structures are usually made with 10 kilovolts less than are used for lateral projections of the cervical vertebrae.

Film: 8″ × 10″ lengthwise.
Position of patient

The patient is asked to sit or stand laterally before the vertical cassette holder. He is then adjusted so that the coronal plane that passes through, or just anterior to, the temporomandibular joints is centered to the midline of the film.

Position of part

Ask the patient to sit or stand straight, with the adjacent shoulder resting firmly against the stand for support. Adjust the body so that its median sagittal plane is parallel with the plane of the film. Depress the shoulders as much as possible and adjust them to lie in the same transverse plane. Extend the patient's head slightly. Immobilize the head with a head clamp or by having the patient fix his gaze on an object in line with his visual axis.

Position of film

1. Center the film 1 inch below the level of the external auditory meatuses for the demonstration of the nasopharynx and for cleft palate studies.

2. Center the film at the level of the mandibular angles for the demonstration of the oropharynx.

3. Center the film at the level of the laryngeal prominence for the demonstration of the larynx, the hypopharynx and the upper end of the esophagus.

Central ray

Direct the central ray perpendicularly to the midpoint of the film.

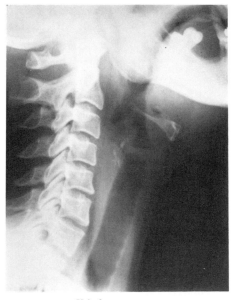

Valsalva maneuver.

608

SOFT PALATE, PHARYNX, AND LARYNX
Lateral position—cont'd

Preliminary studies of the pharyngolaryngeal structures, both lateral and frontal views, are made during the inhalation phase of quiet nasal breathing to ensure filling the passages with air.

According to the site and nature of the abnormality being investigated, further studies may be made in any one or more of the following maneuvers, each of which must be explained to, and performed by, the patient just prior to its actual use:

1. During the phonation of specified vowel sounds for the demonstration of the vocal cords and for cleft palate studies.

2. During the Valsalva maneuver to distend the subglottic larynx and trachea with air.

3. During the modified Valsalva maneuver to distend the supraglottic larynx and the hypopharynx with air.

4. At the height of the act of swallowing a bolus of 1 tablespoon of creamy barium sulfate mixture for the demonstration of the pharyngeal structures.

5. Of the larynx at rest or during phonation following its opacification with an iodinated medium.

6. During the act of swallowing a tuft or pledget of cotton saturated with a barium sulfate mixture for the demonstration of nonopaque foreign bodies located in the pharynx or upper esophagus.

Opaque foreign bodies lodged in the pharynx or upper esophagus can ordinarily be demonstrated in a soft tissue lateral film of the neck or a lateral film of the retrosternal area (page 630). Epstein[1] recommends that a lateral film of the neck be taken at the height of deglutition for the demonstration of opaque foreign bodies lodged in the upper end of the intrathoracic esophagus. Epstein states that this portion of the esophagus is then elevated a distance of two cervical segments, which places it above the level of the clavicles.

[1]Epstein, Bernard S.: A roentgenographic aid to the diagnosis of radiopaque foreign bodies in the upper intrathoracic esophagus, Amer. J. Roentgen. **73**:115-117, 1955.

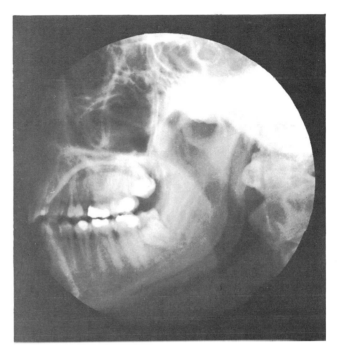

Normal nasopharynx.

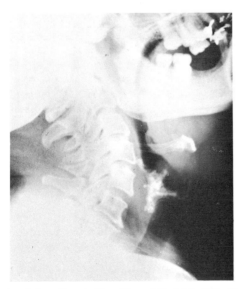

Film made at rest shows the cricoid cartilage at the level of C7 and no evidence of a foreign body.

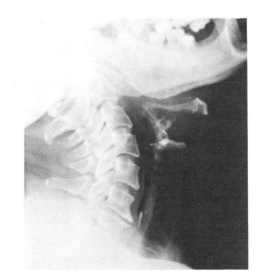

Film of opposite patient made at height of deglutition shows the cricoid cartilage at the level of the C4-C5 interspace and a foreign body in the esophagus at the level of the C6-C7 interspace.

Foreign body studies and diagnostic information courtesy Dr. Bernard S. Epstein.

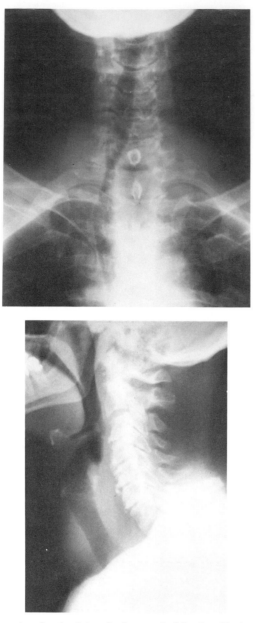

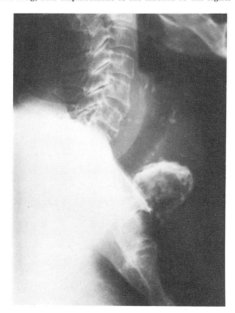

Benign suprasternal and substernal enlargement of the thyroid, showing compression, narrowing, and displacement of the trachea to the right.

Calcified hematoma of thyroid.

Above radiographs and clinical information courtesy Dr. William H. Shehadi.

ANTERIOR PART OF THE NECK
Thyroid gland
Methods of examination

The thyroid gland is enclosed within a capsule and situated in the middle portion of the neck surrounding the front and sides of the upper trachea. It normally extends from the lower third of the thyroid cartilage downward for a distance of two inches to about the level of the first thoracic vertebra. The thyroid is subject to a variety of abnormalities, the most frequently observed change being enlargement, which results in a swelling (called a goiter) in the front part of the neck. The enlargement may be either diffuse or nodular, depending on the nature of the abnormality present; it may be confined to the neck, or a portion of the enlarged gland may protrude into the upper thoracic cavity behind the sternum, in which case it is called an intrathoracic, retrosternal, or substernal goiter. The normal thyroid gland is not discernible on frontal views of the neck, and only the narrow median portion, the isthmus, is visualized on lateral views.

Diffuse enlargement of the thyroid gland usually requires no more than frontal and lateral projections of the neck and of the chest. These studies will demonstrate any intrathoracic extension of the gland, any compression or displacement of the trachea by the enlarged gland, and the presence of any calcium deposits and will indicate whether further studies are needed. The lateral position described on page 630 is used for the demonstration of an intrathoracic extension of the goiter when the shoulders cannot otherwise be rotated backward enough to clear the superior mediastinum. When nodular enlargement is present, oblique studies of the neck are obtained; for these, the patient is adjusted to place the thyroid mass tangent to the film.

Margolin and Steinbach[1] developed a special soft tissue technique and two oblique positions of the neck for the evaluation of thyroid calcifications in selected cases. They recommend the use of this high contrast–maximum detail soft tissue technique for clear differentiation between small calcifications of a benign nature and those of a psammomatous nature.

Exposure technique

With the use of routine mammography equipment, Margolin and Steinbach employ an exposure technique which they based on that used for breast studies: (1) low kilovoltage and a high milliampere-second factor; (2) no added filtration; (3) short part-film distance; (4) fine grain, nonscreen, industrial type films; and (5) manual processing. They use flexible plastic 5″ × 7″ cassettes, each loaded with two films of different speed (Kodak M and AA) in order to obtain two density variations with one exposure in each position. For the neck of average size they use the following exposure factors:

Oblique position: 56 kvp., 300 milliamperes, 3 seconds, 26-inch focal film distance

Off-lateral position: 48 kvp., 300 milliamperes, 3 seconds, 28-inch focal film distance

When the x-ray tube has a beryllium window, the exposure time can be reduced by 50% to 60%.

When the radiologist examines the patient's neck preceding these studies, he tapes a small lead side marker over the clavicular insertion of each sternocleidomastoid muscle to identify the sides.

[1]Margolin, F. R., and Steinbach, H. L.: Soft tissue roentgenography of thyroid nodules, Amer. J. Roentgen. 102:844-852, 1968.

Oblique position

1. The patient is placed prone on the radiographic table so that the neck can be rested on a sandbag and flexed over the end of the table.

2. The sandbag is adjusted to conform to the curvature of the neck. The flexible plastic film holder is inserted lengthwise between the neck and the sandbag, centered to the uppermost thyroid lobe, and the head is allowed to hang over the end of the table to its most dependent position. The rotation of the head is adjusted to place the anterolateral aspect of the neck in contact with the film holder so that the uppermost lobe of the thyroid is brought into relief.

3. The x-ray tube, with an extension cone attached, is adjusted at a double angle of 10 degrees caudally and 15 degrees posteriorly and is then centered to the film.

4. The patient is positioned in a similar manner for the opposite side.

Off-lateral position

1. After the two oblique projections, the patient is rotated to a steep oblique position, with the affected side dependent. A single off-lateral projection is made with the central ray angled 5 degrees caudally and 5 degrees posteriorly.

Margolin and Steinbach state that this method of examination is applicable when (1) the clinical findings indicate that a nodule is malignant and (2) the routine films show hazy calcium deposits that are suspected of having a psammomatous pattern.

• • •

Matoba and Kikuchi[1] describe a lymphographic technique for the delineation of the thyroid gland and cervical lymph nodes. They report that 10 minutes after a percutaneous injection of 2 ml. of Lipiodol Ultra Fluid (Ethiodol) directly into the thyroid, the lobe of the injected side is clearly outlined and that 24 hours later its regional lymph nodes are visualized.

Angiography and radioisotope scanning are other methods used in the investigation of thyroid disease.

[1]Matoba, N., and Kikuchi, T.: Thyroidolymphography; a new technique for visualization of the thyroid and cervical lymph nodes, Radiology 92:339-342, 1969.

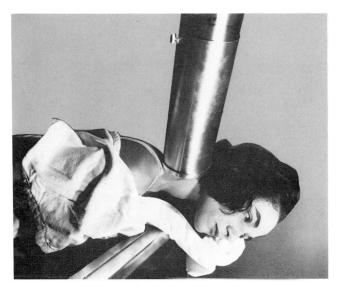

Positioning of patient for oblique projection.

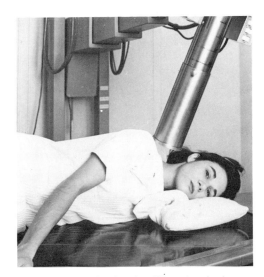

Positioning of patient for off-lateral projection.

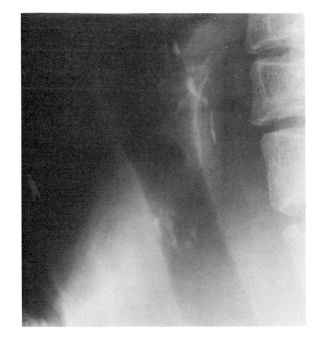

Calcified carcinoma of thyroid. Note clumps of faint calcification arranged in whorl pattern superimposed on tracheal air column.

All illustrations and legends courtesy Dr. Frederick R. Margolin.

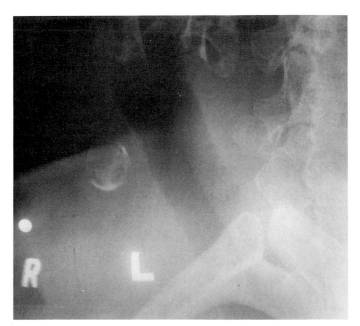

Calcified thyroid nodule projected anterior to trachea. Small R and L markers are taped to patient's skin, and metal dot marks site of clinically palpable nodule in thyroid.

611

Body cavities, surface markings of the abdomen, and bodily habitus

Body cavities

The two great cavities of the body are the posterior, or dorsal, cavity and the anterior, or ventral, cavity. The posterior cavity consists of the tubular vertebral portion, which contains the spinal cord, and the expanded cranial portion, which contains the brain. The anterior cavity is partitioned by the diaphragm into thoracic and abdominal portions, the thoracic cavity being further divided into a pericardial and two pleural portions. While there is no intervening partition, the lower part of the abdominal cavity is called the pelvic cavity.

The principal structures located in the thoracic cavity are the pleural membranes, the lungs, the trachea, the esophagus, the pericardium, and the heart and great vessels.

The principal structures located in the abdominal cavity are the peritoneum, the liver and gallbladder, the pancreas, the spleen, the stomach, the intestines, the kidneys and ureters.

The rectum, the urinary bladder, and parts of the reproductive system are located in the pelvic cavity.

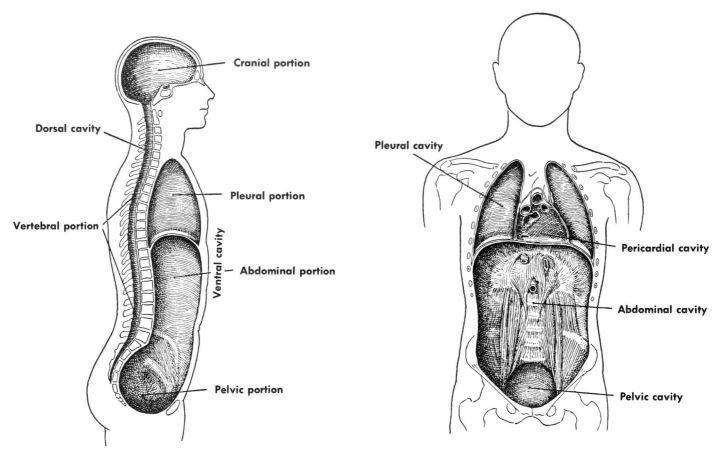

SAGITTAL VIEW OF BODY CAVITIES

ANTERIOR VIEW OF VENTRAL CAVITY

Surface markings of the abdomen

For purposes of convenience in describing the position of the abdominal viscera, the abdomen is divided into nine regions by four imaginary planes known as Addison's[1] planes.

The plane extending transversely midway between the manubrial notch and the upper border of the symphysis pubis is called the *transpyloric plane,* and usually passes through the lower border of the body of the first lumbar vertebra. The second transverse plane passes midway between the transpyloric plane and the upper border of the symphysis pubis. This plane is called the *transtubercular plane,* and usually passes through the ilia at the level of the body of the fifth lumbar vertebra.

[1]Addison, Christopher: In Ellis' demonstration of anatomy, ed. 12, New York, 1906, Wm. Wood & Co.

The two transverse planes divide the abdomen into three regions known as *zones*. The upper division is called the *subcostal,* or *epigastric, zone;* the central, the *umbilical zone;* and the lower, the *hypogastric zone.*

The two sagittal planes pass, one on each side, midway between the anterior superior iliac spines and the median sagittal plane. Each zone is thus divided into three *regions*. From above downward, the three central regions are the *epigastric,* the *umbilical,* and the *hypogastric,* or *pubic*. Each central region is divided into right and left portions by the median sagittal plane of the body. Named from above, the right and left lateral regions are the *hypochondriac,* the *lumbar,* and the *iliac,* or *inguinal.*

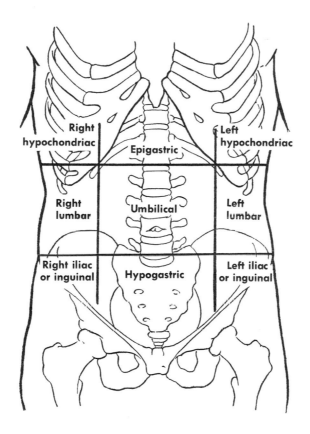

SURFACE MARKINGS OF ABDOMEN

Bodily habitus

The general form, or architecture, of the body, called the habitus, or habit, of the body, determines the size, shape, position, tonus, and motility of the internal organs. Mills,[1] after the study of a large number of subjects, classified numerous types, the hypersthenic, the sthenic, the hyposthenic, and the asthenic being the four major types. Certain organs, such as the gallbladder, vary as much as 6 to 8 inches in position, both transversely and longitudinally, between the two extreme types—the hypersthenic and the asthenic types. For this reason, it is necessary for the technologist to be familiar with the characteristics of the major types and be able to recognize their related intermediate types. The radiographically important characteristics of the two extreme types classified by Mills are outlined below. The illustrations of these two types should be studied and compared with the illustrations of the two dominant intermediate types.

The *hypersthenic* type of body is one of massive build. This type represents the upper extreme, and only a small percentage of subjects (about 5%) fit into this classification. The thorax is broad and deep, the ribs assume an almost horizontal position, and the thoracic cavity is short. The lungs are short, are narrowed above, and are broad at their bases. The heart is squat and wide, and its longitudinal axis is almost transverse. The diaphragm is high, resulting in a long abdomen. The upper part of the abdominal cavity is broad and capacious; the lower part is small. The stomach and gallbladder occupy high, almost horizontal positions, the latter being well away from the midline. The colon is also high in position, and it extends around the periphery of the abdominal cavity.

[1] Mills, Walter R.: The relation of bodily habitus to visceral form, position, tonus, and motility, Amer. J. Roentgen. 4:155-169, 1917.

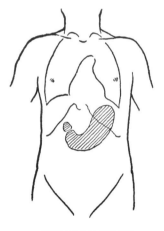

STHENIC HABITUS

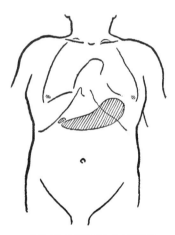

HYPERSTHENIC HABITUS

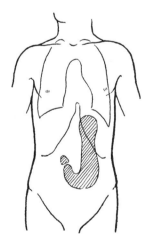

HYPOSTHENIC HABITUS

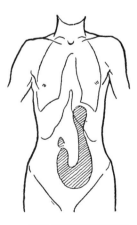

ASTHENIC HABITUS

The *sthenic* habitus is a modification of the hypersthenic type, and, comprising approximately 50% of all subjects, is the predominant type.

The *asthenic* type of body is one of extremely slender build. This type represents the lower extreme, and embraces only about 10% of the subjects. The asthenic thorax is narrow and shallow, the ribs slope sharply downward, and the cavity of the thorax is long. The lungs are long, extend well above the clavicles, and are broader above than at their bases. The heart is long and narrow, and its longitudinal axis is almost vertical. The diaphragm is low in position, and the abdominal cavity is short, its greatest capacity being in the lower portion. The stomach and gallbladder are low, vertical, and near the midline. The colon folds on itself, and occupies a low, median position.

The *hyposthenic* habitus is a modification of the more extreme asthenic type, that is, it is more toward the sthenic type. Approximately 35% of the subjects fit into this classification.

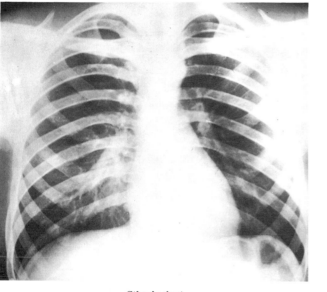

Sthenic chest.

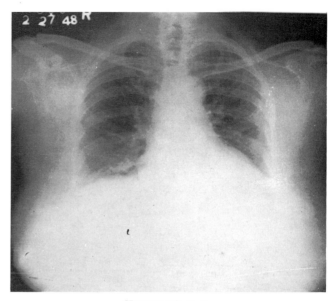

Hypersthenic chest.

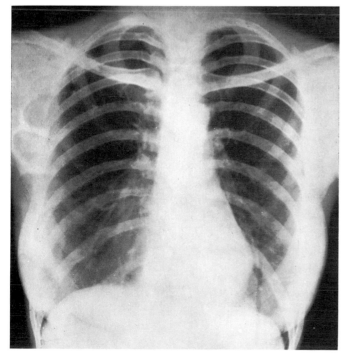

Hyposthenic chest.

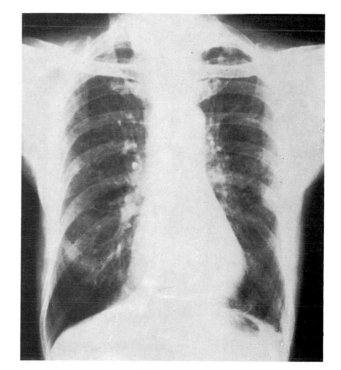

Asthenic chest.

617

Anatomy and positioning of the thoracic viscera

RESPIRATORY SYSTEM AND MEDIASTINAL STRUCTURES

Respiratory system

The thoracic cavity is bounded by the walls of the thorax, extends from the thoracic inlet to the diaphragm, and contains the thoracic viscera. The *thoracic inlet* is bounded laterally by the first pair of ribs, its plane slanting obliquely forward and downward from the level of the superior border of the first thoracic vertebra to the manubrial notch.

The *thoracic viscera* consist of the lungs and the mediastinal structures, the mediastinum containing all the thoracic organs except the lungs.

The *mediastinum* is the potential space between the lungs. It extends from the upper aperture of the thorax, the thoracic inlet, downward to the diaphragm, and is bounded anteriorly by the sternum and posteriorly by the vertebral column. The portion lying above the heart is called the *superior mediastinum*. The lower portion is subdivided into the *anterior mediastinum*, the shallow space in front of the heart; the *middle mediastinum*, which is the largest part and is occupied by the heart; and the *posterior mediastinum*, which lies behind the heart. The radiographically important mediastinal structures are the heart and the great blood vessels (the anatomy of which is described in the discussion on the circulatory system), the trachea, the esophagus, and the thymus gland.

The *respiratory system proper* consists of the larynx (described in the preceding discussion), the trachea, the bronchi, and the two lungs. The air passages of these organs communicate with the exterior through the pharynx, the mouth, and the nose, each of which, in addition to other, previously described functions, is considered a part of the respiratory apparatus.

The *trachea* is a fibrous, muscular tube and has sixteen to twenty C-shaped cartilaginous rings embedded in its walls for greater rigidity. The tube is flattened behind,

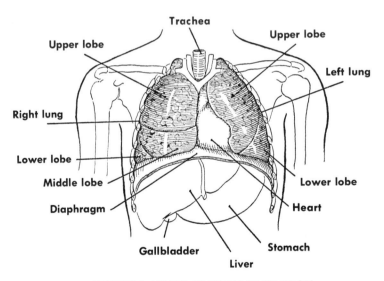

ANTERIOR ASPECT OF LUNGS IN RELATION TO SURROUNDING STRUCTURES

the incomplete cartilaginous rings extending around its anterior two-thirds. It measures approximately ¾ inch in diameter and about 4½ inches in length. The trachea is situated in the median sagittal plane in front of the esophagus, and following the curve of the vertebral column, it extends from its junction with the larynx at the level of the sixth cervical vertebra downward through the mediastinum to about the level of the interspace between the fourth and fifth thoracic vertebrae. At its lower extremity the trachea divides, or bifurcates, into two lesser tubes, the *primary*, or main stem, *bronchi*, one of which enters the right lung and the other the left lung.

The *primary bronchi* slant obliquely downward to their entrance into the lungs, where they branch out to form the right and left bronchial branches. The right bronchus is shorter and wider than the left, and is more vertical in

position. Because of the more vertical position and greater diameter of the right main bronchus, foreign bodies entering the trachea are more likely to pass into the right bronchus than into the left.

The primary bronchus, after entering the *hilus* (also called the *hilum*), divides into a main *stem* for each lobe of the lung, the right bronchus having three stem branches and the left two stem branches. The *stem bronchus*, diminishing in size as it subdivides, branches out to all parts of the lobe and ends in minute tubes called the *terminal bronchioles*. Each terminal bronchiole communicates with a unit of lung structure, the *atrium*, the *infundibulum*, and the *alveoli*. The atria are narrow air channels leading from the bronchiole to the infundibula, or sacculated air spaces. Each infundibulum has many air pockets, the alveoli, projecting from its walls.

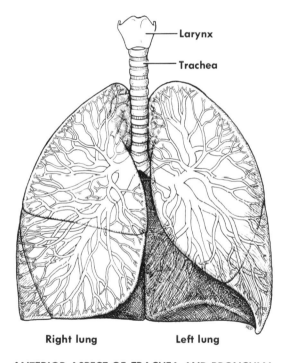

Larynx

Trachea

Right lung   Left lung

ANTERIOR ASPECT OF TRACHEA AND BRONCHIAL
TREE IN RELATION TO LUNGS

The *lungs* are the organs of respiration. They comprise the mechanism for introducing oxygen into, and for removing carbon dioxide from, the blood. The lungs are composed of a light, spongy, highly elastic substance called the *parenchyma*, and are covered by a layer of serous membrane. They are situated, one on each side, in the thoracic cavity, where they fill all of the space not occupied by the mediastinal structures. Each lung presents a rounded *apex* that reaches above the level of the clavicles into the root of the neck, and a broad *base* that, resting upon the obliquely placed diaphragm, reaches lower in back and at the sides than in front. The right lung is about 1 inch shorter than the left lung as a result of the large space occupied by the liver, and is broader than the left lung because of the position of the heart. The outer, or costal, surface of each lung conforms with the shape of the chest wall. The inferior surface of the lung is con-

cave, fitting over the diaphragm, and its outer margins are thin and reach as low as the parietal pleura. The mediastinal surface is concave and presents two depressions, the cardiac fossa for the accommodation of the heart, and the hilus, or hilum, for the accommodation of the root of the lung. The cardiac fossa, which is deeper on the left lung than on the right, lies below and in front of the hilar depression. The structures that comprise the root of the lung enter and leave at the hilus; they are the bronchus, the blood and lymph vessels, and the nerves.

Each lung is enclosed in a double-walled, serous membrane sac called the *pleura*. The inner layer of the pleural sac, called the *visceral*, or *pulmonary*, *pleura*, is closely adherent to the surface of the lung, extends into the *interlobar fissures*, and is continuous with the outer layer at the root of the lung. The outer layer, called the *parietal*

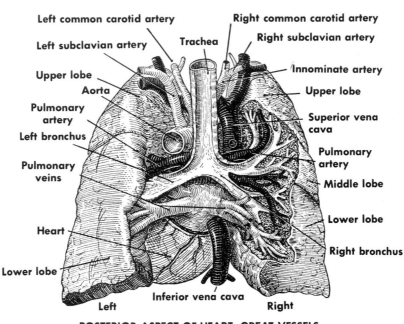

POSTERIOR ASPECT OF HEART, GREAT VESSELS, LUNGS, TRACHEA, AND BRONCHIAL TREES

pleura, lines the wall of the cavity occupied by the lung, being reflected over the adjacent mediastinal structures, and is closely adherent to the upper surface of the diaphragm and the inner surface of the chest wall. The two layers are moistened by serum so that they move easily upon each other and thus prevent friction between the lungs and chest walls during respiratory movements. The space between the two pleural walls is called the *pleural cavity*. The narrow space between the costal and diaphragmatic portions of the parietal pleura, where it dips below the outer margin of the lung, is called the *costophrenic*, or *phrenicocostal*, *sinus*.

The right lung is divided by two deep fissures into three lobes, the upper, middle, and lower lobes. The fissures lie in an oblique plane from above downward and forward so that the lobes overlap each other in the anteroposterior direction. The middle lobe, the smallest of the three, is wedge-shaped and occupies the anterior part of the base and middle portion of the lung. The lower lobe lies below and behind the middle lobe and behind the lower part of the upper lobe. The left lung is divided into two lobes by a deep fissure that also extends in an oblique plane from above downward and forward. The upper lobe lies above and in front of the lower lobe.

Each of the five lobes is composed of closely bound but individual *secondary segments*. Each of these segments is in turn composed of several smaller units called *primary lobules*. The primary lobule is the anatomic unit of lung structure, and comprises a terminal bronchiole with its expanded air spaces, the *atria*, *infundibula*, and *alveoli*, and its blood and lymph vessels and nerves. The walls of the alveoli are thin and delicate, and they support the fine network of pulmonary capillaries in which the blood receives its fresh supply of oxygen.

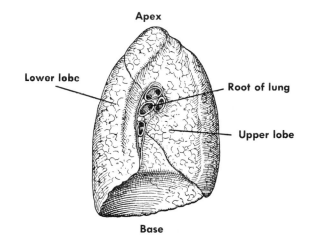

MEDIASTINAL ASPECT OF RIGHT LUNG

MEDIASTINAL ASPECT OF LEFT LUNG

Mediastinal structures

The *esophagus* is that part of the digestive canal which connects the pharynx with the stomach. It is a narrow, musculomembranous tube about 9 inches in length. It begins at the level of the sixth cervical vertebra, where it is continuous with the pharynx, and reaches to the level of about the eleventh thoracic vertebra, where it ends at the esophageal orifice of the stomach. Following the curves of the vertebral column, the esophagus descends through the posterior part of the mediastinum and then runs forward to pass through the esophageal hiatus of the diaphragm. The esophagus normally presents two narrowed areas, one at its upper end, where it enters the thorax, and one at its lower end at the hiatus in the diaphragm. It also presents two indentations, one at the aortic arch, and one where it crosses the left bronchus.

The esophagus lies just in front of the vertebral column with its anterior surface in close relation to the trachea, and to the aortic arch and the heart, which makes it valuable in certain heart examinations. When the esophagus is filled with a barium sulfate mixture, the posterior border of the heart and aorta are well outlined in oblique and lateral projections. Frontal, oblique, and lateral positions are used in examinations of the esophagus. Radiography of the esophagus will be considered with the remainder of the digestive system.

The *thymus gland* is said to be a temporary organ because, after reaching its maximum size at puberty, it gradually decreases until it almost disappears. The function of this gland is not fully known. It consists of two pyramid-shaped lobes that lie in the lower neck and superior mediastinum, just in front of the trachea and the great vessels of the heart. At its maximum development, it rests on the pericardium and reaches as high as the thyroid gland. When the thymus is abnormally enlarged, a condition that may occur in infants and young children, it presses on the retrothymic organs, displacing them backward and causing respiratory disturbances. A roentgenographic examination of the thymus is made in both the posteroanterior and the lateral directions. Using a tenth of a second or less, the exposures are made at the end of full inhalation. When infants and children too young to cooperate are examined, crying should be induced in order to ensure filling the trachea with air.

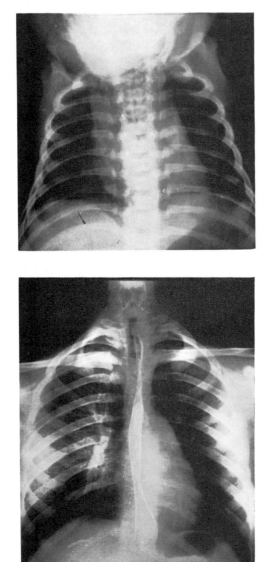

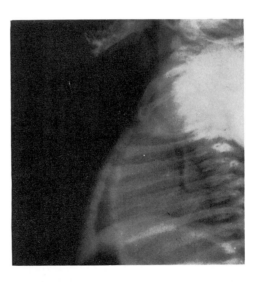

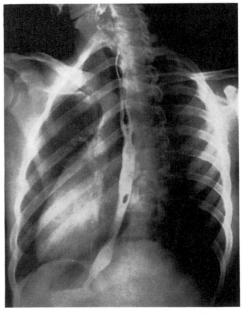

Courtesy W. Wm. Pollino.

624

Radiography of the thoracic viscera

Body position

For radiography of the heart and lungs, the patient is placed in an erect position whenever possible, in order to prevent engorgement of the pulmonary vessels and to allow the diaphragm to move to its lowest position. In the recumbent position, the abdominal viscera and diaphragm move upward, compress the thoracic viscera, and prevent full expansion of the pulmonic fields. While the difference is not great in thin subjects, it is quite marked in obese subjects. The radiographs illustrating the effect of body position were made on the same subject.

Part position

A slight amount of rotation from the posteroanterior position causes considerable distortion of the heart shadow. In order to obviate this, the body must be carefully positioned and immobilized. The patient is instructed to sit or stand erect; if he is standing, the weight of the body must be equally distributed on the feet. The head must be erect and facing directly forward. For oblique views, the hips are rotated with the thorax, and the feet are placed to point directly forward. The shoulders must lie in the same transverse plane on all views. For the anterior view (posteroanterior projection), the shoulders should be depressed to carry the clavicles below the apices, and should be held in contact with the cassette or cassette holder with a compression band when necessary. Except in the presence of an upper thoracic scoliosis, a faulty position in the anterior view can be detected by the asymmetrical projection of the sternoclavicular joints. Compare the clavicular shadows in the illustrations below.

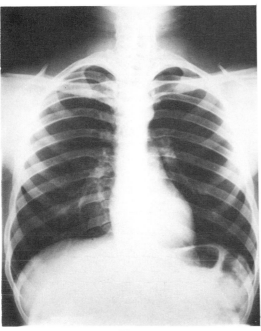

Erect.

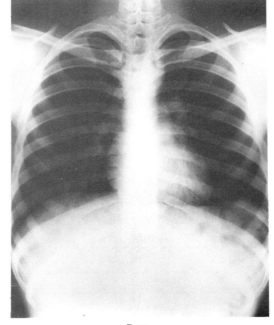

Prone.

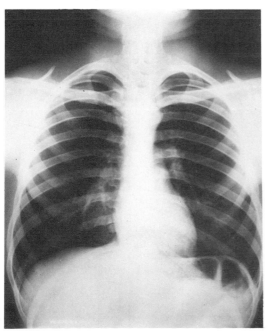

Without rotation.

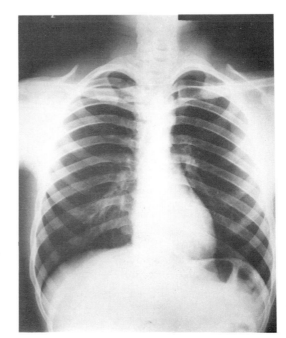

With rotation.

625

Breathing instructions

Exposures for the lungs are made at the end of full inhalation for the purpose of demonstrating the greatest possible area of lung structure. However, the patient must not inhale to the point of strain. More air is inhaled on the second breath, and without strain, than on the first breath. This fact should be taken advantage of when examining obese patients.

When a pneumothorax is suspected, one exposure is made on full inhalation, and then another exposure is made on full exhalation for the purpose of demonstrating small amounts of air that might be obscured on the inhalation film. Inhalation and exhalation films are also used to demonstrate the excursion of the diaphragm, and they are sometimes used to demonstrate the presence of a foreign body. When the projections are being made for the excursion of the diaphragm, both exposures may be made on one film. The penetration must be increased 6 or 8 kilovolts for exhalation films.

Exposures for the heart are made at the end of normal inhalation in order to prevent elongation of the heart by a full downward movement of the diaphragm.

Stereoscopic projections are made with vertical tube shifts, and both exposures must be made on one respiratory movement.

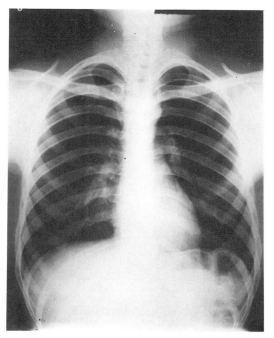

Inhalation.

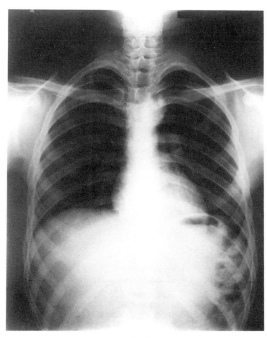

Exhalation.

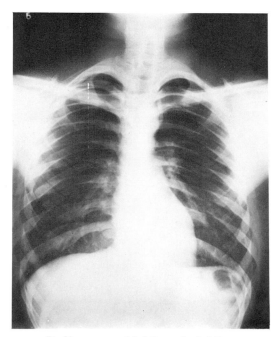

Double exposure—inhalation and exhalation.

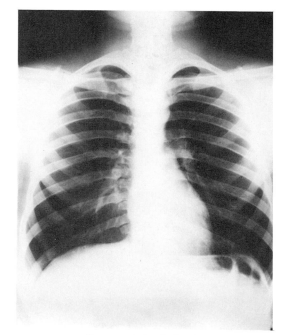

Lower centering for heart.

Technical procedure

The views required for an adequate radiographic demonstration of the thoracic viscera are determined by the radiologist, usually from his radioscopic findings, according to the type and location of the pathologic lesion. The anterior view (posteroanterior projection) is the basic view and is used in all lung and heart examinations. Right and left oblique and lateral views, and views made in the so-called special positions, are employed, as required, as a supplement to the basic anterior view. Furthermore, it is sometimes necessary to improvise variations of the basic positions in order to project an area free of superimposed structures. Wide-angle radiography (described on page 172, Volume I) is used to great advantage for frontal plane separation of lesions that are poorly shown due to foreshortening or that are obscured by superimposition on the basic anteroposterior view.

The technical procedure, that is, the exposure factors and accessories, employed in examining the thoracic viscera depends upon the radiographic characteristics of the existent pathology. When the lung fields are normally aerated, it is customary to use a non-Bucky technique except with obese subjects. The milliampere-second and kilovoltage factors must be balanced in such a way as to obtain sharply defined pulmonary markings from the hilus to the periphery. This cannot be accomplished if the milliampere-second factor is too high; the density gradient will be too short, as indicated by a chalky appearance of the film, with the result that the finer lung markings will be poorly demonstrated, particularly around the periphery. From 5 to 20 milliampere-seconds is the average range used for the posteroanterior and oblique projections, the factor being doubled for lateral projections. The exposure time should be one-tenth of a second or less in order to overcome the vibratory motion transmitted by the heart-beats to the adjacent portions of the lungs. Whenever possible, a focal-film distance of 72 inches is used in order to minimize magnification of the heart shadow and to obtain sharper outlines of the delicate lung structures.

A Potter-Bucky or stationary grid technique is usually employed in the investigation of opaque areas within the lung fields, and to demonstrate the lung structure through thickened pleural membranes. When the exposure required to penetrate the affected side is not too great, if it will not spoil contrast, the radiation reaching the film can be equalized by covering the unaffected side with a filter of semiopaque plastic material, such as that described by Fuchs,[1] so that both sides can be projected simultaneously. Interlobar effusions and pleural effusions are usually well demonstrated with the conventional non-Bucky technique by placing the patient in the required positions.

Radiation protection

The beam of radiation should, as in every roentgenographic examination, be closely coned to the part size. The gonadal area, particularly of pregnant women, should be further shielded by a lead apron extending from the level of the iliac crests or slightly higher to the mid-thighs. Such a shield can be mounted on a height-adjustable, two-pole stand, or it can be attached to the sides of the cassette carriage.

[1]Fuchs, Arthur W.: A radiographic view-finder, Radiogr. Clin. Photogr. 12:2-7, 1936.

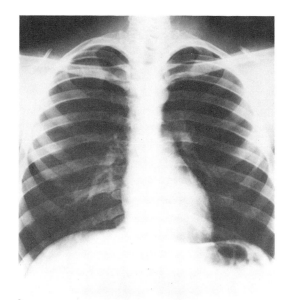

36″ distance. Compare with film to left—on opposite page.

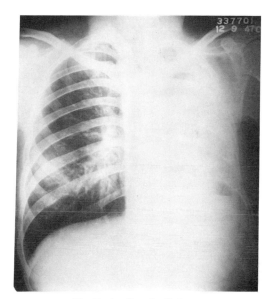

Non-Bucky film of pathology.

Courtesy Dr. Ross Golden.

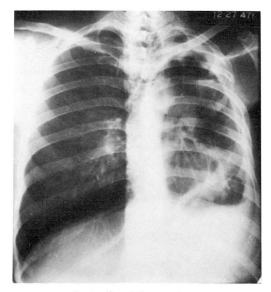

Bucky film of above patient.

Courtesy Dr. Ross Golden.

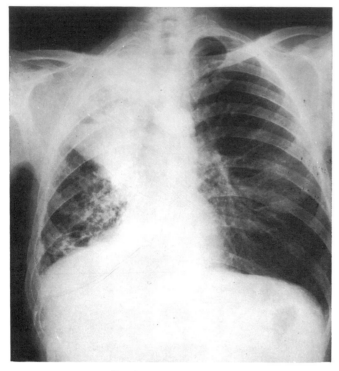

Routine stationary radiograph.

Specialized equipment

Body-section radiography is the term applied to the technical method of recording an unobscured view of a specific body plane on the film through diffusing the shadows of the superjacent and subjacent structures by simultaneously moving the x-ray tube and the film in opposite directions. This method of examination is a valuable adjunct to the conventional methods employed in the investigation of such conditions as bronchogenic tumors and lung abscesses, and in the differential diagnosis of renal tumors and cysts, to name but a few of its uses. The principles and the more common uses of body-section techniques are discussed in Volume I (pages 284 to 314).

Kymography is the term applied to the technical procedure of recording the movements of the heart, the diaphragm, or other body organs by means of special apparatus. The patient is placed before the kymograph in the erect position, either seated or standing, and adjusted as for a conventional radiograph. The milliampere-second factor is converted so that the time of exposure will be long enough to cover several movements of the organ being examined. The reader is referred to the bibliography for a list of papers giving a full description of kymographic equipment and its diagnostic application.

Electrokymography is a special type of examination in which a fluoroscopic pulsation is picked up and amplified by electronic devices, passed through an electrocardiographic apparatus, and recorded on electrocardiographic paper. Heart sounds and/or pulse waves may be recorded simultaneously.

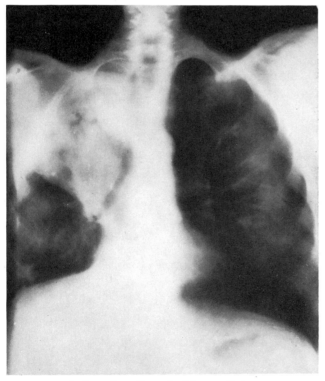

Body-section radiograph of above patient.

Courtesy Dr. Hugh M. Wilson.

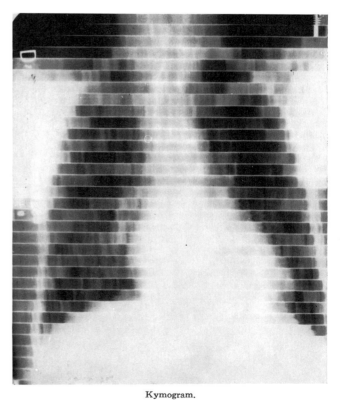

Kymogram.

Courtesy Dr. Marcy L. Sussman.

TRACHEA
Anteroposterior projection
Posteroanterior view
Film: $10'' \times 12''$ lengthwise.

Position of patient

The patient may be examined in either the supine or the erect position. When examining the trachea in the anteroposterior position, it is desirable to use the Potter-Bucky diaphragm to minimize secondary radiation since the kilovoltage must be high enough to penetrate both the sternum and the cervical vertebrae.

Position of part

Center the median sagittal plane of the body to the midline of the Potter-Bucky table or stand. Adjust the shoulders to lie in the same transverse plane. Extend the head slightly and adjust it so that its median sagittal plane is perpendicular to the plane of the film. Immobilize with a head clamp or a weighted band.

Center the film at the level of the manubrium.

Instruct the patient to inhale slowly during the exposure in order to ensure filling the trachea with air.

Central ray

With the central ray perpendicular to the plane of the film, direct it through the manubrium.

Structures shown

An anteroposterior projection showing the outline of the air-filled trachea, which, under normal conditions, is superimposed on the shadow of the cervical vertebrae.

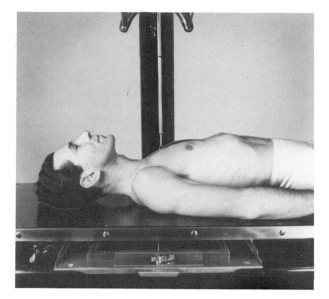

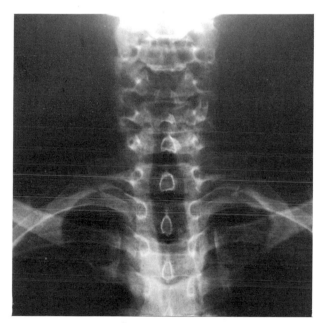

During respiration.

629

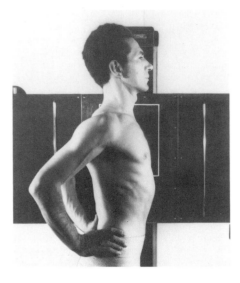

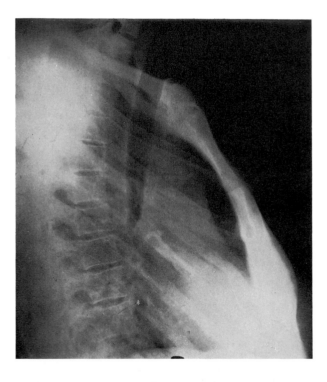

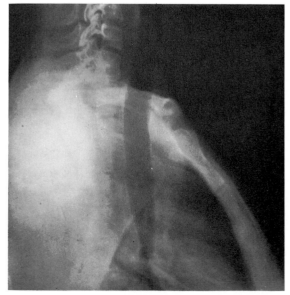

TRACHEA AND SUPERIOR MEDIASTINUM
Lateral (retrosternal) projection

Film: $10'' \times 12''$ or $11'' \times 14''$ lengthwise.

Position of patient

Place the patient in a lateral position, either seated or standing, before a vertical cassette stand. Have the patient sit or stand erect; if he is standing, the weight of the body must be equally distributed on the feet.

Adjust the height of the cassette so that the upper border of the film is at or above the level of the laryngeal prominence. Adjust the patient's position to center the trachea to the midline of the film; the trachea lies in the coronal plane that passes approximately midway between the manubrial notch and the midaxillary line.

Position of part

The shoulders must be rotated well backward in order to prevent their superimposed shadows from obscuring the structures of the superior mediastinum. The patient may place his hands as shown in the accompanying photograph, or he may clasp them behind his body and then rotate his shoulders backward as far as possible. When it is necessary to have the arms held in position, it must be done by a person who is rarely exposed to x-radiation. When such a person is not available, the arms can be tied in close proximity with a wide bandage.

Readjust the position of the body, being careful to have the median sagittal plane vertical and parallel with the plane of the film. Extend the head slightly.

The exposure is made during deep inhalation to ensure filling the trachea with air.

Central ray

Direct the central ray horizontally through a point midway between the manubrial notch and the anterior border of the head of the humerus for the superior mediastinal structures, and from 4 to 5 inches lower for the demonstration of the entire chest.

Structures shown

A lateral projection demonstrating the air-filled trachea and the regions of the thyroid and thymus glands. This projection, first described by Eiselberg and Sgalitzer,[1] is used extensively to demonstrate retrosternal extensions of the thyroid gland, thymic enlargement in infants (in the recumbent position), the opacified pharynx and upper esophagus, as well as the trachea and bronchi.

[1]Eiselberg, A., and Sgalitzer, D. M.: X-ray examination of the trachea and the bronchi, Surg. Gynec. Obstet. **47**:53-68, 1928.

TRACHEA AND PULMONARY APEX
Transshoulder lateral projection
Twining position

This position is used to obtain a lateral view of the apex of the lung nearer to the film, and a lateral view of the trachea and superior mediastinum on patients who cannot rotate their shoulders backward enough for a direct lateral projection.

Film: $10'' \times 12''$ lengthwise.

Position of patient

Place the patient before a vertical cassette stand, either seated or standing, with the affected side toward the film.

Position of part

Elevate the arm adjacent to the film in extreme abduction, flex the elbow, and place the forearm across the head. Center the film to the region of the trachea at the level of the axilla, and have the patient rest the shoulder firmly against the cassette for support. Depress the opposite shoulder as much as possible. Adjust the body in a true lateral position, with its median sagittal plane parallel with the plane of the film.

For the trachea, instruct the patient to inhale slowly during the exposure. For the lung apex, make the exposure at the end of full inhalation.

Central ray

Direct the central ray through the adjacent supraclavicular fossa at an angle of 15 degrees toward the feet; it emerges through the axilla adjacent to the film.

Structures shown

A lateral view of the air-filled trachea and of the apex of the lung adjacent to the film.

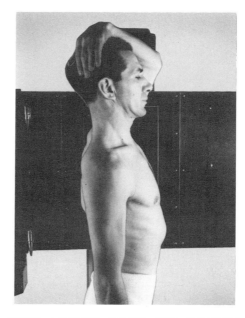

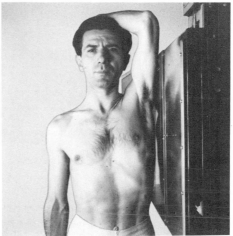

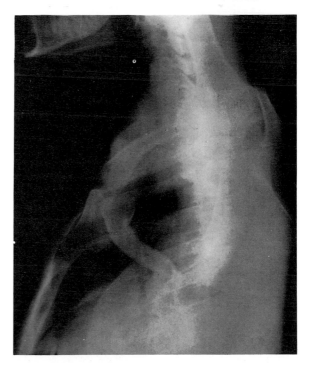

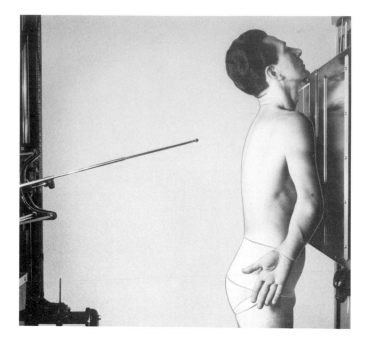

PULMONARY APICES
Posteroanterior projection
Anteroposterior view

Film: $8'' \times 10''$ or $10'' \times 12''$ crosswise.

Position of patient

Place the patient in the posteroanterior position, either seated or standing, before a vertical cassette stand. Ask the patient to sit or stand erect; if he is standing, the weight of the body must be equally distributed on the feet. Adjust the height of the cassette so that the film is centered at the level of the manubrial notch.

Position of part

Center the median sagittal plane of the body to the midline of the film and extend the chin over the top of the cassette. Adjust the head so that its median sagittal plane is vertical. Flex the elbows and place the hands, palms out, on the hips. Depress the shoulders, rotate them forward, and adjust them to lie in the same transverse plane. Instruct the patient to keep his shoulders in contact with the cassette.

The exposure may be made at the end of either full inhalation or full exhalation. Inhalation elevates the clavicles and exhalation depresses them, while the apices move little, if at all, on either phase of respiration.

Central ray

When the exposure is to be made on inhalation, direct the central ray through the third thoracic vertebra at an upward angle of 10 or 15 degrees toward the head.

When the exposure is to be made on exhalation, direct the central ray perpendicularly to the plane of the film and center at the level of the third thoracic vertebra.

Structures shown

An anterior view (posteroanterior projection) of the apices projected above the shadows of the clavicles.

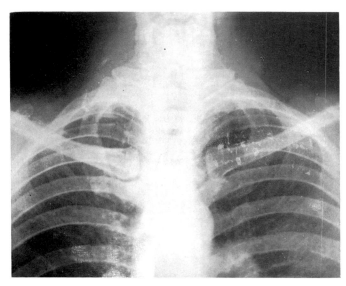

Inhalation with central ray angulated.

NOTE: Barsony and Koppenstein[1] described an axial projection for the demonstration of the pulmonary apices. The patient is placed in the erect position, facing the film and standing some distance from it. He is then asked to lean forward and rest the vertex of his head against the film. The arms hang down along the thighs. The central ray is directed horizontally through the apices. For a unilateral projection, the shoulder of the affected side is placed in contact with the film, as described for the lordotic positions shown on pages 141 and 149, Volume I.

[1]Barsony, T., and Koppenstein, E.: Röntgenuntersuchung des Lungenspitzenfeldes mit axialer Strahlenrichtung, Röentgenpraxis 2:326-330, 1930.

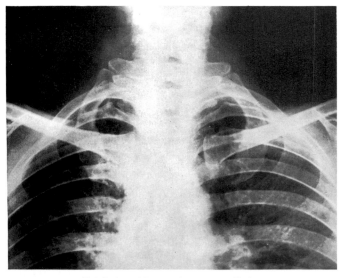

Exhalation with central ray perpendicular.

PULMONARY APICES
Anteroposterior projection
Posteroanterior view

Film: $8'' \times 10''$ or $10'' \times 12''$ crosswise.

Position of patient

The patient may be examined in the erect position, or in the supine position with the shoulders either horizontal or elevated on an angle block. In the latter case, a 20- or 25-degree angle block is most satisfactory.

Position of part

Center the film to the median sagittal plane at the level of the second thoracic vertebra and then adjust the body in a true anteroposterior position. Flex the elbows and place the hands on the hips with the palms out, or pronate the hands beside the hips. Rotate the shoulders forward and adjust them to lie in the same transverse plane.

The exposure is made at the end of full inhalation.

Central ray

With the patient in either the erect or the fully recumbent position, direct the central ray to the second thoracic vertebra at an angle of 15 or 20 degrees toward the head.

If the patient is in a semirecumbent position and the film is elevated on an angle block, direct the central ray vertically through the lower neck.

Structures shown

A posterior view (anteroposterior projection) of the apices lying below the shadows of the clavicles when the erect or the fully recumbent positions are used, and lying above the shadows of the clavicles when the semirecumbent position and the angle block are used.

NOTE: The anteroposterior position is used in preference to the posteroanterior position for subjects whose clavicles occupy a high position, and for obese subjects, in order to separate the apical and clavicular shadows without undue distortion of the apices.

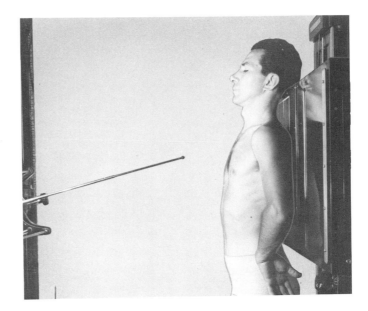

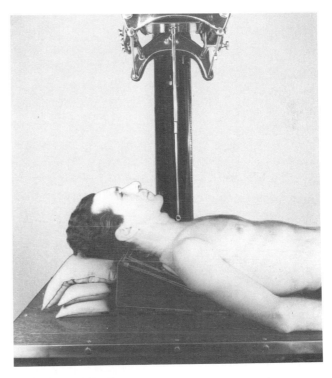

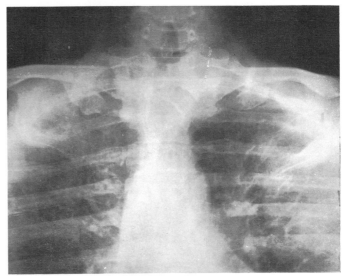

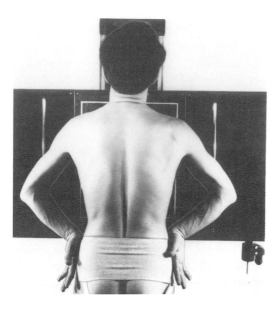

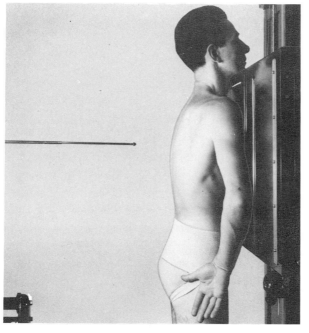

CHEST
Lungs and heart
Posteroanterior projection
Anteroposterior view

Film: 14″ × 17″ lengthwise.

Position of patient

If possible, the patient should be examined in the erect position, either standing or seated, so that the diaphragm will be at its lowest position and so that engorgement of the pulmonary vessels is avoided. The central ray–part-film relationship is the same for the prone position as for the erect position.

Place the patient, with his arms hanging by his sides, before a vertical cassette holder. Adjust the height of the cassette so that the upper border of the film is about 1½ inches above the shoulders.

Position of part

Center the median sagittal plane of the body to the midline of the film, and have the patient stand straight, with the weight of the body equally distributed on the feet. Extend the chin over the top of the cassette and adjust the head so that its median sagittal plane is vertical. When positioning a female subject who has pendulous breasts, spread them upward and outward to prevent them from casting a dense shadow over the lower part of the lung fields, and have the patient hold them in place by leaning against the cassette.

With the palms of the hands facing upward to rotate the scapulae outward, place the hands low on the hips so that they will not be superimposed on the costophrenic angles. Adjust the shoulders to lie in the same transverse plane, depress them to carry the clavicles below the apices, and then rotate them forward. Instruct the patient to keep his shoulders in contact with the cassette. The patient who is unduly unsteady due to age and/or illness may be aided in maintaining the position by placing his arms around the cassette. When this placement of the arms is necessary, care must be exercised to adjust them so as to rotate the scapulae away from the lung fields as much as possible.

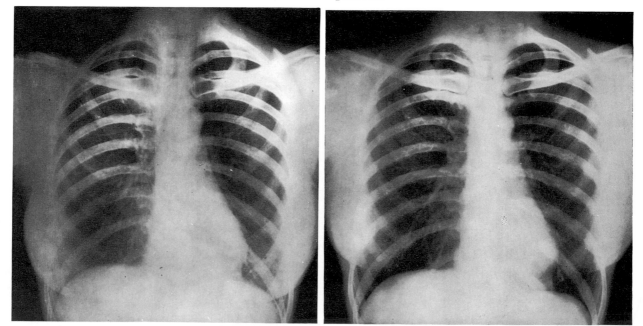

Note breast shadows.   Correct placement of breasts.

CHEST
Lungs and heart
Posteroanterior projection
Anteroposterior view—cont'd

If an immobilization band is used, care must be exercised to avoid rotating the body when applying the band. The least amount of rotation will result in considerable distortion of the heart shadow.

Breathing instructions

General survey films are made at the end of full inhalation to show the greatest possible area of lung structure. The lungs will expand more, and without strain to the patient, on the second breath than on the first. For certain conditions, such as pneumothorax, the presence of a foreign body, and fixation of the diaphragm, films are sometimes made on both inhalation and exhalation. For the exhalation film, the penetration must be increased 6 or 8 kilovolts, according to the habitus of the subject.

For stereoscopic projections, the x-ray tube is shifted in the longitudinal direction, and both exposures must be made on one respiratory movement.

Central ray

The central ray is directed in the median sagittal plane (1) at the level of the fourth thoracic vertebra for the lungs, and (2) at the level of the sixth thoracic vertebra for the heart and aorta.

Structures shown

A posteroanterior projection, anteroposterior view, of the thoracic viscera, showing the air-filled trachea, the lungs, the diaphragmatic domes, the heart and aortic knob, and, if enlarged laterally, the thyroid or thymus gland. The vascular markings are much more prominent on the projection made on exhalation. The bronchial tree is shown from an oblique angle. The esophagus is well demonstrated when filled with a barium sulfate mixture. Unless a high kilovoltage technique is used routinely in these examinations, it is necessary to increase the frontal plane exposure by some 8 or 10 kilovolts in order to demonstrate the opacified esophagus through the superimposed spinal, sternal, and heart shadows.

Lesions that are poorly shown due to foreshortening or that are obscured by superimposition on the basic anteroposterior view can be clearly delineated by the wide-angle technique described on page 172, Volume I.

NOTE: The posteroanterior projection of the heart should be dark enough to show a faint outline of the thoracic vertebrae for the differentiation of the heart contour and any curvature of the vertebral column, and to show calcifications within the heart shadow.

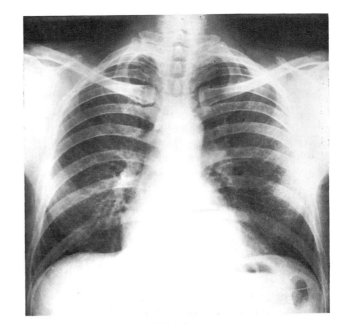

Inhalation.

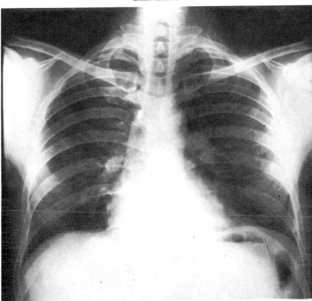

Exhalation.

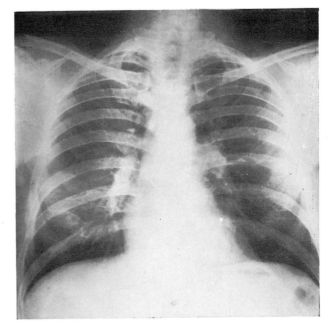

Heart film.

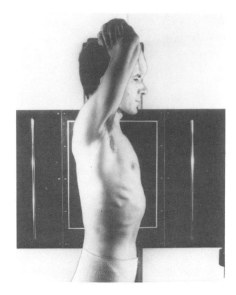

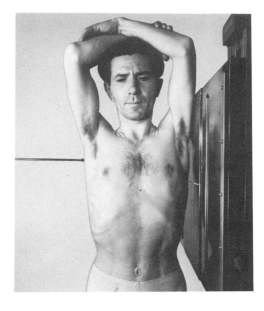

CHEST
Lungs and heart
Lateral projections

Film: 14″ × 17″ lengthwise.

A stationary grid or a high-speed movable grid should be used for this view with hypersthenic and obese subjects.

Position of patient

Turn the patient to a lateral position, arms by the sides. The left lateral position, left side to the film, is used to demonstrate the heart and left lung; the right lateral position is used to demonstrate the right lung. Adjust the height of the cassette so that the upper border of the film is about 1½ inches above the shoulders.

Position of part

Adjust the position of the patient so that, with the median sagittal plane of the body vertical, the adjacent shoulder rests against the cassette or the front of the cassette holder. Center the thorax to the film; the mid-axillary line will lie about 2 inches posterior to the midline of the film. Have the patient sit or stand straight, extend the arms directly upward, flex the elbows, and, with the forearms resting on his head, grasp the elbows to hold the arms in position. If the patient is unsteady, place an enema standard directly in front of him and have him extend his arms and grasp the standard for support.

Recheck the position of the body; *the median sagittal plane must be vertical.* Depending upon the breadth of the shoulders, the lower part of the thorax will be some distance from the film, but this is necessary in order to obtain true structural outlines. (Compare lower left radiograph with upper radiograph on facing page.) Having the patient lean in against the cassette results in great distortion of all the thoracic structures. Forward leaning also results in distorted structural outlines (see radiograph below).

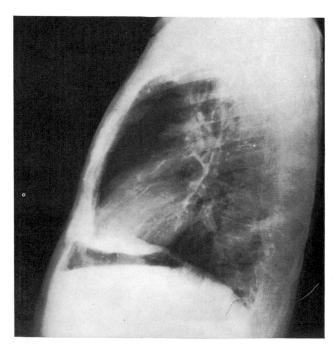

Foreshortening.

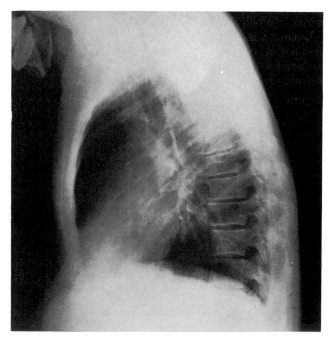

Forward bending.

CHEST
Lungs and heart
Lateral projections—cont'd
Breathing instructions

The exposure is made at the end of full inhalation, preferably at the end of the second breath, to show the greatest possible area of lung structure.

Barium studies

The barium sulfate mixture used in heart examinations should be approximately three times as thick as that used for the stomach so that it will descend more slowly and will adhere to the esophageal walls. Have the patient take two or three swallows and then hold a large bolus of the barium mixture in his mouth until you are ready to make the exposure. The usual exposure technique need not be altered for barium studies in the lateral and oblique positions.

Central ray

Direct the central ray horizontally and center (1) at the level of the fourth thoracic vertebra for the lungs, (2) at the level of the sixth or seventh thoracic vertebra for the heart.

Structures shown

The left lateral projection is used to demonstrate the heart and aorta, and left-sided pulmonary lesions; the right lateral projection is used to demonstrate right-sided pulmonary lesions. The lateral positions are used extensively to demonstrate the interlobar fissures, to differentiate the lobes, and to localize pulmonary lesions.

NOTE: The exposure factors used for the lateral view of the chest should be balanced in such a way as to maintain the contrast-density standard established for the frontal view, a comparable demonstration of the lower half of the humeral head adjacent to the film being the usual criterion. An increase from the frontal view factors of 14 kilovolts and double the milliampere-second factor proves satisfactory for a majority of patients.

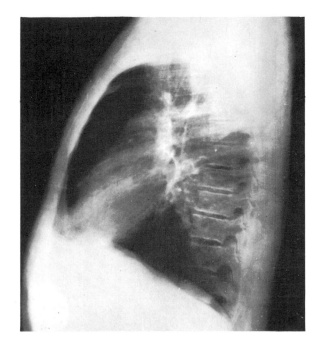

Left lateral. Compare heart shadows with film on opposite page.

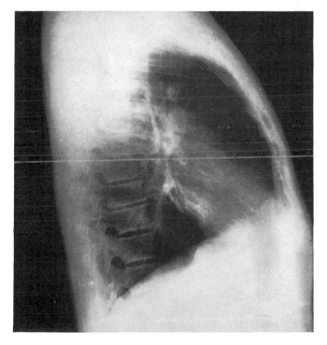

Right lateral.

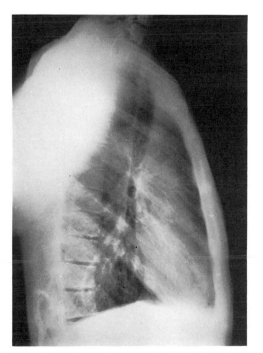

Shoulder placement for superior mediastinum. (Positioning described on page 630.)

637

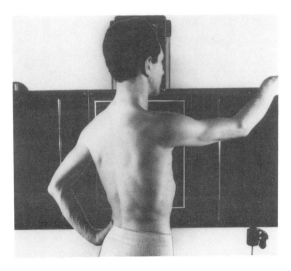

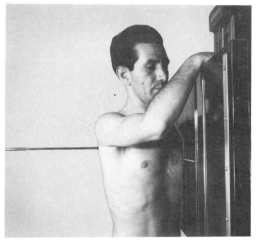

Position for left anterior oblique view, left posteroanterior oblique projection.

CHEST
Lungs and heart
Posteroanterior oblique projections
Left and right anterior oblique views

Film: $14'' \times 17''$ lengthwise.

Grid technique, stationary or high-speed movable grid, should be used with patients who are exceptionally heavy.

Position of patient

The patient is maintained in the same position, standing or seated erect, that was used for the posteroanterior projection. Ask the patient to let his arms hang free and, unless otherwise specified, have him turn approximately 45 degrees toward the right side for a left oblique projection, and approximately 45 degrees toward the left side for a right oblique projection. Ask the patient to stand or sit straight; when he is standing, the weight of the body must be equally distributed on the feet to prevent unwanted rotation. Check the film centering used for the frontal view to be certain that the film projects far enough above the upper border of the shoulders to clear the identification marker.

Position of part

Left anterior oblique view. Rotate the patient so as to place the left shoulder and breast in contact with the cassette, and then center the chest to the film. Ask the patient to place his left hand on the hip with the palm down. Adjust the rotation of the body to the desired degree of obliquity, usually 45 degrees for routine examinations of the chest and, for the purpose of separating the shadows of the aorta and the spine, 55 to 60 degrees for studies of the heart and great vessels. Ask the patient to raise his right arm to shoulder level and to grasp the side of the cassette stand for support. In order to prevent rotation of the spine, adjust the shoulders to lie in the same transverse plane and have the patient face straight ahead.

Right anterior oblique view. Reverse the above position, and unless otherwise instructed, the patient is here adjusted to place the thorax at an angle of 45 degrees.

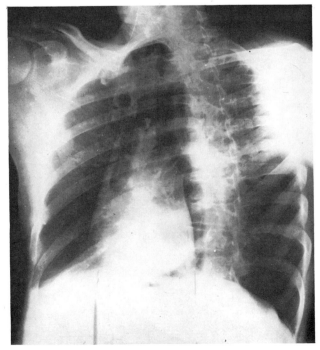

Left anterior oblique view.

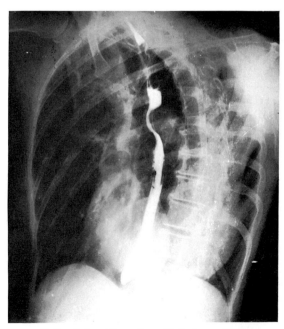

Left anterior oblique view with barium swallow.
Courtesy Dr. Francis H. Ghiselin.

638

CHEST
Lungs and heart
Posteroanterior oblique projections
Left and right anterior oblique views—cont'd

Central ray

Direct the central ray horizontally, and center (1) at the level of the fourth thoracic vertebra for the lungs, and (2) at the level of the sixth or seventh thoracic vertebra for the heart.

An increase of 12 to 14 kilovolts from the frontal view exposure will maintain the established contrast-density standard, and will correctly penetrate the chest of average shape.

Breathing instructions

The exposure is made at the end of full inhalation.

Barium studies

The barium sulfate mixture used in heart studies should be about the consistency of cooked cereal so that it will descend slowly and will adhere to the esophageal mucosa. With the patient in position and briefed on the procedure, have him swallow two or three mouthfuls of the mixture and then hold a bolus of one tablespoonful in his mouth until he is signaled to take a deep breath and then to swallow the bolus in one movement immediately before the exposure.

The usual exposure technique need not be increased for barium studies in the oblique position.

Structures shown

Left anterior oblique view. The maximum area of the left lung field, with its posterior part lying behind the shadow of the spine and its anterior part lying under the superimposed shadows of the spine and the mediastinal structures. The trachea and its bifurcation, the entire right branch of the bronchial tree, and a foreshortened view of the right lung. The heart, the descending aorta, lying just in front of the spinal shadow, the arch of the aorta, and the pulmonary artery and its main right branch.

Right anterior oblique view. The maximum area of the right lung field, with its posterior portion lying behind the shadow of the spine and its anterior part under the superimposed shadows of the spine and the mediastinal contents. The trachea and entire left branch of the bronchial tree, and a foreshortened view of the left lung. This projection gives the best view of the left atrium, the left main branch of the pulmonary artery, the anterior portion of the apex of the left ventricle, and the right retrocardiac space. When filled with a barium sulfate mixture, the esophagus is well shown in the right anterior oblique view.

NOTE: Stead[1] states that he and his associates have found what he calls the "pulmonary oblique" projection to be of particular value in the study of pulmonary diseases. For this purpose the patient is turned only slightly (10 to 20[1,2] degrees to the right or left) from the posteroanterior position. It was found that this slight degree of obliquity rotates the superior segment of the respective lower lobe from behind the hilum and displays the medial part of the right middle lobe or the lingula of the left upper lobe free from the hilum. These areas are not clearly shown in the standard "cardiac oblique" of 45- to 60-degree rotation, due largely to superimposition of the spine.

[1]Stead, William W.: Personal communication.
[2]Zizmor, Judah: Personal communication.

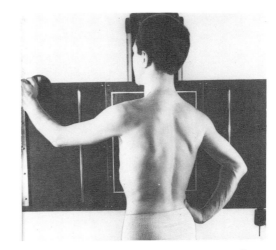

Position for right anterior oblique view, right posteroanterior oblique projection.

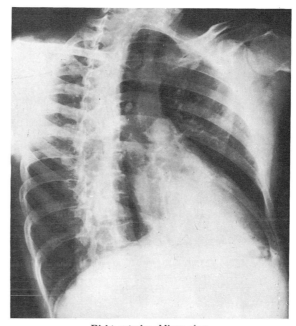

Right anterior oblique view.

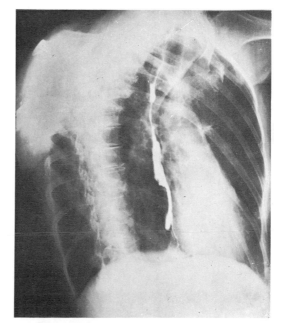

Right anterior oblique view with barium swallow.
Courtesy Dr. Francis H. Ghiselin.

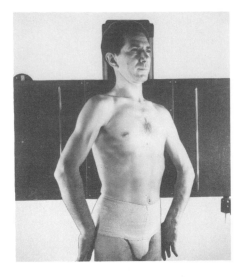

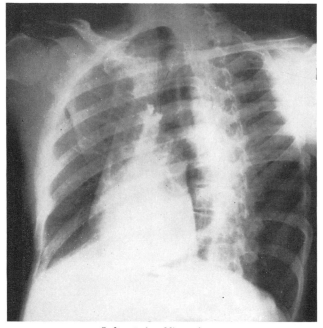

Left anterior oblique view.

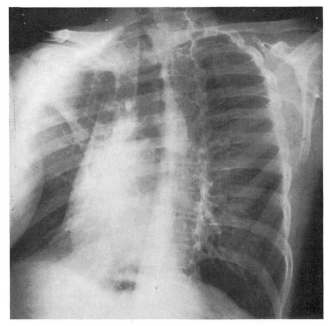

Right posterior oblique view.

CHEST
Lungs and heart
Anteroposterior oblique projections
Right and left posterior oblique views

Posterior oblique views (anteroposterior oblique projections) are used when the patient is too ill to be turned to the prone position, and sometimes as supplementary views in the investigation of specific lesions. They are also employed with the recumbent patient in contrast studies of the heart and great vessels.

One point the technologist must bear in mind is that the *right posterior oblique view* corresponds to the *left anterior oblique view*, and the *left posterior oblique view* to the *right anterior oblique view*.

Film: 14″ × 17″ lengthwise.

Position of patient

With the patient in the anteroposterior position, either erect or recumbent, adjust the cassette so that the upper border of the film is about 1½ inches above the shoulders.

Position of part

Rotate the patient toward the correct side, adjust the thorax at the desired degree of obliquity, and center the chest to the film. If the patient is recumbent, support the elevated hip and arm on sandbags or firm pillows.

Flex the elbows and place the hands on the hips with the palms facing outward, or pronate the hands beside the hips. Adjust the shoulders to lie in the same transverse plane in a position of forward rotation.

The exposure is made at the end of full inhalation.

Central ray

Direct the central ray perpendicularly and center (1) at the level of the fourth thoracic vertebra for the lungs, or (2) at the level of the sixth or seventh thoracic vertebra for the heart.

Structures shown

A posterior oblique view of the thoracic viscera is similar to the corresponding anterior oblique view; that is, a right posterior oblique view is comparable to a left anterior oblique view. However, the lung fields usually appear shorter due to magnification of the shadow of the diaphragm. The heart and great vessels also cast magnified shadows as a result of being farther from the film.

640

CHEST
Lungs and heart
Anteroposterior projection
Posteroanterior view

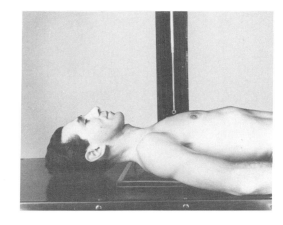

The anteroposterior position is used when the patient is too ill to be turned to the prone position, and it is sometimes used as a supplementary view in the investigation of certain pulmonary lesions.

Film: 14″ × 17″ lengthwise.

Position of patient

Place the patient in the anteroposterior position, either erect or recumbent. In the latter case, the thorax should be elevated, if possible, to a semirecumbent position in order to depress the diaphragm.

Position of part

Center the cassette to the median sagittal plane of the chest and adjust it so that, depending upon the focal-film distance to be used, the upper border of the film is 1½ to 2½ inches above the shoulders.

Flex the elbows, pronate the hands at the level of the hips, and then elevate the elbows on pillows or other suitable supports in order to draw the scapulae outward. The hands are placed, palms outward, near the trochanteric region of the hips when the patient is in the erect position. Adjust the shoulders to lie in the same transverse plane.

The exposure is made at the end of full inhalation.

Central ray

With the central ray perpendicular to the plane of the film, direct it to the sternal angle for the lungs, and to the midsternum for the heart.

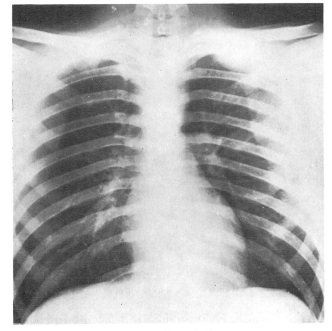

Anteroanterior projection.

Structures shown

An anteroposterior projection of the thoracic viscera, giving a view somewhat similar to the posteroanterior projection. Being farther from the film, the heart and great vessels cast magnified shadows, and the lung fields appear shorter due to the magnification of the shadow of the diaphragm. The shadows of the clavicles are projected higher, and the ribs assume a different angle.

NOTE: Resnick[1] recommends an angulated anteroposterior projection to free the basal portions of the lung fields from superimposition by the anterior diaphragmatic, abdominal, and cardiac structures. He reports that this projection also differentiates middle lobe and lingular processes from lower lobe disease. For this projection the patient may be either erect or supine, and the central ray is directed to the midsternal region at an angle of 30 degrees toward the feet. Resnick states that a more suitable angulation may be chosen by studying the preliminary films.

[1]Resnick, D.: The angulated basal view: a new method for evaluation of lower lobe pulmonary disease, Radiology **96**:204-205, 1970.

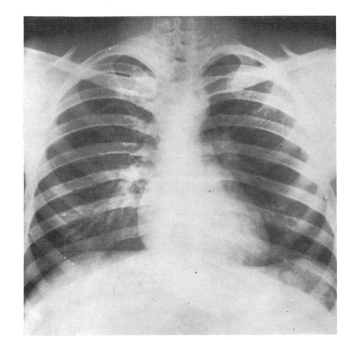

Posteroanterior projection

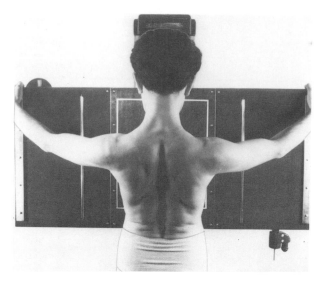

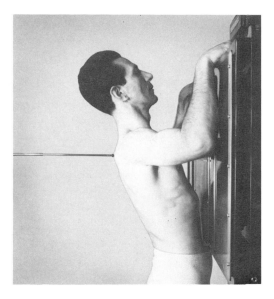

LUNGS
Posteroanterior lordotic projection
Anteroposterior lordotic view
Fleischner position

Film: $14'' \times 17''$ lengthwise.

Position of patient

Place the patient in the posteroanterior position before a vertical cassette stand. Adjust the height of the cassette so that the upper margin of the film is about 1 inch below the upper border of the shoulders.

Position of part

Center the median sagittal plane of the body to the midline of the film. Have the patient grasp the sides of the cassette stand near the top, brace his abdomen against the stand, and then lean backward in a position of extreme lordosis. The thorax should be inclined backward approximately 45 degrees.

The exposure is made at the end of full inhalation.

Central ray

Direct the central ray horizontally to the fourth thoracic vertebra.

Structures shown

An anterior semiaxial view of the lungs, used to demonstrate interlobar effusions.

A similar view can be obtained by adjusting the patient in the prone position and directing the central ray 45 degrees toward the feet.

Kjellberg[1] recommends the prone position with a 30-degree caudal angulation of the central ray for the demonstration of minimal mitral disease.

[1]Kjellberg, S. R.: Importance of prone position in the roentgenologic diagnosis of slight mitral disease, Acta Radiol. **31:**178-181, 1949.

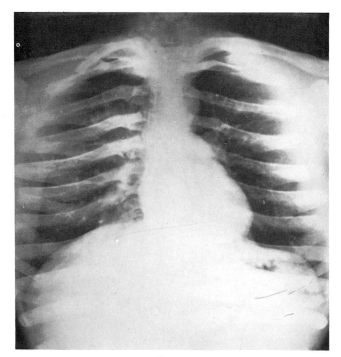

Erect.

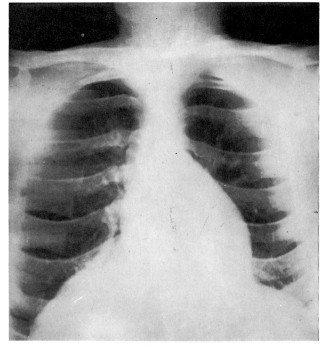

Prone.

LUNGS
Anteroposterior lordotic projections
Posteroanterior lordotic views
Lindblom positions

Film: $14'' \times 17''$ lengthwise.

Position of patient

Place the patient in the anteroposterior position, before, and approximately 1 foot away from, a vertical cassette stand. Adjust the height of the cassette so that the upper margin of the film will be about $1\frac{1}{2}$ inches above the upper border of the shoulders when the patient is adjusted in the lordotic position.

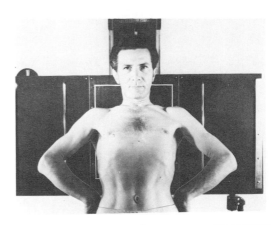

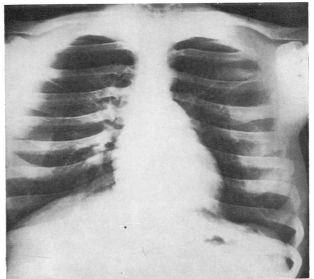

Position of part

Anteroposterior projection. Adjust the body in the anteroposterior position, with the median sagittal plane centered to the midline of the cassette.

Oblique projection. Rotate the body approximately 30 degrees away from the anteroposterior position, with the affected side toward and centered to the film.

With the patient in either of the above positions, flex the elbows and place the hands, palms out, on the hips. Have the patient lean backward in a position of extreme lordosis and rest his shoulders against the cassette.

The exposure is made at the end of full inhalation.

Central ray

With the central ray directed horizontally, center at the level of the midsternum.

Structures shown

Posterior semiaxial views of the lungs, which are used to demonstrate the apices and such conditions as interlobar effusions.

Rundle, de Lambert, and Epps[1] have worked out an exact anteroposterior lordotic position for the localization of cervicothoracic tumor masses, especially for the differentiation of extrathoracic and partially or wholly intrathoracic masses. The authors state that the position is particularly valuable in examinations of the posterosuperior mediastinum, because it is so frequently impossible to obtain a satisfactory lateral projection of this area.

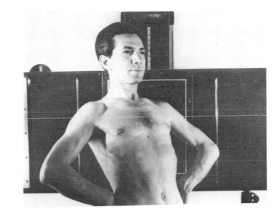

The authors recommend placing a skin-pencil mark just above the vertebra prominens and another over the upper edge of the manubrial notch to aid in adjusting the body position. The patient is then tilted backward until the plane of the thoracic inlet, indicated by the pencil marks, is at right angles to the plane of the film; the anterior ends of the first pair of ribs will be seen to lie in the same horizontal plane as their posterior ends. The central ray is directed perpendicularly and centered to the upper edge of the manubrial notch.

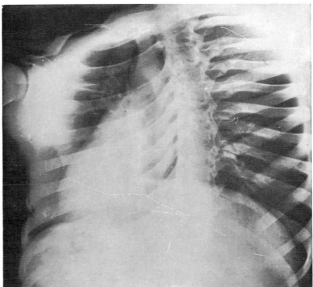

[1]Rundle, F. F., de Lambert, R. M., and Epps, R. G.: Cervicothoracic tumors: a technical aid to their roentgenologic localization, Amer. J. Roentgen. **81:**316-321, 1959.

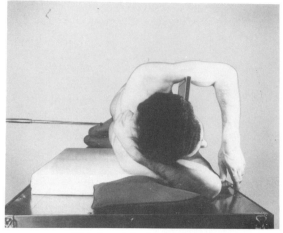

Right lateral decubitus position.

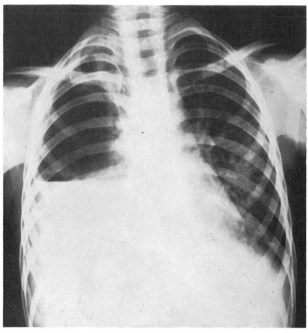

Erect.

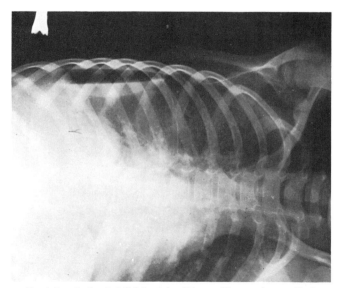

Frontal projection in left lateral decubitus position on above patient.

Radiographs courtesy Dr. Hugh M. Wilson.

LUNGS AND PLEURAE

Frontal projection in lateral decubitus position for fluid levels and small pneumothoraces

Film: 14″ × 17″ lengthwise.

Position of patient

Place the patient in a lateral recumbent position, and so that he is lying on either the affected or the unaffected side, as indicated by the existing condition. A small amount of fluid in the pleural cavity is, in most instances, best shown with the patient lying on the affected side, where the fluid will not be overlapped by the mediastinal shadows. The reverse is true in the case of a small amount of air.

Position of part

If the patient is lying on the affected side, elevate the body several inches with a suitable platform, a firm pad, or folded sheets.

Extend the arms well above the head and adjust the thorax in a true lateral position. Place the cassette vertically against either the anterior or the posterior surface of the chest, adjust it so that the film extends approximately 2 inches beyond the shoulders, and immobilize it with sandbags or another suitable support.

The exposure is made at the end of full inhalation.

Central ray

Direct the central ray horizontally through the fourth thoracic vertebra.

Structures shown

A frontal projection (posteroanterior or anteroposterior), demonstrating the change in fluid position and revealing the previously obscured pulmonary areas, or, in the case of a suspected pneumothorax, the presence of any free air.

This application of the lateral decubitus position was first recommended by Rigler,[1] and more recently by Abo.[2]

NOTE: An exposure made with the patient leaning directly laterally from the erect posteroanterior position is sometimes an advantage in the demonstration of fluid levels in pulmonary cavities. Ekimsky[3] recommends this position, with the patient leaning laterally 45 degrees, for the demonstration of small pleural effusions. He points out that the inclined position is simpler to perform than the decubitus position, and states that it is equally satisfactory.

[1]Rigler, L. G.: Roentgen diagnosis of small pleural effusions, J.A.M.A. **96:**104-108, 1931.
[2]Abo, Stanley: Roentgenographic detection of minimal pneumothorax in the lateral decubitus position, Amer. J. Roentgen. **77:**1066-1070, 1957.
[3]Ekimsky, B.: Comparative study of lateral decubitus views and those with lateral body inclination in small pleural effusions, Vestn. Rentgen. Radiol. **41:**43-49, 1966. (In Russian.) Abst.: Radiology **87:**1135, 1966.

LUNGS AND PLEURAE
Lateral projections for fluid level
Ventral or dorsal decubitus position

Film: $14'' \times 17''$ lengthwise.

Position of patient

With the patient in either a prone or a supine position, elevate the thorax 2 or 3 inches on folded sheets or a firm pad.

Position of part

Adjust the body in a true posteroanterior or anteroposterior position and extend the arms well above the head. Place the cassette vertically against the affected side, adjust it so that the film extends to the level of the laryngeal prominence, and immobilize it with sandbags or other support.

The exposure is made at the end of full inhalation.

Central ray

With the central ray directed horizontally, center to the midaxillary line at the level of the fourth thoracic vertebra.

Structures shown

A lateral view demonstrating the change in the position of the fluid and revealing pulmonary areas that are obscured by the fluid in standard projections.

NOTE: Miller[1] described and illustrated several cassette holder devices, including one bolt-on device, designed to eliminate the all-too-familiar problems of obtaining cross-table projections. The apparatus can be attached to any standard radiographic table, can be rapidly raised and lowered, and does not interfere with the usual functions of the table.

[1]Miller, R. E.: Simple apparatus for decubitus films with horizontal beam, Radiology **97:**682-683, 1970.

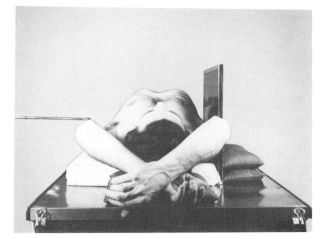

Dorsal decubitus position.

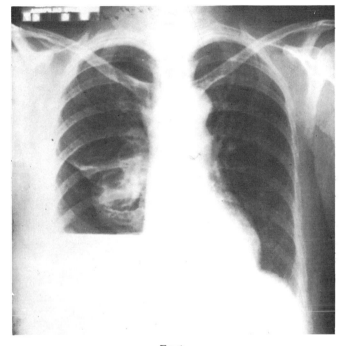

Erect.

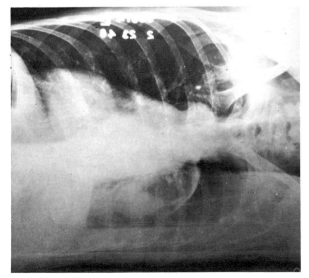

Frontal projection in right lateral decubitus position.

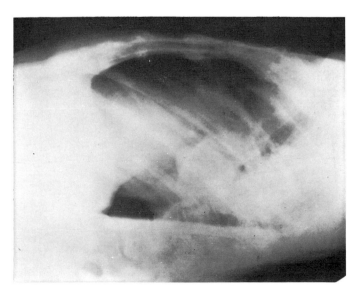

Lateral projection in dorsal decubitus position.

Radiographs courtesy Dr. Dan Tucker.

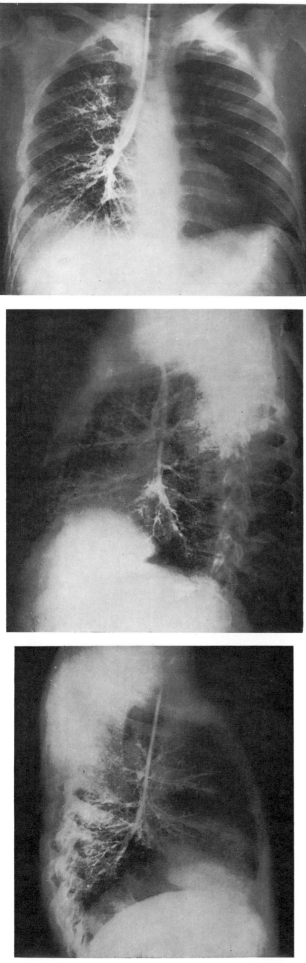

BRONCHOGRAPHY

Bronchography is the term applied to the specialized radiologic examination of the lungs and bronchial tree by means of introducing an opaque contrast medium into the bronchi. This method of examination is employed in the investigation of such conditions as hemoptysis, bronchiectasis, chronic pneumonia, bronchial obstruction, pulmonary tumors, cysts and cavities, and bronchopleural-cutaneous fistulae.

There are numerous iodinated media, both aqueous and oily, available for bronchography. Barium and bismuth suspensions are used by some radiologists, and powdered tantalum by others; however, the oily iodinated media are more generally used.

There are several methods of introducing the contrast substance into the trachea. Once there, by any method of instillation other than by selective catheterization, the distribution of the medium through the bronchial branches depends upon gravity, so that the direction of its flow must be guided by body position. In order to direct the medium into the different bronchial segments, the physician leans and rotates the patient and angles the tilt-table as required; this may be done under radioscopic observation. The success of the examination depends not only upon satisfactory distribution of the contrast agent through the bronchi but also upon suppressing the cough reflex to prevent alveolar filling and/or expulsion of the medium before the filming can be completed. The patient can suppress, to some extent, the urge to cough, but inhibition of this involuntary action depends largely upon premedication—upon moderate sedation and local anesthetization of the throat structures.

PREPARATION AND CARE OF PATIENT

The meal preceding the examination is withheld as a precaution against aspiration of any regurgitated material. Food and fluid are forbidden until the full effect of the local anesthetic has worn off, about two hours after the examination, for the purpose of preventing aspiration on attempted swallowing.

The type of premedication used depends upon the nature of the existent pathology. In the case of an exudative lesion, some doctors prescribe an expectorant drug and postural drainage for a two- or three-day period prior to the examination. This is done to promote the expulsion of mucus or exudate from the lungs and bronchi and thus to clear the air passages for satisfactory opacification.

Immediate medication consists of (1) moderate sedation, administered about one hour prior to the examination, to relax the patient and lessen his sensitivity to the procedure and (2) a drug such as ephedrine or atropine, administered about thirty minutes before the examination, to check secretion of the bronchopulmonary membrane during the examination. Because of the prolonged effect of sedative drugs, the outpatient should be instructed to make arrangements to be escorted home, and to postpone normal activities until the following day.

Before introducing the contrast medium, the physician carefully anesthetizes the throat structures with a topical anesthetic solution to inhibit the gag and cough reflexes. The patient is instructed to breathe rapidly and shallowly during this procedure.

It is important that the patient be acquainted with the several steps of the bronchographic procedure, and that he understand why he must exert real effort to control coughing. The patient's apprehension about having foreign material injected into his air passages is usually considerably relieved when he is assured that he will at all times have adequate breathing space in the airways despite the presence of the contrast substance. He should be assured that the cough reflex will be greatly minimized and largely controlled by the local anesthetic, but that he must help by instituting rapid, shallow breathing in an attempt to suppress each urge to cough.

Upon completion of the bronchographic examination, the patient should be instructed to cough *gently* to avoid forcing contrast substance into the alveoli, from whence its elimination may depend upon absorption. The patient is kept in the radiology department for postural drainage, which is accomplished by reversing the filling positions, a few minutes in each, from the seated position to drain the upper bronchial segments, and from the Trendelenburg position to drain the lower segments. A postdrainage film should be taken within the next day or two.

PREPARATION OF EXAMINING ROOM

In the preparation of the examining room an important point to remember is that bronchographic filming must be carried out as expeditiously as possible. This part of the procedure is best performed by a team of two technologists. An ample number of cassettes and the identification markers should be conveniently placed. Preliminary films are always taken, at which time the postinjection radiographic technique and the pathologic status of the patient's lungs are determined.

The supplies for the care of the patient and for the instillation procedure should be conveniently arranged. The instrument tray is set up, as specified by the examining physician, according to the requirements of each instillation method employed in the department. The technologist should have each listing recorded in his procedure book so that no item will be overlooked, with resultant delay and inconvenience. In the following general list, certain items are common to all methods, whereas others are peculiar to one method.

Sterile items: (1) laryngeal mirror, (2) throat atomizer, (3) medicine glasses, (4) laryngeal syringe, (5) forceps, (6) curved laryngeal cannula, (7) hypodermic syringe and needles, (8) 2 ml. syringe, (9) 5 ml. Luer-Lok syringe, (10) cricothyroid puncture needles of specified type and size, (11) No. 11 knife blade, (12) premeasured Seldinger guide wires, (13) intratracheal catheter of specified type and size, (14) specimen containers, (15) 20 ml. Luer-Lok syringe, (16) sterile gloves for radiologist in the transcricothyroid method.

Nonsterile items: (1) caps, masks, and gowns for the physician and any assistant who must face the patient, (2) head mirror or head lamp, (3) emesis basins, tissues, and disposable towels for the patient's use, (4) waste bag or lined disposal can, (5) waste basin for soiled swabs and applicators, (6) jar of sterile tongue depressors, (7) jar of sterile cotton-tipped applicators or a sterile flexible-tipped metal applicator, (8) dressing bowls or jars containing sterile cotton pledgets and gauze swabs, (9) lubricant for intratracheal catheter, (10) vial of specified local anesthetic, (11) antiseptic solution, usually 70% alcohol, for cleansing skin in the transcricothyroid method, (12) small prepared dressing for application to transcricothyroid puncture site when the needle is removed, (13) vials of contrast agent. Full emergency equipment should be at hand for treatment of the occasional allergic or shock reaction to the local anesthetic drug.

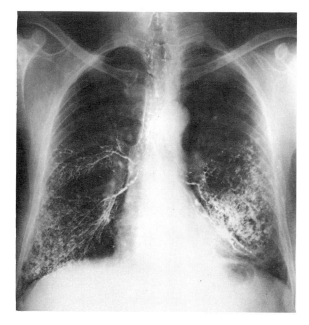

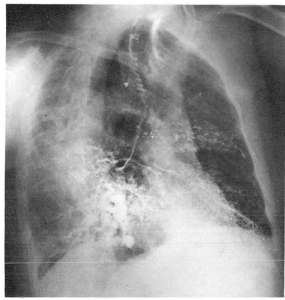

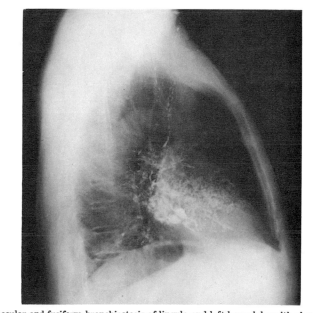

Saccular and fusiform bronchiectasis of lingula and left lower lobe with chronic pneumonia.

Bronchograms and diagnostic information courtesy Dr. Judah Zizmor.

647

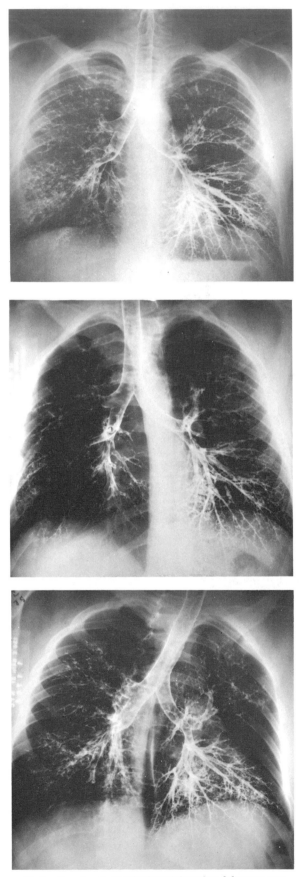

Obstruction of main lingular branch bronchus, left upper lobe.

Bronchograms and diagnostic information courtesy Dr. Judah Zizmor.

BRONCHOGRAPHY—cont'd

Methods of contrast instillation

The *supraglottic* and *intraglottic* methods of instillation are identical except for the placement of the laryngeal cannula, through which the medium is introduced. In the supraglottic method the medium is rapidly dropped from the cannula onto the base of the tongue, from whence it flows into the glottis. In the intraglottic method the cannula or catheter is advanced into the glottis for the introduction of the contrast substance. These two methods are employed most frequently because of their comparative simplicity and because they do not require hospitalization of the patient.

For either method, the patient is seated for the instillation procedure, preferably on the side of the tilt table to expedite subsequent gravity filling of the upper-lobe bronchi. Following anesthetization of the throat structures, the doctor has the patient lean toward the side to be filled and support himself on the outstretched hand or on the forearm, a greater degree of leaning being necessary for the left side. The patient's head must be in the vertical position throughout the supraglottic instillation so that the contrast substance will flow directly backward and thus into the laryngeal orifice.

Immediately upon completion of the instillation, while an adequate amount of the medium is still in the trachea, the patient is placed in the supine position. He is then rotated, and the table is angled as required to distribute the medium through the upper-lobe segments of the bronchi; this procedure may be done under radioscopic observation with spot films exposed as indicated.

Amplatz and Haut[1] describe a technique of rapid and uniform distribution of the contrast medium throughout the bronchial tree without rotation of the patient or angulation of the table. Following routine premedication of the patient, a catheter is passed, transorally or transnasally, through the glottis and trachea into the main stem bronchus of the affected side. A local anesthetic is injected in small amounts until the cough reflex is suppressed. The patient is then turned to the lateral decubitus position with the affected side dependent. He is instructed to exhale forcefully, and then to hold his breath during a rapid bolus injection of contrast medium and the exposure of a single spot film. The patient is then instructed to breathe normally. This aspirates contrast medium into the peripheral bronchial radicles and provides double contrast visualization of the entire bronchial tree. After spot-filming in the lateral and oblique positions, conventional overhead studies are obtained in the following sequence: direct lateral, oblique, and anteroposterior.

In the transglottic *intratracheal intubation* method of instillation, a plastic intratracheal catheter is passed, transorally or transnasally, through the glottis and trachea into the main stem bronchus of the side under investigation. Unless a general anesthetic is indicated, this method does not require hospital admission of adult patients. Children are examined by this method under general anesthesia.

[1]Amplatz, K., and Haut, G.: Lateral decubitus bronchography with a single bolus, Radiology **95**:439-440, 1970.

When the patient is under general anesthesia, or for another reason is placed in the recumbent position for the instillation of the contrast agent, the head end of the table is elevated enough to prevent a backward flow of the medium into the throat. By this method, the catheter passes through the nasopharyngeal secretions so it is not possible to obtain uncontaminated bronchial aspirates for culture.

In the *percutaneous cricothyroid* or *percutaneous transtracheal* method, a suitable puncture needle is inserted into the subglottic tracheal space through the cricothyroid membrane or slightly lower at an intercartilaginous tracheal space. This method requires that the patient be hospitalized.

Since Cope[1] introduced the Seldinger[2] technique of needle, guide wire, catheter replacement for use in percutaneous transtracheal catheterization, this method has come into wide use for nonselective as well as selective bronchial catherization for bronchography and for aspirating sterile bronchial secretions for laboratory examination. Cope reports that this procedure is easy to perform, that it is well tolerated by patients, and that it overcomes most of the disadvantages of transglottic catheterization.

Cope method of percutaneous transtracheal bronchography

Premedication for the average adult patient consists of (1) 100 mg. of pentobarbital and 100 mg. of levopropoxyphene (Novard) administered by mouth one hour prior to the examination and (2) 60 mg. of codeine and 0.4 mg. of atropine administered subcutaneously one-half hour before the procedure.

The patient is placed on the radiographic table in the supine position, and the head end of the table is then elevated about 10 degrees. The radiologist explains the procedure to the patient and gives him explicit instructions to aid him in cooperating during the several phases of the examination.

The patient's head is adjusted in hyperextension to make the larynx and trachea as prominent as possible. The skin over the anterior aspect of the neck is prepared with an antiseptic solution and draped. The doctor then infiltrates the tissues around the puncture site with a local anesthetic solution. Selecting a puncture site in the midline over the cricothyroid membrane or upper trachea, he nicks the skin with a knife blade for easier insertion of the needle. With the syringe disconnected from the needle immediately after each injection to permit the needle to ride free during coughing, lidocaine or other local anesthetic is injected into the trachea in small amounts until the cough reflex is suppressed.

The first needle is now replaced with a curved 17-gauge Teflon needle. This consists of a curved, solid-pointed, 18-gauge metal needle surrounded by a close-fitting Teflon sheath. When correctly placed, the metal needle is removed, leaving the Teflon cannula in position in the trachea.

[1]Cope, C.: Selective bronchial catheterization by a new percutaneous transtracheal technique, Amer. J. Roentgen. **96**:932-935, 1966.
[2]Seldinger, S. I.: Catheter replacement of needle in percutaneous arteriography; new technique, Acta Radiol. **39**:368-376, 1953.

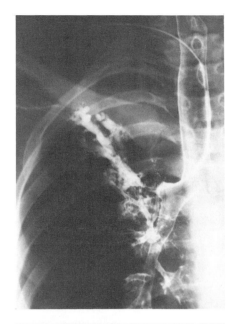

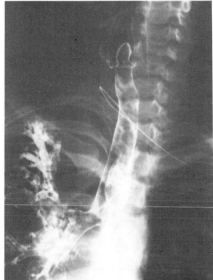

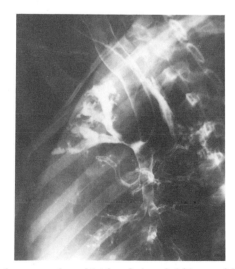

Bronchial adenoma causing subtotal occlusion of right upper-lobe bronchus. Note that because the transcricoid catheter has bypassed the level of obstruction, contrast injection has uncovered postobstruction bronchiectasis.

Above radiographs and clinical information courtesy Dr. Constantin Cope.

BRONCHOGRAPHY—cont'd

Methods of contrast instillation—cont'd

Cope method of percutaneous transtracheal bronchography—cont'd

Nonselective bronchography can now be performed. The contrast medium is injected through the Teflon cannula and, because of the flexibility of the Teflon cannula, the patient can be safely rotated and the table angled to any desired position for gravity filling of the bronchi and for radioscopy and filming.

Selective bronchial filling requires catheterization of the affected bronchial segment. A premeasured Seldinger wire guide is inserted through the Teflon cannula and passed into the lower trachea. The Teflon cannula is then removed, and an intratracheal catheter is threaded over the wire guide and passed to the lower trachea. The wire guide is removed. Under radioscopic guidance, the catheter may be directed into either main-stem bronchus. A premeasured maneuverable wire guide is inserted within the catheter to aid in locating and intubating the desired bronchial segment, after which the wire is removed. Sterile secretions can now be aspirated for pathologic and bacteriologic examination. The contrast medium is then injected under radioscopic guidance, and spot films are exposed as indicated. The catheter may then be removed, or it may be taped to the patient's neck while the conventional films are obtained. These studies are usually made with the patient in the erect position.

Bronchographic filming

Unilateral or bilateral opacification of the bronchial tree may be performed in a single examination. In the latter case, the first side is filmed before the opacification of the contralateral side.

Bronchographic filming may include (1) a supine anteroposterior projection, (2) an erect, single or stereoscopic, posteroanterior projection, (3) right and left oblique projections, and (4) a lateral projection when only one side is injected or, in the case of a bilateral examination, of the first side injected.

Postinjection exposures should be increased by the equivalent of 6 or 8 kilovolts to outline the bronchial segments overshadowed by the heart. For thick-chested subjects, and for the demonstration of consolidated areas, it is necessary to use a stationary grid or a high-speed Potter-Bucky diaphragm. Tomographic studies are sometimes used to advantage.

Anatomy and positioning of the digestive system

Digestive system

The digestive system consists of the alimentary tract and certain accessory organs that contribute to the digestive process.

The alimentary tract is a musculomembranous, tube-like structure, the several regions of which vary in diameter according to functional requirements. The greater part of the tract, which is about 29 or 30 feet in length, lies in the abdominal cavity. The component parts of the alimentary tract are: the mouth, in which the food is masticated and converted into a bolus by insalivation; the pharynx and esophagus, which are the organs of deglutition; the stomach, in which the digestive process begins; the small intestine, in which the digestive process is completed; and the large intestine, an organ of egestion and water absorption, which terminates at the anus.

The radiographically important accessory organs of the digestive system are the teeth, which serve to masticate the food; the salivary glands, which secrete fluid into the mouth for insalivation of the food; and the liver and pancreas, which secrete specialized digestive juices into the small intestine.

The anatomy and positioning of the oral, cervical, and thoracic portions of the digestive system are described under the respective regional headings.

The abdominopelvic cavity is lined by a double-walled, seromembranous sac called the *peritoneum*. The outer, or parietal, layer of the peritoneum is closely adherent to the abdominal and pelvic walls and to the undersurface of the diaphragm. The inner, or visceral, layer is reflected over the contained organs and forms folds called the mesentery and omenta, which serve to support the viscera in position. The narrow space between the two layers, or walls, of the peritoneum is called the peritoneal cavity.

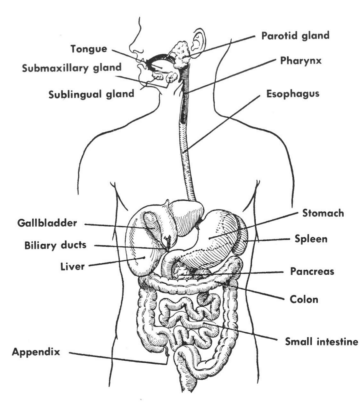

ALIMENTARY TRACT AND ITS ACCESSORY ORGANS

ALIMENTARY TRACT

The *stomach* is the dilated, sacklike portion of the digestive tract extending between the esophagus and the small intestine. Its wall is composed of four layers: (1) a covering layer, the serosa, (2) a muscular layer consisting of oblique, circular, and longitudinal fibers, (3) a submucous layer, and (4) a thick, soft mucosal lining, which is thrown into numerous folds, called *rugae*, when the organ is contracted.

The stomach has two openings, each of which is controlled by a muscular sphincter. The opening between the esophagus and the stomach is known as the *cardiac orifice*, and that between the stomach and the small intestine as the *pylorus*.

The stomach has two surfaces, anterior and posterior, and two borders called *curvatures*. The right border forms the lesser curvature, and the left border forms the greater curvature. The lesser curvature extends from the esophageal orifice to the pylorus, and near its lower end, it presents a notch called the *incisura angularis*. The greater curvature, arching above the cardiac orifice and extending to the pylorus, is considerably longer than the lesser curvature. It presents a dilatation just opposite the incisura angularis of the lesser curvature, and a notch, called the *sulcus intermedius*, about 1 inch from the pylorus. The right border of the esophagus is continuous with the lesser curvature, and its left border joins the greater curvature at a sharp angle called the *cardiac incisura*. The expanded portion of the short abdominal end of the esophagus is called the *cardiac antrum*.

The stomach is divided into cardiac and pyloric portions by a plane passing through the incisura angularis of the lesser curvature and the left limit of the dilatation of the greater curvature. The portion lying between this plane and a plane passing transversely through the cardiac incisura is referred to as the *body* of the stomach, the upper part being called the *fundus*. When the body is in the erect position, the fundus is usually filled with gas and is referred to by radiologists as the gas bubble, or magenblase. In the pyloric end, the portion lying between the pylorus and the sulcus intermedius is called the pyloric antrum. The remainder, the portion lying to the left of the sulcus intermedius, is the lowest, or most dependent, part of the stomach and is referred to as the *pyloric vestibule*.

The size, shape, and position of the stomach depend upon bodily habitus and vary with posture and with the amount of the contents of the stomach. In subjects of the hypersthenic habitus, the stomach is almost horizontal in direction and is high in position, its most dependent portion lying well above the umbilicus. In subjects of the opposite extreme, the asthenic habitus, the stomach is vertical in direction and occupies a low position, its most dependent portion extending well below the interspinous line. Between these two extremes are the many intermediate types of bodily habitus, with corresponding variations in the shape and position of the stomach. For a detailed study of the relationship between body type and the location of the stomach and duodenum, see the papers of Moody, Van Nuys, and Chamberlain,[1,2] and of Vik.[3]

[1]Moody, R. O., Van Nuys, R. G., and Chamberlain, W. Edward: Position of the stomach, liver, and colon, J.A.M.A. **81**:1924-1931, 1923.
[2]Moody, R. O., Van Nuys, R. G., and Chamberlain, W. Edward: Visceral anatomy of healthy adults, Amer. J. Anat. **37**:273-288, 1926.
[3]Vik, Frances L.: Positioning patients for radiography of the stomach according to body habitus, Xray Techn. **12**:85-89, 1940.

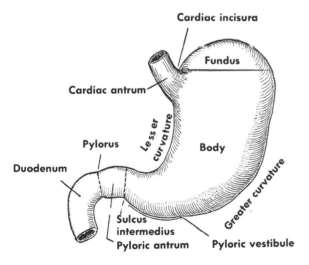

ANTERIOR SURFACE OF STOMACH

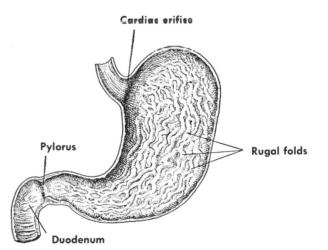

SECTION OF STOMACH SHOWING RUGAE

The *small intestine* extends from the pyloric orifice of the stomach to the ileocecal valve, where it joins the large intestine at a right angle. It averages about 22 feet in length, and its diameter gradually diminishes from approximately 1½ inches in its upper part to approximately 1 inch in its lower part. Its wall is composed of four coats: serous, muscular, submucous, and mucous. The muscular coat consists of an inner layer of circular fibers and an outer layer of longitudinal fibers. The small intestine is divided into three portions, the duodenum, the jejunum, and the ileum.

The duodenum is 8 to 10 inches in length and is the widest portion of the small bowel. Beginning at the pylorus, the duodenum follows a C-shaped course, its several regions being described accordingly as superior, descending, horizontal, and ascending portions. The superior portion passes backward and to the right for a distance of about 2 inches and then bends downward to become the descending portion. The first part of the superior portion is called the duodenal cap because of its roentgen appearance when filled with an opaque medium. The descending portion is about 3 or 4 inches in length. It passes downward along the head of the pancreas and in close relation to the undersurface of the liver. The common bile duct and the pancreatic duct usually unite and open into a common orifice situated in this portion of the duodenum. The horizontal portion passes toward the left at a slight upward inclination for a distance of about 2½ inches and continues as the ascending portion on the left side of the vertebrae.

This portion, which is about 1 inch long, joins the jejunum at a sharp curve called the duodenojejunal flexure, or the angle of Treitz. While the duodenal loop is the most fixed part of the small bowel and normally lies in the upper part of the umbilical region of the abdomen, its position varies with bodily habitus and with the amount of the gastric and intestinal content.

The remainder of the small intestine is arbitrarily divided into two portions, the upper two-fifths being referred to as the jejunum and the lower three-fifths as the ileum. The jejunum and the ileum are gathered into freely movable loops, or convolutions, and attached to the posterior wall of the abdomen by the mesentery. The loops lie in the central and lower part of the abdominal cavity within the arch of the large intestine.

The *large intestine* begins in the right iliac region at the terminus of the ileum, describes an arch surrounding the loops of the small intestine, and ends at the anus. It is about 5 feet long, and is greater in diameter than the small bowel. It is subdivided into the cecum, the colon, and the rectum. Its wall is composed of serous, muscular, submucous, and mucous coats. The muscular coat consists of an inner layer of circular fibers and of an outer layer of longitudinal fibers arranged in three bands over the greater part of the intestine and in two bands over the remaining part. The bands, called taeniae coli, are shorter than the other layers, with the result that the wall of the large intestine is pouched, or sacculated, between them. The recesses of the sacculations are called haustra.

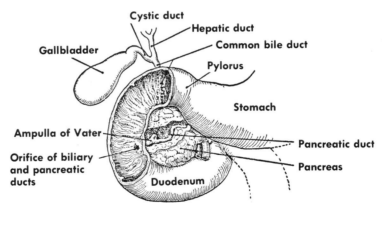

DUODENAL LOOP IN RELATION TO BILIARY AND PANCREATIC DUCTS

The cecum is the dilated, pouchlike portion of the large intestine and is situated below the junction of the ileum and the colon. It is approximately 2½ inches in length and 3 inches in diameter. The appendix, or vermiform process, is attached to the posteromedial side of the cecum. The appendix is a narrow, wormlike tube and averages about 3 inches in length. Its wall is similar to that of the intestine. The ileocecal valve is situated at the junction of the ascending colon and the cecum. The valve projects into the lumen of the tube and guards the opening between the ileum and the colon.

The colon is subdivided into ascending, transverse, descending, and sigmoid portions. The ascending portion passes upward from its junction with the cecum to the undersurface of the liver, where it joins the transverse portion at an angle called the right colic, or hepatic, flexure. The transverse portion, which is the longest and most movable part of the colon, crosses the abdomen to the undersurface of the spleen. It then makes a sharp curve, called the left colic, or splenic, flexure, and ends in the descending portion. The descending portion passes downward and medialward to its junction with the sigmoid portion at the upper aperture of the lesser pelvis. The sigmoid portion curves on itself to form an S-shaped loop and ends in the rectum at the level of the third sacral segment.

The rectum extends from the sigmoid to the anus, the external aperture of the intestine. The rectum is approximately 6 inches in length. Its lower portion, about 1 inch long, is constricted to form the anal canal. Just above the anal canal it presents a dilatation called the rectal ampulla. Following the sacrococcygeal curve, the rectum passes downward and backward to the level of the pelvic floor and then bends sharply forward and downward into the canal portion that extends to the anus. The rectum thus presents two anteroposterior curves, a fact that must be remembered when inserting an enema tube.

Peristalsis is the term applied to the contraction waves by which the digestive tube propels its contents toward the rectum. There are normally about three or four waves per minute in the filled stomach; the waves begin in the upper part of the organ and travel toward the pylorus. The average emptying time of the normal stomach is from two to three hours.

Peristaltic action in the intestines is greatest in the upper part of the tract, showing a gradual decrease toward the lower portion. The duodenum and the jejunum, in addition to the peristaltic waves, undergo localized contractions, which usually occur at three- or four-second intervals during digestion. The head of a barium meal normally reaches the ileocecal valve in two or three hours, and the tail of the meal in four to five hours. The meal usually reaches the rectum in about twenty-four hours.

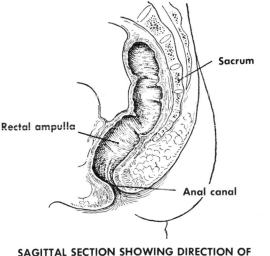

SAGITTAL SECTION SHOWING DIRECTION OF
ANAL CANAL AND RECTUM

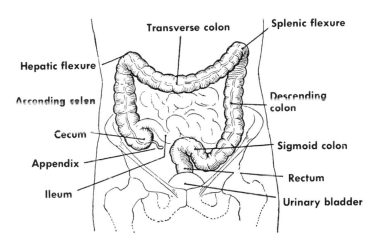

ANTERIOR ASPECT OF LARGE BOWEL

LIVER AND BILIARY SYSTEM

The liver is a massive, irregularly wedge-shaped gland, with its base situated on the right, and its apex directed forward and to the left. It occupies almost all of the right hypochondrium and a large part of the epigastrium; its right portion extends downward into the right lumbar region as far as the fourth lumbar vertebra, and its left extremity extends across the left hypochondrium as far as the mammillary line. The liver measures about 8½ inches transversely at its widest part; 6½ inches vertically at its longest part; and 4½ inches anteroposteriorly at its deepest part, which is just above the right kidney. Its superior surface is convex and is closely fitted to the undersurface of the diaphragm and the anterior wall of the abdomen. Its posterior surface slants downward and forward to the inferior surface, which is concave, and is molded over the subjacent viscera, on which it rests.

The liver is divided into two major lobes, a large right lobe and a small left lobe, and into two minor lobes, which are located on the left portion of the right lobe, the caudate lobe on its posterior surface and the quadrate lobe on its inferior surface. The hilus of the liver, called the porta hepatis, is situated transversely between the two minor lobes. The porta transmits the hepatic artery, the portal vein, and the bile ducts, the branches of these three vessels accompanying each other in their ramifications through the liver substance. A deep groove, through which the inferior vena cava passes, is located on the posterior surface of the liver and separates the caudate lobe from the right lobe proper; the hepatic veins empty into the inferior vena cava. The fossa for the gallbladder lies on the inferior surface of the right lobe, just below the porta and beside the quadrate lobe.

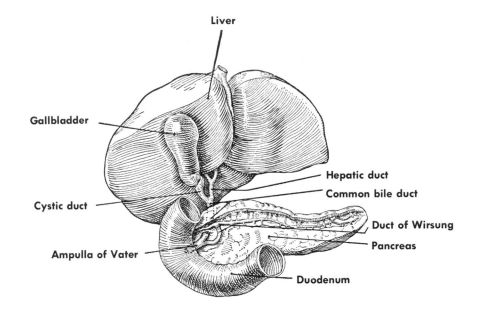

INFEROPOSTERIOR ASPECT OF LIVER AND GALLBLADDER

The liver substance is composed of minute lobules held together by a delicate connective tissue, which transmits the terminal branches of the hepatic artery and the portal vein, and the beginning branches of the hepatic veins and the bile ducts. Each lobule contains a mass of hepatic cells arranged in irregular columns between blood capillaries and capillary-like blood channels called sinusoids. The sinusoids pass from the periphery to the center of the lobule, where they empty into a central vein. The central vein, extending the length of the lobule, opens into a beginning branch of the hepatic vein. The bile capillaries arise from the cells and converge toward the periphery of the lobule, where they unite to form the beginning branches of the bile ducts.

The portal vein and the hepatic artery, both of which convey blood to the liver, enter the porta hepatis and branch out through the liver substance. The portal vein ends in the sinusoids, and the hepatic artery ends in capillaries which communicate with the sinusoids. Thus, in addition to the usual arterial blood supply, the liver receives blood from the portal system. The portal system, of which the portal vein is the main trunk, consists of the veins arising from the walls of the stomach, from the greater part of the intestinal tract and the gallbladder, and from the pancreas and the spleen. The blood circulating through these organs is carried to the liver for modification before being returned to the heart. The hepatic veins convey the blood from the liver sinusoids to the inferior vena cava.

The liver has numerous physiologic functions, but the one of chief interest from the radiographic standpoint is the formation of bile, which the gland secretes to the extent of 1 to 3 pints each day. Bile, being the channel of elimination for the waste products of red cell destruction, is an excretion as well as a secretion. As a secretion, it is an important aid in the emulsification and assimilation of fats. The bile is collected from the liver cells by the ducts and either carried to the gallbladder for temporary storage or poured directly into the duodenum through the common bile duct.

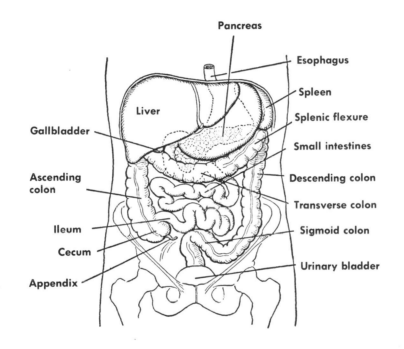

ANTERIOR ASPECT OF ABDOMINAL VISCERA IN RELATION TO SURROUNDING STRUCTURES

657

The biliary, or excretory, system of the liver consists of the *bile ducts* and the *gallbladder*. Beginning within the lobules as bile capillaries, the ducts unite to form larger and larger passages as they converge, finally forming two main ducts, one leading from each major lobe. The two main ducts emerge at the porta hepatis and join to form the *common hepatic duct*, which, in turn, unites with the *cystic duct* to form the *common bile duct*. The hepatic and cystic ducts are each about 1½ inches in length. The common bile duct passes downward for a distance of about 3 inches and, after joining the pancreatic duct, empties into the descending portion of the duodenum through the ampulla of Vater. The lower end of the common bile duct is controlled by a circular muscle called the sphincter of Oddi. During the interdigestive periods the sphincter remains in a contracted state, thus routing most of the bile into the gallbladder for concentration and temporary storage; during digestion, it relaxes to permit the bile to flow from the liver and gallbladder into the duodenum.

The gallbladder is a thin-walled, more or less pear-shaped musculomembranous sac with a capacity of approximately 2 ounces. The gallbladder functions to con-centrate bile by the absorption of the water content, to store bile during interdigestive periods, and by the contraction of its musculature, to evacuate the bile during digestion. The muscular contraction of the gallbladder is activated by a hormone called *cholecystokinin*. This hormone is secreted by the duodenal mucosa and liberated into the blood when fatty or acid chyme passes into the intestine. The organ consists of a narrow neck that is continuous with the cystic duct, of a body, or main portion, and of a fundus, which is its broad lower portion. The gallbladder is usually lodged in a fossa on the inferior surface of the right lobe of the liver, where it lies in an oblique plane from above downward and forward. Measuring about 1 inch in width at its widest part and 3 to 4 inches in length, it extends from the lower right margin of the porta hepatis to a variable distance below the anterior border of the liver. The position of the gallbladder varies with bodily habitus, being high and well away from the midline in hypersthenic subjects, and low and near the spine in asthenic subjects. The gallbladder is sometimes embedded in the liver and is frequently seen to hang free below the edge of the liver.

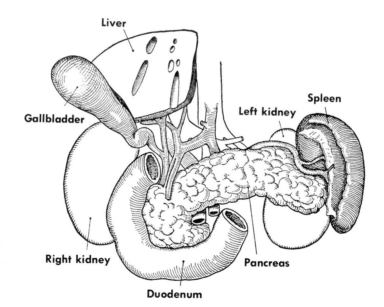

PANCREAS AND SPLEEN

The *pancreas* is an elongated, racemose gland situated across the posterior abdominal wall, where it reaches from the duodenum to the spleen. It is about 5½ inches in length and consists of a head, a neck, a body, and a tail. The head, which is the broadest portion of the organ, extends downward and is enclosed within the curve of the duodenum. The neck is the slightly constricted portion connecting the head and the body; it lies immediately below the pylorus, which rests upon its upper anterior surface. The body and tail of the pancreas pass transversely behind the stomach and in front of the left kidney, the narrow tail terminating near the spleen.

The pancreas is made up of many cell-containing lobules and a highly ramified duct system. The digestive juice secreted by these cells is conveyed into the main pancreatic duct, called the *duct of Wirsung*, and from there into the duodenum. The main pancreatic duct usually unites with the common bile duct to form a single passage, the ampulla of Vater, which opens into the descending duodenum. This arrangement is, however, variable. The two ducts (common bile and pancreatic) sometimes remain divided until their common termination at the sphincter of Oddi.

The pancreatic duct then opens directly into the duodenum instead of communicating with it via the ampulla of the biliary duct. An accessory pancreatic duct is sometimes present; it opens into the duodenum independently. The insulin-secreting cells do not communicate with the ducts but give their secretion directly into the blood through the capillaries. They are arranged in small groups, called the islands of Langerhans, in the spaces between the lobules of the pancreas. The pancreas cannot be visualized on plain film studies.

The *spleen* is included in this section only because of its location. It belongs to the circulatory system. It is a gland-like but ductless organ that functions to produce lymphocytes and to store red blood corpuscles. The spleen is more or less bean-shaped and measures about 5 inches in length, 3 inches in width, and 1½ inches in thickness. It is situated obliquely in the left hypochondrium, just below the diaphragm and behind the stomach. It is in contact with the abdominal wall laterally, with the adrenal gland and left kidney medially, and with the splenic flexure of the colon inferiorly. The spleen is visualized both with and without contrast media.

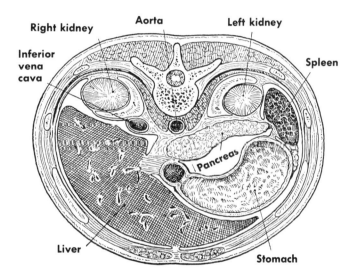

Radiography of the digestive system

A completete roentgenologic investigation of gastro-intestinal disorders may include an examination of (1) the paranasal sinuses and teeth for the detection of lesions of focal infection, (2) the abdomen as a whole for the detection of any condition such as renal stones and tumor masses that might cause referred symptoms, (3) the liver and gallbladder, and (4) the several portions of the alimentary tract for the detection of any local lesion. The extent of the examination of each patient, however, depends upon the site, and the type and extent of the pathologic involvement. A patient usually receives a complete examination, that is, an examination of each of the regions listed above, only when the symptoms are obscure—when the cause of the digestive disturbance has not been localized.

Radiologists differ somewhat on certain details of the procedures they employ in examining the different parts of the gastrointestinal tract and its accessory organs; however, the various methods are basically similar. For a survey examination of the abdomen, it is essential that the intestinal tract be evacuated of gas and fecal material and of any radiopaque medication such as bismuth in order to obtain an unobstructed view of the contained viscera. The method the radiologist employs to clear the intestinal tract depends upon whether the survey films are preliminary to a specialized examination, and upon the condition of the patient.

The demonstration of the thin-walled, hollow organs (the gallbladder and the gastrointestinal tract) requires the use of a contrast medium as well as special preliminary preparation, both of which vary according to the region being investigated. Each radiologist has an established routine covering the preparation of the patient under varying circumstances, the formula of the contrast medium for each of the different regions, and the roentgenographic procedure to be employed in examinations of the gallbladder and other gastrointestinal organs. The roentgenographic procedure necessary for an adequate demonstration of the findings in each gastrointestinal patient is determined by the radiologist during his radioscopic examination, the exact views and the body positions depending upon the habitus of the patient and upon the site and type of the lesion.

The procedures generally employed in examinations of the alimentary tract and its accessory organs will be considered under the following headings:

1. The abdomen
2. The liver and the spleen
3. The biliary tract
    a. The gallbladder
    b. The extrahepatic bile ducts
    c. The pancreas
    d. The biliary and urinary tracts
4. The alimentary tract
    a. The esophagus
    b. The gastrointestinal tract
    c. Retrogastric soft tissues
    d. The stomach and the duodenum
    e. The small intestine
    f. The large intestine

ABDOMEN

PREPARATION

Careful preliminary preparation of the intestinal tract is important in radiologic investigations of the abdominal viscera. In the presence of *nonacute* conditions, the preparation usually consists of the following:

1. The patient is placed on a low-residue diet for two days preceding the examination. This is done to prevent the possibility of gas formation due to excessive fermentation of the intestinal contents.

2. The patient is instructed to take a specified cathartic the night before, and a cleansing enema, usually of normal saline solution, not more than two hours prior to the examination. The patient should be given detailed instructions as to the correct procedure to follow in preparing and taking the enema, and he should be questioned about the results when he reports for the examination. Because swallowed air is quickly dispersed through the small intestine and its nitrogen content is not readily absorbed, patients should be instructed to avoid swallowing before and during examinations of the abdominal viscera.[1,2]

The scout film, an anteroposterior projection, should be processed before proceeding with any required additional views in case the radiologist wishes to order further evacuation of the colon.

While many patients referred for an examination of the abdomen are well enough to undergo routine preparation, a number have, or are suspected of having, some condition that removes them from the "routine" classification even though they are not acutely ill. The radiologist usually consults with the referring physician as to the presumptive diagnosis and may vary the preparation procedure accordingly. Preliminary preparation is never administered to acutely ill patients, to those who have a condition such as intestinal obstruction or perforation, or to those who have a visceral rupture.

[1]Magnusson, W.: On meteorism in pyelography and on passage of gas through the small intestine, Acta Radiol. **12**:552-561, 1931.
[2]Wangensteen, O. H., and Rea, C. E.: Distention factor in simple intestinal obstruction, Surgery **5**:327-339, 1939.

EXPOSURE TECHNIQUE

In examinations of the abdomen without a contrast medium, it is imperative to obtain maximum soft tissue differentiation throughout all its different regions. Because of the wide range in the thickness of the abdomen and the delicate differences in physical density between the contained viscera, it is necessary to use a more critical exposure technique than is required to demonstrate the difference in density between an opacified organ and the structures adjacent to it. The exposure factors should be adjusted to produce a "softer" result, that is, more gray tones and less black-and-white contrast, than is either necessary or desirable when a contrast medium is being employed. The softer result can usually be obtained with a comparatively low milliampere-second technique. When a high milliampere-second technique is employed, or when the machine produces a very soft type of radiation, it is frequently necessary to use additional filtration, particularly for children and for adults of asthenic habitus. A 3 or 4 mm. aluminum filter, cut to cover the distal two-thirds of the radiation aperture, often eliminates the necessity of making two radiographs of patients who have a large, barrel-shaped chest and a narrow, flat abdomen. The upper edge of such filters should be beveled to prevent a line of demarcation between the two regions of the abdomen.

A sharply defined outline of the psoas muscles, the lower border of the liver, the kidneys, the ribs, and the spinous processes of the lumbar vertebrae is the best criterion for judging the quality of an abdominal radiograph from the standpoint of detail. Only the radiologist can determine the proper density and photographic contrast. It may be stated in general, however, that radiographs of the abdomen should have more gray tones and should be approximately 5 kilovolts lighter than those of the lumbar vertebrae.

IMMOBILIZATION

One of the prime requisites in abdominal examinations is the prevention of movement, both voluntary and involuntary. In order to prevent muscle contraction that is caused by tenseness, the patient must be adjusted in a comfortable position so that he can relax. The technologist should explain the breathing procedure and have the patient rehearse it until he understands exactly what is expected of him. A compression band may be applied across the abdomen, but the pressure must be moderate. A large, air-filled gum-rubber bag equalizes the pressure over the whole of the abdomen, thus preventing a "band mark" in the radiograph, and it also improves the quality of the film. The exposure should not be started for one or two seconds after the suspension of respiration, to allow the patient to come to rest and to allow involuntary movement of the viscera to subside.

Voluntary motion is recognized by a blurred outline of the structures that do not have involuntary movement, such as the liver, the psoas muscles, and the spine. Involuntary motion appears as a haziness that may be confined to localized areas or may be generalized if caused by peristalsis; it is usually more exaggerated and is generalized when caused by contraction of the anterior abdominal muscles.

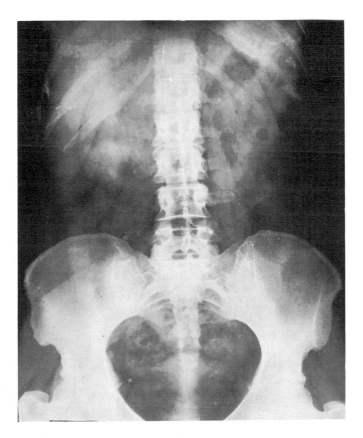

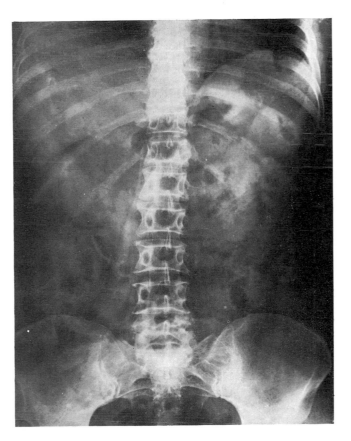

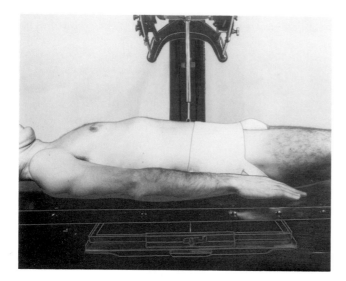

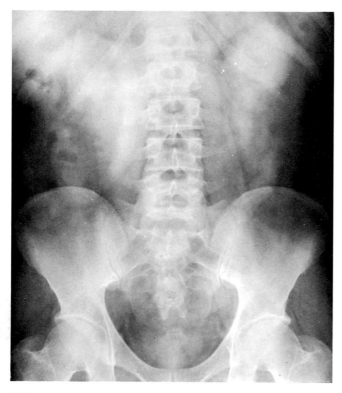

ABDOMEN
Anteroposterior projection
Posteroanterior view

Film: $14'' \times 17''$ lengthwise.

Position of patient

The patient may be placed in either the supine or the erect position, the former being preferable in most instances. When the erect position is used, it is customary to adjust the patient in the posteroanterior position except in kidney examinations.

Position of part

Center the median sagittal plane of the body to the midline of the table or vertical Potter-Bucky stand; if the patient is erect, the weight of the body must be equally distributed on the feet. Adjust the shoulders to lie in the same transverse plane and place the arms where they will not cast shadows on the film. With the patient supine, place sandbags or a folded sheet under his knees to relieve strain. Place one long sandbag under the ankles and immobilize them with another sandbag.

Center the film at the level of the iliac crests, or high enough to include the diaphragm. When examining a patient who is too tall for this centering to include the pelvic area, make a second exposure on a $10'' \times 12''$ film. The film is placed crosswise and is centered about 2 inches above the upper border of the symphysis pubis.

A compression band may be applied across the abdomen with moderate pressure. Respiration is suspended at the end of exhalation.

Local gonadal shielding should be applied in examinations of male patients.

Central ray

Direct the central ray perpendicularly to the midpoint of the film.

Structures shown

An anteroposterior projection of the abdomen, showing the size and shape of the liver, the spleen and the kidneys, and any intra-abdominal calcifications or tumor masses.

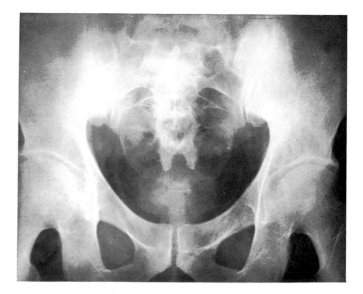

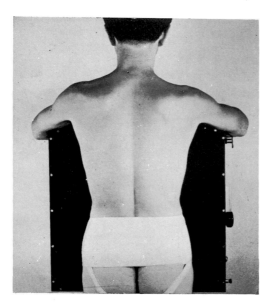

ABDOMEN

Lateral projection

Film: $14'' \times 17''$ lengthwise.

Position of patient

Turn the patient to a lateral recumbent position, having him lie on the right or left side, as indicated.

Position of part

Flex the patient's knees to a comfortable position and adjust the body so that the abdomen is centered to the midline of the table. Place sandbags under and between the knees and the ankles. Flex the elbows, place the lower hand under the head, and have the patient grasp the side of the table with the opposite hand.

Center the film at the level of the iliac crests, or high enough to include the diaphragm. A compression band may be applied across the pelvis. Respiration is suspended at the end of exhalation.

Central ray

Direct the central ray perpendicularly to the midpoint of the film.

Structures shown

A lateral projection of the abdomen, showing the prevertebral space occupied by the abdominal aorta, and any intra-abdominal calcifications or tumor masses.

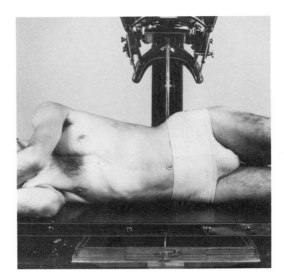

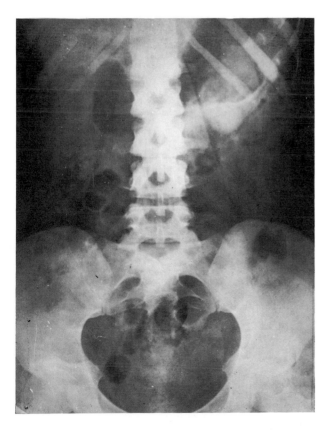

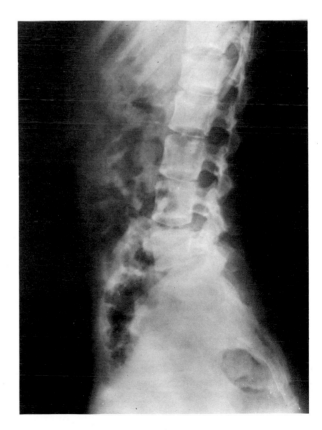

Radiographs courtesy Dr. Dan Tucker.

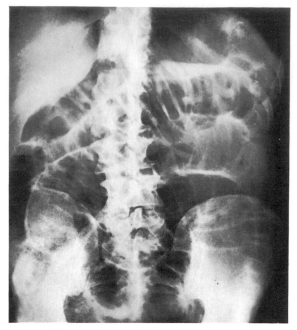

Supine study showing intestinal obstruction.

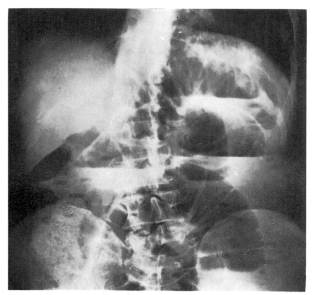

Erect study of above patient.

Radiographs and clinical information courtesy Dr. Hugh M. Wilson.

ABDOMEN
Body positions and specialized procedures

The abdomen is examined as required in anteroposterior, postero-anterior, and lateral directions, with the patient in either a recumbent or an erect position. Anteroposterior and lateral projections made with the patient in the recumbent position are the views usually employed to demonstrate intra-abdominal tumor masses, and for the differentiation of questionable intra-abdominal calcifications.

For the demonstration of a fluid level in the obstructed intestine, and of accumulations of free air in the abdomen (spontaneous pneumoperitoneum) as a result of a perforated peptic ulcer or other rupture of a hollow viscus, the examination usually consists of two frontal views. The first film is exposed with the patient in the supine position. The second film is exposed with the patient in either a lateral recumbent position (for a decubitus anteroposterior or postero-anterior projection) or in a seated erect position. The patient must not be placed in the erect position without the express permission of the radiologist. Acutely ill patients must be handled carefully and must not be moved unnecessarily, and the examination must be completed as quickly as possible. Hospital radiology departments should have an established high-speed exposure technique for both Bucky and non-Bucky examinations of patients with acute abdominal symptoms, in order to obviate any possible mistake because of hasty conversion of the standard exposure factors.

For a decubitus projection, the patient is adjusted in the required recumbent position, the cassette is placed in the vertical position, and the central ray is directed horizontally. When fluid is present, the body must be elevated on a special platform or a firm pad to demonstrate the dependent side of the abdomen. In the presence of air, elevation of the body is not necessary.

Semierect positions are not usually employed for the demonstration of air-fluid levels. When the patient is so adjusted, it is important that the central ray be directed horizontally so that it will parallel the air or fluid level; otherwise, the outline of the air or fluid will be diffused if not obliterated. This effect is demonstrated with a coconut on page 489, Volume II.

For the demonstration of small amounts of intraperitoneal gas in acute abdominal cases, Miller[1,2] recommends that the patient be kept in the left lateral position on a stretcher for ten to twenty minutes prior to the examination. This position allows the gas to rise into the area under the right hemidiaphragm where it will not be superimposed by the gastric gas bubble. Films are then taken in the following sequence:

1. Left lateral decubitus projection (anteroposterior or postero-anterior) of the chest and upper abdomen with the stretcher positioned against the vertical Potter-Bucky table. Chest exposure technique is used for this film.

[1]Miller, R. E., and Nelson, S. W.: The roentgenologic demonstration of tiny amounts of free intraperitoneal gas: experimental and clinical studies, Amer. J. Roentgen. 112:574-585, 1971.
[2]Miller, R. E.: The technical approach to the acute abdomen, Seminars Roentgen. 8:267-279, 1973.

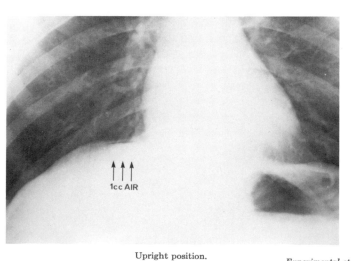

Upright position.

Experimental studies courtesy Dr. Roscoe E. Miller.

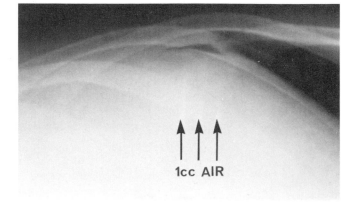

Left lateral decubitus position.

2. Maintain the patient in the left lateral position while he is moved to the horizontally placed table and tilted to the erect position. The patient is then turned to a frontal position (anteroposterior or posteroanterior) for (a) a chest film, and (b) a conventional film of the abdomen.

3. The table is then brought back to the horizontal position for a supine film of the abdomen.

For an evaluation of abdominal stab wounds, Bowerman and Smithwick[1] use a positive contrast technique. Following the introduction of a water-soluble iodinated contrast medium, films are obtained in anteroposterior, cross-table lateral, and, when possible, erect lateral directions.

When the usual signs of splenic injury are not shown on the conventional supine and erect films, Schorr and Danon[2] administer 200 ml. of barium sulfate mixture by mouth and then obtain supine and left lateral decubitus films of the left upper quadrant, both to include the entire stomach, the left dome of the diaphragm, and the lower end of the esophagus. Leigh[3] recommends a right lateral decubitus film with gas in the stomach.

ABDOMINAL FISTULAE AND SINUSES

For the radiographic demonstration of the origin and extent of fistulae and sinuses, the tract is filled with a radiopaque contrast medium, usually under radioscopic control, and right-angle projections are made. Many radiologists have one or both views made stereoscopically. Oblique views are occasionally required to demonstrate the full extent of a sinus tract.

For the exploration of fistulae and sinuses in the abdominal region, it is desirable to have the intestinal tract as free of gas and fecal material as possible. Unless the radiologist is making the injection under radioscopic control, it is customary to make a scout film of the abdomen in order to check the condition of the intestinal tract and to establish the desired film density.

When more than one sinus opening is present, each accessory opening is occluded with a sterile gauze packing or a collodion dressing in order to prevent reflux of the contrast substance and is identified by a specific lead marker placed over the dressing. The primary sinus opening is dressed and identified in a similar manner if the catheter is removed after the injection. When a reflux of the contrast medium occurs, the skin must be thoroughly cleansed before making an exposure.

When radioscopy is not employed, the patient is placed in position for the first view before the physician makes the injection, in order to obviate drainage of the opaque substance by unnecessary movement. The first film is then processed and submitted to the radiologist for further instructions before changing the patient's position.

A modified gastrointestinal procedure is usually employed to detect the origin of fecal fistulae. An iodized oil is frequently used in conjunction with a thin suspension of barium sulfate because the oil breaks up into clearly visible globules as soon as it reaches the watery barium mixture in the lumen of the intestine. For the demonstration of a colonic fistula, the colon is filled with an enema consisting of the full amount of water, but only about one-third the amount of barium ordinarily used. The radiologist then injects an iodized oil through the fistulous tract and localizes its origin at the intestinal wall by the globulation of the oil. For the demonstration of a fistula of the small intestine, the patient ingests a thin barium meal, which the radiologist follows radioscopically or radiographically until it reaches the suspected region; he then injects the fistulous tract with the iodized oil. These examinations are carried out under radioscopic control, films being exposed as indicated.

[1]Bowerman, J. W., and Smithwick, W.: Contrast examination of abdominal stab wounds, Radiology **97**:619-624, 1970.
[2]Schorr, S., and Danon, J. Rupture of the spleen; a new roentgen sign, Amer. J. Roentgen. **99**:616-624, 1967.
[3]Leigh, P. A. A.: Ruptured spleen: a radiological pitfall and a suggested modification, Brit. J. Radiol. **60**:289-291, 1973.

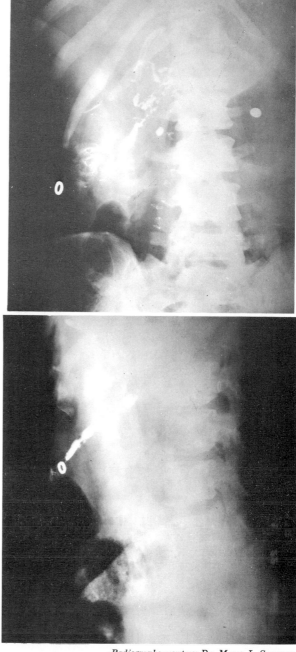

Radiographs courtesy Dr. Marcy L. Sussman.

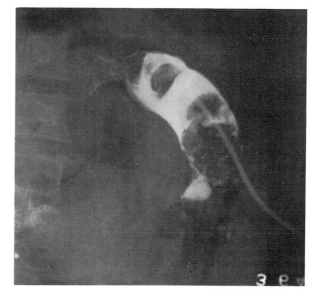

Courtesy Dr. Ross Golden.

665

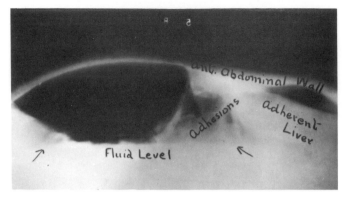

Dorsal decubitus projection.

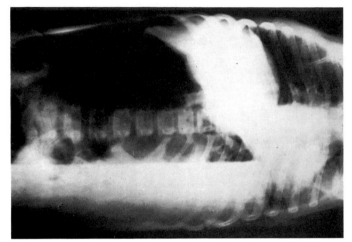

Left lateral decubitus projection.

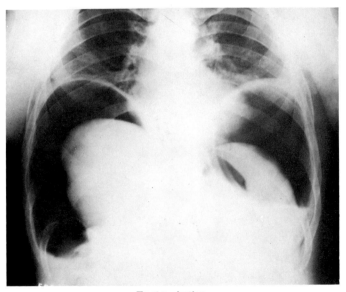

Erect projection.

Radiographs courtesy Dr. William H. Stewart.

ABDOMEN—cont'd
Body positions and specialized procedures—cont'd

ABDOMINAL PNEUMORADIOGRAPHY

Abdominal pneumoradiography is a general term covering the several procedures employed in radiologic examinations of the abdominopelvic organs by means of a gaseous contrast medium. The gas is introduced into the cavity, or space, surrounding the organs or organ under investigation. The radiographically negative background provided by the gas makes it possible to demonstrate clearly the contour, position, and mobility of the various organs and to delineate any space-occupying lesion.

These procedures are performed in the radiology department, usually with the patient on a radioscopic-radiographic tilt table. The gaseous medium is introduced, under strict aseptic conditions, by percutaneous puncture with a hollow needle.

1. Into the *peritoneal cavity* by way of the anterior abdominal wall, for the demonstration of the intraperitoneal abdominal and pelvic organs. This procedure is called *pneumoperitoneum*, or sometimes *artificial* pneumoperitoneum, to distinguish the diagnostic procedure from *spontaneous* pneumoperitoneum—the release of gas into the cavity from a ruptured hollow viscus.

2. Into the *retroperitoneal space* by way of the presacral space, for bilateral delineation of the kidneys and other retroperitoneal structures. This procedure is called *presacral pneumoretroperitoneum* or *presacral pneumoradiography*.

3. Into the *perirenal space* by way of the adjacent flank, for the delineation of the kidney and the adrenal gland of the injected side. This procedure is called *perirenal pneumoradiography* or *perirenal gas insufflation*.

The two latter procedures are described in further detail in the discussion on the urinary system (pages 782 and 783). The injection procedure usually employed to introduce gas into the peritoneal cavity is described in the discussion on the nongravid female patient (pages 840 to 843).

The gases most frequently used for abdominal pneumoradiography are air, oxygen, and nitrous oxide. Carbon dioxide is so rapidly absorbed that it is suitable for use only when this characteristic of the medium will not interfere with the examination procedure to be employed.

Preparation of patient

The intestinal tract must be free of fecal material and gas in order to obtain an unobstructed view of the abdominopelvic organs and of space-occupying lesions. Thorough preliminary cleansing of the intestinal tract is, therefore, important in these examinations. The patient is usually given a nongas-forming cathartic on the preceding evening and a cleansing enema one or two hours before the examination. The preceding meal is withheld.

Peritoneal and presacral retroperitoneal injections are made under local anesthesia. The physician may have a mild sedative administered a half hour before the examination.

ABDOMINAL PNEUMORADIOGRAPHIC POSITIONS

Because gaseous media rise to the highest level, the organ or region of interest must be placed uppermost for

666

each view taken. This is done by adjusting the patient's position and/or the angulation of the radiographic table.

1. The anterior abdominal wall and any adhesions between it and the underlying organs are demonstrated by placing the patient in the supine position. A *dorsal decubitus projection* (horizontally projected lateral view) is taken.

2. For negative contrast delineation of the walls of the stomach, the peritoneal cavity and the lumen of the stomach are simultaneously filled with gas.[1,2] Following the establishment of pneumoperitoneum, the stomach is inflated by the administration of 1.5 grams of tartaric acid followed by 2 grams of sodium carbonate. Each powder is dissolved in a small amount of water. The stomach walls are then examined radioscopically and by stationary projections and/or tomographic sections.

3. The prevertebral region and any tumor mass located in this area are demonstrated by adjusting the patient in the prone position, with suitable supports placed under his chest and thighs to remove pressure from the abdomen and thus to allow full forward movement of the abdominal viscera. A *ventral decubitus projection* (cross-table lateral view) is made.

4. For pressure distribution of the gas around all the abdominal organs to show their contour and relationship, the chest and thigh supports are removed, and a conventional posteroanterior projection is made.

5. The right abdominal wall and subphrenic space and the right-sided organs are demonstrated by placing the patient on his left side for a *left lateral decubitus projection* (horizontally projected frontal view, anteroposterior or posteroanterior).

6. The left abdominal wall and subphrenic space and the left-sided organs are demonstrated by placing the patient on his right side for a *right lateral decubitus projection* (horizontally projected frontal view, anteroposterior or posteroanterior).

7. The lower surface of the diaphragm, the upper abdominal organs (particularly the adrenal glands), and any space-occupying lesion in this region are demonstrated by placing the patient in the *erect position*.

The body position and the views taken for pneumoradiographic demonstration of the female pelvic organs are described on pages 840 to 843.

EXPOSURE DECREASE FOR AIR STUDIES

Depending upon the volume of gas introduced, the habitus of the patient, and the decree of body fat present, air studies of the abdominopelvic organs require the equivalent of a 10- to 20-kilovolt decrease in the routine exposure technique.

NOTE: Gelfand[3] recommends the use of positive contrast peritoneography in selected cases of abdominal abnormalities. Gelfand uses a 25% sodium diatrizoate solution (75 grams of Hypaque in 300 ml. of sterile water) for this method of peritoneography.

[1]Saito, Makoto: La radiographie des parois de l'estomac, "pneumo-gastro-pariétographie," Bull. Soc. Chir. Paris **59**:910-912, 1933.

[2]Köhler, Rolf: Parietography of the stomach, Acta Radiol. [Diagn.] 3:393-406, 1965.

[3]Gelfand, D. W.: Positive contrast peritoneography: the abnormal abdomen, Amer. J. Roentgen. **119**:190-197, 1973.

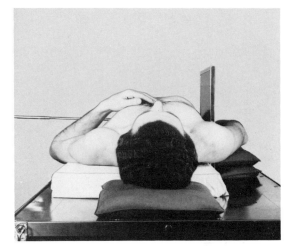

Dorsal decubitus position.

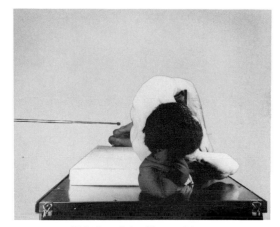

Right lateral decubitus position.

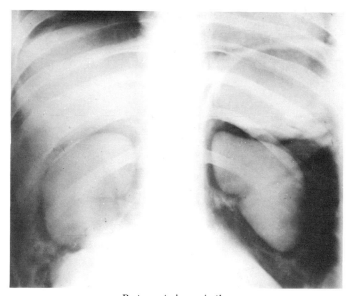

Posteroanterior projection.

Courtesy Dr. William H. Stewart.

667

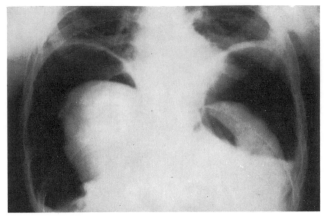

Erect peritoneal pneumoradiogram.

Courtesy Dr. William H. Stewart.

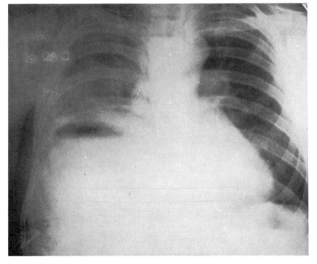

Erect position.

Courtesy Dr. Ross Golden.

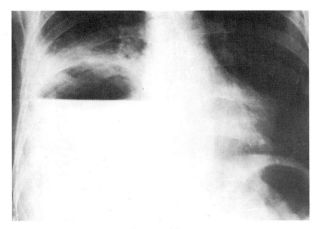

Erect position.

Courtesy Dr. William H. Shehadi.

LIVER AND SPLEEN
Specialized procedures

Radiologic investigations of the liver and the spleen are conducted to detect such conditions as abnormal variations in size or contour, calcifications, subphrenic abscesses, cysts, tumor masses, and vascular lesions. Some of these conditions are demonstrable by simple roentgenographic means, while others require specialized procedures involving the use of contrast media.

Because the physical density of the liver is such that its shadow is cast through those of the surrounding structures, this organ is usually well outlined on all abdominal films. The spleen is a comparatively small structure, so that its outline is well visualized only in moderately thin subjects.

The surfaces of the liver and spleen, and any peripherally located cysts or tumor masses, are well demonstrated by means of artificial pneumoperitoneum. In cases of subdiaphragmatic (or subphrenic) abscess, for the purpose of detecting a free gas pocket, one film is exposed with the patient either erect or laterally recumbent.

The blood vessels of the liver and spleen are investigated by means of *abdominal aortography* (described in the discussion on angiography) and by *portal* or *splenoportal venography*. *Portal venography* is performed in the operating room during surgery, the contrast solution being injected directly into the exposed vein. *Splenoportal venography* is performed in the radiology department where the radiopaque contrast solution is injected percutaneously into the pulp of the spleen. The procedure may be performed with the patient under either local or general anesthesia. Among others, Moore[1] and Child[2] described the procedure employed in portal venography, and Rousselot[3] and Evans[4] described the procedure employed in percutaneous splenoportal venography with the patient in the supine position. Moskowitz and associates[5] recommend that splenoportography be carried out with the patient in the prone position to ensure contrast filling of the more anteriorly directed left portal vein. Exposures are usually made at one-second intervals for the visualization of the entire portal system.

[1]Moore, G. E., and Bridenbaugh, R. B.: Roentgen demonstration of the venous circulation in the liver; portal venography, Radiology **57**:685-690, 1951.

[2]Child, C. G., O'Sullivan, W. D., Payne, M. A., and McClure, R. D.: Portal venography, Radiology **57**:691-701, 1951.

[3]Rousselot, L. M., Ruzicka, F. F., and Doehner, G. A.: Portal venography via the portal and percutaneous splenic routes, Surgery **34**:557-569, 1953.

[4]Evans, J. A., and O'Sullivan, W. D.: Percutaneous splenoportal venography, Med. Radiogr. Photogr. **31**:98-107, 1955.

[5]Moskowitz, H., Chait, A., Margulis, M., and Mellins, H. Z.: Prone splenoportography, Radiology **90**:1132-1135, 1968.

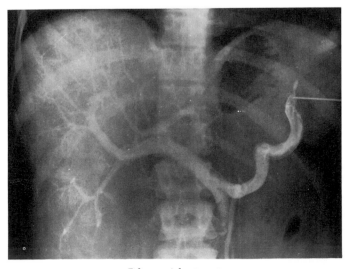

Splenoportal venogram.

Courtesy Dr. Henry K. Taylor.

LIVER AND SPLEEN
Anteroposterior projection
Posteroanterior view

Film: $14'' \times 17''$ crosswise or lengthwise, depending upon the build of the patient.

Position of patient

The patient is placed in the supine position for a general survey examination and for the determination of the size and shape of the liver and the spleen.

Position of part

Center the median sagittal plane of the body to the midline of the table. Adjust the shoulders to lie in the same transverse plane; flex the elbows and abduct the arms enough to clear the film area. Support the ankles and knees on sandbags or folded sheets to relieve strain.

With the cassette placed crosswise in the Potter-Bucky tray, adjust its position so that approximately 1 inch of the iliac bones is included on the lower border of the film. If the patient is too tall for this centering to include the diaphragm, place the cassette lengthwise. Exceptionally broad subjects who are also tall require two exposures: one with the film placed crosswise to include the entire diaphragm, and one with the film placed lengthwise to include the iliac crests.

In order to obviate contour distortion, compression is not applied in liver and spleen examinations. Respiration is suspended at the end of exhalation.

Central ray

Direct the central ray vertically through the xiphoid process.

Structures shown

An anteroposterior projection showing the size and shape of the liver, the spleen, and the kidneys.

NOTE: Unless the routine abdominal film density is fairly dark, the penetration should be increased approximately 5 kilovolts for liver and spleen examinations.

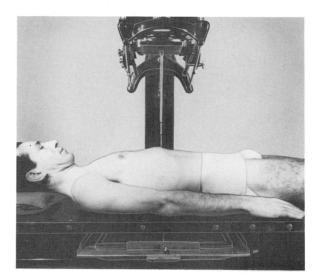

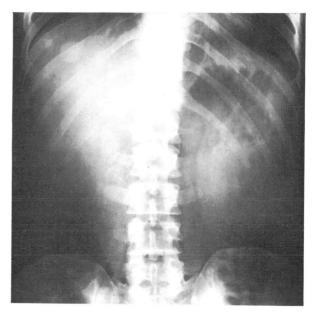

Courtesy Dr. William H. Shehadi.

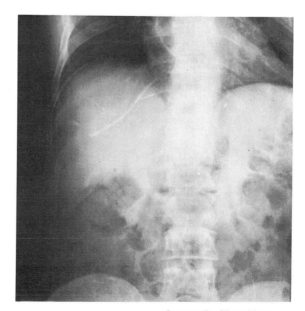

Courtesy Dr. Henry K. Taylor.

669

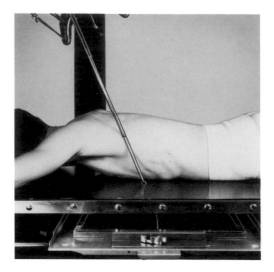

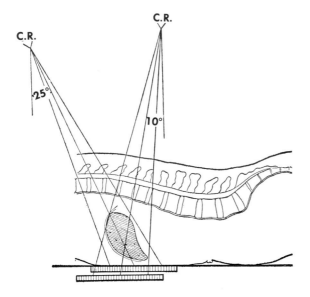

LIVER
Posteroanterior projections
Anteroposterior view
Benassi method

Film: Two 14″ × 17″ films.

Position of patient

The patient is adjusted in the prone position so that the broad anterior surface of the liver is nearer the film.

Position of part

Center the median sagittal plane of the body to the midline of the table. Flex the patient's elbows, and adjust his arms in a comfortable position. Adjust the shoulders to lie in the same transverse plane. Support the ankles on sandbags to prevent the weight of the feet from resting on the toes.

With the cassette placed crosswise or lengthwise, according to the build of the patient, adjust the position of the Potter-Bucky tray so that the midpoint of the film will coincide with the central ray.

Compression is not applied. Respiration is suspended at the end of exhalation.

Central ray

Direct the central ray through the xiphoid process (1) at an angle of 25 degrees toward the feet for the first radiograph and (2) at an angle of 10 degrees toward the head for the second radiograph.

For a general survey examination, the central ray is directed perpendicularly.

Structures shown

Two posteroanterior projections demonstrating the greater surface of the liver.

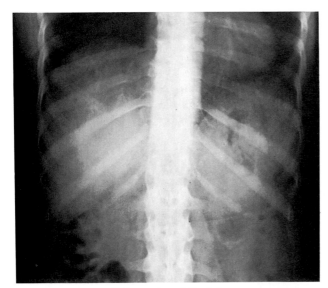

25 degrees toward the feet.

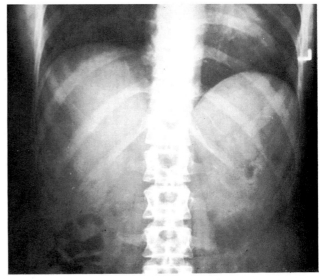

10 degrees toward the head.

SPLEEN
Oblique anteroposterior projection
Oblique posteroanterior view
Benassi position

Film: $11'' \times 14''$ lengthwise.

Position of patient

The patient is adjusted in the supine position so that the spleen is nearer the film.

Position of part

Elevate the right side of the patient's body about 40 to 45 degrees, and center the left side to the midline of the table. Support the elevated shoulder and hip on sandbags or firm pillows. Place the arms in a comfortable position, and adjust the shoulders to lie in the same transverse plane.

With the cassette in the Potter-Bucky tray, adjust its position so that the film is centered at, or just below, the level of the xiphoid process.

Compression is not applied. Respiration is suspended at the end of exhalation.

Central ray

Direct the central ray vertically to the midpoint of the film.

Structures shown

An oblique projection demonstrating the greater surface of the spleen.

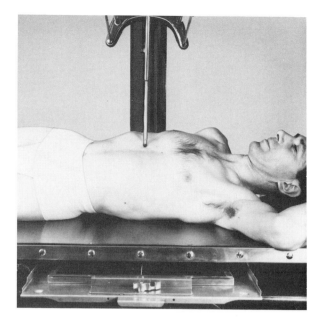

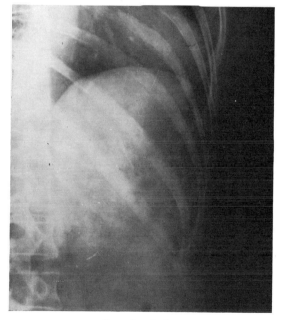

Benassi projection.

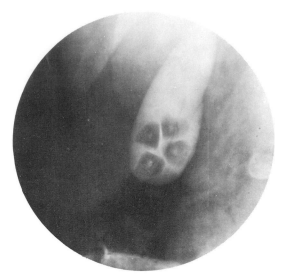

Oral cholecystogram.

Courtesy Dr. Max Dannenberg.

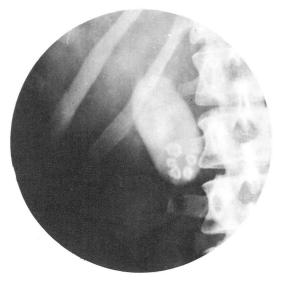

Oral cholecystogram.

Courtesy Dr. Max Dannenberg.

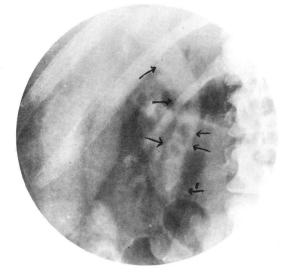

Intravenous cholangiogram.

Courtesy Dr. William H. Shehadi.

BILIARY TRACT
Cholecystography and Cholangiography (Cholegraphy)

Cholegraphy is the general term used to denote specialized radiologic examinations of the biliary tract with the use of a radiopaque contrast material. The contrast medium may be administered (1) by mouth (*oral*), (2) by injection into a vein in a single bolus or by drip infusion (*intravenous*), or (3) by direct injection into the ducts (a) through *percutaneous transhepatic puncture*, (b) during biliary tract surgery (*operative* or *immediate*), or (c) through an indwelling drainage tube (*postoperative, delayed*, or *T tube*). Each method of examination is named according to (1) the route of entry of the medium, italicized above, and (2) the portion of the biliary tract examined. Thus, designated by the route of entry, *cholecystangiography*, or *cholecystocholangiography*, indicate the demonstration of both the gallbladder and the bile ducts; *cholecystography*, of the gallbladder; and *cholangiography*, of the bile ducts.

The contrast substance can be delivered to the liver by either the oral or the venous route due to the double blood supply to this organ. When given by mouth, the contrast medium is absorbed through the intestines and carried to the liver through the portal vein; when given by intravenous injection, it passes through the blood circulation and enters the liver through the hepatic artery. From the hepatic cells, the contrast substance is excreted with the bile and conveyed to the gallbladder by the system of ducts. The contrast-carrying bile is stored and concentrated in the gallbladder, rendering it radiopaque.

Biliary tract examinations are employed to determine (1) the function of the liver—its ability to remove the contrast medium from the bloodstream and excrete it with the bile; (2) the patency and condition of the biliary ducts; and (3) the concentrating and emptying power of the gallbladder. Thus the presence of such lesions as biliary calculi, neoplasms, stenosis, and, indirectly, lesions of the head of the pancreas may be detected. The greatest number of biliary tract examinations are probably performed in quest of gallstones. The calculi, or stones, formed in the biliary tract are widely variable in composition, in size, and in shape. Pure cholesterol stones appear as negative filling defects within the opacified bile. Calcium-containing deposits, either as solitary calculi or in the form of milk of bile, can be readily detected on the plain film.

Cholecystography was developed by Graham, Cole, and Copher in 1924-1925,[1] first with the use of sodium tetrabromophenolphthalein as the contrast medium, and then with sodium tetraiodophenolphthalein. Iodine has greater radiopacity and proved to be less toxic than bromine. When administered orally, however, it caused marked nausea, vomiting, and diarrhea. Because of these side effects, many radiologists preferred to use the intravenous method; however, extreme precautions had to be taken to prevent extravasation because the medium was irritating and damaging to the soft tissues. The phenolphthalein derivatives were discarded when improved contrast media became available.

[1]Graham, E. A., Cole, W. H., and Copher, G. H.: Cholecystography: the use of sodium tetraiodophenolphthalein, J.A.M.A. 84:1175-1177, 1925.

Oral cholegraphic contrast media appeared in the sequence listed below. Prior to Telepaque, the first of the three-iodinated compounds, preoperative visualization of the biliary tract was limited to the gallbladder. In addition to permitting visualization of the bile ducts, the three-iodinated compounds resulted in a decrease in side reactions. Most of the present-day contrast media are supplied in 0.5-gram tablets or capsules. The usual dose is 3 grams (6 tablets or 6 capsules).

		Visualization
Two-iodinated compounds		
1924-1925	Tetrabromophenolphthalein	Gallbladder
	Tetraiodophenolphthalein	Gallbladder
1940	Priodax	Gallbladder
1944	Monophen	Gallbladder
Three-iodinated compounds		
1949	Telepaque	Gallbladder and ducts
1952	Teridax	Gallbladder and ducts
1960	Biloptin	Gallbladder and ducts
	Oragrafin	Gallbladder and ducts
1962	Bilopaque	Gallbladder and ducts
Six-iodinated compounds		
1952-1953	Biligrafin forte	Gallbladder and ducts
	Cholografin	Gallbladder and ducts
1956	Duografin (Cholografin	Gallbladder and ducts
	methylglucamine plus	Urinary tract
	Renografin)	

Courtesy Dr. William H. Shehadi.

Cholografin methylglucamine is the contrast medium now employed in the intravenous method. This medium produces few side effects and causes practically no irritation when a chance extravasation occurs. It is supplied in 20 ml. vials of a 52% sterile solution, this amount constituting the usual dose. Injected directly into the bloodstream, and thus bypassing the digestive tract, it reaches the liver quickly and is excreted with the bile in an amount sufficient to opacify the hepatic, cystic, and common ducts in ten to twenty minutes.

The contrast agent selected for use in the direct injection methods (percutaneous transhepatic, operative, T-tube) may be any one of the water-soluble, iodinated compounds employed for intravenous urography.

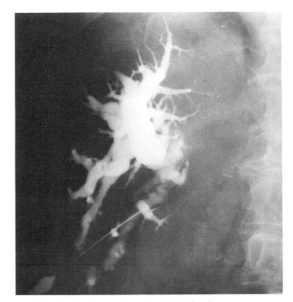
Percutaneous transhepatic cholangiogram.

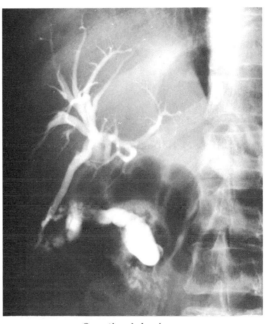
Operative cholangiogram.

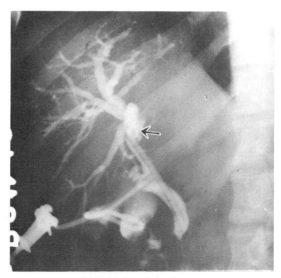
Postoperative cholangiogram.
Radiographs courtesy Dr. William H. Shehadi.

UNTOWARD SIDE REACTIONS TO IODINATED MEDIA

The present-day iodinated media compounded for intravenous injection have a relatively low degree of toxicity, so that severe reactions such as chills, rigors, acute respiratory distress, fainting, and shock are few if not rare. In a majority of patients the reaction is both mild and brief. The usual symptoms are a hot flush, possibly a few patches of urticarial rash, mild nausea and vomiting, sneezing, and possible rhinitis. However, in an occasional patient severe reactions, immediate or delayed, may appear that require treatment. It is therefore necessary to have at hand an emergency cart with drugs and equipment. The typical emergency cart is equipped with (1) an assortment of sterile syringes and needles; (2) sterile forceps; (3) containers of sterile gauze squares and cotton balls; (4) 70% alcohol or other skin-cleansing agent; (5) a tourniquet; (6) antihistaminic drugs such as diphenhydramine hydrochloride (Benadryl), chlorpheniramine (Chlor-Trimeton), and promethazine hydrochloride (Phenergan); (7) adrenergic or sympathomimetic drugs such as epinephrine (Adrenalin), ephedrine, cortisone, and levarterenol (Levophed); (8) a flask containing a sterile solution of 5% dextrose in distilled water or saline solution; (9) an oxygen tank fitted with a mask; (10) a sphygmomanometer (blood pressure apparatus) and a stethoscope; (11) amyl nitrite (crushable ampules) or aromatic spirit of ammonia.

A sensitivity test, usually consisting of an intravenous injection of 1 ml. of the iodinated medium, is sometimes performed just prior to the examination. When this is done, the patient is kept under observation for some ten minutes to allow for the development of any systemic or skin reaction. Radiologists in general consider this test to be an unreliable means of determining whether a patient will react unfavorably to the injected contrast agent.

INSTRUCTIONS TO PATIENT

The purpose of the preliminary preparation and the procedure to be followed should be explained to the patient in order to secure his full cooperation. He should be told the approximate time required for the examination, allowing for the possibility of delay should the colon require further cleansing or the emptying time of the gallbladder be delayed.

The patient should be given clearly written, typed, or mimeographed instructions covering (1) preliminary preparation of the intestinal tract and, if an enema is ordered, how to prepare and take it; (2) preliminary diet; (3) the exact time to ingest the oral medium, and how to prepare it when mixing is required; (4) the avoidance of laxatives for twenty-four hours prior to the ingestion or injection of the medium; (5) the avoidance of all food, both solid and liquid, after taking an oral medium (water may be taken as desired before the oral examination, but it is withheld following the evening meal if the patient is to be dehydrated for an intravenous examination); (6) the time to report for the examination.

When the patient reports for the examination, he should be questioned as to how he followed each step of the preparation procedure. If the oral method is being used, he should be asked whether he experienced any reaction such as vomiting or diarrhea. Vomiting may be important if it occurs within two hours after the ingestion of the contrast medium. Mild catharsis may do no harm, but diarrhea can result in egestion of a majority of the contrast substance, so that only a faint shadow, if any, of the gallbladder will be visualized.

Because prolonged fasting causes the formation of gas, as well as a possible headache, patients should be given early-morning appointments if at all possible.

SCOUT FILM OF ABDOMEN

A general survey film of the abdomen preceding preparation for a biliary tract examination serves a double purpose. First, if the intestinal tract is found to be clean, and if the contrast medium is to be administered orally, preparation for the examination can be shortened by one day; if the intestinal tract is not clean, this film usually serves to indicate what measure must be taken to cleanse it. Second, it sometimes demonstrates a gallbladder filled with radiopaque stones, and this finding may terminate the examination.

According to the preference of the radiologist, the scout film of the abdomen may be made with the patient in either the supine or the prone position. Some radiologists like to have an anteroposterior projection of the abdomen and a localized posteroanterior projection of the gallbladder area. In view of the fact that the part being examined should be closest to the film, most radiologists have both the scout film of the abdomen and the localization film of the gallbladder made with the patient in the prone position.

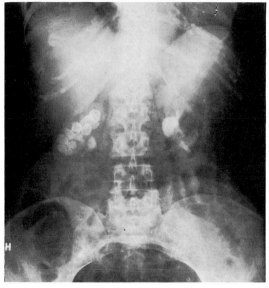

Multiple biliary and bilateral renal stones.

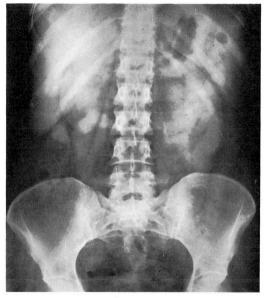

Prepared.

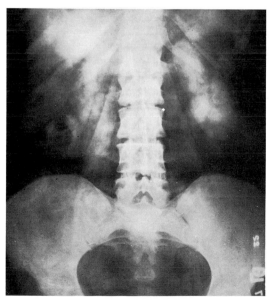

Unprepared.

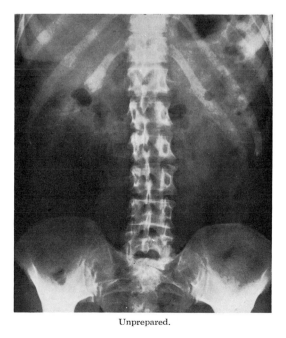

Unprepared.

675

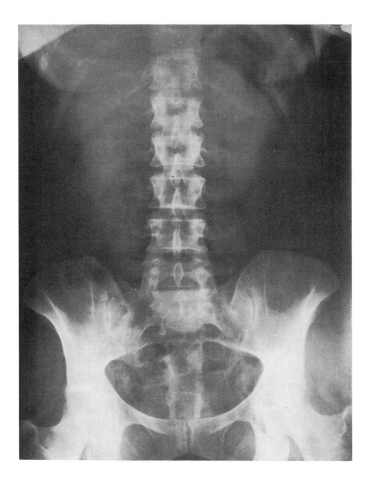

PREPARATION OF INTESTINAL TRACT

Much of the success of biliary tract examinations depends upon a clear view of the right upper quadrant of the abdomen, that is, upon a clean colon. As indicated by the scout film of the abdomen, the bowel content may be light to moderate, so that it can be eliminated with one or two cleansing enemas, or it may be so heavy as to require a cathartic. Often, no preparation is needed.

Many radiologists order two enemas, one to be given on the evening preceding the examination and one on the morning of the examination. Unless otherwise specified, the cleansing enemas employed in radiography usually consist of a normal saline solution (1¾ teaspoonfuls of common table salt to 1 quart of water). When ordered for the morning of the examination, the enema should be no more than lukewarm in order to prevent gas formation, and it should be administered not more than two hours and not less than one hour prior to the examination. When the fecal return is large, the enema should be repeated to ensure adequate cleansing of the bowel. The patient should be given careful instructions as to the correct procedure to follow in preparing and taking a self-administered enema, and the time or times should be specified.

When a cathartic is required, a nongas-forming compound such as castor oil or licorice powder is usually ordered, 1½ ounces of either drug being generally considered the optimum dose. (The kindest way to administer castor oil is in a heavy red wine such as port, with which it is immiscible. When the castor oil is sandwiched between two layers of wine and swallowed in one gulp, patients even report enjoying the cocoction.) Cathartics are administered twenty-four hours preceding the ingestion or injection of a contrast agent to allow irritation of the intestinal mucosa to subside and, in the oral method, to prevent egestion of the medium with the fecal material.

The patient who has painful hemorrhoids will appreciate being given a medicated suppository to insert into the rectum fifteen or twenty minutes before taking an enema. Patients required to take a cathartic should be given a medicated ointment for application to the sorely irritated area around the anus. Sample-sized containers of these preparations are obtainable at a nominal cost.

PRELIMINARY DIET

There is a diversity of medical opinion on the subject of the preliminary diet. The disagreement pertains largely to the oral procedure. The diets most frequently recommended are (1) an evening meal that is rich in fatty content (simple fats such as eggs, butter, cream, and milk, but no fried food) in order to empty the gallbladder and thus to have it ready to receive the opacified bile; (2) an evening meal that is fat-free to prevent the possibility of continued emptying of the gallbladder during the time the liver is excreting the opacified bile; and (3) a noon meal that is rich in simple fats, and an evening meal that is fat-free. Oral media are usually administered about three hours after the evening meal. With the exception of small amounts of water as desired, the patient is permitted nothing by mouth after taking the oral medium. Breakfast is usually withheld in all methods.

FATTY MEAL

After obtaining satisfactory visualization of the gall-bladder by the oral or the intravenous method of cholegraphy, either a meal high in fatty content or a suitable substitute for the meal is administered. This is done for the purposes of (1) testing the emptying power of the gallbladder, (2) examining, in the oral method, the extrahepatic bile ducts as they fill with the opacified bile flowing from the gallbladder, and (3) detecting nonopaque gallstones and/or papillomas too small to be visible through the large amount of opacified bile contained in the filled gallbladder.

During the gastric phase of digestion, foodstuff is converted into a creamy, semifluid material called *chyme*, in which the fatty content of the food has been changed into fatty acids and glycerol. Chyme is released into the duodenum by the intermittent relaxation of the pyloric sphincter. In the presence of fatty acid in the duodenum, the mucosa secretes a hormone called *cholecystokinin*, which, when carried in the bloodstream, causes contraction and, usually, emptying of the gallbladder. The time required for gallbladder reaction depends upon how quickly the fat can go through the stomach for delivery to the duodenum. For this reason, only highly emulsified, easily digested fats such as those found in egg yolk, butter, and cream are selected for the high-fat meal given to activate gallbladder motility.

A fatty meal may consist of two eggs (cooked any way), buttered toast, and a glass of milk or other beverage with cream. Obtaining satisfactory filling of the cystic and common ducts with this meal is somewhat a matter of chance because of the delays involved in having the patient dress and leave the radiology department for the meal.

An eggnog, made of two egg yolks and half-and-half cream and milk, produces prompt and excellent results. Commercially prepared concentrated eggnog substitutes are usually just as effective and are more convenient in the absence of a diet kitchen. Following the ingestion of either of these preparations, duct studies are taken at ten- to fifteen-minute intervals until satisfactory visualization is obtained. A delayed film is taken forty-five to sixty minutes post cibum to check the degree of emptying of the gallbladder.

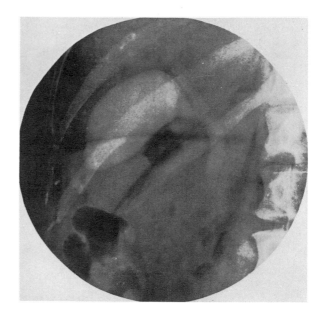

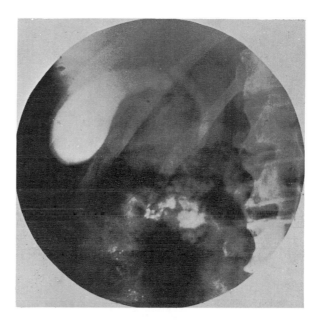

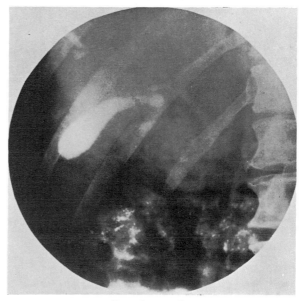

Post cibum studies.

Courtesy Dr. William H. Shehadi.

677

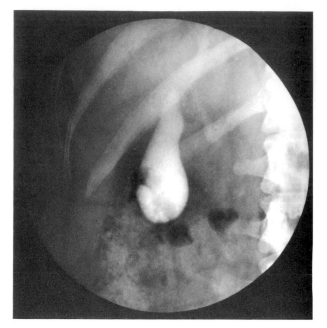

Prone position.

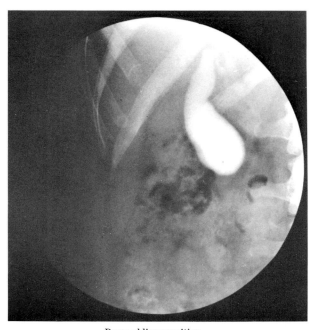

Prone oblique position.
Radiographs courtesy Dr. William H. Shehadi.

BILIARY TRACT—cont'd

Oral cholegraphy

The success of cholecystography and cholangiography by the oral method depends upon the integrative function (1) of the intestinal mucosa to absorb the contrast substance and liberate it into the portal bloodstream for conveyance to the liver, (2) of the liver to remove the opaque substance from the blood and excrete it with the bile, and (3) of the gallbladder (a) to concentrate the inflowing opacified bile by removing a large part of its approximately 90% water content, (b) to store the concentrated bile during the interdigestive period, and (c) to empty its contents when activated to this function by a fatty meal. Because it is dependent upon each of these functions, the oral method is not attempted when there are acute abdominal symptoms or gastrointestinal disturbances that would prevent retention and absorption of the contrast medium.

The greatly improved oral contrast media now available are generally well tolerated, and they permit satisfactory visualization of the extrahepatic bile ducts as well as of the gallbladder in a large percentage of patients so examined. Because of these factors, and because of the comparative simplicity of the examination, the oral method has become the basic procedure in radiologic investigations of the biliary tract.

Oral media differ in the rate of their absorption and liberation into the portal bloodstream. The time allowed between the ingestion of the medium and the examination is determined accordingly. This time varies from ten to twelve hours for most of the present-day oral agents. It is claimed that one of the newer oral media, ipodate calcium (Oragrafin calcium), is so rapidly absorbed and liberated into the portal bloodstream that it begins to appear in the extrahepatic ducts in one hour or less after ingestion. This contrast medium is supplied in single-dose packets containing 3 grams of ipodate calcium granules. The contents of the packet are rapidly mixed in a small amount (one-fourth glass) of lukewarm water for administration. A single or double dose (one or two packets) ingested one hour prior to the examination is said to afford satisfactory visualization of the extrahepatic ducts in an average of one and one-half to two and one-half hours, and of the gallbladder in an average of three to four hours, after ingestion.

GENERAL ROUTINE PROCEDURE

In the procedure generally employed, any one of the contrast media available for oral cholegraphy is given in a single dose, consisting of 3 grams or more, on the evening preceding the examination. The time of ingestion is set to allow ten to twelve hours for maximum concentration in the gallbladder prior to the examination.

Filming begins with studies of the opacified gallbladder. When satisfactory cholecystograms have been obtained, some form of a fatty meal is administered to induce emptying of the gallbladder. At specified intervals, films are then taken to demonstrate the extrahepatic ducts and the emptying rate of the gallbladder. Following a rapid-acting meal such as an eggnog or a commercially prepared substitute, duct studies are usually taken at ten-minute intervals until satisfactory visualization is obtained. Faster and more complete filling of the ducts can be obtained by placing the patient on the radiographic table in the right anteroposterior oblique position as soon as he has ingested the eggnog. This position places the gallbladder at a higher level, which permits more rapid emptying of the opacified bile, with improved bile duct opacification. The termination of the examination depends upon the emptying rate of the gallbladder.

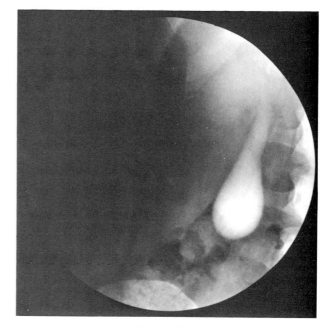

Erect position.

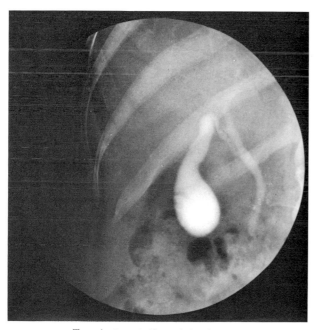

Ten-minute post cibum cholangiogram.

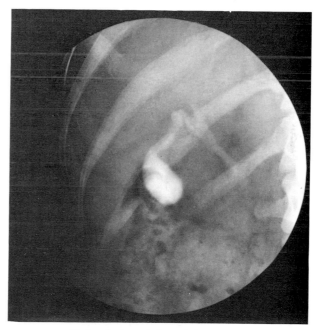

Forty-minute post cibum cholecystogram.

Radiographs courtesy Dr. William H. Shehadi.

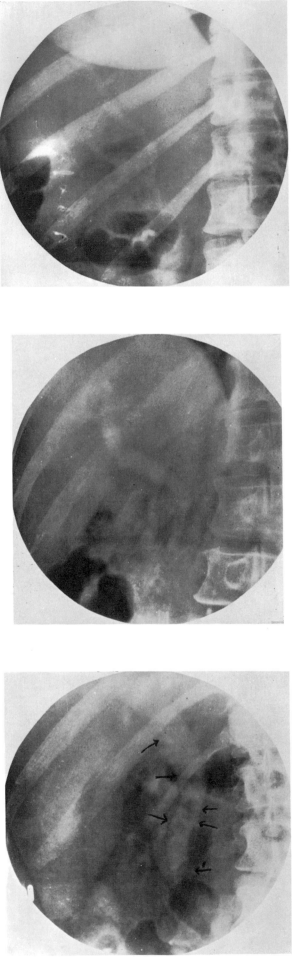

BILIARY TRACT—cont'd

Intravenous cholegraphy

The intravenous method of cholegraphy is employed in the investigation of (1) the biliary ducts of cholecystectomized patients, and (2) the biliary ducts and gallbladder of noncholecystectomized patients (a) in cases of nonvisualization by the oral method, and (b) in cases where, due to vomiting or diarrhea, the patient cannot retain the orally administered medium long enough for its absorption. In cases of nonvisualization, the intravenous procedure may be instituted at once. This is done to save time for the radiology department as well as for the patient, and to spare the patient the rigors of having the intestinal tract prepared again.

Preliminary cleansing of the colon for this procedure usually consists of administering castor oil or another nongas-forming cathartic on the evening preceding the examination. Specifications for the evening meal vary. Shehadi[1] recommends that the evening meal of noncholecystectomized patients be high in simple fats such as eggs, butter, cream, and milk, but that it contain no fried food. He further recommends that both cholecystectomized and noncholecystectomized patients be dehydrated by withholding fluids for at least twelve hours prior to the examination in order to obtain better concentration of the contrast agent.

Breakfast is usually withheld for the same reasons as in oral cholegraphy, but in intravenous cholegraphy, withholding the meal becomes of paramount importance since vomiting is one of the anticipated side reactions to the intravenous contrast agent. When vomiting occurs, there is a possibility that food may be aspirated, which may have serious consequences.

The intravenously administered medium reaches the liver rapidly and consequently is excreted rapidly, so that filming is started shortly after the injection. It therefore behooves the technologist to make as many of the preliminary preparations as possible before the patient is brought into the examining room. A part of this preparation includes making ready the basic identification markers. A postinjection time-interval marker is placed on each of the duct studies, and a postcibal-interval marker is placed on the functional studies of the gallbladder. Body position (supine, prone, erect, decubitus, Trendelenburg) is also indicated on the film.

The items required for the injection should be conveniently arranged on a small, movable table. A more or less standard setup for this procedure includes (1) a tourniquet, and a towel or other pad to be placed under the elbow; (2) a jar of sterile gauze squares or cotton balls; (3) sterile sponge forceps; (4) 70% alcohol for cleansing the skin; (5) sterile 2 ml. syringes and needles for injecting the test dose of the medium and, possibly, an antihistaminic; (6) a sterile 30 ml. syringe and intravenous needles for the injection of the contrast agent; (7) blood pressure apparatus; (8) emesis basins and tissues; and (9) the emergency cart.

The patient is placed in the supine position for a preliminary film of the abdomen. When a sensitivity test is

[1]Shehadi, William H.: Clinical radiology of the biliary tract, New York, 1963, McGraw-Hill Book Co.

performed, the patient is observed for ten to fifteen minutes to allow for the development of any unfavorable reaction. If the patient manifests no untoward reaction, as in a vast majority of cases, the technologist can utilize the waiting time to make the final preparations for the injection of the full dose of the contrast medium and for the first postinjection duct study.

The patient is adjusted in the right anteroposterior oblique position (page 690) for the duct studies. A scout film should be made at this time to check the centering and the exposure factors. Arrange a chair or stool for the physician's comfort; he makes the injection slowly during a period of ten minutes, in order to minimize reaction and to avoid injecting more of the medium than necessary, in case of a sudden severe reaction. However mild the usual hot flush, the patient feels better cared for when an effort is being made to ease his discomfort. This may be the simple act of placing a damp, cold towel on his forehead or throat for the five minutes or so required for the hot flush to subside.

Timed from the completion of the injection, duct studies are ordinarily made at ten-minute intervals until satisfactory visualization is obtained. Maximum opacification usually requires thirty to forty minutes. The films are processed as exposed and are immediately presented to the radiologist so that he can make any change required to adapt the examination to the individual patient. Lateral films of the opacified ducts may reveal valuable information about their anatomy and pathology. Tomography is also utilized in examinations of the biliary tract.

In noncholecystectomized patients the gallbladder frequently becomes visible within thirty minutes, but it is usually not maximally opacified until about two hours following the injection. As in the oral method, the patient is adjusted in the positions required for adequate demonstration of the gallbladder. Following satisfactory cholecystograms, the patient is given a fatty meal to test the emptying power of the gallbladder. Since satisfactory cholangiograms are already in hand, the post cibum examination in this method usually consists of one film unless emptying is found to be slow.

In a more recently developed method of intravenous cholangiography, the contrast medium is diluted in an isotonic saline solution or in a 5% glucose solution and is then administered by slow intravenous infusion. The recommended time for the infusion is ten minutes, but some examiners extend the time to as much as one hour. The consensus appears to be that (1) indications and contraindications for the infusion method are essentially the same as those for the single bolus (20 ml.) method, (2) opacification of the gallbladder and ducts may be improved, and (3) the chief advantage of the drip infusion is the appreciable decrease in the incidence of adverse (side) reactions.

Renal excretion may occur in a high percentage of cases regardless of whether the single bolus or drip infusion injection is used. The supine right oblique position (page 690) obviates superimposition of the opacified ducts and the upper urinary tract.

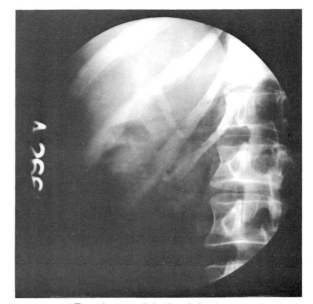

Ten-minute postinjection cholangiogram.

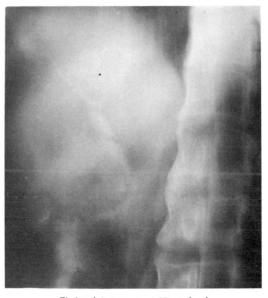

Cholangiotomogram at 10 cm. level.

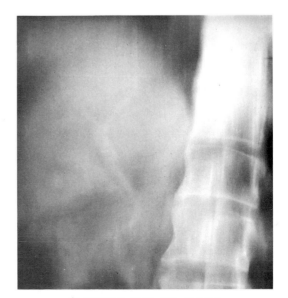

Cholangiotomogram at 11 cm. level.

Radiographs courtesy Dr. William H. Shehadi.

BILIARY TRACT—cont'd
Oral and intravenous cholegraphy

TECHNICAL REQUIREMENTS

For the technical quality of cholecystograms and cho-langiograms to be above question, the following requisites must be met:

1. The focal spot of the x-ray tube must be small and unpitted.

2. The intensifying screens must be clean, unblemished, and in perfect contact.

3. The Potter-Bucky diaphragm must be in perfect condition and its timing device accurate.

4. The examination area must be closely coned.

5. Immobilization with a broad compression band should be employed to aid in the control of movement, preferably with an air-filled, gum-rubber bag to improve contrast.

6. The patient must be taught to relax as well as to suspend respiration during the exposures.

7. The exposure time must be short, preferably no more than a half second, in order to eliminate blurring of the gallbladder and/or duct shadows as a result of vibratory movement caused by peristaltic action in the adjacent segments of the intestine.

8. The exposure factors must be adjusted to produce maximum soft tissue differentiation. The films must show a sharp outline of the lower border of the liver, the right kidney, and the margin of the right psoas muscle, and it must show a degree of intrastructural detail of the included bony parts that is commensurate with the thickness of the abdomen, that is, with the part-film distance.

9. The scout film of patients of asthenic habitus must be dark enough to demonstrate the shadow of the gallbladder through the vertebral shadow, lest the gallbladder and the vertebrae be superimposed.

10. Following the scout film, the exposure should be adjusted so that it will just penetrate the gallbladder. This means that the surrounding soft tissues will be under-exposed when the shadow of the gallbladder is faint, and overpenetrated when it is dense.

11. Finally, the films must be correctly processed. Ideally, soft tissue films should not be processed at temperatures higher than 68° F.; the best results are obtained at 65° F.

POSITION OF PATIENT

The comfort of the patient is one of the most important factors in the prevention of motion. Elevated parts must be supported, and pressure points must be relieved with suitable padding. The body must be adjusted in a comfortable, unstrained position in order to prevent movement of the viscera by unintentional contraction of the abdominal muscles as a result of tenseness. For the scout, or localization, film of the gallbladder, the patient is placed in the prone position and adjusted for a direct postero-anterior projection. The head should be rested on the left cheek to avoid rotating the vertebral column toward the right side. The right arm should be placed as shown in the photograph below and the left arm extended along the side of the body, further to aid in rotating the vertebral column slightly away from the right side. When a thin patient is examined, a folded towel or other soft pad should be placed under the iliac spines to relieve pressure. The ankles should be supported on sandbags so that the weight of the feet will not rest on the toes.

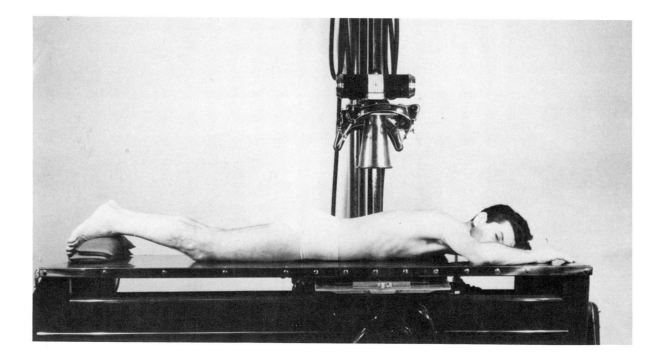

IMMOBILIZATION

The patient should be carefully immobilized, preferably with a large, air-filled, gum-rubber bag as well as with a broad compression band. The inflated bag not only aids in compression but also prevents the protrusion of soft tissue folds above and below the band and improves the quality of the radiograph. When the patient is rotated to an oblique position, the inflated bag or a radioparent wedge should be placed under the abdomen to compress the viscera and thus to aid in eliminating movement.

RESPIRATION

Exposures are routinely made at the end of exhalation because this phase of respiration places the patient under less strain. The patient must never be asked either to exhale or to inhale to the point of strain, because spasmodic contraction of the abdominal muscles will occur. The breathing instructions should be carefully explained, and the patient should then be requested to rehearse them until he is able to suspend respiration and relax. By keeping his hand on the patient's back during the rehearsal procedure, the technologist can detect tenseness easily and can also judge the time interval needed for the individual patient to relax after the cessation of respiration. When the instructions are not understood, breathing can usually be controlled by having the patient close his mouth and hold his nose.

According to the habitus of the subject and the degree of body fat present, the gallbladder moves lateralward and upward 1 to 3 inches on full exhalation, and conversely, it moves medialward and downward 1 to 3 inches on full inhalation. This should be remembered and utilized when the gallbladder shadow on the scout film is partially obscured by rib shadows or by small amounts of gas. When cholecystograms are made on inhalation, they should be so marked.

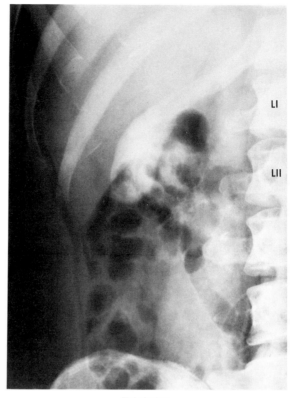

Exhalation.

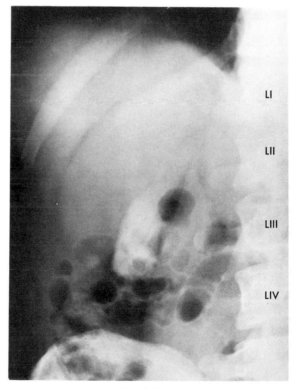

Inhalation.

BILIARY TRACT—cont'd
Oral and intravenous cholegraphy—cont'd
INITIAL GALLBLADDER FILMS

Anatomic descriptions of the gallbladder are based on the average. They usually state that the gallbladder is a pear-shaped organ situated in an oblique plane in the right upper quadrant of the abdomen, where, from the neck end, its long axis slants downward and slightly forward. In practice we encounter many deviations from this arrangement. The shape of the gallbladder varies considerably from the classic pyriform configuration. Depending upon bodily habitus and the arrangement of its attachment to the liver, it may, in its usual right-sided position, be located anywhere from the level of the eighth rib down to well within the iliac fossa, and anywhere from the median sagittal plane to near the lateral wall of the abdomen. It is sometimes found in the left side of the abdomen, even though the liver is in normal position. Because of the possibility of the latter location, the initial study includes a 14″ × 17″ film of the abdomen in addition to a 10″ × 12″ film of the right side. The wide range in the right-sided location of the gallbladder can be covered with the 10″ × 12″ film by centering at the level of the ninth costal cartilage for patients of average build, about 2 inches higher for those approaching the hypersthenic type, and 2 inches lower for asthenic patients.

In order to ensure accurate centering for closely coned studies, a transverse wax pencil mark may be made on the side of the body to indicate the centering of the 10″ × 12″ film, and after the gallbladder is localized, an X mark may then be made on the skin to indicate its exact level in the prone position. Depending upon the habitus of the patient, the centering will be several inches higher than the X mark for anteroposterior and anteroposterior oblique projections, and several inches lower for posteroanterior oblique and erect projections.

INSPECTION OF INITIAL FILMS

As soon as the two scout films have been processed, they are carefully inspected for the following information: (1) the presence or absence of the gallbladder shadow, and (2) if present, (a) whether the concentration of the contrast medium is sufficient for adequate visualization, (b) whether it is overlapped by intestinal and/or bony shadows, (c) its exact location, and (d) whether a change in the exposure factors is needed for proper penetration of the organ.

When the gallbladder is not visualized, and only a 10″ × 12″ scout film was made, transposition of the viscera or of the gallbladder only must be ruled out with a 14″ × 17″ film of the abdomen. On slender patients, the region of the vertebral column and that of the iliac fossa must be carefully scrutinized for evidence of the gallbladder shadow in one of these areas. When the gallbladder region is obscured by intestinal content, the colon should be evacuated with a cleansing enema of normal saline solution (see illustrations below). It is frequently necessary to administer more than one enema in order to clear the hepatic flexure. Some radiologists administer an injection of neostigmine (Prostigmin) or vasopressin (Pitressin) to clear the colon. When this is done, a period of about forty-five minutes is allowed for the drug to take effect before making the follow-up film. When the gallbladder shadow is nowhere visible, the patient should again be questioned, particularly about diet. Many patients will confess at this point that they did break fasting or that they did not take all of the contrast medium.

In the intravenous method, because the contrast agent is introduced directly into the bloodstream and is thus delivered to the liver in a known quantity, it is not usual to inject a second dose in "no shadow" or "faint shadow" cases. In the oral method, however, whether the contrast medium reaches the bloodstream depends upon (1) the condition of the gastrointestinal mucosa, (2) the giving of explicit instructions to the patient, and (3) the cooperation of the patient in following the instructions. For the purpose of ruling out any possible error in the technique of administering the medium or, as is sometimes the case, the patient's failure to comply with the instructions, patients are usually kept on a fat-free diet, a second dose of the contrast agent is administered that evening, and the examination is reattempted on the following morning.

When it is established that the patient followed instructions, or that he could not retain the contrast medium due to vomiting or diarrhea, many radiologists immediately proceed with the intravenous medium. In the presence of diarrhea, some radiologists administer paregoric with a second dose of the oral medium. In the absence of diarrhea, oral media are reabsorbed by the intestinal mucosa in a quantity sufficient to produce fair reopacification of the gallbladder on the following day, as is frequently noted on follow-up examinations of the gastrointestinal tract. The cumulative effect of reabsorption of the first dose plus a second dose sometimes succeeds in a satisfactory visualization.

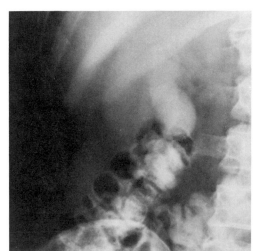

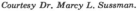
Courtesy Dr. Marcy L. Sussman.

INSPECTION OF INITIAL FILMS—cont'd

When an unobstructed and satisfactorily opacified shadow of the gallbladder is revealed, no special procedure is required. The routine projections used for the precibal demonstration of the gallbladder are the posteroanterior projections, one of which is made either in the erect position[1-3] or in the right lateral decubitus position, and several posteroanterior oblique projections, which are made in varying degrees of obliquity.

When only the fundus of the gallbladder is obscured by intestinal content, the shadows can usually be separated with suitably rotated posteroanterior oblique projections made in the recumbent position. Lindblom[4] recommended a semiaxial projection for this purpose (page 689). Kirklin,[5] crediting Whelan with this application of the position, recommended the use of the right lateral decubitus position (page 689).

When the shadow of the gallbladder is superimposed by shadows of the ribs, subsequent exposures in the recumbent position should be made on full inhalation for the purpose of pushing the viscera downward. In order to separate the shadows of the gallbladder and of the vertebrae, it is necessary to rotate the body to an oblique position. For exceptionally thin patients, it is frequently necessary to use the lateral position and, for oblique studies, the supine position. When the gallbladder is located in the iliac fossa, it is necessary to use the supine position to draw the organ upward. In extreme cases it is necessary to use a cranial angulation of either the table or the central ray. The right lateral decubitus position is used for stratification studies of the low-placed gallbladder.

Biliary tract films should be carefully inspected with standard white-light illumination as they are processed, in order to ensure a satisfactory examination. Regardless of how sharp the detail of contiguous structures, each film not showing sharp, clean-cut outlines of the biliary structures must be considered as having been taken during involuntary motion, and it should therefore be repeated immediately.

The wide range of variation in both the location and the pathology of the gallbladder makes it imperative that each patient receive individual attention. Some radiologists routinely radioscope gallbladder patients and take spot films in addition to the conventionally projected studies. When it is not possible for the radiologist personally to inspect the films as they are processed and to determine the procedure necessary for an adequate demonstration of the biliary tract, the technologist must be capable of doing so. This requires a knowledge of biliary tract examinations that can be gained only through careful training and long experience.

[1]Marinot, J.: La radiographie de la vésicule biliare en position debout, Théses de la Faculté de Médecine de Paris, No. 229, Paris, 1924, Louis Arnette.

[2]Akerlund, A.: Beobachtungen bei Cholezystogrammen in aufrechter Korperstellung, Acta Radiol. 14:74-81, 1933.

[3]Ettinger, Alice: Visualization of minute gallstones, Amer. J. Roentgen. 35:656-661, 1936.

[4]Lindblom, K.: Axial projection of the gallbladder, Acta Radiol. 32:189-190, 1949.

[5]Kirklin, B. R.: A new position for cholecystography, Amer. J. Roentgen. 60:263-268, 1948.

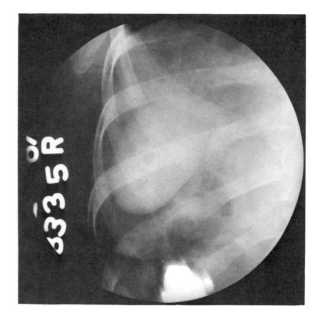

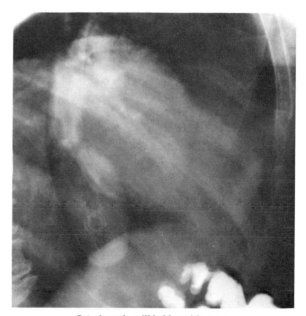

Intrahepatic gallbladder with stones.

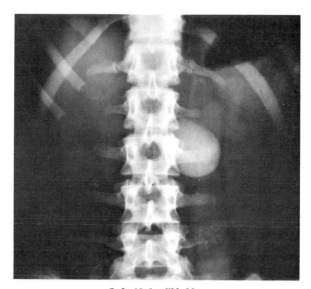

Left-sided gallbladder.

Radiographs courtesy Dr. William H. Shehadi.

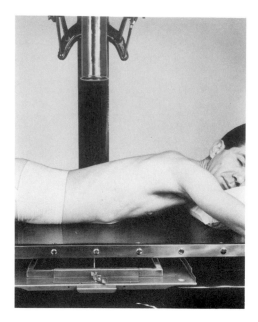

GALLBLADDER
Posteroanterior projection
Anteroposterior view

Film: $10'' \times 12''$ for scout film, $8'' \times 10''$ for subsequent exposures.

Position of patient

Place the patient in the prone position with a pillow under the head; if the patient is thin, place the pillow lengthwise and adjust it so that it extends downward as far as, or a little below, the transmammillary line.

Position of part

Adjust the body so that the right side of the abdomen is centered to the midline of the table. Rest the head on the left cheek in order to rotate the vertebrae slightly toward the left side. Flex the right elbow and adjust the arm in a comfortable position. Place the left arm along the side of the body. Elevate the ankles on sandbags to relieve pressure on the toes.

When examining a female subject who has pendulous breasts, spread the breasts upward and outward to ensure clearing the gallbladder region.

Center the film according to the habitus of the patient. Make a transverse mark on the side of the body with a wax skin pencil to indicate the centering of the scout film. After localization, indicate the exact site of the gallbladder by making an X mark on the skin.

Immobilize with a compression band and an air-filled, gum-rubber bag, applied tightly across the upper abdominal region. Respiration is suspended at the end of exhalation in the routine procedure. Have the patient rehearse the breathing instructions until he is able to relax as well as to suspend respiration. Watching carefully for an indication of tenseness, allow about two seconds to elapse after the cessation of respiration before making the exposure; this is to permit any peristaltic action to subside and to give the patient time to relax.

Central ray

Direct the central ray perpendicularly to the midpoint of the film.

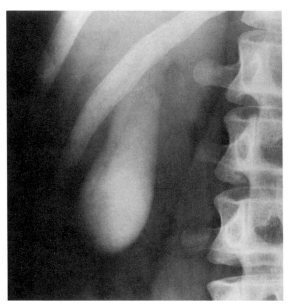

Prefatty meal.

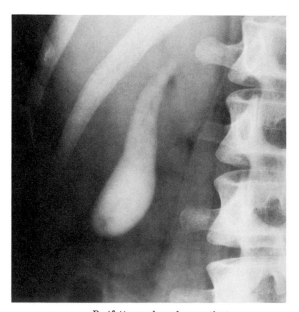

Postfatty meal on above patient.

Courtesy Dr. Marcy L. Sussman.

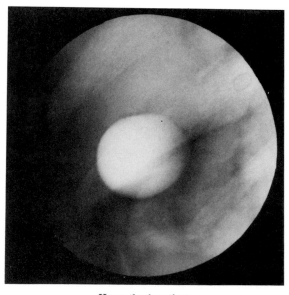

Hypersthenic patient.

Courtesy Dr. Max Dannenberg.

GALLBLADDER
Posteroanterior projection
Anteroposterior view—cont'd
Erect position

When the patient is placed in the upright position, adjust the body so that the previously localized gallbladder is centered to the midline of the Potter-Bucky grid. The gallbladder can be elevated to, or almost to, the location it assumed in the prone position, indicated by the X mark, by having the patient fully extend his arms. He may rest them, with the elbows either flexed or extended, against the table. Otherwise, depending upon the habitus of the patient, center the film 2 to 4 inches below the level of the X mark to allow for the change in the position of the gallbladder. The remainder of the procedure is the same as for the prone position.

Structures shown

The posteroanterior projection gives a semiaxial view of the opacified gallbladder. The foreshortening of its shadow in the posteroanterior position is due to the angle between the long axis of the obliquely placed gallbladder and the plane of the film. The degree of angulation and, consequently, the amount of foreshortening vary according to bodily habitus and are influenced by body position, being less in the erect position.

The gallbladder is directed anteriorly at a downward angle that ranges from an almost horizontal position in the hypersthenic patient to an almost vertical position in the asthenic patient. As a result, foreshortening of the shadow of the gallbladder is negligible in asthenic patients. On the other hand, in patients of the hypersthenic type, the neck, body, and fundus of the gallbladder are superimposed and thus cast an irregularly circular or triangular shadow, the shape depending upon the degree of lateral displacement. In subjects of average build, the gallbladder casts a pear-shaped shadow that is somewhat foreshortened but does not show actual superimposition of the different regions of the gallbladder.

In the erect position the gallbladder assumes a more vertical angle as it moves downward, backward, and medialward. The extent of the change in both angle and location depends upon habitus and abdominal fat. The upright position is used to demonstrate the mobility of the gallbladder, to detect the presence of stones that are too small to cast individual shadows, and to differentiate papilloma or other tumor shadows from cholesterol calculi shadows, as determined by the mobility of the latter. Small stones that are heavier than bile gravitate to the fundic portion of the gallbladder, where the aggregate has either sufficient radiopacity or sufficient radiparency to cast a shadow. Due to the fact that the opacified bile layers out according to concentration, that is, according to specific gravity, or weight, minute stones will float at the surface of a certain bile layer, depending upon the relative specific gravity, and cast a shadow that has the appearance of a horizontal band (note lower radiograph).

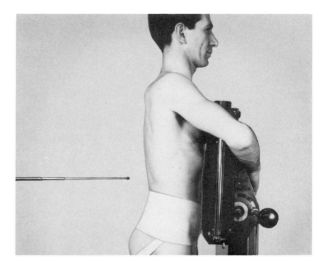

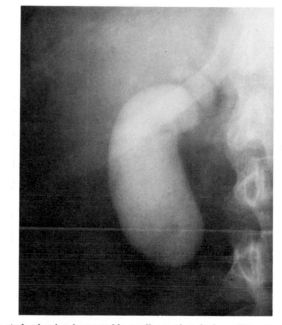

Prone study showing innumerable small negative shadows filling the greater portion of the gallbladder and representing bile pigment calculi.

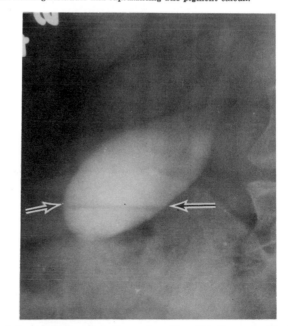

Film of above patient made in the erect position. Note linear stratification of the bile pigment calculi (arrows) in the lower portion of the gallbladder.

Radiographs and clinical information courtesy Dr. William H. Shehadi.

687

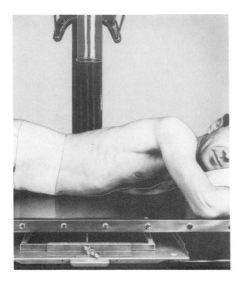

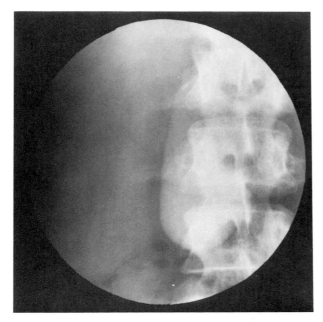

Prone position.

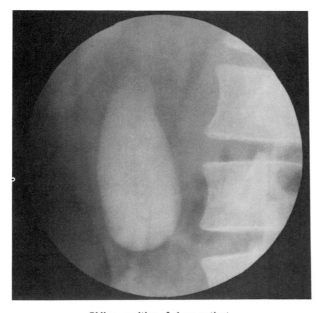

Oblique position of above patient.
Radiographs courtesy Dr. Marcy L. Sussman.

GALLBLADDER
Left posteroanterior oblique projection
Left anteroposterior oblique view

Film: $8'' \times 10''$ lengthwise.

Position of patient

In the routine procedure the patient is adjusted in the recumbent position for oblique and lateral projections of the gallbladder.

Position of part

The degree of rotation necessary for a satisfactory demonstration of the gallbladder depends upon the location of the organ with reference to the vertebrae (thin subjects requiring more rotation than obese subjects), upon the angulation of the long axis of the organ, and upon whether the hepatic flexure is clear. It is common practice to make several oblique projections, changing the rotation of the body 10 or 15 degrees between exposures. A direct right lateral view is sometimes required to differentiate gallstones from renal stones or calcified mesenteric nodes. The lateral position is also required to separate the shadows of the gallbladder and the vertebrae in exceptionally thin patients, and to place the long axis of a transversely placed gallbladder parallel with the plane of the film.

With the patient in the prone position, elevate the right side to the desired degree of obliquity, and have the patient support himself on the flexed knee and elbow. Adjust the body to center the previously localized gallbladder to the midline of the table. Place the air-filled gum-rubber bag or a foam wedge under the side of the abdomen, and after centering the film, apply the compression band.

Unless otherwise indicated by the scout film, respiration is suspended at the end of exhalation.

Central ray

Direct the central ray vertically to the midpoint of the film.

Structures shown

An oblique or lateral view of the opacified gallbladder projected free of self-superimposition or foreshortening, and of the structures adjacent to the gallbladder.

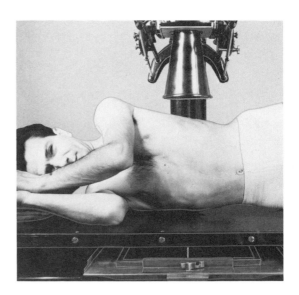

GALLBLADDER

Right lateral decubitus projection

The use of the right lateral decubitus projection for the demonstration of the gallbladder was evolved by Whelan.[1] The position, with the use of a large film for the inclusion of the entire abdomen, is shown on page 667. The patient may be placed on a stretcher or a movable table before a vertical Potter-Bucky diaphragm, or with the use of a stationary grid or a grid-front cassette, he may be positioned on the horizontal table. The patient is placed on his right side with his body elevated 2 or 3 inches on a suitable radioparent support, in order to center the gallbladder region to a vertically placed 8″ × 10″ film. The central ray is directed horizontally.

The right lateral decubitus position, as well as the erect position, is used to demonstrate (1) stones that are heavier than bile and that are too small to be visible other than when accumulated in the dependent portion of the gallbladder, and (2) stones that are lighter than bile and that are visualized only by stratification. This position has the further advantage of permitting the gallbladder to gravitate toward the dependent right side, where it will lie below any adjacent gas-containing loops of the intestine, and away from bony superimposition when it occupies a low and/or medial position.

Lordotic projection

The use of the posteroanterior lordotic projection in cholecystography was described by Lindblom.[2] This position, with the use of a large film centered to the chest, is illustrated on page 642. For the demonstration of the gallbladder, the right side of the abdomen is centered to the midline of a vertical Potter-Bucky diaphragm. The patient is asked to grasp the sides of the stand or table, to brace his abdomen against the grid or table, and then to lean his thorax backward in a forced lordotic position. The film is centered to the gallbladder region, and the central ray is directed horizontally.

The lordotic position is used primarily for drawing the gallbladder upward, where its shadow will not be superimposed by those of the intestinal contents.

[1]Whelan, Frank J.: Special cholecystographic technique, Xray Techn. **19:**230-234, 1948.
[2]Lindblom, K.: Axial projection of the gallbladder, Acta Radiol. **32:**189-190, 1949.

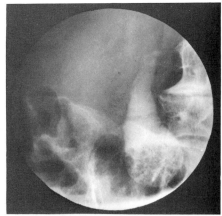

Erect projection.

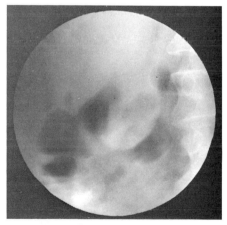

Decubitus projection on above patient.

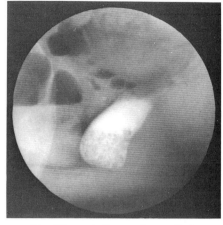

Prone projection.

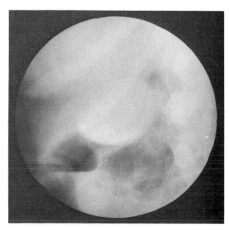

Lordotic projection an above patient.
Radiographs courtesy Dr. William H. Shehadi.

689

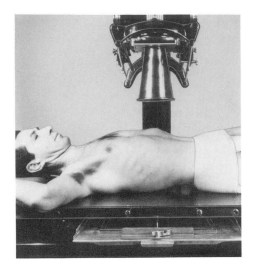

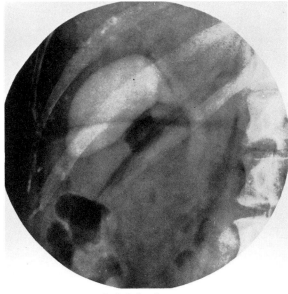

Oral cholangiogram.

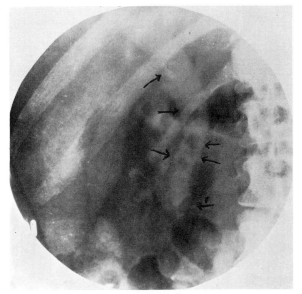

Intravenous cholangiogram.

Radiographs courtesy Dr. William H. Shehadi.

EXTRAHEPATIC BILE DUCTS
Right anteroposterior oblique projection
Right posteroanterior oblique view

The use of the right anteroposterior oblique position for the demonstration of the extrahepatic bile ducts was introduced by Stenström[1] in 1940. This position places the plane of the extrahepatic duct system approximately parallel with the plane of the film, and it rotates the ducts somewhat lateralward, where they can be projected free from superimposition by the vertebral shadow. The gallbladder is placed at a higher level, where it is possible for it to empty more rapidly and in a more continuous flow, which results in denser opacification of the ducts in the oral method.

Oral cholangiography is undertaken only when the gallbladder shows moderately dense opacification, because visualization of the small-caliber bile ducts requires that they be filled with a fairly heavy concentration of radiopaque contrast material. In order to ensure the best possible filling, the patient should be adjusted in position as soon as he has ingested the fatty meal and so kept until the duct studies have been completed. The demonstration of these passages by the oral method also depends upon taking the films as the largest quantity of opacified bile is flowing from the gallbladder to the duodenum. Oral cholangiograms are made at ten-minute intervals after the ingestion of the fatty meal until satisfactory visualization is obtained, maximum opacification usually occurring in the twenty- to thirty-minute postcibal interval.

Film: $8'' \times 10''$ or $10'' \times 12''$ crosswise.

Position of patient

The patient is placed in the supine position, with the right side of the body centered to the midline of the table.

Position of part

Elevate the left side of the body 15 to 20 degrees, and support the elevated shoulder, hip, and knee on sandbags or another suitable support. The patient's hips and knees should be fully extended for the purpose of arching the back and, thereby, drawing the gallbladder and the ductal tree upward and outward to the fullest extent, usually placing them above the hepatic flexure. Make any necessary readjustment that is required to center the right side of the body to the midline of the table.

Depending upon the habitus of the patient, the film is centered 2 to 4 inches higher than for the prone position.

A compression band may be applied with moderate pressure. Respiration is suspended for the exposure.

Central ray

Direct the central ray vertically to the midpoint of the film.

[1]Stenström, B.: Ueber Cholangiographie, Acta Radiol. **21**:549-570, 1940.

BILIARY TRACT

Percutaneous transhepatic cholangiography

Percutaneous transhepatic cholangiography[1] and *transabdominal cholangiography*[2] are terms applied to the third method employed for preoperative radiologic exploration of the biliary tract. This method is utilized for selected patients only; specifically, for patients with jaundice when the ductal system cannot be demonstrated by the other preoperative methods of cholangiography.

A water-soluble, iodinated medium, one of those used for intravenous urography, is employed. The contrast agent is introduced directly into one of the intrahepatic ducts by way of a long needle inserted through the abdominal wall and liver. Because of the possibility of copious internal bleeding and/or bile escape into the peritoneal cavity, this examination is performed shortly before scheduled surgery, either definite or on standby in case the need arises.

This procedure is carried out in the radiology department. The patient is placed on a combination radioscopic-radiographic table. A qualified nurse is usually in attendance and is responsible for the preparation of the sterile tray. General anesthesia is administered when indicated; otherwise the examination is performed following suitable sedation and local anesthesia.

Following the introduction of the needle and the withdrawal by syringe of as much bile as possible, the contrast medium is injected under radioscopic observation, and spot-film studies are made after each of several fractional injections. Where the equipment is available, television monitoring is used to direct the needle and control bile duct filling. Conventional studies are made as directed by the radiologist. The puncture needle is usually left in situ for the purpose of removing as much bile and contrast solution as possible upon completion of the examination. When this is not done, a delayed film or films may be made to evaluate absorption of the contrast medium.

[1]Evans, J. A., Glenn, F., Thorbjarnarson, B., and Mujahed, Z.: Percutaneous transhepatic cholangiography, Radiology **78**:362-370, 1962.
[2]Carter, F. R., and Saypol, G. M.: Transabdominal cholangiography, J.A.M.A. **148**:253-255, 1952.

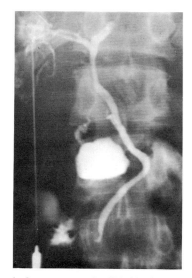

Normal extrahepatic duct system and gallbladder in a patient with hepatitis. Note needle positioned in one of the small intrahepatic bile radicles.

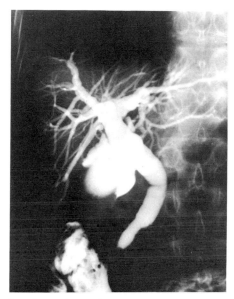

Jaundiced patient. Cholangiogram demonstrates cause of jaundice to be impacted stone at the ampulla.

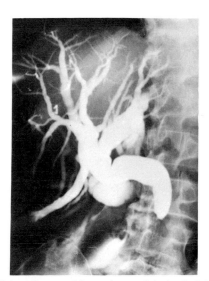

Patient with jaundice caused by carcinoma of the head of the pancreas.

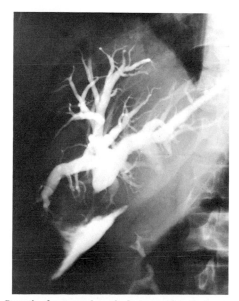

Stenosis of common hepatic duct secondary to trauma.

Radiographs and diagnostic information courtesy Dr. John A. Evans.

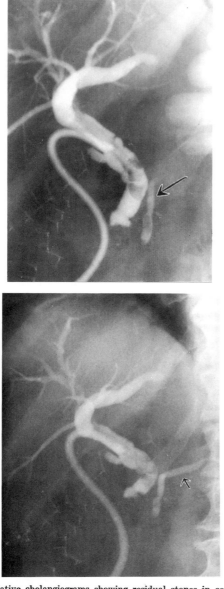

Delayed operative cholangiograms showing residual stones in common duct. Note reflux into pancreatic duct (arrow).

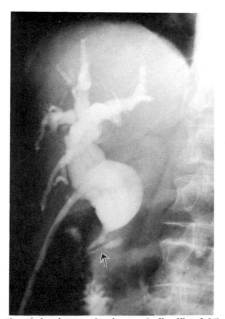

Delayed operative cholangiogram showing markedly dilated bile ducts. Note reflux into pancreatic duct (arrow).

Radiographs and diagnostic information courtesy Dr. William H. Shehadi.

BILIARY TRACT—cont'd
Operative (or immediate) cholangiography

Operative cholangiography, introduced by Mirizzi[1] in 1932, is carried out during biliary tract surgery, as its title indicates. Following drainage of the bile, and in the absence of obstruction, this method permits contrast filling of the major intrahepatic ducts as well as of the extrahepatic ducts. The value of operative cholangiography is such that it has become an integral part of biliary tract surgery. It is used in the investigation of the patency of the bile ducts and of the functional status of the sphincter of Oddi, to reveal the presence of calculi that cannot be detected by palpation, and to demonstrate such conditions as small intraluminal neoplasms and stricture or dilatation of the ducts. When the pancreatic duct shares a common channel with the distal common bile duct before emptying into the duodenum, it is sometimes seen, on operative cholangiograms, to be partially filled by reflux.

The production of films of diagnostic quality in operative cholangiography depends not only upon a skilled technologist but upon the capacity of the mobile radiographic unit. A transformer with high electrical output (200 to 300 milliamperes) is a necessity, as is also a high-speed Potter-Bucky diaphragm or grid-front cassettes and a cassette tunnel.

During the preparation of the operating room, and in cooperation with the nursing staff, the technologist should adjust the grid or the cassette tunnel on the operating table. He should clean the mobile unit with a damp (not wet) cloth and place the machine in a convenient and easily maneuverable position. The machine should be connected and tested, and the controls should be adjusted according to predetermined exposure factors. An adequate number of cassettes should be on hand, and arrangements should be made for immediate processing of the films as they are exposed.

The patient is adjusted on the operating table so that the right upper quadrant of the abdomen is centered to the movable grid or to the film area of the tunnel. The left side of the body is elevated 15 to 20 degrees and is supported on folded sheets; this position prevents the possibility of superimposing the bile ducts on the vertebrae.

[1]Mirizzi, P. L.: La colangiografía durante las operaciones de las vías biliares, Bol. Soc. Cir. B. Air. **16**:1133-1161, 1932.

After exposing, draining, and exploring the biliary tract, and frequently after excision of the gallbladder, the surgeon instills the contrast agent. This is usually introduced into the common bile duct, through either a needle, a small catheter, or, after cholecystectomy, an inlying T tube. When the latter route is used, the procedure is referred to as *delayed operative*, or *operative T tube*, *cholangiography*.

The exposure time used for operative cholangiography must be as short as possible, and the exposures must be made during temporary respiratory arrest, which the anesthetist induces for the purpose. Films are exposed at the direction of the surgeon. The total volume of contrast solution is usually introduced in small amounts in two or three stages, with one or more films being exposed after each injection.

While it is no longer common practice because of the generally excellent quality of present-day operative cholangiograms, an occlusal, or a dental, film is sometimes encased in a sterile surgical glove or other aseptic envelope and is placed directly under the exposed common bile duct for better delineation of this important passage. This procedure is termed *choledochography* (of the ductus choledochus, or common bile duct), and the resultant films are called *choledochograms*.

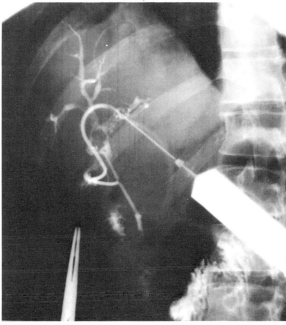

5 ml. injection.

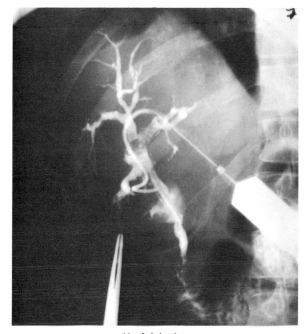

10 ml. injection.

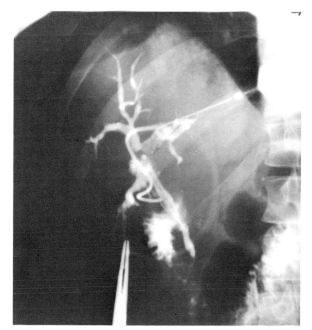

15 ml. injection.

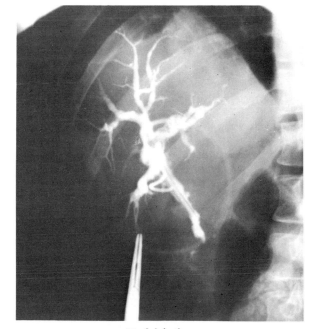

20 ml. injection.

Radiographs courtesy Dr. Robert L. Pinck.

693

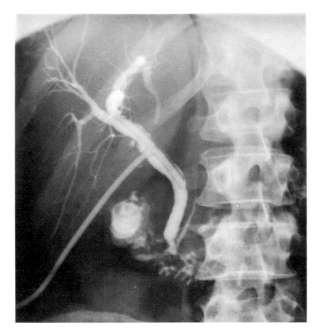

BILIARY TRACT—cont'd

Postoperative cholangiography

Postoperative, *delayed*, and *T-tube* cholangiography are radiologic terms applied to the biliary tract examination that is performed by way of the T-shaped rubber tube left in the common bile duct for postoperative drainage. This examination is performed to demonstrate the caliber and patency of the ducts, the status of the sphincter of Oddi, and the presence of residual or previously undetected stones or other pathology.

Postoperative cholangiography is carried out in the radiology department. Preliminary preparation usually consists of the following:

1. The drainage tube is clamped the day preceding the examination. This is done to let the tube fill with bile as a preventive measure against air bubbles entering the ducts, where they would simulate cholesterol stones.

2. The preceding meal is withheld.

3. When indicated, a cleansing enema is administered about one hour before the examination. Premedication is not required.

The contrast agent used is one of the water-soluble, organic contrast media such as methiodal (Skiodan), or one of those used in intravenous urography. The medium should be warmed to body temperature by placing the ampules in a basin of warm water. Other items required for the injection are sponges soaked with 70% alcohol, for cleansing the injection area of the T tube, and a sterile 30 ml. syringe and needle for the introduction of the contrast solution.

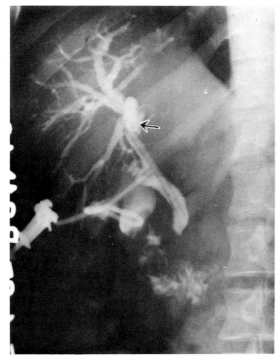

Postoperative cholangiograms.
Courtesy Dr. William H. Shehadi.

After a preliminary film of the abdomen has been obtained, the patient is adjusted in the right anteroposterior oblique position (page 690), with the right upper quadrant of the abdomen centered to the midline of the table.

The radiologist may inject the contrast medium under radioscopic control, with spot and conventional films exposed as indicated. Otherwise, $10'' \times 12''$ films are exposed serially after each of several fractional injections of the medium and then at specified intervals until most of the contrast solution has entered the duodenum. At this point, while the common bile duct is still filled, an erect study consisting of one or more films may be made. Stern and associates[1] stress the importance of making a lateral study to demonstrate the anatomic branching of the hepatic ducts in this plane and to detect any abnormality not demonstrable in other views. The clamp is not removed from the T tube before the completion of the examination, so that the patient may be turned onto his right side for this study.

[1]Stern, W. Z., Schein, C. J., and Jacobson, H. G.: The significance of the lateral view in T-tube cholangiography, Amer. J. Roentgen. **87:**764-771, 1962.

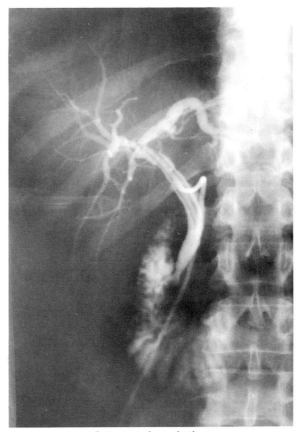

Anteroposterior projection.

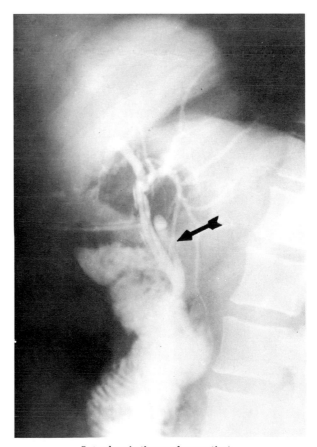

Lateral projection on above patient.

Radiographs courtesy Dr. William Z. Stern.

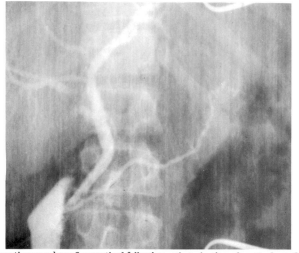

Pancreaticogram by reflux method following catheterization of cystic duct. Overflow into duodenum occurs when intraductal pressure exceeds resistance of sphincter of Oddi.

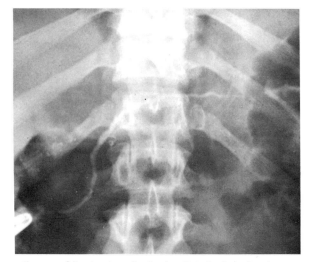

Pancreaticogram following transduodenal catheterization of main pancreatic duct and injection of contrast material.

Radiographs and legends courtesy Dr. Arthur R. Clemett.

PANCREAS

Operative pancreatography

Operative (or direct) *pancreatography* is the surgico-radiologic procedure wherein a water-soluble, iodinated contrast medium is introduced into the main pancreatic duct (duct of Wirsung) for the investigation of abnormalities of the pancreas. This may be done (1) by reflux filling from an injection made into the common bile duct when these two passages share a common channel before emptying into the duodenum or (2) by direct injection through transduodenal catheterization of the duct.

The production of high-quality films depends not only upon close teamwork between the surgeon, the anesthetist, and the technologist but upon having a high-capacity mobile unit and a high-speed Potter-Bucky diaphragm or grid-front cassettes and a cassette tunnel. The exposure field should be closely coned to further reduce secondary radiation. The exposure factors should be adjusted so that the shortest possible exposure time is used, in order to obviate vibratory movement transmitted by the pulsating aorta.

The technologist should be present when the operating room is being prepared so that, in cooperation with the nursing staff, he can adjust the grid or the cassette tunnel so that it will be centered to the median sagittal plane of the patient's body at the level of the xiphoid process. The mobile unit should be cleaned with a damp (not wet) cloth and placed in a convenient and easily movable position. The machine should be connected and tested, and the controls should be adjusted according to predetermined exposure factors. An ample supply of films should be on hand, and arrangements should be made for immediate processing of the films as they are exposed.

The patient is placed on the operating table in the direct supine position and adjusted so that the xiphoid process is centered over the Potter-Bucky diaphragm or the exposure area of the cassette tunnel.

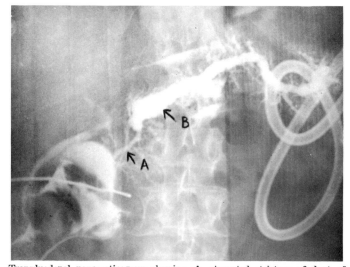

Transduodenal pancreaticogram showing, **A,** elongated stricture of duct of Wirsung secondary to carcinoma, and, **B,** dilation of duct proximal to stricture.

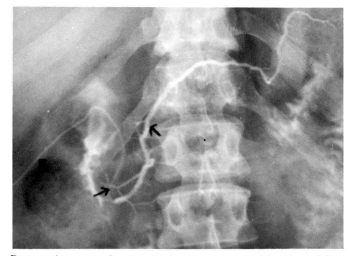

Postoperative pancreaticogram showing (two lower arrows) catheter left in duct of Wirsung and exteriorized via ampulla of Vater, common bile duct, and cystic duct stump. Hypaque was slowly injected through tube and showed pancreatic duct (upper arrow) to be of about average diameter for normal glands.

Radiographs and legends courtesy Dr. M. H. Worth, Jr.

REFLUX METHOD

Operative pancreatography performed by the reflux method, described by Hays[1] and Clemett,[2] differs from operative cholangiography (pages 692 and 693) only in that the sphincter of Oddi is closed by an intravenous injection of morphine sulfate administered about ten seconds before the injection of the contrast medium into the cystic or common bile duct. Satisfactory reflux filling of the pancreatic duct system is reported to have occurred in over two-thirds of the examinations that were attempted by this method.[1, 2] One or more contrast studies (called *pancreaticograms*) are exposed at the direction of the surgeon and during temporary respiratory arrest, which the anesthetist induces for the purpose.

TRANSDUODENAL METHOD

Transduodenal pancreatography, first performed by Doubilet,[3, 4] requires that the duodenum be incised (duodenotomy) to expose the duodenal papilla for transpapillary catheterization of the main pancreatic duct. An ampullar sphincterotomy is performed routinely by some surgeons but is performed by others only when required for localization of the orifice of the duct. A fine plastic catheter is passed into the distal end of the duct for a distance of 3 or 4 cm. Following intubation, a syringe containing the contrast medium is attached to the catheter, and the contrast medium is slowly injected. The anesthetist induces temporary respiratory arrest for the exposures, which are made as directed by the surgeon while he maintains injection pressure with the syringe. When the catheter is left in situ for postoperative drainage, follow-up studies are usually made.

Doubilet and associates stated that in the presence of acute inflammation of the pancreas, the contrast medium extravasates through the duct walls, so that the acinar tissue of the involved area, as well as the duct system, becomes opacified. In the absence of inflammation, only the ducts are visualized unless the parenchyma is deliberately opacified by serial injections of the contrast medium.

[1]Hays, Mark A.: Operative pancreatography, Surg. Gynec. Obstet. **110**:404-408, 1960.
[2]Clemett, Arthur R.: Examination of the pancreas. In Margulis, A. R., and Burhenne, H. J., editors: Alimentary tract roentgenology, St. Louis, 1967, The C. V. Mosby Co.
[3]Doubilet, H., Poppel, M. H., and Mulholland, J. H.: Pancreatography: techniques, principles, and observations, Radiology **64**:325-339, 1955.
[4]Doubilet, H., Poppel, M. H., and Mulholland, J. H.: Pancreatography, Ann. N. Y. Acad. Sci. **78**:829-851, 1959.

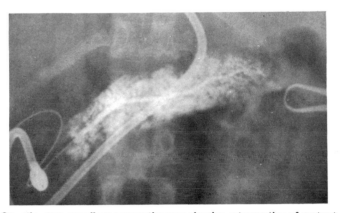

Operative transampullary pancreaticogram showing extravasation of contrast material into parenchymal tissue due to inflammation.

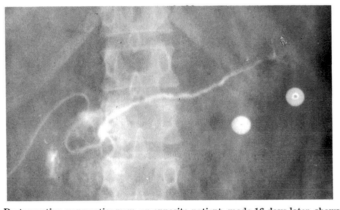

Postoperative pancreaticogram on opposite patient, made 16 days later, shows dramatic reduction in extravasation due to recovery from pancreatitis.

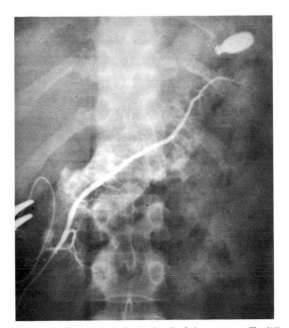

This patient had a discrete mass in the head of the pancreas. To differentiate carcinoma from pancreatitis, pancreas was deliberately opacified by three serial injections of 4 ml. of 50% Hypaque.

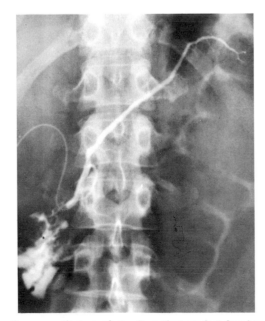

Postoperative pancreaticogram of opposite patient, made 5 days later, demonstrates subsidence of inflammation and a normal duct of Wirsung.

Radiographs and diagnostic information courtesy Dr. M. H. Worth, Jr.

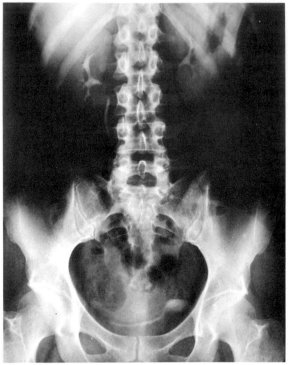

Three-minute urogram.

BILIARY AND URINARY TRACTS
Simultaneous cholegraphy and urography

Simultaneous cholecystocholangiography (cholegraphy) and urography is the term used to denote the single-stage radiologic examination of the biliary and urinary tracts. For this procedure, two of the iodinated organic compounds selectively excreted by the liver and the kidneys are combined for simultaneous intravenous administration. A commercially prepared combination of two such media is now available under the trade name of Duografin. This preparation is a combination of Renografin and Cholografin methylglucamine, and is supplied in 50 ml. ampules, which is the usual adult dose.

Shehadi[1] recommends this combined examination of the biliary and urinary tracts for general survey purposes, for a differential diagnosis of right upper quadrant masses, and for the investigation of ill-defined right-sided symptoms.

The preparation of the patient requires a combination of the measures used for intravenous urography and those for cholangiography. That is, the patient receives one or two fatty meals on the preceding day and a vegetable cathartic in the evening, and undergoes a 12- to 14-hour period of dehydration; breakfast is omitted.

The examination is preceded by an anteroposterior projection of the abdomen on a 14″ × 17″ film, and a posteroanterior projection of the gallbladder region on a 10″ × 12″ film. The injection procedure is the same as for an individual examination of either tract.

[1]Shehadi, William H.: Clinical radiology of the biliary tract, New York, 1963, McGraw-Hill Book Co.

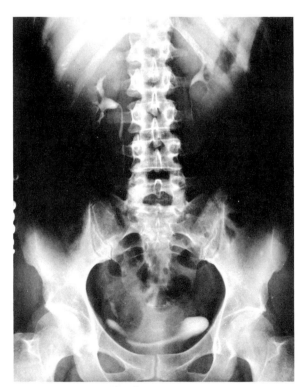

Six-minute urogram.

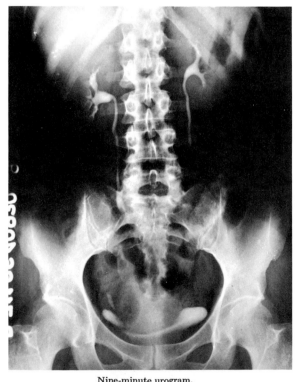

Nine-minute urogram.

Radiographs courtesy Dr. William H. Shehadi.

Urograms are exposed at postinjection intervals of three, six, and nine minutes. An erect film and a postmicturition film of the bladder are conveniently made between the serial studies of the biliary ducts. Unless renal excretion is delayed, this usually completes the urographic series.

Cholangiograms, with the patient adjusted in the right anteroposterior oblique position, are exposed at ten-minute postinjection intervals until satisfactory visualization is obtained.

Upon satisfactory visualization of the gallbladder, the examination is completed in the usual manner. Opacifica-

tion of the gallbladder usually requires two hours, but it may occur as early as thirty minutes after the injection.

Opacification of the two tracts normally occurs with the filling of the upper urinary tract preceding that of the bile ducts by a few minutes. Any overlapping shadows of the anteriorly placed biliary ducts and those of the posteriorly placed renal structures can be readily separated by suitable rotation. Separation is usually accomplished with the right anteroposterior oblique position. Additional views of either tract may be made, as required by the findings, while the examination is in progress.

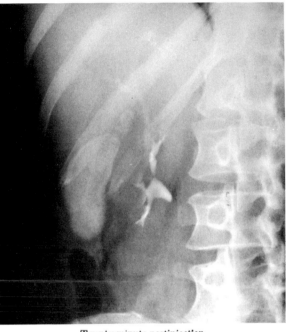

Twenty-minute postinjection.

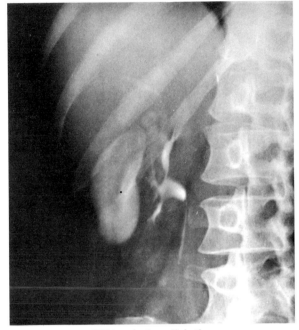

Thirty-minute postinjection.

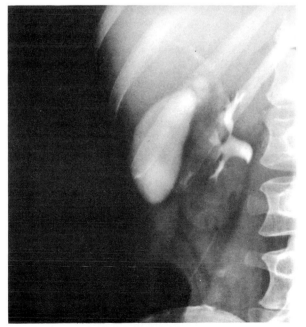

Forty-minute postinjection.

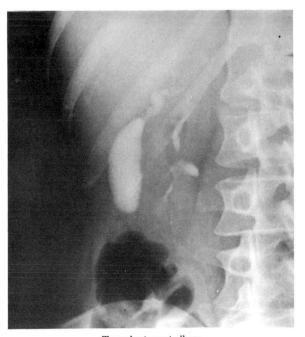

Ten-minute post cibum.

Radiographs courtesy Dr. William H. Shehadi.

699

ALIMENTARY TRACT

The specialized procedures commonly employed in radiologic examinations of the esophagus, the stomach, and the intestines will be discussed in this section. The esophagus extends between the pharynx and the cardiac end of the stomach and occupies a constant position in the posterior part of the mediastinum, where its roentgenographic demonstration presents little difficulty beyond requiring an artificial contrast medium. On the other hand, the stomach and intestines vary in size, shape, position, and muscular tonus according to the patient's habitus. In addition to the normal structural and functional differences, there is an extensive variety of gastrointestinal abnormalities, many of which cause further changes in location and motility. These variations make the investigation of each gastrointestinal patient an individual study, and meticulous attention must be given to each detail in the examination procedure.

The radiologist carries out examinations of the alimentary tract by a combination of radioscopy and radiography. The radioscopic examination enables him to observe the tract in motion, to make special mucosal studies, and to determine the subsequent procedure required for a complete examination. Films are exposed, as indicated, during and after the radioscopic examination for a permanent record of the findings.

CONTRAST MEDIA

Since the thin-walled alimentary tract does not have sufficient density to cast its shadow through those of the surrounding structures, its roentgenographic demonstration requires the use of an artificial contrast medium. *Barium sulfate*, which is a highly insoluble salt of the metallic element barium, is the contrast substance universally employed in examinations of the alimentary tract. The barium sulfate used for this purpose is a specially prepared, chemically pure product and is supplied in sealed drums clearly labeled "barium sulfate for x-ray diagnosis." All the salts of barium that are soluble in water, or that can be brought into solution by the acids of the gastric secretions, are poisonous. Therefore, it is essential that the barium sulfate introduced into the body be specially prepared, and that it contain no trace of the soluble salts of barium, since these preparations are active poisons. For this reason, when a patient is required to take a contrast meal at home in preparation for a double-meal examination, the barium sulfate should be dispensed by the radiology department.

The powdered, chalklike barium sulfate is mixed with a dispersion, or suspension, medium, usually plain water, in a ratio by volume that depends upon the region to be examined and upon the preference of the radiologist. It should be explained to the student that the term *solution* is frequently but erroneously applied to these fluid preparations. A solution is composed of two or more soluble substances that have been dissolved and molecularly dispersed through one another, the active ingredients of the solutes being released for absorption. To bring barium sulfate particles into solution would be to release their poisons. The student should, therefore, understand that barium sulfate particles are *not dissolved* but are *merely suspended* in the dispersion medium.

There are a number of special barium sulfate products on the market. Those with finely divided barium sulfate particles tend to resist settling out, to stay in suspension longer, than the regular preparation. These micro-divided bariums are generally referred to as colloidal preparations, although it is doubtful whether the particles are fine enough to fall within the colloidal range of 0.1 micrometer to 1 picometer. The special preparations contain gums or other suspending or dispersing agents, and are referred to as suspended, or flocculation-resistant, preparations. Most radiologists favor the special preparations; others prefer to formulate their own preparations, and still others prefer to use plain barium sulfate–water mixtures.

The rate of speed with which the barium mixture passes through the alimentary tract depends upon the suspending medium, the temperature, and the consistency of the

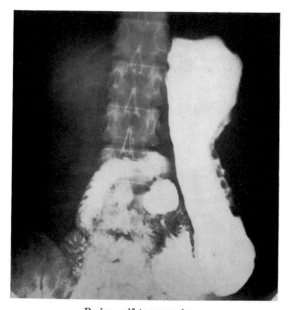

Barium sulfate suspension.
Courtesy Dr. Marcy L. Sussman.

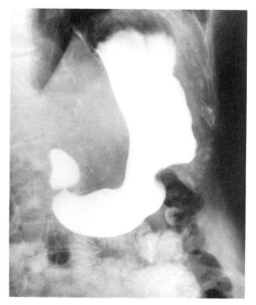

Water-soluble iodinated solution.
Courtesy Dr. William H. Shehadi.

preparation as well as upon the motile function of the tract. For this reason, it is important that the barium sulfate and the suspending medium be measured according to the radiologist's formula for the given region, and that there be no variation of the formula between cases, so that motility comparisons will be accurate. Barium preparations must be mixed thoroughly to keep the heavy barium powder in suspension, and must be stirred just before ingestion or injection. A more stable suspension of plain barium sulfate–water mixtures can be obtained by preparing them a day in advance of their use. This can be done with complete safety because chemically pure barium sulfate particles are insoluble in water, so that the mixtures can be stored several days without deterioration. Preparing the mixtures in advance has the further advantage of freeing time for other activities during the usual early morning rush. When the mixture is chilled overnight in a refrigerator, its chalky taste is less unpalatable. Where it is the practice to administer cold barium enemas (41° F.), the full amount of water can be added and the mixture can then be chilled overnight.

When a barium sulfate mixture contains any agent other than plain water, the importance of discarding leftover mixtures and of thoroughly cleansing the mixing equipment cannot be overstressed. This precaution is necessary because suspending and flavoring agents form a rich culture medium for the growth of bacteria.[1]

The barium sulfate formula commonly used for the different portions of the alimentary tract will be discussed under the respective regional headings.

Because of inspissation in the colon, barium sulfate may become hardened and caked and thus difficult to evacuate. For this reason, each patient should be instructed to take a suitable laxative upon completion of the examination. When a laxative is contraindicated, he should be instructed to take mineral oil and/or to force fluids until his stools are free of all traces of white.

Water-soluble, iodinated contrast media suitable for opacification of the alimentary tract have been in the process of development during the past decade. The iodinated preparations that are now available for this purpose are modifications of basic intravenous urographic media such as diatrizoate sodium (Hypaque) and diatrizoate methylglucamine (Renografin). The alimentary tract forms of these two agents are termed, respectively, oral Hypaque and Gastrografin. Gastrografin is supplied in liquid form; oral Hypaque is available in both liquid and powder form, the powder being preferable where storage space is limited. Mixing directions accompany the packages.

Since the basic urographic compounds are thin, nonadherent solutions, their adaptation to examinations of the alimentary tract is improved by the addition of an emulsifier (a wetting agent or Tween) to render them sufficiently cohesive for satisfactory mucosal delineation. These iodinated preparations may be used for both oral[2] and rectal[3] administration. They are reported to be nontoxic and practically nonabsorbable from the gastrointestinal mucosa. Shehadi[3] reported that out of over 1,500 patients examined with the iodinated media, he noted renal visualization in only two patients. In these two, because of an obstruction in the small bowel, there was prolonged stasis of the medium in the presence of abnormal intestinal mucosa.

The iodinated solutions move through the gastrointestinal tract more quickly than do barium sulfate suspensions. The iodinated solution normally clears the stomach in one to two hours; the entire contrast column reaches and outlines the colon in about four hours. Radiologists report

[1]Amberg, J. R., and Unger, J. D.: Contamination of barium sulfate suspension, Radiology 97:182-183, 1970.
[2]Shehadi, William H.: Orally administered water-soluble iodinated contrast media, Amer. J. Roentgen. 83:1033 041, 1060.
[3]Shehadi, William H.: Studies of the colon and small intestines with water-soluble iodinated contrast media, Amer. J. Roentgen. 89:740-751, 1963.

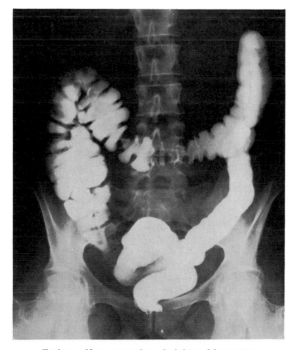

Barium sulfate suspension administered by rectum.
Courtesy Dr. Marcy L. Sussman.

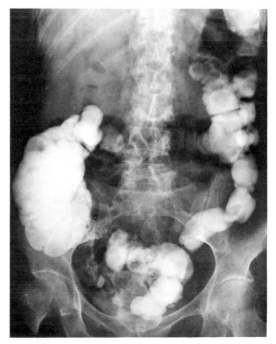

Water-soluble iodinated solution administered by mouth.
Courtesy Dr. William H. Shehadi.

701

that the orally administered iodinated medium has the following additional advantages:

1. It satisfactorily outlines the esophagus, although it does not adhere to the mucosa as well as a barium sulfate suspension does.

2. It affords an entirely satisfactory examination of the stomach and duodenum, including mucosal delineation.

3. It permits an excellent rapid survey of the entire small bowel, although it fails to provide clear anatomic detail of this portion of the tract because, due to the medium's property of absorbing water, it here undergoes dilution, with considerable decrease in opacification. Because of this water-absorbing property, Shehadi[1] recommends that caution be exercised in administering these iodinated media orally to infants, to elderly people, and to patients who are seriously ill and/or dehydrated.

4. Due to the normal function of rapid water absorption through the colonic mucosa, it again becomes densely concentrated, with the result that it delineates the entire large bowel almost as well as does a retrograde filling with a barium sulfate suspension. Because of this result and its accelerated transit time, a reasonably rapid investigation of the large bowel by the oral route can be performed when

[1]Shehadi, William H.: Personal communication.

a patient cannot cooperate for a satisfactory enema study.

A great advantage of the water-soluble media, one that makes them highly satisfactory for presurgical explorations, is that they are easily removable by aspiration either before or during surgery. Furthermore, if the water-soluble, iodinated medium escapes into the peritoneum through a preexisting perforation of the stomach or intestine, no ill effects will result, and the medium is readily absorbed from the peritoneal cavity and excreted by the kidneys. This is a definite advantage when investigating perforated ulcers. Another advantage is that water-soluble media are not subject to inspissation in the colon. This feature eliminates the all-too-familiar concern with prompt egestion of barium sulfate suspensions in order to prevent the occurrence of a serious barium impaction.

The chief drawback of the iodinated preparations is their strongly bitter taste. It can be masked to some extent, however, by using a carbonated soft drink such as ginger ale to dilute the liquid and to dissolve the powder. The patient should be forewarned, so that, knowing what to expect, he will be better able to tolerate the bitter taste. A second drawback is that the rectally administered iodinated medium is not evacuated completely enough to permit a double-contrast study of the colon mucosa.

RADIOLOGIC APPARATUS

Revolutionary advances have been made in the design and scope of modern radiologic equipment. The radioscopic image intensifier with cine camera and miniature still camera attachments, remote control of the patient's position as well as of the equipment, and a television viewing arrangement permit the radiologist to conduct both the radioscopic and the filming phases of examinations from an adjoining room. Intensification of the radioscopic image by 3,000 to 5,000 times is achieved with a low current, which appreciably reduces radiation to the patient. Conventional radioscopy requires the use of 3 to 5 milliamperes in a totally darkened room, whereas the image intensifier produces a clear, bright image with the use of 0.5 to 1.5 milliamperes in a partially lighted room. Unfortunately, these units are not yet in general use; therefore, the following comments on standard equipment will be retained.

Most radiology departments have a combination radioscopic-radiographic unit with a spot-film device and an automatic change-over switch that permits instantaneous exposures of small areas during radioscopy. The spot-film device is attached to the radioscopic screen, and depending upon its design, as many as four exposures can be made on one 8″ × 10″ film. The device has a small radioparent compression cone so that, by manual pressure over the desired region of the stomach or intestinal tract, the bulk of the contained barium sulfate mixture can be displaced for localized mucosal studies. The cone is detachable or displaceable to permit a shorter part-film distance for noncompression studies. The commercially designed spot-film devices incorporate a special switch that automatically changes the current-voltage settings from radioscopy to predetermined radiographic values when the cassette is shifted into exposure position.

There are many types of serialographs (also called polygraphs and multigraphs) for making localized serial studies on one film either with or without compression. These devices are used with the overhead tube. They consist of a large leaded shield with a central exposure aperture, over which is attached a small, gum-rubber bag enclosed in a canvas band (called a Chaoul pneumatic compression apparatus). The leaded shield may be placed on the table for Potter-Bucky exposures, as first described by Taylor,[1] or the device may be built onto a cassette-changing tunnel. The radiologist, using radioscopic control, positions the patient over the serialograph, centers the desired area to the exposure aperture, and applies the desired degree of pressure by inflating the compression bladder with the attached hand bulb.

The technologist should be familiar with both the routine and the specialized examination procedures, and the equipment and the compression devices employed by his radiologist, so that, with adequate preparation, he can prevent unnecessary delays during an examination.

PREPARATION OF EXAMINING ROOM

The examining room should be completely prepared, a careful check should be made for any light leaks, and the patient should be brought into the room before the radiologist is called to start the examination. In the preparation of the room, the technologist should (1) test the apparatus and adjust the controls to the usual settings, (2) have the footboard and shoulder support ready for attachment when needed, (3) check the mechanism of the spot-film device and see that there are sufficient films ready for use, (4) prepare the required amount of each barium mixture formula to be used, and (5) set up the utility table with the items likely to be needed according to the condition of the patient or patients to be examined.

Where a large volume of this work is done, it is convenient to place the basic creamy barium sulfate mixture in a large pitcher so that the mixture can be stirred and dispensed as needed. The thicker mixtures, especially the paste, are best placed in individual containers. It is desirable to have disposable cups in sizes of 4 or 6 ounces, and of 10 or 12 ounces. When nondisposable containers are used, they must be carefully washed and scalded after each use, and, in addition, they must be boiled after they have been used for infectious patients. The utility table should be stocked with (1) long-handled spoons of the iced

[1]Taylor, Henry K.: Potter-Bucky table adapted for multiple exposures, Radiology 10:506-509, 1928.

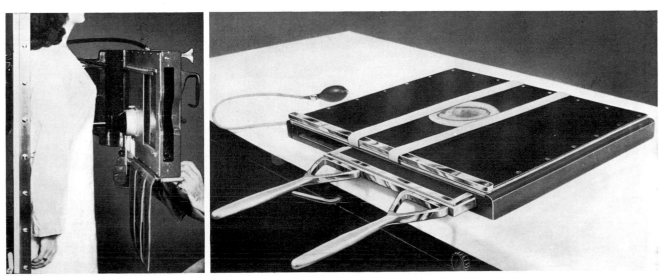

Spot-film device.   Polygraph.

PREPARATION OF EXAMINING ROOM—cont'd

tea and dessert variety, for stirring and for feeding the heavy mixtures by spoon, (2) flexible drinking straws for use when the patient is recumbent (they are safer than glass tubes and are disposable), (3) a dressing jar of small cotton tufts or pledgets for pharyngoesophageal studies, (4) a small decanter of water (before making the "toe touch" test on patients with hiatal hernia or esophageal regurgitation, the patient is given several swallows of water to clear the esophagus of barium), (5) a box of tissues for the patient's use and to pick up small spills, (6) emesis basins and disposable towels, and (7) waste basins or paper waste bags.

Either before or when the patient is brought into the examining room for the preliminary film of his abdomen, the technologist should explain that the barium sulfate meal he is to drink will taste neither good nor bad, just chalky. The patient should also be informed that the room may be darkened during radioscopy and that the doctor may enter wearing colored goggles for the purpose of protecting the dark adaptation of his eyes. Further explanations of the procedure are best made by the physician as the need arises.

When the radiologist enters the examining room, and before the white light is turned off or dimmed, the patient and the doctor should be introduced to each other.

The technologist may be required to be present during radioscopy to administer the contrast medium as directed, to take care of the patient, and otherwise to assist as needed. Where this is the practice, the technologist must wear a leaded apron.

RADIATION PROTECTION

During radioscopy, spot filming, and conventional filming in either a partial or a complete gastrointestinal examination, radiation to the patient is at best, but of necessity, considerable. It is taken for granted that proper added filtration is at all times in place under every x-ray tube in the radiology department. It is further assumed that, based upon the capacity of the machines and the best available accessory equipment, the exposure factors are adjusted to deliver the least possible radiation to the patient. The technologist's responsibility, then, lies in the application of local gonadal shielding when feasible and in avoiding repeat exposures through accurate positioning and close coning and through clearly instructing the patient.

EXPOSURE TIME

One of the most important considerations in gastrointestinal radiography is the elimination of motion. The highest degree of motor activity is normally found in the stomach and the upper part of the small intestine, the activity gradually decreasing along the intestinal tract until it becomes fairly sluggish in the lower part of the large bowel. Peristaltic speed also depends upon the individual patient's habitus, and it is influenced by the presence of pathology, by body position, and by respiration. The choice of the exposure time for each region must be based upon these factors.

In esophageal examinations the exposure time should be 0.1 second or less for erect projections. The time may be slightly longer for recumbent projections because, moving against gravity, the barium meal descends more slowly. The rate of passage of the meal through the esophagus is fairly slow if the meal is swallowed at the end of full inhalation, is increased if the meal is swallowed at the end of moderate inhalation, and passes through the upper part rapidly but is delayed in the lower part for several seconds if the meal is swallowed at the end of full exhalation. Respiration is inhibited for several seconds after the beginning of deglutition, thus allowing sufficient time for the exposure to be made without instructing the patient to hold his breath after swallowing.

In examinations of the stomach and small intestine, the exposure time for patients who have normal peristaltic activity should be 0.2 second, in no case more than 0.5 second, and it should be 0.1 second for those who have hypermotility. In examinations of the large bowel, exposure times of 0.5 to 1 second may be used for frontal and oblique projections of the entire colon, and exposure times of 1.5 to 2 seconds may be used for lateral and axial (Chassard-Lapiné) projections of the rectosigmoid region. Exposures of the stomach and intestines are made at the end of exhalation in the routine procedure.

Mucosal studies are usually made without the use of a Potter-Bucky diaphragm in order to obtain better soft tissue detail, secondary radiation being minimized with a small cone. Where the exposure field cannot be limited with a small cone, contrast is unquestionably improved with the Potter-Bucky diaphragm.

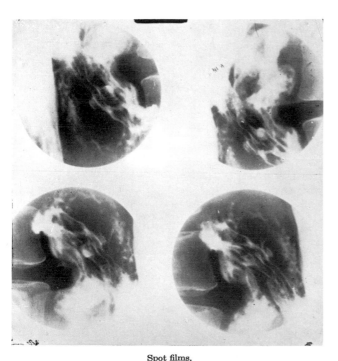

Spot films.

Courtesy Dr. Marcy L. Sussman.

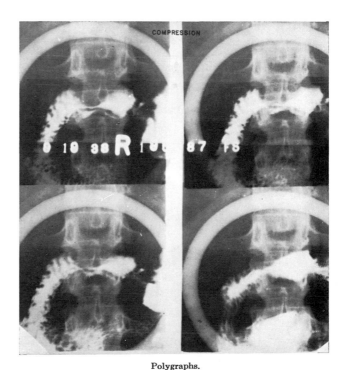

Polygraphs.

Courtesy Dr. Francis H. Ghiselin.

705

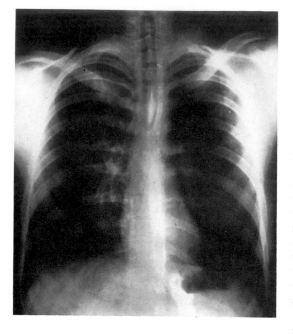

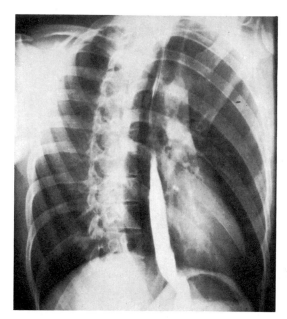

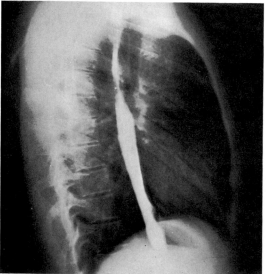

Erect studies.

Radiographs courtesy Dr. Ross Golden.

ESOPHAGUS

When only the esophagus is to be examined, which requires a procedure frequently referred to as a "barium swallow," no preliminary preparation of the patient is required.

BARIUM SULFATE PREPARATIONS

The radiologist usually begins the radioscopic examination of the esophagus with a thin barium sulfate mixture for the detection of strictures, and then completes the investigation with a heavy barium paste for the detection of intraluminal lesions. The thin meal ordinarily contains barium sulfate and water in equal parts by volume, the consistency of the mixture being about that of cream. The heavy meal must be considerably thicker, about the consistency of cooked cereal, so that it will descend slowly, and adhere to and coat the esophageal mucosa. This requires three or four parts of barium sulfate to one part of water. Gelatin capsules (sizes 0 and 00) filled with barium sulfate are sometimes used to demonstrate an obstruction. Tufts or pledgets of cotton saturated with a thin barium mixture are used for the same purpose and also for the detection of nonopaque foreign bodies in the pharynx and upper esophagus.

A double-contrast effect can be obtained by following up a swallow of thick barium mixture with a swallow of water or of heavy mineral oil. The "perforated straw technique" suggested by Amplatz[1] is used by many examiners. For this method, a perforation is made in a paper or plastic drinking straw so that air will be swallowed with the barium mixture. According to the thickness of the barium suspension, the size of the hole should be as small as possible to allow the formation of only small air bubbles within the barium meal.

Opaque foreign bodies lodged in the pharynx or in the upper part of the esophagus can usually be demonstrated without the use of a contrast medium. A soft tissue lateral film of the neck (page 608) and/or a lateral film of the retrosternal area (page 630) is taken for this purpose. Epstein[2] recommends that a lateral neck film be taken at the height of deglutition for the delineation of opaque foreign bodies in the upper end of the intrathoracic esophagus. This portion of the esophagus is then elevated a distance of two cervical segments, which places it above the level of the clavicles (see illustrations on page 609).

EXAMINATION PROCEDURE

The radioscopic and spot-film examination is started with the patient in the erect position whenever possible; afterward, the horizontal and Trendelenburg positions are used as indicated. After the radioscopic examination of the heart and lungs, and when the patient is in the erect position, he is asked to take the glass containing the thin meal in his left hand and to drink it as directed by the radiologist.

The radiologist has the patient swallow several mouthfuls of the meal as he observes the act of deglutition and determines whether there is any abnormality demonstrable with the thin mixture. He may have the patient perform the "toe-touch" maneuver[3] for the demonstration of esophageal regurgitation or of a suspected hiatal hernia; because this test causes only momentary displacement of the contrast medium, the result is not easily recorded other than by spot films or by cineradiography. The technologist administers the thick meal as directed, feeding it to the patient a spoonful at a time. The physician has the patient perform most of the breathing maneuvers under radioscopic observation so that he can make spot film studies of areas and/or lesions not otherwise easily demonstrated.

[1]Amplatz, K.: A new and simple approach to air-contrast studies of the stomach and duodenum, Radiology **70**:392-394, 1958.

[2]Epstein, Bernard S.: A roentgenographic aid to the diagnosis of radiopaque foreign bodies in the upper intrathoracic esophagus, Amer. J. Roentgen. **73**:115-117, 1955.

[3]Lawler, N. A., and McCreath, N. D.: Gastroesophageal regurgitation, Lancet **2A**:369-374, 1951.

ESOPHAGUS

Film: 14″ × 17″ placed lengthwise and centered at the level of the fifth or sixth thoracic vertebra for the inclusion of the entire esophagus.

Positions employed

The routine chest positions (posteroanterior, oblique, and lateral, pages 634 to 639) are employed in examinations of the esophagus. Because it is possible to obtain a wider clear space for an unobstructed view of the esophagus between the vertebrae and the heart with a 35- to 40-degree right posteroanterior oblique position (right anteroposterior oblique view), this is usually used in preference to the left oblique position.

Unless another position is specified, the patient is placed in the recumbent position for esophageal studies. This body position is used for the purpose of obtaining more complete contrast filling of the esophagus, especially of the upper part, by means of having the barium column flow against gravity. The recumbent position is always used for the demonstration of variceal distentions of the esophageal veins because the best filling of the varices is obtained by having the blood flow against gravity. Variceal filling is more complete during increased venous pressure, which may be applied by full exhalation or by the Valsalva maneuver.

Filming procedure

The barium sulfate mixture is fed to the patient either by spoon or through a drinking straw, depending upon its consistency. The patient is asked to swallow several mouthfuls of the meal in rapid succession and then to hold a mouthful until immediately before the exposure.

1. For the demonstration of esophageal varices the patient is asked (a) to *exhale fully*, and then to swallow the barium bolus and avoid inhaling until the exposure has been made, or (b) to take a deep breath and, while holding the breath, to swallow the bolus and then perform the Valsalva maneuver (page 603).

Feist and Riley[1] recommend dynamic studies (cinefluorography) as being more accurate in the identification of early or small varices, and in the differentiation of vascular and nonvascular abnormalities. They state that the minimal mucosal irregularities produced by small abnormalities can be missed by radioscopy and static (still-film) exposures but that they can be clearly defined against a moving stream of contrast medium.

2. For other conditions, the patient is simply instructed to swallow the barium bolus, which he normally does on moderate inhalation. Because respiration is inhibited for about two seconds following deglutition, it is not necessary to instruct the patient to hold his breath for the exposure. Two or three exposures can be made in rapid succession before the contrast meal passes into the stomach if it is swallowed at the end of full inhalation. On the other hand, the demonstration of the entire esophagus sometimes requires that the exposure be made while the patient is drinking the barium mixture through a tube in rapid and continuous swallows.

Central ray

The central ray is directed perpendicularly to the midpoint of the film.

[1]Feist, J. H., and Riley, R. R.: Diagnosis of esophageal varices, Radiology **93:**861-866, 1969.

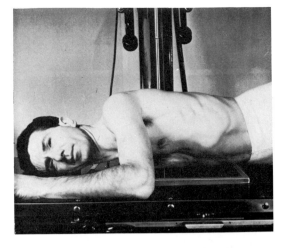

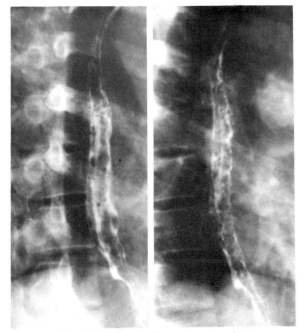

Spot-film studies showing esophageal varices.

Courtesy Dr. Robert L. Pinck.

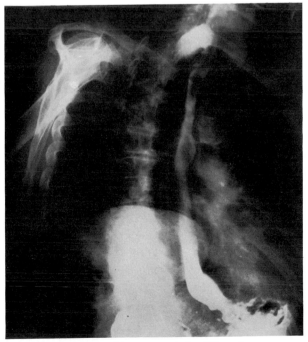

Recumbent right anteroposterior oblique view.

Courtesy Dr. William H. Shehadi.

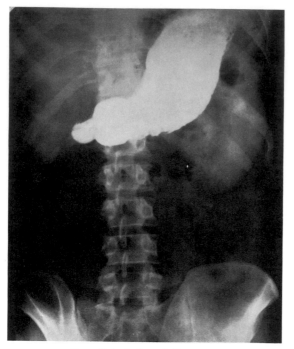

Immediate single-meal film.

Courtesy Dr. Henry K. Taylor.

GASTROINTESTINAL TRACT

G.I. series

A routine gastrointestinal examination, usually called a G.I. series, includes the following:

1. A supine film of the abdomen, to delineate the liver, the spleen, the kidneys, the psoas muscles, and the included bony structures, and to detect any abdominal or pelvic calcifications or tumor masses. The detection of calcifications and tumor masses requires that the survey film of the abdomen be taken following any preliminary cleansing of the intestinal tract and that it be taken after micturition.

2. An initial examination consisting of radioscopic and serial radiographic studies of the esophagus and the stomach and duodenum with an injested opaque meal, usually a barium sulfate meal.

3. When indicated, a small-intestine study consisting of films made at frequent intervals during the passage of the contrast column.

A routine gastrointestinal examination may also include (1) a gastric motility study several hours after the ingestion of the meal, at which time the appendix and the ileocecal region may be examined, and (2) a large-intestine study made about twenty-four hours after the ingestion of the meal. The heart and lungs and the diaphragm are examined radioscopically, and conventional film studies are made when indicated. Progress studies and examinations of patients with a clinically localized lesion may be restricted to any part of the alimentary tract, and the examination procedure is adjusted accordingly.

The radiologist usually examines acutely ill patients, such as those with a bleeding ulcer, in the supine position by a radioscopic and spot-film procedure that is similar to that described by Hampton.[1] Because these examinations are emergencies, everything possible must be done to expedite the procedure. Any special contrast preparation must be ready, and the examination room must be fully prepared before the patient is brought into the radiology department.

[1]Hampton, A. O.: A safe method for the roentgen demonstration of bleeding duodenal ulcers, Amer. J. Roentgen. **38**:565-570, 1937.

PREPARATION OF PATIENT

Before assigning an appointment to a patient, especially for an examination so time-consuming as a gastrointestinal series, he should be told the approximate time required for the procedure so that he will be able to arrange his schedule accordingly. It is also important that the patient understand the reasons for preliminary preparation so that he will give his full cooperation.

The stomach must be empty for an examination of the upper gastrointestinal tract (the stomach and small intestine). It is also desirable to have the colon free of gas and fecal material. In the presence of costive bowel action, a nongas-forming cathartic may be administered thirty-six hours before the examination. When a cathartic is contraindicated, several cleansing enemas may be ordered. The usual preparation consists of placing the patient on a soft or low-residue diet for two days to prevent gas formation as a result of excessive fermentation of the intestinal contents, and of having him take an enema of normal saline solution or of plain warm water the evening before the examination. To ensure an empty stomach, both food and water are withheld after midnight, for a period of eight or nine hours prior to the examination. When a small-intestine study is to be made, food and fluid are withheld after the evening meal.

Because it is believed that nicotine stimulates gastric secretion as well as salivation, many radiologists withhold smoking after midnight. This restriction is made to prevent an excessive accumulation of fluid in the stomach from diluting the barium suspension enough to interfere with its coating property. When an excessive amount of fluid is present it may be withdrawn with a nasogastric tube before proceeding with the examination.

Patients who are released from the radiology department between the initial examination and the motility studies must be cautioned to take nothing by mouth in the interim.

Upon completion of any examination involving the administration of barium sulfate suspensions, the radiologist usually has the patient instructed to cleanse his intestinal tract of the medium in order to prevent the occurrence of a barium impaction. When a cathartic is contraindicated, the patient may be advised to drink water freely (the equivalent of eight glassfuls per day) and to take mineral oil each night until his stools are clear of all traces of white. He should also be advised to take a cleansing enema if the stools become costive.

BARIUM SULFATE MIXTURE

The formula that is generally used in routine gastrointestinal examinations is barium sulfate and water in equal parts by volume, the consistency of the preparation being about that of cream. Some radiologists add a flavoring substance to render the mixture more palatable. Others add a little powdered gum acacia to sustain the suspension. The preparation must be mixed thoroughly, preferably with an electric mixer, and must be stirred just before ingestion.

Many radiologists prefer to use one of the commercially prepared barium meals. These products are obtainable in several flavors, and some are conveniently packaged in individual plastic cups containing the dry ingredients. One has only to add water, recap the cup, and shake it to obtain a smooth mixture and the meal is ready for use.

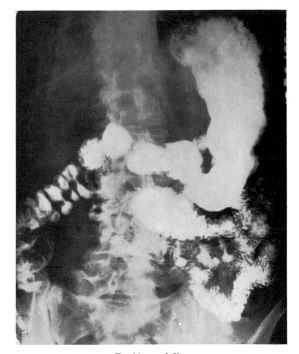

Double-meal film.

Courtesy Dr. Sidney S. Weintraub.

EXAMINATION PROCEDURE

Of the two general gastrointestinal examination procedures, the single-meal method is more widely used than the double-meal method. In the latter procedure, which will be only briefly described, the patient is given the first barium sulfate meal four to six hours preceding, and the second meal during, the initial radioscopic examination. The emptying time of the stomach and the progress of the contrast column through the small intestine are determined by interval studies made following the first meal. The series of stomach and duodenal films and the esophageal study are usually made after the radioscopic examination. The main objection to this method is that portions of the stomach and duodenum are frequently obscured by loops of the small intestine that are filled by the first meal.

In the single-meal method, the barium sulfate meal is administered during the initial radioscopic examination. Following the immediate films of the stomach and duodenum and the esophageal study, the progress of the meal through the gastrointestinal tract is observed at specified intervals.

The radioscopic examination is started with the patient in the erect position whenever possible. The radiologist first makes a radioscopic examination of the heart and lungs, checks the excursion of the diaphragm, and observes the abdomen to determine whether there is food or fluid in the stomach. A glass of barium mixture is then placed in the patient's left hand, and he is instructed to drink it as directed by the radiologist. If the patient is in the recumbent position, the meal is administered through a drinking straw.

The radiologist has the patient swallow two or three mouthfuls of the meal, during which time he examines and makes any indicated spot films of the esophagus. By manual manipulation of the stomach through the abdominal wall, he then coats the gastric mucosa and, utilizing the gastric gas bubble, he performs a double-contrast examination of the stomach and duodenal bulb. In order to obtain more air than is normally present in the stomach, some examiners use the Amplatz "perforated straw technique" (page 706). Pochaczevsky[1] suggests carbonating the barium suspension for double-contrast delineation of the stomach. For this method, the barium suspension is poured into a soda-making dispenser, and then one or two CO_2 cartridges are released into the dispenser. Compression films, made with either a spot-film device or a polygraph, may be required at this time to demonstrate a mucosal lesion of the stomach or duodenum before further filling of the stomach.

Following the study of the rugae, and as the patient drinks the remainder of the barium meal, the radiologist observes the filling of the stomach and further examines the duodenum. He is able to determine the size, shape, and position of the stomach, to examine its changing contour during peristalsis, to observe the filling and emptying of the duodenal bulb, to detect any abnormal alteration in the function or contour of these organs, and to make spot-film studies as indicated. The nonfood contrast meal normally begins to pass into the duodenum almost im-

[1]Pochaczevsky, R.: "Bubbly barium"; a carbonated cocktail for double-contrast examination of the stomach, Radiology 107:465-466, 1973.

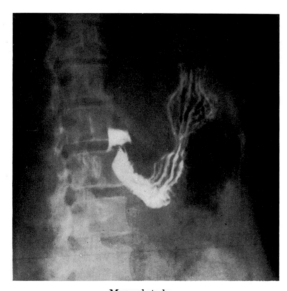

Mucosal study.

Courtesy Dr. Francis H. Ghiselin.

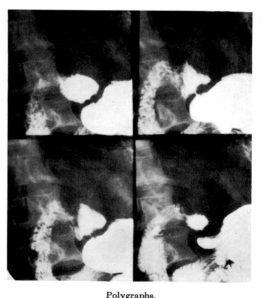

Polygraphs.

Courtesy Dr. Marcy L. Sussman.

mediately. There is sometimes a delay due to nervous tension, which can usually be relieved by having the patient suck on a hard candy drop. Radioscopy is done with the patient in both the erect and the recumbent positions, while his body is rotated and the table is angled so that all aspects of the esophagus, stomach, and duodenum are demonstrated. Spot films are exposed as indicated by the findings. If esophageal involvement is suspected, a study is made with a thick barium mixture.

The subsequent radiographs of the stomach and duodenum should be made immediately following radioscopy, before any considerable amount of the barium meal passes into the jejunum.

The radiologist can ensure accurate centering of the stomach and duodenum on small films (10″ × 12″) by making a wax pencil mark on the patient's back at the level of the pylorus. All patients should be marked in the same position, erect or prone, so that the technologist will be able to make the correct allowance for visceral movement in other body positions.

The stomach and the duodenum are examined in posteroanterior, anteroposterior, oblique, and lateral directions, with the patient in the erect and the recumbent positions, as indicated by the radioscopic findings. The following basic positions are employed:

1. An *erect* posteroanterior projection on a 14″ × 17″ film to demonstrate the type and relative position of the stomach.

2. An *erect* left lateral projection to demonstrate the left retrogastric space.

3. A *recumbent* posteroanterior projection to demonstrate the gastroduodenal surfaces situated in the frontal plane. In order to obtain this view of the transversely placed stomach, the central ray is angled toward the head (a) from 20 to 25 degrees in infants, and (b) from 35 to 45 degrees in adults.

4. One or more *recumbent* right posteroanterior oblique projections (right anteroposterior oblique views). Because gastric peristalsis is usually more active in this position, serial studies are sometimes exposed at thirty- to forty-second intervals for the delineation of the pyloric canal and the duodenal cap.

5. A *recumbent* right lateral projection. This view is used to demonstrate the duodenal loop in profile, the duodenojejunal junction, and the right retrogastric space.

6. Recumbent anteroposterior projections, usually on 11″ × 14″ films. In the supine position, sometimes aided by slight rotation toward the left, the contrast meal flows into and outlines the fundic end of the stomach, and the air bubble rises into the antral portion of the stomach and the duodenum, where it affords a double-contrast study for the investigation of lesions of the posterior wall. This body position also demonstrates the retrogastric portion of the duodenum and jejunum due to the displacement of the stomach.

Variations of the supine positions are (a) lowering the head end of the table 25 to 30 degrees to demonstrate a hiatal hernia, and (b) lowering the head end of the table 10 to 15 degrees, and rotating the patient slightly toward the right side to place the gastroesophageal junction in profile to the right of the spine. The latter position is used to demonstrate esophageal regurgitation and hiatal hernias.

Special supplemental studies for the delineation of areas and/or lesions not demonstrable in the basic projections are usually made by spot filming during radioscopy.

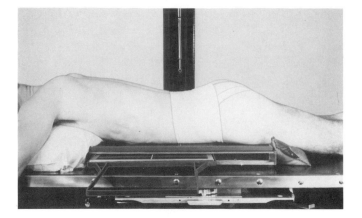

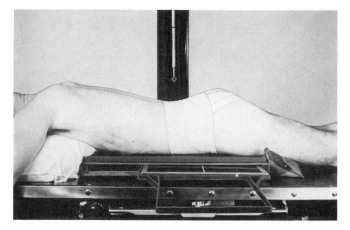

GASTROINTESTINAL TRACT
Serial and mucosal studies

Film: Depending upon the design of the polygraphic apparatus, it is possible to make four views on one 8″ × 10″ or 10″ × 12″ film, six views on one 11″ × 14″ film, and nine or twelve views on one 14″ × 17″ film.

Position of patient

The polygraphic cassette-changing tunnel or Potter-Bucky shield is placed in position, with the exposure aperture centered to the midline of the radioscopic-radiographic table, and is then immobilized. If a tunnel is used, the tray must be removed for radioscopy.

The patient is placed in the prone position, and the region to be studied is approximately centered to the exposure aperture of the polygraph.

Position of part

Using radioscopic control, the radiologist adjusts the position of the patient so that the area being examined is centered to the polygraphic aperture, and for a mucosal study, he inflates the compression bladder enough to give the desired degree of pressure. In the latter examination (the mucosal study) an immobilization band may be required to prevent rotation and thus to ensure a constant degree of pressure.

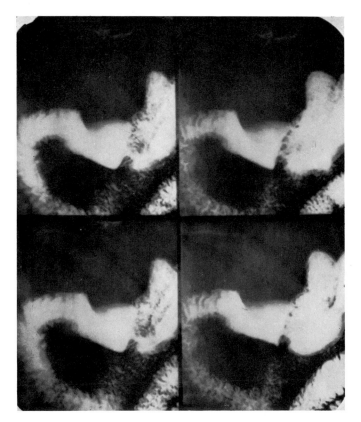

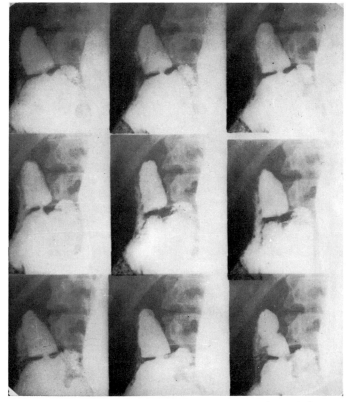

Radiographs courtesy Dr. Marcy L. Sussman.

712

GASTROINTESTINAL TRACT
Serial and mucosal studies—cont'd

Central ray

Following the radioscopic adjustments, the radioscopic screen and tube are displaced. With the central ray directed vertically, the overhead tube is centered to the exposure aperture of the polygraph.

Sequence of exposures

Place the cassette in the tray of the tunnel or Potter-Bucky diaphragm and center the right upper exposure area of the film to the polygraphic aperture. For subsequent exposures, the cassette is manually shifted in a definite order so that the sequence of views on the finished radiograph will read from above downward and from left to right.

The exposures are made at the end of exhalation unless otherwise requested by the radiologist.

Structures shown

A noncompression study of the pyloric end of the stomach and the duodenal bulb at several different stages of filling and emptying, or a compression study of the mucosa of any localized area of the gastrointestinal tract.

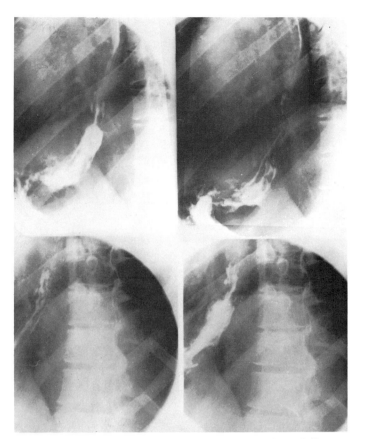

Courtesy Dr. Marcy L. Sussman.

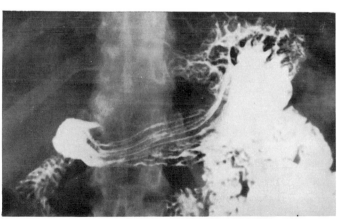

Courtesy Dr. Judah Zizmor.

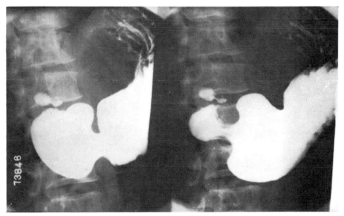

Courtesy Dr. Marcy L. Sussman.

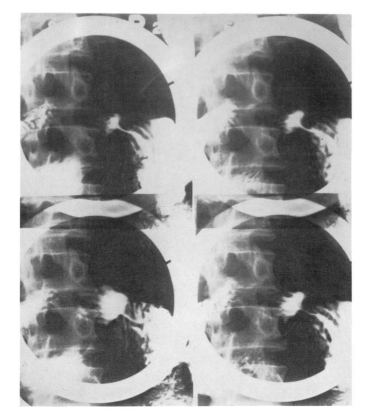

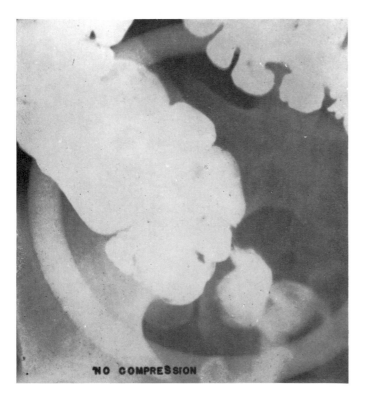

NO COMPRESSION

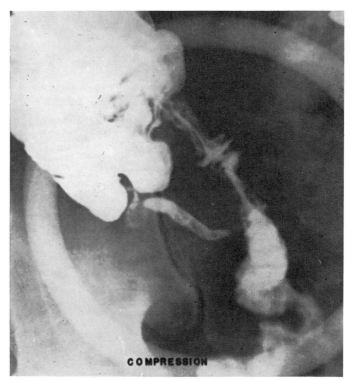

COMPRESSION

Radiographs courtesy Dr. Francis H. Ghiselin.

714

RETROGASTRIC SOFT TISSUES
Poppel method for biplane projections in supine position

Poppel[1] has recommended biplane projections of the supinely placed, barium-filled stomach, for the purpose of detecting any space-occupying lesion of the pancreas as shown by an increase in the normal width of the midline retrogastric soft tissues. Poppel specified that the stomach be completely filled so that its posterior wall will, by the weight of the barium, be placed as close as possible to the spine. In order to prevent gravitation of the barium mixture into the cardia, the projections must be made in rapid succession immediately after placing the patient in the supine position.

Poppel recommended that the lateral view, projected from left to right, be made first. Then, as quickly as possible, without moving the patient, and on the same phase of suspended respiration as was used with the lateral view, the anteroposterior projection is made.

The frontal view serves to identify the vertebral body crossed by the stomach, and the lateral view serves to demonstrate the width of the soft tissues located between that vertebral body and the segment of the stomach lying anterior to it.

Film: $10'' \times 12''$ or $11'' \times 14''$.

Exposure procedure

Because both of the views required for this examination must be made as quickly as possible after placing the patient in the supine position, all preparations for the exposure procedure must be made in advance. Without special biplane equipment, the lateral view is made by adjusting the tube to project the central ray horizontally across the table to a vertically placed cassette and wafer grid: the patient must be placed so that this projection can be made from left to right.

1. Adjust the tube in position for the horizontal projection, and have the cassette and wafer grid ready to be placed.

2. When the radiologist has filled the stomach and indicated the localization point, adjust the patient in the supine position. Center the left side of the body to the midline of the table in readiness for the second (anteroposterior) projection.

3. Place the cassette and wafer grid vertically against the right side of the body, center them to the localization point, and support them with sandbags. Center the tube, have the patient suspend respiration, and make the first exposure.

4. Place a cassette in the Potter-Bucky tray and center it to the localization mark. Readjust the position of the tube and direct the central ray vertically to the midpoint of the film.

Respiration must be suspended at the same phase for each exposure.

[1]Poppel, M. H.: Roentgen manifestation of pancreatic disease, Springfield, Ill., 1951, Charles C Thomas, Publisher.

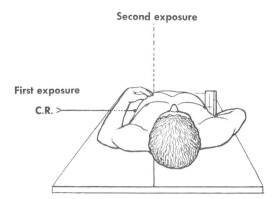

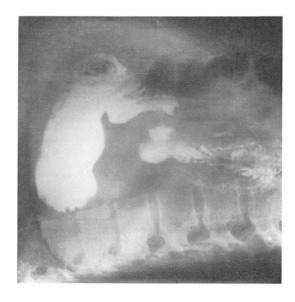

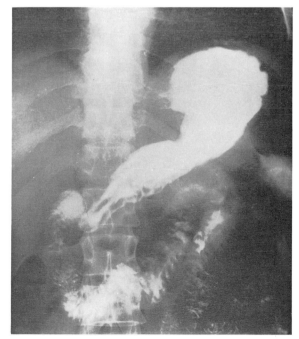

Radiographs courtesy Dr. M. H. Poppel.

715

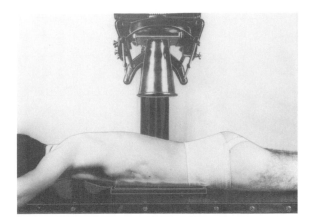

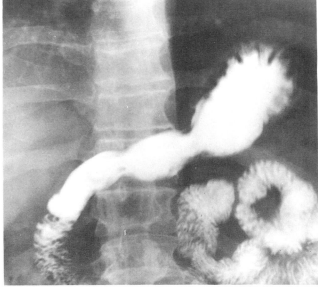

Direct posteroanterior projection.

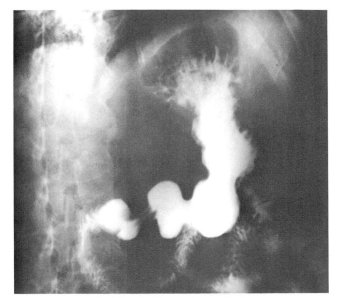

Angled projection on above patient.

Radiographs courtesy Dr. Sewell S. Gordon.

STOMACH AND DUODENUM
Posteroanterior projection
Anteroposterior view

Film: 10″ × 12″ lengthwise for recumbent projections of the average subject, 14″ × 17″ lengthwise for erect study.

Position of patient

Routine studies of the stomach and duodenum are made with the patient in the recumbent position. An erect posteroanterior projection is sometimes made to demonstrate the relative position of the stomach.

In adjusting thin patients in the prone position, the weight of the body should be supported on pillows or other suitable pads adjusted under the thorax and pelvis. This is done to prevent the stomach or duodenum from pressing against the vertebrae, with resultant pressure-filling defects.

Position of part

With the patient in the posteroanterior position, either recumbent or erect, adjust his position so that the midline of the cassette or the Potter-Bucky diaphragm will coincide (1) with a sagittal plane passing approximately 2½ inches to the left of the mark that localizes the pylorus when a 10″ × 12″ film is used, or (2) with the median sagittal plane of the body when a 14″ × 17″ film is used.

The film is centered longitudinally at the marked level, or at the estimated level, of the pylorus when the patient is prone. The centering will be 3 to 6 inches lower for erect projections. The greatest visceral movement between the prone and the erect positions occurs in asthenic patients.

Angled posteroanterior projection

Gordon[1] developed this projection to "open up" the high, transverse (hypersthenic type) stomach for the demonstration of the greater and lesser curvatures, the antral portion of the stomach, the pyloric canal, and the duodenal cap. The resultant projection gives this type of stomach much the same configuration as the average sthenic type of stomach.

The patient is placed in the prone position, with the median sagittal plane of the body centered to the midline of the table. A 14″ × 17″ film is placed lengthwise and is adjusted so that its upper edge is placed at the level of the patient's chin. The central ray is then directed to the midpoint of the film at an angle of 35 to 45 degrees toward the head. Gugliantini[2] recommends a cranial angulation of 20 to 25 degrees for the demonstration of the stomach of infants.

[1]Gordon, S. S.: The angled posteroanterior projection of the stomach; an attempt at better visualization of the high transverse stomach, Radiology **69**:393-397, 1957.

[2]Gugliantini, P.: Utilità delle incidenze oblique caudocraniali nello studio radiologico della stenosi congenita ipertrofica del piloro, Ann. Radiol. [Diagn.] **34**:56-69, 1961. Abst.: Amer. J. Roentgen. **87**:623, 1962.

STOMACH AND DUODENUM
Posteroanterior projection
Anteroposterior view—cont'd

Immobilization

Respiration is suspended at the end of exhalation unless otherwise requested by the radiologist.

An immobilization band is not employed for the routine radiographic projections of the stomach and intestines because the pressure is likely to cause filling defects, and because it interferes with the emptying and filling of the duodenal cap, which is important in serial studies.

Central ray

Except for the angled projection of the high, transverse stomach, the central ray is directed perpendicularly to the midpoint of the film.

Structures shown

An anteroposterior view (posteroanterior projection) of the contour of the barium-filled stomach and the duodenal bulb. The erect projection shows the size and shape and the relative position of the filled stomach, but it does not give an adequate demonstration of the unfilled fundic end of the organ. In the prone position, the stomach moves upward 1½ to 4 inches, according to the patient's habitus, and spreads transversely, with a comparable decrease in its length, and, except in thin subjects, the fundus usually fills.

The pyloric canal and the duodenal cap are well demonstrated in patients ranging from the asthenic to the hyposthenic type, are frequently partially obscured in patients of the sthenic type, and, except in the angled projection, are completely obscured in those of the hypersthenic type by the prepyloric portion of the stomach.

NOTE: When both body positions are to be used, the variation in the thickness of the abdomen between the erect and the prone position must be measured or accurately estimated and the exposure adjusted accordingly. The thickness change is usually 3 or 4 cm. in patients of average build, is less in thin subjects, and is considerably more in obese subjects.

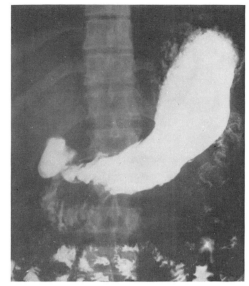
Sthenic.

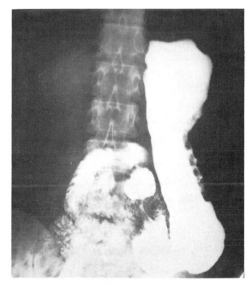
Hyposthenic.

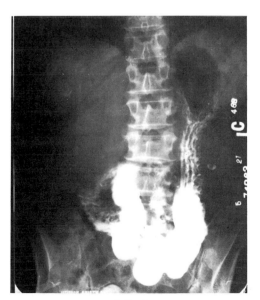
Asthenic.
Courtesy Dr. Marcy L. Sussman.

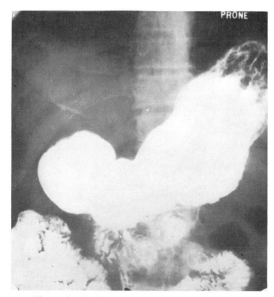
Hypersthenic (direct posteroanterior projection).
Above radiographs courtesy Dr. Francis H. Ghiselin.

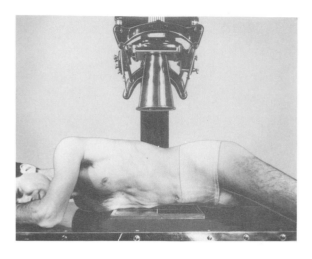

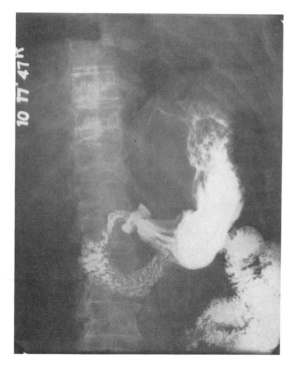

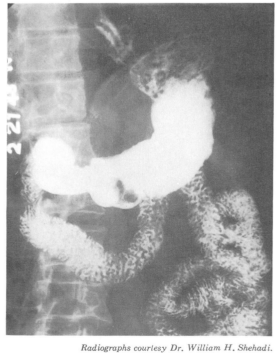

Radiographs courtesy Dr. William H. Shehadi.

STOMACH AND DUODENUM
Right posteroanterior oblique projection
Right anteroposterior oblique view
Film: 10″ × 12″ lengthwise.

Position of patient

Right posteroanterior oblique projections of the stomach and duodenum are made with the patient in the recumbent position.

Position of part

After the posteroanterior study or studies are made, ask the patient to rest his head on his right cheek and to place his right arm along the side of his body. Have him turn toward his left and support himself on the left forearm and the flexed knee. Before making the final adjustment in body rotation, adjust the patient's position so that a longitudinal plane passing approximately midway between the vertebrae and the forward surface of the elevated side will coincide with the midline of the Potter-Bucky diaphragm or the cassette. If using non-Bucky technique, center the film at the level, or at the estimated level, of the pylorus.

The approximate degree of rotation required to give the best view of the pyloric canal and the duodenum depends upon the size, shape, and position of the stomach. Hypersthenic patients will, in general, require a greater degree of rotation than less massively built patients. In the usual routine procedure, several studies are made with 10- to 15-degree changes in the obliquity of the body.

The right posteroanterior oblique position is used for serial studies of the pyloric canal and the duodenal cap because gastric peristalsis is usually more active when the patient is in that position. The exposures are made at 30- to 40-second intervals.

Respiration is suspended at the end of exhalation unless otherwise specified by the radiologist.

Central ray

Direct the central ray perpendicularly to the midpoint of the film.

Structures shown

A right anteroposterior oblique view of the stomach and the entire duodenal loop. This projection, with a rotation of 40 to 70 degrees, according to the type of stomach, gives the best view of the pyloric canal and the duodenal cap in patients who approximate the sthenic type of habitus.

STOMACH AND DUODENUM

Lateral projection

Film: $10'' \times 12''$ or $11'' \times 14''$ lengthwise, the longer film being required for the erect position.

Position of patient

The patient is placed in the erect left lateral position for the demonstration of the left retrogastric space, and in the recumbent right lateral position for the demonstration of the right retrogastric space, the duodenal loop, and the duodenojejunal junction.

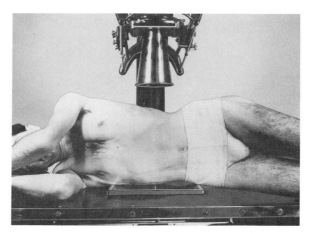

Position of part

With the patient in either the erect or the recumbent position, adjust the body so that a coronal plane passing approximately midway between the midaxillary line and the anterior surface of the abdomen will coincide with the midline of the cassette or the Potter-Bucky diaphragm. The film is then centered at the level of the pylorus or at its estimated level, depending on whether the mark indicating its site was made in the same body position. Adjust the body in a true lateral position, and have the patient grasp the side of the table or stand for support.

Respiration is suspended at the end of exhalation unless otherwise requested by the radiologist.

Central ray

Direct the central ray perpendicularly to the midpoint of the film.

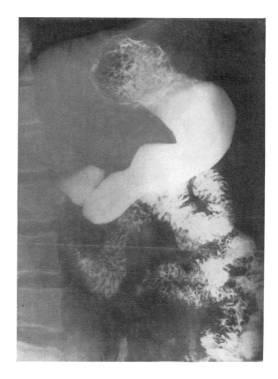

Structures shown

A lateral projection showing the anterior and posterior aspects of the stomach, the pyloric canal, and the duodenal bulb. The right lateral projection frequently affords the best view of the pyloric canal and the duodenal cap in obese patients as well as in patients of hypersthenic habitus.

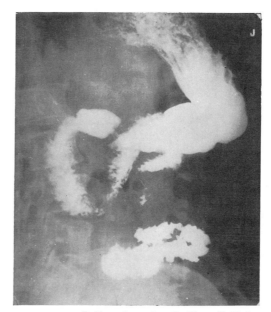

Radiographs courtesy Dr. Henry K. Taylor.

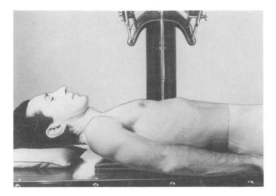

STOMACH AND DUODENUM AND DIAPHRAGMATIC HERNIAS

Anteroposterior projections
Posteroanterior views

Film: $11'' \times 14''$ crosswise for stomach and duodenum, lengthwise for small hiatal hernias; $14'' \times 17''$ lengthwise for gross diaphragmatic herniations.

Position of patient

The patient is placed in the supine position. The stomach moves upward and to the left in this position, and except in thin subjects, its pyloric end is elevated so that the barium mixture flows into and fills its cardiac or fundic end. The filling of the fundus displaces the gas bubble into the antral end of the stomach, where it affords double-contrast delineation of posterior wall lesions. When the patient is thin, the intestinal loops do not move upward enough to tilt the stomach for fundic filling. It is therefore necessary to rotate the body toward the left or to angle the head end of the table downward.

The table is tilted to full Trendelenburg angulation for the demonstration of diaphragmatic herniations. In the Trendelenburg position, the involved organ or organs, which may appear to be normally located in all other body positions, shift upward and protrude through the hernial orifice (most frequently through the esophageal hiatus). A lateral study, by either vertical or horizontal projection, may be made.

For unobstructed visualization of small hiatal hernias and esophageal regurgitation, the patient is rotated slightly to the right to place the gastroesophageal junction to the right of the vertebral shadow.

Position of part

Adjust the position of the patient so that the midline of the table will coincide (1) with the median sagittal plane of the body when a $14'' \times 17''$ film is used, or (2) with a sagittal plane passing midway between the median sagittal plane and the left side of the thorax when an $11'' \times 14''$ film is used. Longitudinal centering of the large film depends upon the extent of the hernial protrusion into the thorax, and is determined during radioscopy. For the stomach and duodenum, the smaller film is centered at the estimated level of the pylorus. The greatest upward movement of the viscera between the prone and supine positions occurs in obese subjects.

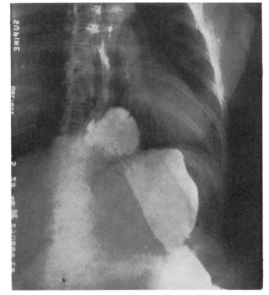

Supine. Diaphragmatic hernia.
Courtesy Dr. Francis H. Ghiselin.

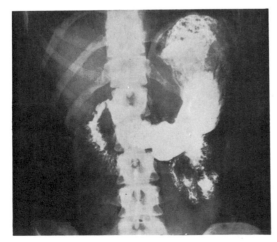

Stomach prone.

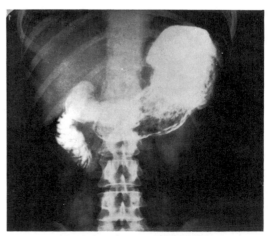

Stomach supine on opposite patient.
Courtesy Dr. Henry K. Taylor.

STOMACH AND DUODENUM AND DIAPHRAGMATIC HERNIAS
Anteroposterior projections
Posteroanterior views—cont'd
Position of part—cont'd

Depending upon the area to be demonstrated, the body is adjusted in a direct anteroposterior position or in a slightly oblique position, as directed by the radiologist.

Respiration is suspended at the end of exhalation unless otherwise specified by the radiologist.

Central ray

The central ray is directed perpendicularly to the midpoint of the film.

Structures shown

Stomach. A posteroanterior view (anteroposterior projection) of the stomach, showing a well-filled fundic portion and, usually, double-contrast delineation of the body, the antral portion, and the duodenum. Because of the elevation and upward displacement of the stomach, this position affords the best frontal view of the retrogastric portion of the duodenum and jejunum.

Diaphragm. A posteroanterior view of the abdominothoracic region, demonstrating the organ or organs involved in, and the location and extent of, any gross hernial protrusion through the diaphragm.

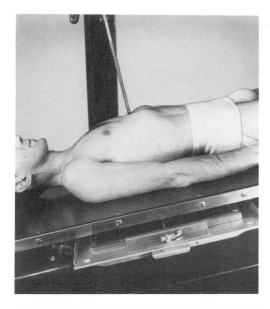

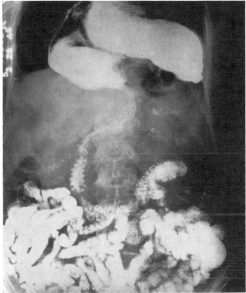

Supine.

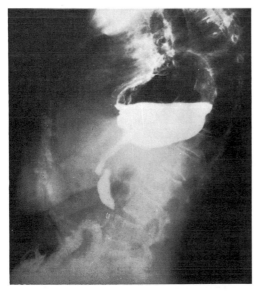

Lateral erect.

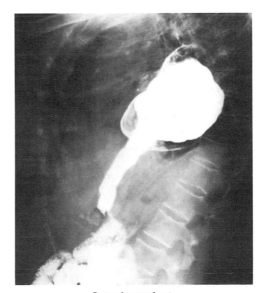

Lateral recumbent.

Radiographs courtesy Dr. Dan Tucker.

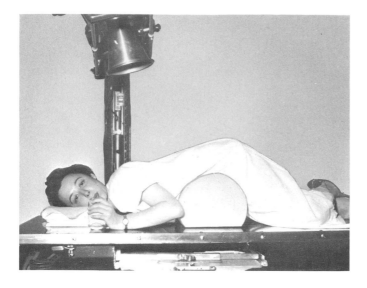

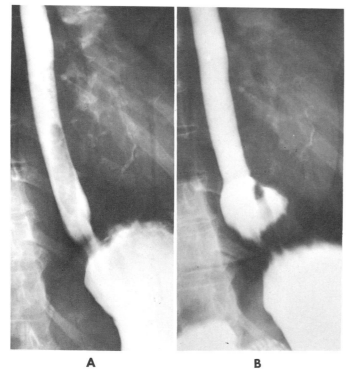

| **A** | **B** |

Comparison RAO views on one patient. **A,** Without abdominal compression; no evidence of hernia. **B,** With abdominal compression; large sliding hernia obvious.

Illustrations and diagnostic information courtesy Dr. Bernard S. Wolf.

RADIOGRAPHIC DEMONSTRATION OF MINIMAL HIATAL HERNIAS

Wolf method[1]

The procedures described on this and the facing page are modifications of the Trendelenburg position. These techniques were evolved for the purpose of applying greater intra-abdominal pressure than is provided by body angulation alone and thereby ensuring more consistent results in the radiographic demonstration of small, sliding gastroesophageal herniations through the esophageal hiatus.

The Wolf method requires the use of a semicylindrical (one flat side), radioparent compression device measuring 22 inches in length, 10 inches in width, and 8 inches in height. This compression device, which is shown in position under the patient in the photograph to the left, may be made of a material such as balsa wood or foam rubber.

Wolf[2] states that this device not only provides Trendelenburg angulation of the patient's trunk but increases intra-abdominal pressure enough to permit adequate contrast filling and maximum distention of the entire esophagus. A further advantage of this device is that it does not require angulation of the table; thus the patient is able to hold the barium container and to ingest the barium mixture through a tube with comparative ease.

Film: 14″ × 17″ lengthwise.

Position of patient

The patient is placed on the examining table and is asked to assume a modified knee-chest position during the placement of the compression device. This device is placed transversely under the abdomen and just below the costal margin. The patient is then adjusted in a 40- to 45-degree right posteroanterior oblique position, with the thorax centered to the midline of the table.

The film is adjusted so that its midpoint will coincide with the angulation of the central ray.

Central ray

The central ray is directed at right angles to the long axis of the patient's back and is centered at the level of either the sixth or the seventh thoracic vertebra.

Instructions for exposure

A container holding the barium mixture and a drinking tube is placed in the patient's left hand. He is instructed to ingest the mixture in rapid, continuous swallows. To allow for complete filling of the esophagus, the exposure is made during the third or fourth swallow.

[1]Wolf, B. S., and Guglielmo, J.: Method for the roentgen demonstration of minimal hiatal herniation, J. Mt. Sinai Hosp. N. Y. **23**:738-741, 1956.
[2]Wolf, B. S., and Guglielmo, J.: The roentgen demonstration of minimal hiatus hernia, Med. Radiogr. Photogr. **33**:90-92, 1957.

RADIOGRAPHIC DEMONSTRATION OF MINIMAL HIATAL HERNIAS

Sommer-Foegelle method

The Sommer-Foegelle method of demonstrating minimal hiatus hernias requires the use of a specially constructed, 34-degree angle board over which the patient is flexed to place his trunk in a Trendelenburg position. The upper edge of the board is thickly padded to exert pressure on the lower abdomen and to further increase intra-abdominal pressure. Sommer[1] states that the angle board technique provides highly accurate diagnostic results.

The angle board incorporates a 10″ × 12″ stationary grid and a cassette tray. (See Foegelle's paper[2] for detailed information on the construction of the angle board.)

Film: 10″ × 12″ lengthwise.

Position of patient

The angle board is placed on the examining table, and the film area is centered to the midline of the table. The patient is assisted in getting onto the table in the kneeling position. He is then adjusted so that his thighs are placed against the board, with the median sagittal plane of the body centered to the film area of the device. The patient is now asked to lean straight forward and to rest his full weight on the board. The xiphoid process should be centered over the film.

Central ray

The tube is angled so that the central ray is directed at right angles to the midpoint of the film.

[1]Sommer, A. W., and Stevenson, C. L.: Hiatal hernia; an evaluation of diagnostic procedures, Amer. J. Dig. Dis. **6:**412-422, 1961.
[2]Foegelle, E. F.: Stomach radiography, special emphasis on hiatal hernia, Xray Techn. **30:**167-171, 1958.

Instructions for exposure

No additional contrast medium is administered in this procedure. The patient is asked to inhale deeply and slowly and to exhale completely three or four times. At the end of the last complete exhalation, he is asked to close his mouth, to hold his nostrils together, and then, against the closed mouth and nostrils, to try to inhale deeply (Müller maneuver). The exposure is made during the maneuver.

NOTE: Because small hiatal herniations are always superimposed by the vertebrae in this position (direct posteroanterior), a high-kilovoltage technique is recommended.

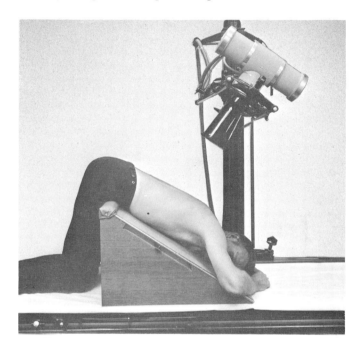

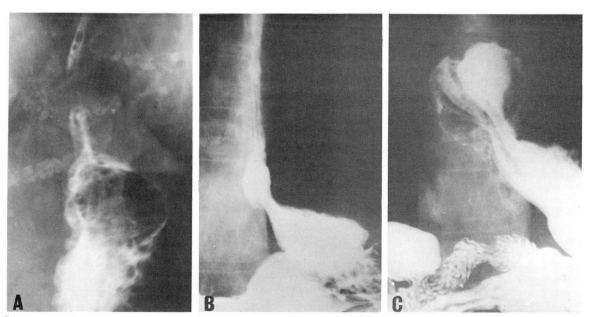

Comparison studies on one patient. **A,** Recumbent RAO view; no evidence of hernia. **B,** Supine Trendelenburg; small hiatus hernia demonstrated. **C,** Angle board position plus Müller maneuver; compare size of hernia with that shown in **B.**

Illustrations and diagnostic information courtesy Dr. A. W. Sommer and Mr. E. F. Foegelle.

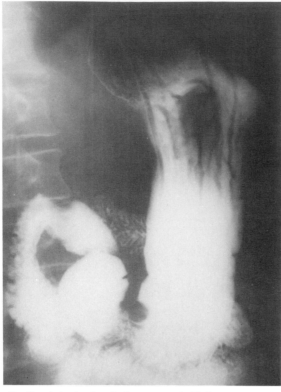

Routine study showing shadow suspected of being gastric mass.

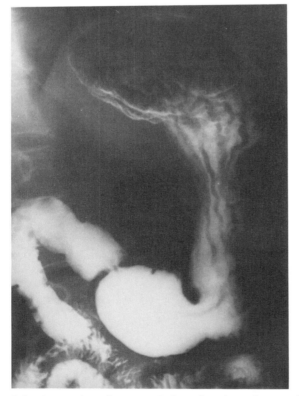

Film of the above patient after gas-producing pellets shows the stomach to be normal.

Radiographs and clinical information courtesy Dr. Herbert F. Hempel.

STOMACH, DUODENUM, AND PANCREAS
Special procedures

In routine gastrointestinal procedures, the radiologist coats the stomach wall with a small amount of barium mixture and then utilizes the gas contained in the magenblase (gastric air bubble) to obtain double-contrast delineation of the gastric and duodenal mucosa. He controls the distribution of the barium and air by gravity (patient position), by palpation, and by localized compression. Abnormalities of the head of the pancreas are demonstrated by characteristic irregularities in the gastric and/or duodenal mucosal pattern, and by an increase in the thickness of the retrogastric and retroduodenal space. The routine techniques are generally considered to be adequate in a majority of cases. Selected cases are examined by one of the special techniques.

Various radiologic examination techniques have been developed to improve visualization of the walls of the stomach and duodenum, and the irregularities in these structures produced by pathology in the head of the pancreas. (Abnormalities of the body and tail of the pancreas are not shown by gastroduodenography.) In the special procedures utilizing negative contrast or double contrast, the stomach and/or duodenum are inflated with enough gas to smooth out the mucosal folds for the detection of small lesions that might otherwise be obscured. The inflated organ presses against the head of the pancreas and thus outlines any abnormality in its contour.

A colloidal barium sulfate suspension is used in the double-contrast techniques. The barium-to-water proportions must be carefully measured to the specifications of the radiologist. In most of these techniques, inflation of the stomach is obtained with ingestible gas-producing preparations. These agents are fast acting, generating large amounts of gas within two to three minutes and dissipating within fifteen to twenty minutes.

Hypotonic duodenography requires the use of a spasmolytic (anticholinergic) drug, which is also used in some double-contrast gastroduodenal studies. Propantheline bromide (Pro-Banthine) is widely used for these examinations. Hanelin[1] reports that the side effects of Pro-Banthine include drying of salivary, gastric, and upper respiratory tract secretions, tachycardia, loss of bladder tone with resulting inability to urinate for several hours, and pupillary dilatation and blurred vision. The last two of these effects require that the patient's bladder be emptied just prior to the procedure and that he not be allowed to drive his car until his eye accommodation returns to normal, about two hours later. Hanelin stated that Pro-Banthine is contraindicated in cases of glaucoma, cardiac disease, and prostatism. Miller[2,3] states that none of the above listed side effects and contraindications apply to the drug glucagon, and he reports that he has found an intramuscular injection of 2 mg. of glucagon to be a more effective intestinal relaxant than either 1 mg. of atropine or 30 mg. of Pro-Banthine.

[1]Hanelin, J.: Some technical aspects in the demonstration of gastric lesions, Seminars Roentgen. 6:235-253, 1971.

[2]Miller, R. E., Chernish, S. M., Rosenak, B. D., and Rodda, B. E.: Hypotonic duodenography with glucagon, Radiology 108:35-42, 1973.

[3]Dr. Roscoe E. Miller: Personal communication.

Because the patient can be positioned under radioscopic control for optimal visualization of minimal lesions, spot films replace most of the usual postradioscopic filming. Tomography, using the linear sweep at a 15- or 20-degree arc, is utilized in some of the techniques. The technologist must keep in mind that the gas generated in the stomach by the gas-forming preparations dissipates rapidly, so that postradioscopic filming must be carried out without delay.

Examination of the stomach wall by the visual (endoscopic) and gastrocamera method is usually performed by the attending gastroscopist, a procedure now being performed by some radiologists. Hines and associates[1] state that because of the premedication requirements and the discomfort to the patient, the gastrocamera method can be used only in selected cases.

Negative contrast techniques

1. Some radiologists introduce gas into the stomach with a carbonated beverage such as ginger ale or Coca-Cola, or with an effervescent powder (Seidlitz powder) and then obtain conventional and/or tomographic studies of the gas-filled stomach. Others administer one of these preparations after coating the gastric mucosa with a barium mixture; some reports state that this method is not entirely satisfactory because the mucosal coating is frequently washed away by the large amount of liquid.

2. Gastric parietography, first reported by Saito,[2] utilizes simultaneous perigastric and endogastric gas. After establishing pneumoperitoneum (pages 666 to 667), the patient is rotated alternately onto his right and left sides for twenty to 30 minutes to allow the gas to contact and surround the stomach wall. The stomach is then inflated by the ingestion of 1.5 grams of tartaric acid followed by 2 grams of sodium bicarbonate, each dissolved in a small amount of water. Filming must be carried out immediately because this gas dissipates within fifteen to twenty minutes; the dosage can, however, be repeated when necessary. Saito recommended that filming be carried out by cross-table projections.

Saito reported that he and his associates use a similar peristructural and endostructural gas technique for examinations of the colon. Virtana[3] described the use of rectal parietography in cases of ulcerative colitis. He injects 200 to 400 ml. of oxygen into the presacral space (pneumoretroperitoneum, page 782) with the patient prone in the Trendelenburg position. The rectum is then filled with a barium suspension or occasionally with barium and air, for double contrast. Films are obtained in posteroanterior, both oblique, and lateral positions, and the examination is concluded with lateral tomography.

[1]Hines, W. B., Kerr, R. M., Meschen, I., and Martin, J. F.: Roentgenologic and gastrocamera correlation in lesions of the stomach, Amer. J. Roentgen. 113:129-138, 1971.

[2]Saito, M.: La radiographie des parois de l'estomac, "pneumo-gastro-parietographie," Bull. Chir. Paris 59:910-912, 1933.

[3]Virtana, P.: Rectal parietography in ulcerative colitis, Acta Radiol. [Diagn.] 4:344-348, 1966.

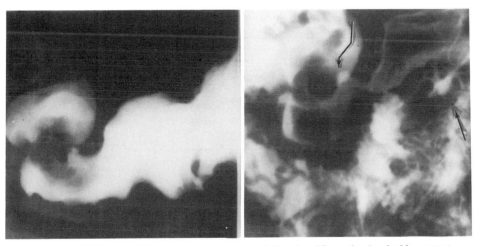

Right prone oblique.   Left supine oblique, showing double contrast.
Two gastric ulcers (arrows) in a 45-year-old woman.

Radiographs and clinical information courtesy Dr. Joseph Hanelin.

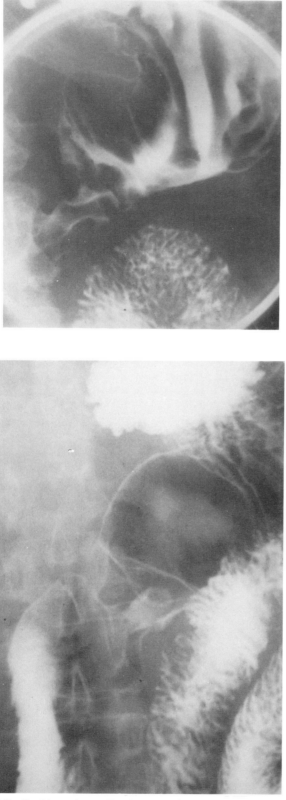

STOMACH, DUODENUM, AND PANCREAS—cont'd

Special procedures—cont'd

Double-contrast techniques

1. Many examiners introduce both contrast media by way of a nasogastric tube because this method enables them to control the amount of barium and air in the stomach. The patient may be premedicated with a mild sedative. The nasopharynx and throat are sprayed with a local anesthetic for the insertion of the tube, which the patient then swallows with the aid of sips of cold water. Following the positive contrast study, any excess of barium mixture is withdrawn through the tube before air is injected for the double-contrast study.

2. Double-contrast studies of the stomach have been greatly simplified by the use of the gas-producing pellets and granules developed in Japan.[1] These preparations, designed to be administered with the liquid barium sulfate mixture, contain tartaric acid, sodium bicarbonate, and a silicone antifoaming agent. Each of the small pellets releases 13 cc. of CO_2 within three minutes after contact with the water in the barium mixture. Since they are administered without additional water, these preparations do not interfere with the coating action of the barium. The specified dose of pellets or granules is placed on the patient's tongue, and he then swallows it with the specified amount of barium mixture.

Following the radioscopic and spot-film examination of the gastric wall, the examiner allows barium to pass into the duodenum. He then elevates the patient's right side to allow gas to pass into and distend the duodenum. This maneuver often results in satisfactory double-contrast delineation of the duodenum. To ensure satisfactory demonstration of the duodenum and the head of the pancreas, a spasmolytic drug is used to induce temporary (fifteen to twenty minute) gastric and duodenal atony. The anticholinergic drug is administered before the gas-producing preparation so that it will take effect before the gas dissipates.

[1]Hanelin, J.: Some technical aspects in the demonstration of gastric lesions, Seminars Roentgen. 6:235-253, 1971.

Use of Pro-Banthine and gas pills. The upper film shows a narrowed antrum. In the lower film the Pro-Banthine has caused gastric and duodenal atony. The short, fixed, tubular, prepyloric narrowing is disclosed with double-contrast. Diagnosis: cancer.

Radiographs and clinical information courtesy Dr. Joseph Hanelin.

Hypotonic duodenography

Hypotonic duodenography was first described by Liotta.[1] The procedure is used for the evaluation of post-bulbar duodenal lesions and for the detection of pancreatic disease. It requires duodenal intubation and temporary drug-induced duodenal paralysis so that a double-contrast examination can be performed without interference from peristaltic activity. During the atonic state, when distended with the contrast media to two or three times its normal size, the duodenum presses against and outlines any abnormality in the contour of the head of the pancreas.

After rapid, radioscopically controlled intubation of the duodenum, the radiologist administers an intramuscular injection of a spasmolytic drug. This induces gastric and duodenal atony within three or four minutes and lasts about twenty minutes. A barium sulfate mixture and air are injected through the tube and the examination is carried out under radioscopic observation, usually being recorded with spot films only.

Rapid duodenal intubation

Rapid, radioscopically controlled intubation of the duodenum with the use of a flexible guide wire inserted into the intestinal tube was first described by Gianturco.[2] This technique is an extension of Seldinger's technique for the introduction of vascular catheters, and the procedure requires about ten minutes.

After local anesthetization of the nasopharynx and throat, a soft plastic duodenal tube is passed into the stomach as the patient sips cold water. A maneuverable guide wire is then inserted into the side of the tube, and under radioscopic control, the tube is gently guided through the pylorus. The guide wire is withdrawn as the tube is advanced to the transverse duodenum.

This method of rapid small intestine intubation is also used for small intestine enemas and for rapid decompression of small bowel obstructions,[3] as well as for hypotonic duodenography. The conventional method of gastrointestinal intubation is described on pages 732 and 733.

[1]Liotta, D.: Pour le diagnostic des tumeurs du pancréas: la duodénografie hypotonique, Lyon Chir. **50**:445-460, 1955.

[2]Gianturco, C.: Rapid fluoroscopic duodenal intubation, Radiology **88**:1165-1166, 1969.

[3]Sargent, E. N., and Meyers, H. I.: Wire guide and technique for Cantor tube insertion; rapid small bowel intubation, Amer. J. Roentgen. **107**:150-155, 1969.

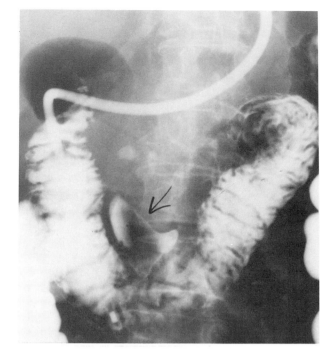

Hypotonic duodenogram showing deformity of a duodenal diverticulum by a small carcinoma of the head of the pancreas.

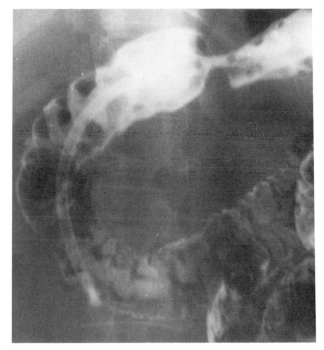

Hypotonic duodenogram showing multiple defects in the duodenal bulb and proximal second duodenum due to hypertrophy of Brunner's glands.

Radiographs and clinical information courtesy Dr. Arthur R. Clemett.

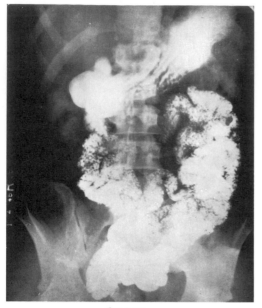

One hour.

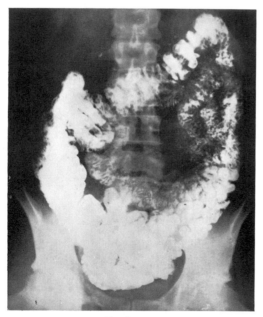

Two hours.

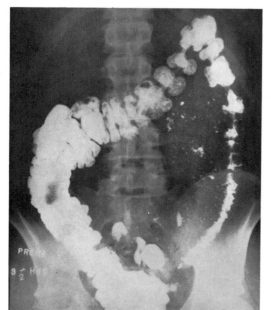

Three and one-half hours.

GASTROINTESTINAL MOTILITY STUDIES

Following the ingestion of a barium sulfate meal for a gastrointestinal series, *motility*, or *delayed*, studies of the gastrointestinal tract are usually made. This is done for the purpose of investigating the peristaltic function of the digestive tract and detecting any abnormality outlined by the advancing column of contrast material. The patient is allowed nothing to eat or drink until the emptying time of the stomach has been determined. Gastric emptying of the nonfood-containing contrast meal usually occurs in one to four hours, peristaltic activity being greatest in patients of hypersthenic habitus. The rate of speed with which the barium meal progresses also depends upon its consistency, a thin mixture progressing faster than a thick mixture, and upon the presence of any functional or pathologic disturbance of the normal motility of the tract.

Gastrointestinal motility studies of adults are made on 14″ × 17″ films. The films are centered high enough to include the stomach until it is empty, and then low enough to include the pubic symphysis for the intestinal studies. The patient is usually placed in the supine position for small-intestine studies and in the prone position for gastric motility studies. A time-interval marker is placed on each film to indicate the time lapse between the ingestion of the opaque meal and the exposure of the film.

Many radiologists include, in their routine procedure, one or two films for the delineation of the small bowel. These studies are taken at specified intervals preceding the gastric-motility study.

The time interval between the immediate films of the stomach and duodenum and the gastric-motility film is usually six hours. This period is generally considered the maximum normal emptying time of the stomach. However, because some radiologists consider a four-hour residue just as significant as a six-hour residue, the time varies. Six hours after ingestion, the head of the barium column is usually at the hepatic flexure, and the tail of the barium column is usually in the terminal portion of the ileum. Frequently the appendix is well filled. A compression study of the ileocecal region and of the appendix may be performed at this time.

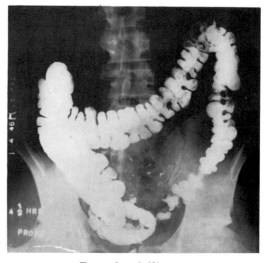

Four and one-half hours.
Radiographs courtesy Dr. Francis H. Ghiselin.

728

The large intestine may be examined approximately twenty-four hours after the ingestion of the barium mixture, and again at forty-eight—and seventy-two—hour intervals when indicated, to check the progress of the meal and to detect any abnormality demonstrable with the ingested medium.

An ingested barium meal demonstrates the function and certain pathologic conditions of the large bowel, but it is not sufficient in quantity to fill the lumen completely. Because of the presence of fecal masses, the meal may not coat all portions of the bowel wall. In order to demonstrate the luminal contour of the entire bowel, it is necessary to distend the bowel with a contrast enema. Many radiologists follow up each gastrointestinal series with a barium enema. This makes it necessary to evacuate the bowel with a cleansing enema.

When a contrast enema is included in the routine gastrointestinal series, an evacuation of the large bowel that is as complete as possible can be ensured by preparing the patient and by making the large-intestine examination first. The patient is usually given a cathartic thirty-six hours before the examination, is put on a low-residue diet the preceding day, and is given a cleansing enema on the night before, and another on the morning of, the examination. Immediately following completion of the contrast enema examination, the gastrointestinal series is started.

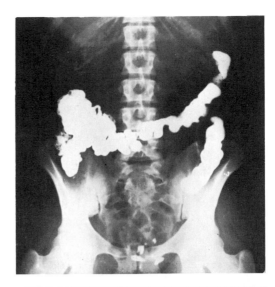

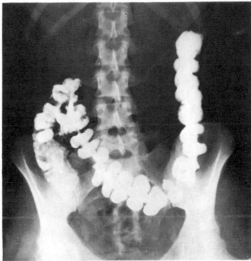

Twenty-four-hour studies.

Courtesy Dr. William H. Shehadi.

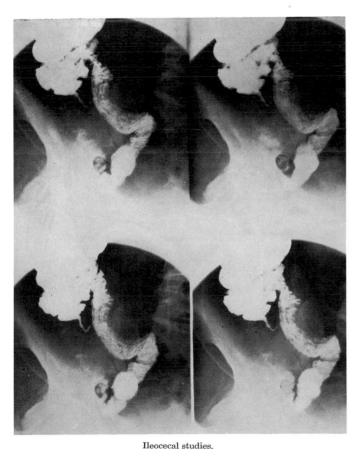

Ileocecal studies.

Courtesy Dr. Marcy L. Sussman.

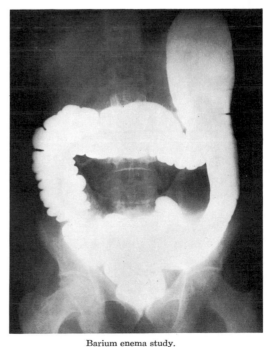

Barium enema study.

Courtesy Dr. Marcy L. Sussman.

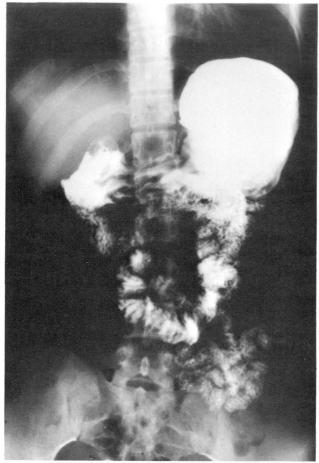

Immediate film.

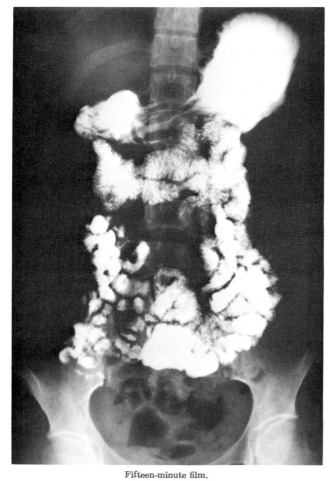

Fifteen-minute film.

Radiographs courtesy Dr. John A. Evans.

SMALL INTESTINE

Oral methods of examination

Radiologic examinations of the small bowel are performed by administering a barium sulfate preparation (1) by mouth, (2) by complete reflux filling with a large volume barium enema, or (3) by direct injection into the bowel by way of an intestinal tube for what is called a *small-intestine enema*. The two latter methods are usually used only when the oral method fails to provide conclusive information.

In preparation for a small-intestine study, a soft or low-residue diet is instituted for two days preceding the examination, unless the patient is already on such a diet. Food and fluid are withheld after the evening meal, and breakfast is withheld. A cleansing enema is administered to clear the colon when necessary. Because these patients usually have either diarrhea, tarry stools (indicating bleeding), or fairly severe abdominal pain, cathartics are never given unless expressly ordered.

The barium formula is the same as for a gastrointestinal series because, even though not in question, the esophagus, stomach, and duodenum are usually investigated.

The examination is preceded by a preliminary film of the abdomen. Each small-bowel study is identified by a time marker indicating the interval between its exposure and the ingestion of the barium meal. These studies are made with the patient adjusted in the supine position (1) to take advantage of the upward and lateralward shift of the barium-filled stomach for visualization of the retrogastric portions of the duodenum and jejunum, and (2) to prevent possible compression overlapping of loops of the bowel. When thin subjects are examined, it is usually necessary to angle the table to the Trendelenburg position for the later films in order to "unfold" low-lying and superimposed loops of the ileum.

The first small-bowel study is usually taken at the fifteen-minute postingestion interval. The basic routine that is established for the following interval exposures varies from fifteen to thirty minutes, according to the average transit time peculiar to the barium sulfate preparation employed—that is, whether the medium is one of the faster transit time–suspended preparations or the usual nonsuspended preparation. It also depends upon whether the medium is mixed with plain water or with normal saline solution and at what temperature. Regardless of the barium preparation used, however, the radiologist inspects the films as they are processed and varies the basic procedure according to the requirements of the individual patient. Radioscopic and film studies, spot and/or conventional, may be made of any segment of the bowel as the loops become opacified.

Howarth and associates[1] administer a cholinergic type drug (metoclopramide) to increase peristalsis. They administer 20 mg. of this drug prior to the ingestion of the barium meal, and they report that the small bowel transit time is reduced to about one-third the normal transit time. They state that this drug is also valuable for evaluation of the stomach when gastric atony or pylorospasm is present.

Goldstein and associates[2] accelerate peristalsis for small bowel studies by adding 10 ml. of Gastrografin to the barium meal, reporting that by this method the head of the meal reaches the cecum in 45 minutes.

Many radiologists administer a glassful of ice water (or other routinely used food stimulant) to the patient with hypomotility at the three- or four-hour interval to accelerate peristalsis. Other radiologists routinely stimulate peristalsis by administering a glassful of ice water or normal saline solution upon completion of the filming of the stomach and duodenum, and by administering a second glassful thirty minutes later. Still others administer one of these peristalsis stimulants every fifteen minutes throughout the transit time. By these methods, the transit of the medium is followed radioscopically, with spot and conventional films exposed as indicated, and the examination is usually completed in thirty to sixty minutes.

Saline solution is not used with patients who are on a salt-free diet.

Saline solution sometimes causes nausea, especially in repeated doses. Its purpose should be explained to the patient, and everything possible should be done to prevent or allay nausea. The patient should be allowed to rinse his mouth after drinking the salty solution, he should be instructed to lie on his right side between films, and he should be given a bottle of smelling salts or a pledget of cotton moistened with aromatic spirit of ammonia.

Complete reflux method

For complete reflux filling of the small bowel, Miller[3,4] administers 2 mg. of glucagon to relax the intestine, and from 2 to 10 mg. of diazepam (Valium) to diminish discomfort during the initial portion of the filling. A 20% weight/volume barium suspension is used, and a large amount of the mixture (about 4,500 ml.) is required to fill the gut. A retention enema tip is used, and the patient is placed in the supine position for the examination. The barium suspension is allowed to flow until it is observed in the duodenal bulb. The enema bag is then lowered to the floor to drain the colon before filming of the small bowel.

[1]Howarth, F. H., Cockel, R., Roper, B. W., and Hawkins, C. F.: The effect of metoclopramide upon gastric motility and its value in barium progress meals, Clin. Radiol. 20:294-300, 1969.

[2]Goldstein, H. M., Poole, G. J., Rosenquist, C. J., Friedland, G. W., and Zboralske, F. F.: Comparison of methods for acceleration of small intestinal radiographic examination, Radiology 98:519-523, 1971.

[3]Miller, R. E.: Complete reflux small bowel examination, Radiology 84:457-462, 1965.

[4]Miller, R. E.: Localization of small bowel hemorrhage; complete reflux small bowel examination, Amer. J. Dig. Dis. 17:1019-1923, 1972.

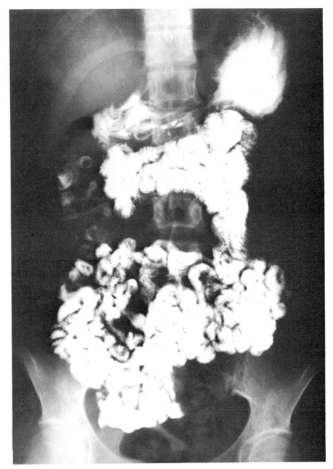

Thirty-minute film.

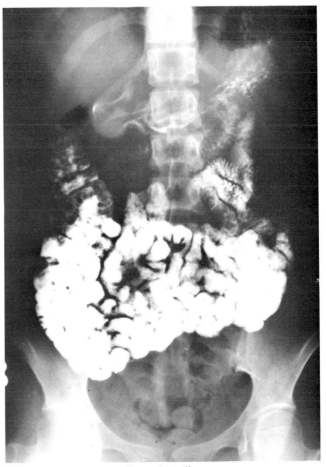

Sixty-minute film.

Radiographs courtesy Dr. John A. Evans.

SMALL INTESTINE—cont'd

Intubation examination procedures

The term *gastrointestinal intubation* denotes the procedure in which a long, specially designed tube is inserted through the nose and passed into the stomach, from whence the tube is carried downward by peristaltic action. Gastrointestinal intubation is employed for both therapeutic and diagnostic purposes.

When used therapeutically, the intestinal tube is connected to a suction system, usually a three-bottle arrangement, for continuous siphoning of the gas and fluid contents of the gastrointestinal tract. The purpose of the measure is to prevent or relieve postoperative distention, or to deflate or decompress an obstructed small bowel.

For diagnostic purposes, intestinal intubation is utilized in radiologic investigations of the small bowel. An opaque medium is injected through the tube directly into the bowel under radioscopic observation. When the intestinal tube is inserted for the express purpose of delineating and inspecting the jejunum and ileum in their entirety, the procedure is termed a *small-intestine enema*. More frequently, radiologic examinations are made through a previously installed tube for the investigation of a localized section of the bowel, usually to determine the nature of an obstruction when the passage of the tube is arrested at the obstructed site. Golden[1] termed this latter procedure a *Miller-Abbott tube study* to differentiate it from the small-intestine enema procedure.

The Miller-Abbott double-lumen, single-balloon tube (or a similar one) is usually used to intubate the small intestine. Some radiologists use a triple-lumen, double-balloon tube for the examination of localized areas, the two balloons being inflated to enclose the area under investigation. Intestinal tubes are available in rubber and also in a polyvinyl plastic material. The plastic material is said to be much less irritating to the mucosa of the nose and throat. Neither tube should be sterilized by heat.

Just above the metal tip of the tube is a small, thin-rubber balloon that is used only once and then replaced. There are marks on the tube, beginning at the tip, or distal, end, to indicate the extent of its passage as read from the edge of the nostril. The marks are indicated in centimeters to 85 cm., and in feet thereafter. The lumen of the tube is asymmetrically divided into the following two lumina, or channels: (1) a small *balloon lumen* that communicates with the balloon only, and that is used for the inflation and deflation of the balloon and for the injection of mercury to weight the balloon, and (2) a large *aspiration lumen* that communicates with the gastrointestinal tract through perforations near and at the distal end of the tube. It is by way of the aspiration lumen that gas and fluid are withdrawn and that liquids are injected. At the proximal end of the tube, the aspiration lumen and the balloon lumen are brought out into separate tubes, or arms. *The proximal end of each lumen must be accurately identified and so prominently labeled as to obviate error in their use in the dark of the radioscopic room.*

Gastrointestinal intubations are performed by, or under the direction of, the referring physician or the radiologist. Because the manipulation of the tube into the stomach does not require the advanced knowledge and skill of a physician and is likely to be time-consuming, this initial part of intubation is entrusted, in some hospitals, to a nurse or a nurse-technologist who has been specially instructed in the technique of the procedure. (See Golden[1]

for an excellently detailed, step-by-step description of the gastrointestinal intubation technique he employs.) Only the information considered necessary to equip the non-nurse technologist to assist at intubations that are performed in the radiology department will be included here.

The following list of items represents an approximately standard layout (the instruments are obtainable from the central supply room): (1) a double-lumen intestinal tube, the balloon of which *must*, just before use, be inflated and tested under water to be sure that it has no leak; (2) a water-soluble lubricating medium such as K-Y jelly; (3) a suction apparatus, usually a three-bottle system mounted on a standard; (4) an atomizer containing the specified local anesthetic solution; (5) sterile Luer syringes of the specified sizes for the aspiration and lavage of the stomach, for inflating and deflating the balloon, and for injecting mercury into the balloon lumen; (6) a test tube containing 2 ml. of mercury for weighting the balloon; (7) a pitcher of ice water, a drinking glass, and a drinking tube or straw; (8) a flask of normal saline solution or plain water, as specified, for lavage of the stomach; (9) tissues for the patient's use; (10) emesis basins, disposable towels, waste basins, and paper waste bags; (11) a roll of adhesive tape; (12) a crushable ampule of amyl nitrite.

The introduction of an intestinal tube is an unpleasant experience for the patient, especially if he is acutely ill. Depending upon the condition of the patient, explain that the tube is more readily passed, and will cause him less discomfort, if he can sit erect and lean slightly forward, or if he can be elevated almost to a sitting position. Because the passage of the tube frequently induces vomiting, the patient and the radioscopic table should be protected with rubber sheeting that is suitably covered, preferably with an absorbent paper sheet. Have the patient blow his nose to clear the passages of mucus.

The physician selects the larger nasal passage (the septum is often deviated from the midline) and sprays it with a local anesthetic solution. The balloon must be fully deflated and then lubricated well with K-Y jelly. The technologist should be ready to begin giving the patient ice water through a drinking tube as soon as the radiologist indicates that he has passed the tube into the nasopharynx. As the patient swallows, the tube is passed through the nasopharynx and esophagus into the stomach. The physician then inflates the balloon, and the patient is adjusted in a semisupine position with the left side elevated. The stomach is now aspirated through the large lumen of the tube with a syringe. If the physician lavages the stomach, the arm of the aspiration lumen is attached to the suction apparatus.

When the above step has been completed, the patient is turned to a right posteroanterior oblique position. A syringe is connected to the balloon lumen, the mercury is poured into the syringe and is allowed to flow into the balloon, and then the air is slowly withdrawn. As the patient is given more water, the radiologist advances the tube under radioscopic observation, guiding it along the anterior wall of the greater curvature and into the pyloric canal. In this position the tube has enough slack to permit it to pass into the duodenum but not enough slack to permit it to coil in the stomach. The tube is secured with an adhesive strap beside the nostril to prevent regurgitation or advance. The stomach is again aspirated, either by syringe or by attaching the large lumen arm to the suction apparatus.

[1]Golden, Ross: Radiologic examination of the small intestine, ed. 2, Springfield, Ill., 1959, Charles C Thomas, Publisher.

With the tip of the tube in approximation to the pyloric sphincter and the patient in the right posteroanterior oblique position, where gastric peristalsis is usually more active, the tube should pass into the duodenum in a reasonably short time. Without intervention, however, this process sometimes takes many hours. Having the patient drink ice water to stimulate peristalsis and inhale amyl nitrite to relax the pyloric sphincter frequently is successful. When these measures fail, the radiologist guides the tube into the duodenum by manual manipulation under radioscopic observation. After the tube enters the duodenum, it is again inflated to provide a bolus, which the peristaltic waves can more readily move along the intestine.

When the tube is inserted for decompression of an intestinal obstruction and possible later radiologic investigation, the adhesive strap is removed and replaced with an adhesive loop attached to the forehead. The tube can slide through the loop without tension as it advances toward the obstructed site. The patient is then returned to his room. Films of the abdomen may be taken to check the progress of the tube and the effectiveness of decompression. Simple obstructions are sometimes relieved by suction; others require surgical intervention.

If the passage of the intestinal tube is arrested, the suction is discontinued and the patient is returned to the radiology department for a Miller-Abbott tube study. The contrast medium employed for studies of a localized segment of the small bowel may be either a water-soluble iodinated solution (oral Hypaque or Gastrografin) or a thin barium sulfate suspension. Under radioscopic observation, the contrast agent is injected through the large lumen of the tube with a Luer syringe. Spot and conventional films are exposed as indicated.

When the intestinal tube is introduced for the purpose of performing a small-intestine enema, the tube is advanced into the proximal loop of the jejunum and then secured at this level with an adhesive strap beside the nose. The contrast agent is usually a thin preparation (2:10 ratio by volume) of barium sulfate and water. Although medical opinion varies as to the quantity of barium mixture required for this examination, the recommended amounts range from 8 ounces to as much as 1 quart. The medium is injected through the aspiration lumen of the tube in a continuous, low-pressure flow from a suitable container mounted on a standard, as for a large-intestine enema. Spot and conventional films are exposed as indicated. Except for the presence of the tube in the upper jejunum, the resultant films resemble those obtained by the oral method.

NOTE: See page 727 for a description of rapid, radioscopically controlled small-bowel intubation.

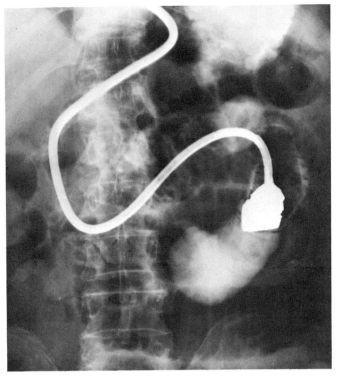

Miller-Abbott tube study. Water-soluble medium.

Courtesy Dr. William H. Shehadi.

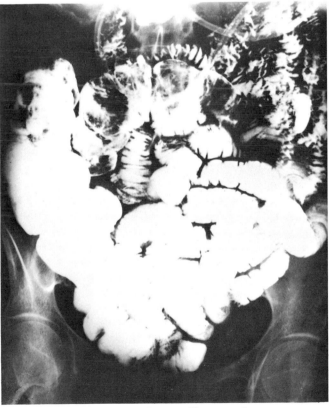

Small bowel enema. Barium sulfate suspension.

Courtesy Dr. Stanley M. Wyman.

733

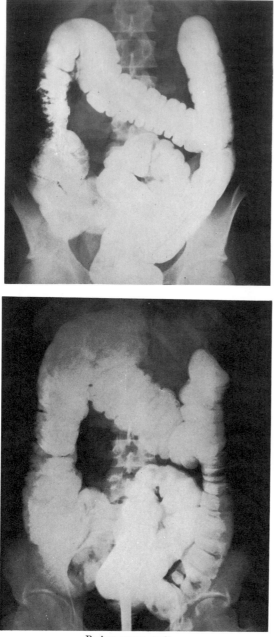

LARGE INTESTINE

Examination procedure in diagnostic enema studies

There are two basic radiologic methods of examining the large intestine by means of diagnostic or contrast enemas: (1) the single-contrast method, in which the colon is examined with a barium sulfate suspension only, and (2) the double-contrast method, which may be performed (a) in a two-stage procedure, in which the colon is first examined with a barium sulfate mixture and then, immediately following evacuation of the barium suspension, is examined with an air enema or another gaseous enema, or (b) in a single-stage procedure, in which, with the use of a three-way valve, the radiologist selectively injects the barium mixture or the gas.

The opaque medium demonstrates the anatomy and tonus of the colon and most of the abnormalities to which it is subject. The gaseous medium serves to distend the lumen of the bowel and to render visible, through the transparency of its shadow, all parts of the barium-coated mucosal lining of the colon and any small intraluminal lesions, such as polypoid tumors.

CONTRAST MEDIA

Chemically pure barium sulfate is the opaque medium in general use for routine retrograde examinations of the large bowel, although some radiologists prefer the commercially prepared barium sulfate products. There are many of the latter on the market, and some of them are referred to as colloidal preparations because they have finely divided barium particles that tend to resist settling out, while others are referred to as suspended or flocculation-resistant preparations because they contain some form of suspending or dispersing agent.

Barium enema studies.

Courtesy Dr. Francis H. Ghiselin.

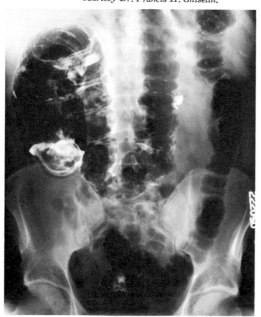

Double-contrast enema studies.   *Courtesy Dr. Robert L. Pinck.*

CONTRAST MEDIA—cont'd

Air, which is a mixture of one part oxygen, four parts nitrogen, and small amounts of other gases, is the gaseous medium commonly used in double-contrast enema studies. Carbon dioxide is also used because it is more rapidly absorbed than is the nitrogen of air when evacuation of the gaseous medium is incomplete.

Specially prepared solutions (oral Hypaque and Gastrografin) that are ingestible, water-soluble, and iodinated are used for retrograde filling of the colon in selected cases. A disadvantage of the iodinated solution is that evacuation is often insufficient for satisfactory double-contrast visualization of the mucosal pattern. A great advantage of these agents is that when a patient is for some reason unable to cooperate for a successful enema study, the colon can be satisfactorily examined with an ingested dose of an oral iodinated medium because (1) the transit time from ingestion to colonic filling is fast (averaging three to four hours); (2) being practically nonabsorbable from the gastrointestinal mucosa, the oral dose reaches and outlines the entire large bowel; and (3) unlike ingested barium sulfate suspensions, these media are not subject to drying, flaking, and unequal distribution in the colon, so that the oral dose frequently delineates the colon almost as well as does a barium enema.

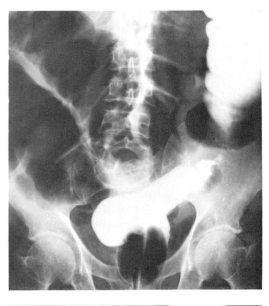

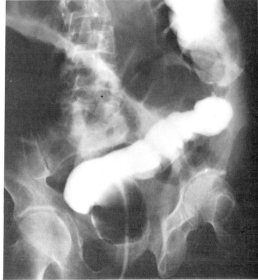

Retrograde filling with water-soluble medium showing obstructing lesion not shown with barium enema.

Radiographs and diagnostic information courtesy Dr. William H. Shehadi.

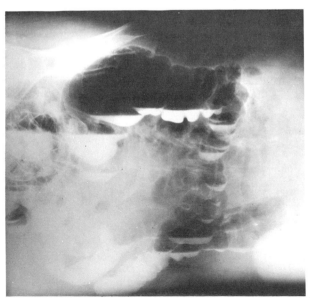

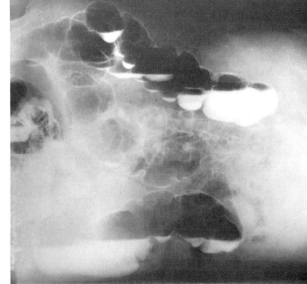

Double-contrast enema studies.

Right lateral decubitus projection.   Left lateral decubitus projection.

Courtesy Dr. William H. Shehadi.

735

LARGE INTESTINE—cont'd
Examination procedure in diagnostic enema studies—cont'd
PREPARATION OF INTESTINAL TRACT

There is a diversity of medical opinion about preparation measures. However, members of the profession commonly agree that the large bowel must be completely emptied of its contents in order to render all portions of its inner wall visible for inspection. When coated with a barium sulfate suspension, any retained fecal masses are likely to simulate the appearance of polypoid or other small tumor masses. This makes thorough cleansing of the entire colon a matter of prime importance. Any preliminary preparation of the intestinal tract of patients who have a condition such as severe diarrhea, gross bleeding, or symptoms of obstruction is, of course, limited if possible. Other patients are prepared, with modifications where indicated, according to the specifications established by the examining radiologist. In the usual procedure, preliminary preparation includes dietary restrictions as well as a cathartic and cleansing enema or a laxative suppository.

Diet. The patient may be placed on a soft or low-residue diet for two or three days preceding the examination, and he may be further restricted to clear liquids on the day before the examination. This is done to prevent gas formation due to excessive fermentation of the contents of the small intestine, and to obviate the possibility of masses of residual material passing from the small bowel into the proximal colon before the examination can be performed. A light breakfast of toast and black coffee or clear tea an hour or so before the examination is usually permitted because this meal is not likely to reach the cecum before the examination.

Cathartics. The physiologic effect of vegetable cathartics is, briefly, irritation of the intestinal mucosa with resultant semiliquefaction of the bowel contents and, by neuromuscular excitation, acceleration of peristaltic activity. These cathartics are effective in evacuating the small intestine and proximal colon, but cleansing enemas are usually required to clear the pelvic colon of residual material.

Castor oil, usually 1½ to 2 ounces taken in the early afternoon, is the most effective and most frequently prescribed purgative agent. The physiologic action of castor oil is primarily on the small bowel, causing only slight irritation of the colon, so that it must be supplemented by cleansing enemas. Some examiners administer two types of cathartic, one that acts primarily on the small intestine and is administered at or before noon and one that acts primarily on the large intestine and is administered at five or six o'clock in the evening. The first drug may be castor oil or, because it is more acceptable to the patient, an emulsified castor oil (Neoloid), and the second may be bisacodyl (Dulcolax; bis-(p-acetoxyphenyl)-2-pyridylmethane) or senna. Even the combination of cathartics is supplemented by cleansing enemas or a bisacodyl (Dulcolax) suppository on the following morning, the morning of the examination. Other cathartics in common use are licorice powder, phenolphthalein, and sodium phosphate (Phospho-soda). For a comprehensive description of cathartic drugs and various methods of preparing the colon for radiologic examination the reader is referred to pages 77 to 129 and 227 to 228 in *Detection of Colon Lesions* (American College of Radiology, 1973).

Patients should be given a small amount of salve containing a mild anesthetic for application to the sorely irritated area around the anus. When hemorrhoids are present, the patient should be given several medicated suppositories for use as needed before and after the cleansing enemas.

Cleansing enemas. Preceding a retrograde examination of the colon, cleansing enemas are administered at intervals of about fifteen minutes until the return flow is clear. This procedure is carried out two or three hours before the examination in order to allow an adequate interval for any retained fluid to be absorbed through the colon mucosa. Where this method is employed, 1 quart of solution is generally considered to be the maximum volume for a cleansing enema. Many examiners are now recommending the use of one cleansing enema and that it consist of 2 quarts of solution.

One quart of solution is generally considered to be the maximum volume for a cleansing enema; frequently, ½ to 1 pint will suffice to stimulate evacuation of the already semifluid contents of the pelvic colon. Because of the possibility of perforation of a weakened or diseased area in the bowel wall, the injection should never be forced beyond the point of comfortable tolerance. If the solution is injected slowly at a low pressure gradient, the patient will not feel undue discomfort or pain without reason.

Cleansing enema solutions should be warm (100° to 105° F.) since the aim is to stimulate peristalsis and the defecation impulse; they should never exceed 105° F., because higher temperatures are not only unpleasant and debilitating but may injure the tissues.

Due to the possibility of water intoxication from the use of hypotonic solutions,[1] normal (isotonic or physiologic) saline solution is generally used. The normal saline solution is also considered to be less irritating. It is made by adding 6 grams (1¾ teaspoonfuls) of common table salt to 1 quart of water. This solution is considered to be isotonic with human blood (to have the same salt concentration), and thus it will not interfere with the equilibrium of the body fluids. The isotonic solution should be used for patients who have chronic constipation because a large part of the injected fluid is likely to be absorbed.

Tannic acid, 2.5 grams per quart of water, was long used as an evacuant in cleansing enemas. This agent evacuates the colon effectively, but it sometimes causes such side effects as intestinal cramps, nausea, and faintness. Govoni and associates[2] recommend the use of hydrogen peroxide (H_2O_2) in both cleansing and barium sulfate enemas, stating that it has all the advantages claimed for tannic acid and none of its disadvantages. The cleansing enema consists of 10 ml. (40 vol.) of H_2O_2 per quart of water, and is administered at body temperature. These authors recommend that the solution be injected slowly while the patient is rotated from the prone position, to his left side, to the supine position, and to his right side. They stress the importance of permitting the patient to evacuate the enema on the first vague symptoms of abdominal colic, because this symptom is quickly followed by diffuse colonic atony, with resultant inadequate evacuation of the gases. When the preliminary film shows a heavy accumulation of fecal

[1]Gillespie, J. B., Miller, G. A., and Schlereth, J.: Water intoxication following enemas for roentgenographic preparations, Amer. J. Roentgen. **82:**1067-1069, 1959.
[2]Govoni, A., Brailsford, J. F., and Mucklow, E. H.: The use of hydrogen peroxide for the elimination of gas from the intestine during roentgenography of the abdominal viscera, Amer. J. Roentgen. **71:**235-238, 1954.

material, it is recommended that the material be eliminated with a plain water enema. The gas content is then eliminated with an H_2O_2 enema of lesser concentration— 25 minims of hydrogen peroxide (20 vol.) per pint of water.

Whatever measures are employed to prepare the intestinal tract, the efficacy of the procedure should be determined by a scout film of the abdomen before the examination is started. When residual gas and/or fecal material is found in the colon, the radiologist may order another cleansing enema, or he may administer an intramuscular injection of vasopressin (Pitressin) to stimulate further evacuation. Defecation usually occurs thirty to forty-five minutes after the injection. Possible side reactions to Pitressin are intestinal cramps, uterine cramps, nausea, faintness, dizziness, and headache.

STANDARD BARIUM ENEMA APPARATUS

An enema can made of stainless steel or another boilable material should be used for all colonic injections. The barium enema can should have a capacity of 2 to 3 quarts (1) to prevent complete emptying of the can, which draws air into the rectum, and (2) to allow for full distension of the colon. (While the radiologist may fill the colon to capacity under radioscopic observation, unless directed to do so, the technologist should never inject more than 1 quart of solution when administering cleansing enemas because of the danger of perforation in the presence of a pathologic lesion.)

The tubing, preferably of disposable plastic, should be 5 or 6 feet in length, and if opaque (rubber), should have a glass connection tube set in at the lower third, so that, by pinching the tubing a foot or so above the connection, the flow of the barium mixture can be checked without removing the can from the standard. The tubing should be equipped with a reliable, easy-to-operate cut-off clip, or with a hemostat.

Carmen metal enema nozzles and rectal tubes are obtainable in three sizes. Disposable soft-plastic rectal tubes are also available in several sizes and, for obvious reasons, are preferable to other tubes of this type. A soft-rubber rectal catheter of small caliber should be used for patients who have inflamed hemorrhoids, fissures, a stricture, or other abnormalities of the anus.

Rectal retention catheters are available in several sizes. These tubes (Bardex, Foley, Weber, Franklin, Virden) are used with patients who have a relaxed anal sphincter, and with those who cannot, for some other reason, retain an enema. The retention catheter is a double-lumen tube with a thin rubber balloon at its distal end. It is not easy to insert, and the condition of the patient with whom it is used is usually poor. Because of the danger of rupture,[1,2] retention catheters should not be inserted by the non-nurse technologist.

There is now available a disposable retention tip, the rubber balloon of which fits snugly against the enema nozzle both before inflation and after deflation, so that it can be inserted and removed with no discomfort to the patient. A reusable squeeze inflator is included in each carton of four dozen tips. The inflator has an air capacity of 90 cc. One complete squeeze of the inflator provides adequate distention of the retention balloon without danger of overinflation.

CLEANSING AND STERILIZATION OF ENEMA APPARATUS

Reflux from the bowel into the enema apparatus always contaminates the tubing, and usually the can as well. In order to obviate the possibility of spreading disease from patient to patient, enema apparatus must be thoroughly cleaned and then sterilized.

1. Remove any fecal masses from the rectal tube with the paper toweling placed around it when it was withdrawn from the rectum.

2. Run cold water from the hopper tap over and through the can, tubing, and rectal tube or catheter at high pressure until all traces of fecal matter and barium are removed.

3. Fill the can with hot, soapy water and wash the entire set carefully, allowing the soapsuds to drain through the tubing and nozzle.

4. Rinse with hot water, allowing it to flow over and through the apparatus. Disconnect the tubing and loosely coil it to prevent kinking.

5. Place the can, tubing, and rectal tube or catheter into a suitable container and boil for five minutes.

6. After boiling, hang the tubing and catheter to drain and dry before putting them away.

Boiling is destructive to rubber, but failure to sterilize these items can hardly be justified on economic grounds.[3,4]

[1]Nathan, M. H., and Kohen, R.: The Bardex tube in performing barium enemas: evaluation of its use and safety, Amer. J. Roentgen. **84**:1121-1124, 1960.

[2]Rosenberg, L. S., and Fine, A.: Fatal venous intravasation of barium during a barium enema, Radiology **73**:771-773, 1959.

[3]Meyers, P. H.: Contamination of barium enema apparatus during its use, J.A.M.A. **173**:1589-1590, 1960.

[4]Steinbach, H. L., Rousseau, R., McCormack, K. R., and Jawetz, E.: Transmission of enteric pathogens by barium enemas, J.A.M.A. **174**:1207-1208, 1960.

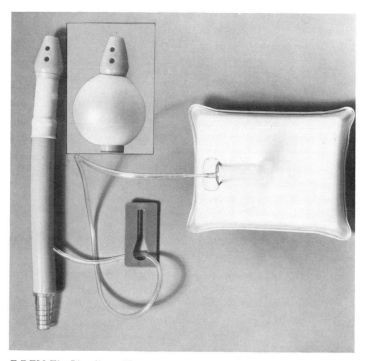

E-Z-EM Slim Line disposable retention tip. Note the snug fit of the uninflated balloon. The inset shows the balloon when inflated with 90 cc. of air, one complete squeeze of the inflator.

LARGE INTESTINE—cont'd
Examination procedure in diagnostic enema studies—cont'd
PREPARATION OF BARIUM SUSPENSION

The concentration of the barium sulfate mixtures employed for colonic enemas varies considerably, the recommended barium-to-water proportions ranging from 1:4 to 1:8 by volume. Heavier concentrations are generally preferred when an air study is to follow the barium study, the purpose being to obtain a better mucosal coating. A thin, or dilute, mixture used in conjunction with high kilovoltage penetration is advocated by some radiologists for the purpose of demonstrating intraluminal lesions situated in overlapped loops of the bowel.

The barium sulfate is mixed in warm water or, especially for patients with chronic constipation, in an isotonic saline solution (1¾ teaspoonfuls of common table salt to each quart of water).

Many radiologists add to their formula powdered gum acacia (usually 2 teaspoonfuls) or methylcellulose jell (2 tablespoonfuls) to sustain the suspension, and to render it somewhat viscid in order to obtain better mucosal coating. Before being added to the barium mixture, the acacia powder must be *completely dissolved* in 7 or 8 ounces of water. An electric mixer may be used to aid in the dissolving, or, preferably, the water and powder mixture may be allowed to stand overnight.

Tannic acid has been widely used because it not only produces more complete evacuation of the colon but is said to leave a better mucosal coating. Unfortunately, this agent sometimes causes unpleasant side effects. Hydrogen peroxide (H_2O_2) has been found to be just as effective and to cause no unpleasant side effects.[1] Govoni and associates recommend that it be used in the proportion of 10 ml. (40 vol.) of H_2O_2 to each quart of barium mixture or, if preferred, in a lesser concentration of 25 minims of H_2O_2 to each pint of fluid.

It is important that each ingredient be accurately measured according to the specifications of the radiologist, and that they be mixed in a pitcher or another suitable vessel, *never in the enema can.* The suspension should be stirred for any necessary reconstitution just before it is poured into the enema can and, lest there be enough settling out to clog the tubing, the suspension should be poured into the enema can just before the examination.

An electric mixer is a necessity for mixing some of the mucilaginous barium sulfate preparations, but it is not required for mixing ordinary barium sulfate suspensions. High-speed rotary mixers whip a large amount of air into the barium suspension. Unless enough time is allowed for the air to settle out, it causes radiolucencies within the barium column and, when enough air is present in the mixture, an irregular peripheral fading in the opacity of the column. Where an electric mixer is used, it is advisable to prepare the suspensions several hours in advance of their use, preferably on the preceding day.

A thermometer rather than the forearm should be used to determine the temperature of barium enema mixtures as well as of cleansing enema solutions. Where it is the practice to administer warm enemas, the temperature should be somewhat below body heat, about 85° to 90° F.

(29° to 32° C.), to avoid irritation, with resultant stimulation of peristalsis and the defecation impulse. In addition to being unpleasant and debilitating, an enema that is too warm is injurious to the tissues and produces so much irritation that it is difficult, if not impossible, for the patient to retain the enema long enough for a satisfactory examination.

Cold barium enema suspensions (41° F., 5° C.) have been recommended[2,3] on the basis that the colder temperature produces less irritation, has a mild anesthetic effect that relaxes the colon, and stimulates tonic contraction of the anal sphincter. These effects result in greater comfort and ease of retention for the patient, and permit less difficult and more rapid filling of the colon. The patient not only feels no sensation of chill but finds the cold suspension soothing and easy to retain. The cold temperature is most easily obtained by preparing the barium mixture a day in advance for overnight storage in a refrigerator.

PREPARATION AND CARE OF PATIENT

There is no radiologic examination in which the full cooperation of the patient is more essential to success than in retrograde examinations of the colon. Few patients who are physically able to do so fail to retain the enema when they understand the procedure and realize that in large measure the success of the examination depends upon them. Time must be taken to explain the procedural differences between an ordinary cleansing enema and a diagnostic enema: (1) the radiologist examines all portions of the bowel as he fills it with the opaque medium under radioscopic observation; (2) this part of the examination involves palpation of the abdomen, rotation of the body as required to visualize the different segments of the colon, and the taking of spot films without and, where indicated, with compression; and (3) a series of large films are then taken before the colon can be evacuated.

The patient should be assured that retention of the diagnostic enema will be comparatively easy because of its cooler temperature, and because its flow is controlled under radioscopic observation. He should be instructed (1) to keep the anal sphincter tightly contracted against the rectal tube to hold it in position and to prevent leakage, (2) to relax the abdominal muscles to prevent intra-abdominal pressure, and (3) to concentrate on deep oral breathing to reduce the incidence of colonic spasm and resultant cramps. The patient should be assured that the flow of the enema will be stopped for the duration of any cramping, and that the fluid will be siphoned back for his relief if necessary. This is done simply by lowering the enema can. The patient, especially if he has inflamed hemorrhoids or another anal abnormality, can be spared much discomfort throughout the examination by having him apply a local anesthetic (medicated suppository and/or salve) fifteen to twenty minutes before the examination.

Patients who have not had a previous colonic examination are usually fearful of being embarrassed by inadequate draping as well as by failure to retain the enema for the

---

[1]Govoni, A., Brailsford, J. F., and Mucklow, E. H.: The use of hydrogen peroxide for the elimination of gas from the intestine during roentgenography of the abdominal viscera, Amer. J. Roentgen. 71:235-238, 1954.

[2]Levene, G., and Kaufman, S. A.: An improved technic for double contrast examination of the colon by the use of compressed carbon dioxide, Radiology 68:83-85, 1957.

[3]Levene, G.: Low temperature barium-water suspensions for roentgenologic examination of the colon, Radiology 77:117-118, 1961.

required time. These anxieties can be dispelled or greatly relieved by assuring the patient that he will be properly covered, and that while there is little chance of mishap, he will be well protected so that he need feel no embarrassment should one occur. A bedpan should be kept in the examining room for patients who cannot or may not be able to make the trip to the toilet. The preliminary preparation required for a retrograde study of the colon is strenuous. The examination itself further depletes the patient's strength. Enfeebled patients, particularly elderly people, are likely to become quite weak and faint from the exertion of the preparation, the examination, and the effort made to expel the enema. A bell should be kept in each toilet so that patients can summon help when needed. While the patient's privacy must be respected, the technologist or an aide should make frequent inquiry to make sure that the patient is all right, in case he is not able to call for help.

Gown and underpadding. Patients who are to have a large intestine enema should be clothed in a cotton gown that has an overlapping back with a tie fastening, so that no patient will ever be subjected to the repulsive experience of having to remove a massively soiled gown by pulling it over his head. Patients should be supplied with disposable paper slippers and advised to remove their hose to protect them from possible splatter.

When a gown becomes soiled, the patient should be allowed to wash and change into a clean gown before proceeding with the examination; this must be done for disabled patients. Any extensive cleaning of the examining table and room should be done while the patient is in the lavatory; if he must remain on the table, the cleaning should be done pleasantly, and as unobtrusively as possible.

The preparation of the patient includes protection of the examining table, a step that increases the patient's sense of security. Pulp-filled disposable underpadding with a waterproof backing is satisfactory for this purpose. Disposable pads are available in several sizes, and they are considerably less expensive than commercial laundry of a sheet. A further advantage is that they eliminate the problem of disinfecting contaminated nondisposable padding.

Insertion of rectal tube. In preparation for the insertion of the rectal tube, instruct the patient to turn onto his left side, lean forward some 35 to 40 degrees, and rest his flexed right knee on the table, above and in front of the slightly flexed left knee (Sims' position). This position relaxes the abdominal muscles, which decreases

intra-abdominal pressure on the rectum and makes relaxation of the anal sphincter less difficult. With the patient in position, make any necessary adjustment in the temperature of the barium mixture, stir it well, and then fill the enema can and hang it on the standard. The standard should be adjusted so that the fluid level is 18 to 24 inches above the level of the anus. The rectal tube should be placed in the fold of several sheets of paper toweling, which are again used to wrap the tube when it is removed from the rectum.

Adjust the overlapping back of the gown or other draping to expose the anal region only, keeping the patient otherwise well covered. The anal orifice is frequently partially obscured by distended hemorrhoids or by a fringe of undistended hemorrhoids. Not infrequently, there is a contraction or other abnormality of the orifice. It is therefore necessary that the anus be exposed and sufficiently well lighted for the orifice to be clearly visible, so that the correct rectal tube can be selected and inserted without injury or discomfort.

Run a little of the barium mixture into a waste basin to free the tubing of air, and then lubricate the rectal tube well with a water-soluble lubricant such as K-Y jelly. During this time explain to the patient that the rectal tube is considerably smaller in diameter than a normally formed stool, and that if he will relax and concentrate on deep oral breathing, he will feel no discomfort when the tube is inserted.

Push the right buttock upward to open the gluteal fold. As the abdominal muscles and anal sphincter are relaxed during the exhalation phase of a deep breath, gently and slowly insert the rectal tube into the anal orifice: (1) following the angle of the anal canal, direct the tube forward 1 to 1½ inches, and (2) following the curve of the rectum, direct the tube slightly backward. Insert the tube for a total distance of no more than 3½ to 4 inches; a greater distance is not only unnecessary, but it involves possible injury to the rectum. When the tube does not enter easily, call the radiologist. The technologist should never forcibly insert a rectal tube; the patient may have distended internal hemorrhoids or another condition that would make a forced insertion dangerous.

After the insertion of the rectal tube, hold it in position to prevent it from slipping while the patient is turning to the frontal position for radioscopy, supine or prone, according to the preference of the radiologist. Adjust the protective underpadding, and relieve any pressure on the tubing so that the enema mixture will flow freely.

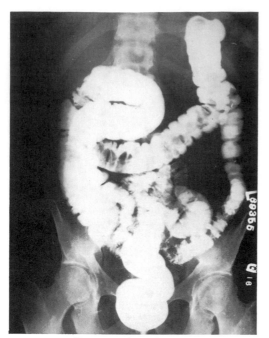

Posteroanterior projection.

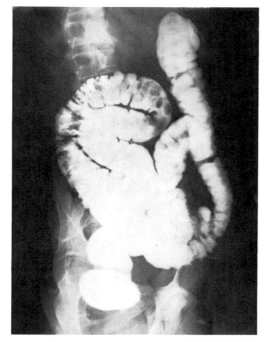

Right posteroanterior oblique projection.

Courtesy Dr. Marcy L. Sussman.

LARGE INTESTINE—cont'd
Examination procedure in diagnostic enema studies—cont'd
ADMINISTRATION OF OPAQUE ENEMA

The radiologist is notified as soon as everything is in readiness for the examination. This should be done before the room lights are dimmed or extinguished, unless the doctor has previously met and interviewed the patient. At the radiologist's indication, release the control clip and make sure that the rectal tube is not occluded with fecal material—that the enema is flowing. When occlusion occurs, soft material can be displaced by withdrawing the rectal tube about 1 inch and, before reinserting it, temporarily elevating the enema can to increase fluid pressure.

The rectal ampulla fills slowly, and unless the flow is stopped for a few seconds at this point, the barium mixture then flows through the sigmoid and descending portions of the colon at a fairly rapid rate of speed, frequently causing a severe cramp and acute stimulation of the defecation impulse. The flow of the enema is usually stopped for several seconds at frequent intervals during the radioscopically controlled filling of the colon. The flow can be stopped more quickly by making a kink in the tubing than by operating the control clip. Where the technologist is not required to perform this service, the radiologist can operate a hemostat with greater ease than the usual cutoff clip.

ADMINISTRATION OF OPAQUE ENEMA—cont'd

During the radioscopic examination, the radiologist rotates the patient so as to inspect all segments of the bowel. He makes spot films as indicated, and determines the positions to be used for the subsequent radiographic studies. Upon completion of the radioscopic examination, the rectal tube is usually removed for easier maneuverability of the patient and to prevent its accidental displacement during the filming procedure. A retention tube is not removed until the patient is placed on a bedpan or on the toilet stool.

After the immediate films have been exposed, the patient is escorted to a toilet or placed on a bedpan, and instructed to expel as much of the enema as possible. A postevacuation film is then made. When this film shows evacuation to be inadequate for satisfactory delineation of the mucosa, the patient may be given a hot beverage (tea or coffee) to stimulate further evacuation.

NOTE: The decrease in the frontal thickness of the abdomen from preevacuation to postevacuation is approximately 5 cm., which requires an exposure decrease equivalent to 10 kilovolts for the latter film.

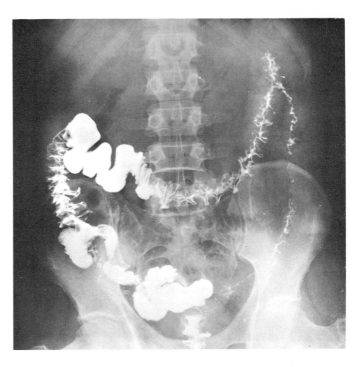

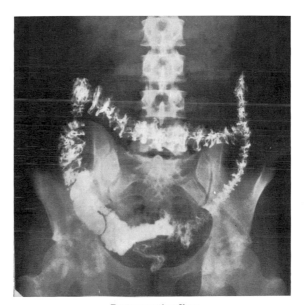

Postevacuation films.

Courtesy Dr. Francis H. Ghiselin.

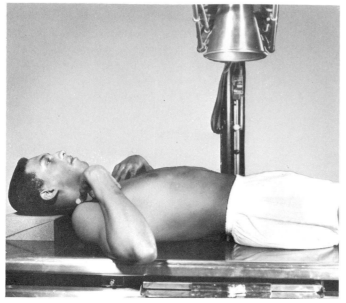

Central ray perpendicular to film.

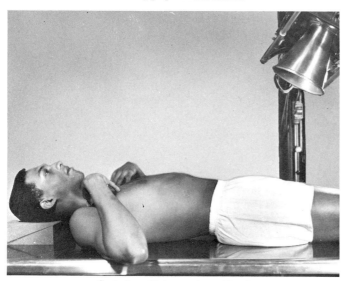

Central ray 35 degrees toward head.

LARGE INTESTINE—cont'd
Radiography of the opacified colon

Radiographic studies of the adult colon are made on 14″ × 17″ films. Except for angled projections, these films are centered at the level of the iliac crests on patients of average build, somewhat higher for hypersthenic patients, and somewhat lower for asthenic patients. The frontal view of the colon in the wide, capacious abdomen requires two exposures, with the films placed crosswise; the first is centered high enough to include the diaphragm, and the other low enough to include the rectum. Localized studies of the rectum and rectosigmoid junction are made on 10″ × 12″ or 11″ × 14″ films centered at the level of, or just slightly above the level of the upper border of the pubic symphysis.

SUPPLEMENTAL POSITIONS

In addition to the direct frontal projection, which is usually made with the patient supine rather than prone, preevacuation filming includes one or more supplemental projections for the demonstration of otherwise obscured flexed and curved areas of the bowel. With the central ray directed perpendicularly, except where otherwise specified, the following are the supplemental positions most frequently employed:

1. With the patient supine or obliqued, as required, the Trendelenburg position is used to separate redundant and overlapping loops of the bowel by "spilling" them out of the pelvis. The central ray is directed vertically for these studies.

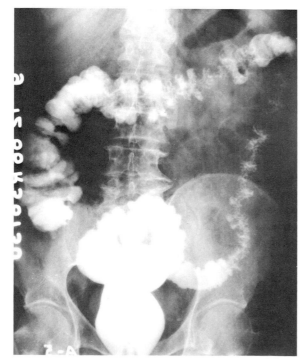

Central ray perpendicular to film.

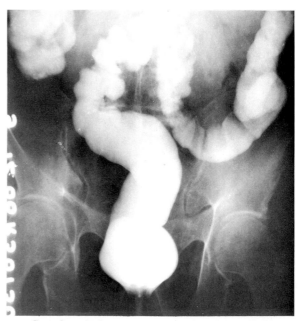

Central ray 35 degrees toward head on opposite patient.

Radiographs courtesy Dr. William H. Shehadi.

2. With the patient supine, the central ray is directed at an angle of 35 to 45 degrees toward the head and centered at the level of the anterior superior iliac spines. This projection, described by Billing,[1] is used to demonstrate the rectosigmoid and sigmoid areas. A similar view can be obtained by reversing the above central ray angulation when the patient is being examined in the prone position.

[1]Billing, L.: Zur Technik der Kontrastuntersuchung des Colon sigmoideum, Acta Radiol. 25:418-422, 1944.

3. With the patient supine, the central ray is directed at an angle of 12 degrees toward the feet and centered to a point about 1 inch proximal to the upper border of the pubic symphysis. This projection, suggested by Oppenheimer,[2] is employed for the demonstration of the rectosigmoid area.

[2]Oppenheimer, A.: Roentgen diagnosis of incipient cancer of the rectum, Amer. J. Roentgen. 52:637-646, 1944.

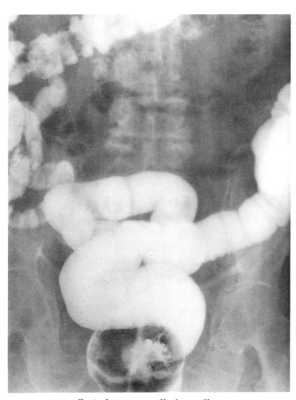

Central ray perpendicular to film.

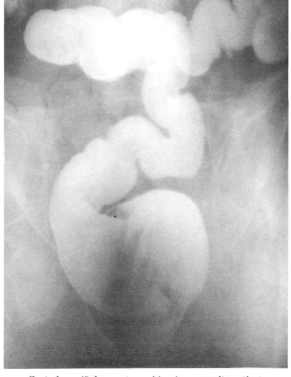

Central ray 45 degrees toward head on opposite patient.

Radiographs courtesy Dr. William B. Seaman.

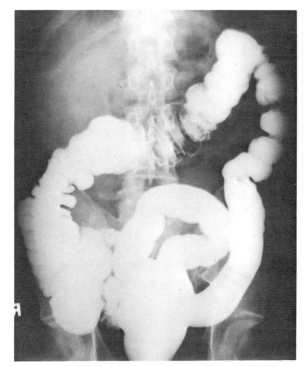

Central ray perpendicular to film.

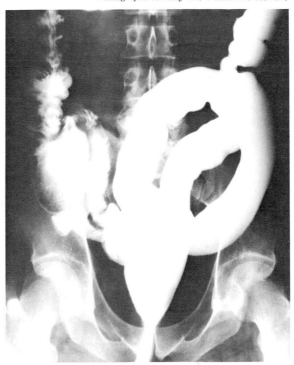

Central ray 12 degrees toward feet on opposite patient.

Radiographs courtesy Dr. Herbert F. Hempel.

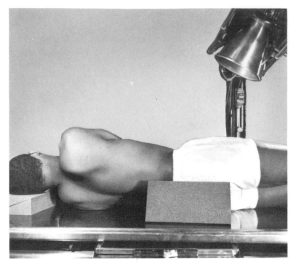

30- to 35-degree LAO position with central ray 30 to 35 degrees toward head.

LARGE INTESTINE—cont'd
Radiography of the opacified colon—cont'd
SUPPLEMENTAL POSITIONS—cont'd

4. The patient is placed in a 30- to 35-degree left anteroposterior oblique position (left posteroanterior oblique view), and the central ray is directed through a point 2 inches medial to the elevated right anterior superior iliac spine at an angle of 30 to 35 degrees toward the head. This projection, described by Fletcher,[1] is used for the demonstration of the rectosigmoid junction and the sigmoid.

5. A 45-degree left anteroposterior oblique position (left posteroanterior oblique view), described by Oppenheimer,[2] is used to demonstrate the hepatic flexure and the adjacent portions of the proximal colon. The reverse (right) anteroposterior oblique position is used to demonstrate the splenic flexure and the adjacent transverse and descending portions of the colon.

6. A 45-degree right posteroanterior oblique position (right anteroposterior oblique view) is used to demonstrate the hepatic flexure and adjacent portions of the colon, and the reverse (left) posteroanterior oblique position is used to demonstrate the splenic flexure and the left-sided portions of the colon when the frontal projection was made with the patient in the prone position.

7. A direct lateral projection, suggested by Robins,[3] is used to demonstrate the rectum and rectosigmoid. The coronal plane passing about 2 inches posterior to the midaxillary line of the body is centered to the table, and the film and central ray are centered 2 inches proximal to the level of the pubic symphysis.

[1]Fletcher, G. H.: An improved method of visualization of the sigmoid, Amer. J. Roentgen. **59:**750-752, 1948.

[2]Oppenheimer, A., and Saleeby, G. W.: Proctography: roentgenologic studies of the rectum and sigmoid, Surg. Gynec. Obstet. **69:**83-93, 1939.

[3]Robins, S. A., and Altman, W. S.: The significance of the lateral view of the rectum, Amer. J. Roentgen. **40:**598-605, 1938.

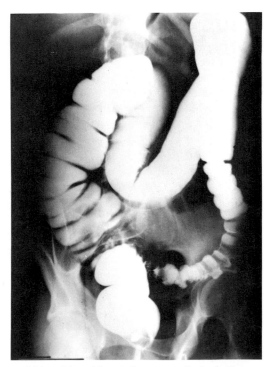

LAO position with central ray perpendicular to film.

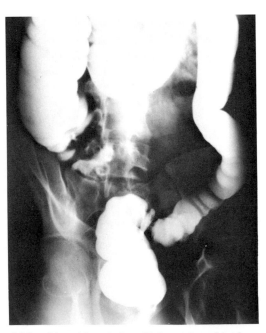

LAO position with central ray 30 degrees toward head.

Radiographs courtesy Dr. Herbert F. Hempel.

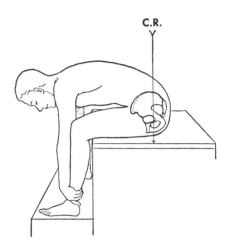

8. The Chassard-Lapiné axial projection is used for the demonstration of the rectum, the rectosigmoid junction, and the sigmoid. It was found[1-3] that this projection, being made at almost a right angle to the frontal projection, demonstrates the anterior and posterior surfaces of the lower portion of the bowel, and permits the coils of the sigmoid to be projected free from overlapping. This projection may be made after evacuation, although, as Raap[1] stated, a preevacuation film can be made when the patient has reasonable sphincteric control.

Chassard-Lapiné position. Seat the patient well back on the side of the table so that the midaxillary plane of the body is as near as possible to the midline of the table. If necessary, shift the transversely placed 11″ × 14″ film forward in the tray so that its transverse axis will coincide as nearly as possible with the midaxillary plane of the body.

Ask the patient to abduct his thighs as far as the edge of the table permits, so that they will not interfere with flexion of the body. Center the film to the median sagittal plane of the pelvis, and then have the patient lean directly forward as far as possible.

Ask the patient to grasp his ankles for support. Respiration is suspended for the exposure.

The exposure required for this projection is approximately the same as that required for a lateral view of the pelvis.

Direct the central ray vertically through the lumbosacral region at the level of the greater trochanters.

[1]Raap, Gerard: A position of value in studying the pelvis and its contents, Southern Med. J. 44:95-99, 1951.

[2]Cimmino, C. V.: Radiography of the sigmoid flexure with the Chassard-Lapiné projection, Med. Radiogr. Photogr. 30:44-46, 1954.

[3]Ettinger, Alice, and Elkin, Milton: Study of the sigmoid by special roentgenographic views, Amer. J. Roentgen. 72:199-208, 1954.

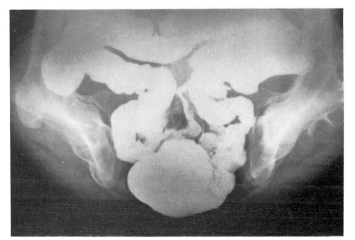

Chassard-Lapiné projection.

Courtesy Dr. William H. Shehadi.

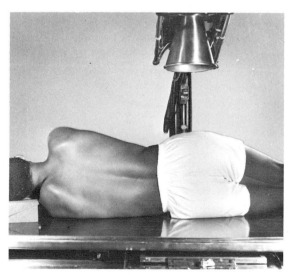

Position for lateral view of rectum.

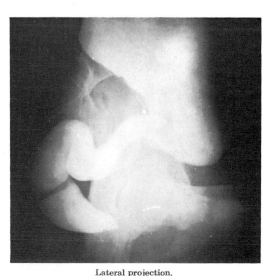

Lateral projection.

Courtesy Dr. Francis H. Ghiselin.

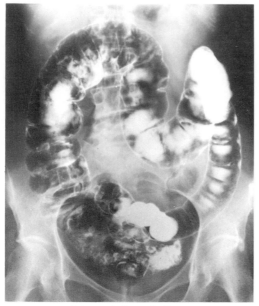

Anteroposterior projection.

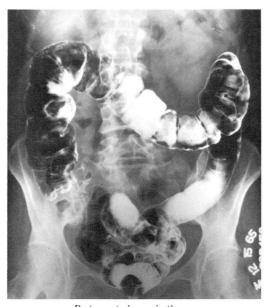

Posteroanterior projection.

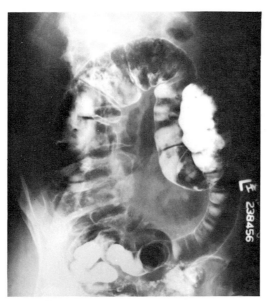

Right posteroanterior oblique projection.
Radiographs courtesy Dr. Robert L. Pinck.

746

LARGE INTESTINE—cont'd

Administration of air enema

In order to prevent drying and flaking of the thin layer of barium suspension adhering to the colonic mucosa, it is important that as little time as possible elapse between the evacuation of the barium mixture and the administration of the gaseous enema. The postevacuation film should be processed expeditiously, during which time the insufflation apparatus should be prepared and the patient adjusted in the Sims' position, ready for the insertion of the rectal tube as soon as the radiologist has determined whether evacuation of the opaque medium was adequate.

The colon is insufflated under radioscopic control by a procedure not unlike the opaque filling. It should be explained to the patient that he will experience much the same sensation with the gaseous filling as he did with the fluid filling, and that he will return to the lavatory to expel it in the same manner.

A hand blower apparatus, similar to the Weber device illustrated below, is widely employed for colonic insufflations. Because the device is operated by hand, this method has the disadvantage of being slow. The apparatus shown in the second illustration is not only simple to construct but makes it possible to introduce a smooth flow of warm air into the colon. This device consists of a 1 gallon bottle with a rubber stopper, through which are inserted two glass connection pipes, one of which is short, while the other extends almost to the bottom of the bottle. The glass connector is removed from the tubing of the enema can, and the end of the hose that is attached to the rectal tube is then connected to the short pipe of the insufflation bottle and the tubing that is attached to the enema can is connected to the long pipe. The enema can is filled with warm water, which is allowed to flow into the bottle to displace the air at an even rate of flow for insufflation of the bowel.

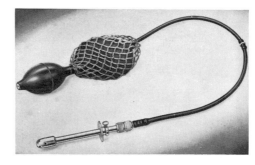

Radiography of the insufflated colon

Both vertical ray and horizontal ray projections are employed for double-contrast studies of the large bowel. Any excess of the barium suspension drains onto the dependent wall of each segment of the colon, leaving a thin, opaque coating on the gas-enveloped uppermost walls. This makes it possible to clearly delineate, by horizontal ray projection, areas that may be obscured in the vertical ray studies.

With vertical ray projection, supine, prone, and 40- to 45-degree right and left oblique positions are used. A direct lateral projection of the rectum and the rectosigmoid junction may be included.

The right and left lateral decubitus positions are the ones most frequently used for horizontal ray studies. These projections require the use of grid-front cassettes or a stationary grid. The patient's trunk is not elevated, since the uppermost side of the colon is the point of interest. The erect position is used for the delineation of the hepatic and splenic flexures.

While the thickness of the abdomen is as great when the colon is distended with gas as when it is distended with a barium suspension, the radioparency of the gaseous medium makes it necessary to decrease the exposure technique for double-contrast studies. Depending upon the amount of gas injected, the exposure should be decreased 10 to 15 kilovolts.

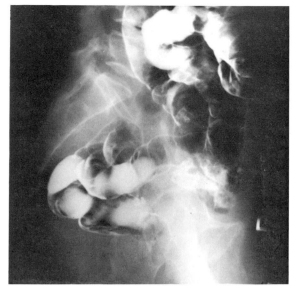

Lateral projection.

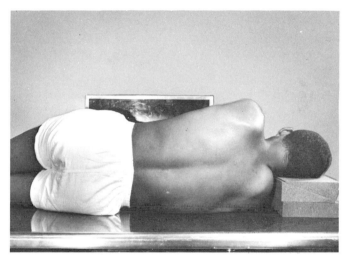

Right lateral decubitus position.

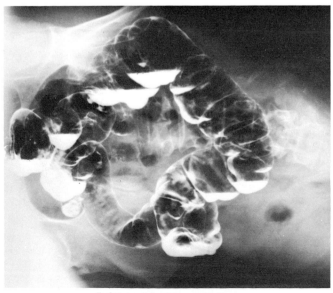

Left lateral decubitus projection.

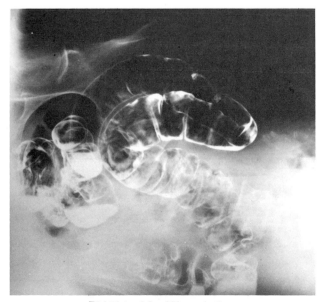

Right lateral decubitus projection.

Radiographs courtesy Dr. Robert L. Pinck.

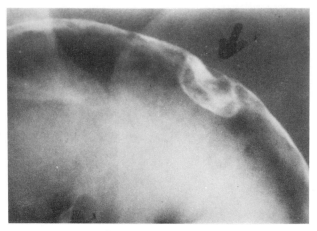

Small carcinoma with intubation.

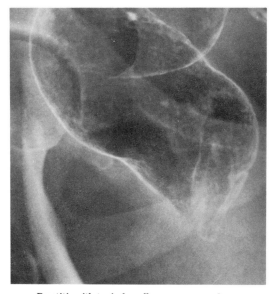

Proctitis with typical swollen mucous membrane.

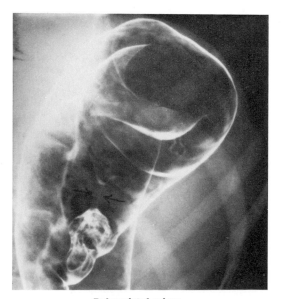

Pedunculated polyps.

Radiographs and diagnostic information courtesy Dr. Sölve Welin.

LARGE INTESTINE—cont'd

Welin technique for double-contrast enemas

Welin,[1,2] who is an internationally acknowledged expert in radiologic examinations of the large bowel, developed a technique for double-contrast enemas that reveals even the smallest intraluminal lesions. Welin states that this method of examination has been extremely valuable in the early diagnosis of such conditions as ulcerative colitis, regional colitis, and polyps.

Welin stresses the importance of preparing the intestine for the examination, stating that (1) the colon must be cleansed as thoroughly as possible and (2) the colonic mucosa must be prepared in such a way as to permit the adhesion of an extremely thin and even coating of barium on the colonic wall. He recommends that evacuation be regulated so that the two stages of the examination can be carried out at short intervals to avoid unnecessary waiting time, and states that it should not be necessary for the patient to be in the examining room more than a total of twenty to twenty-five minutes.

Preliminary preparation

1. On the day preceding the examination:
   a. The patient is placed on a low-residue or a non-residue diet.
   b. Two tablespoonfuls (1 ounce) of castor oil are given before noon, usually at 10 A.M.
   c. A plain water enema is administered in the evening.
2. On the morning of the examination:
   a. Toast and a cup of coffee or tea are permitted.
   b. On arrival in the radiology department, at least thirty minutes before the examination, the patient is given atropine by mouth, 0.25 to 1 mg. according to age. The atropine is administered to inhibit the action of the secretory glands of the colon. Drying the mucosa has two advantages: (1) it prevents a layer of mucus from concealing small lesions, and (2) the dry surface permits better adhesion of the barium mixture. Welin states that the atropine also diminishes the distress of the strong colonic contractions produced by the drugs used in the cleansing and barium enemas, and because it relaxes the bowel, it prevents discomfort when the bowel is distended with air.
   c. After the administration of the atropine, the colon is irrigated with a solution consisting of lukewarm water in which has been dissolved one packet (2.5 grams) of bisacodyl tannex (Clysodrast). This compound contains 1.5 mg. of the laxative drug bisacodyl and 2.5 grams of tannic acid. The bisacodyl acts on contact with the colonic mucosa to increase peristaltic contractions, and the tannic acid further inhibits the secretion of mucus as well as strongly stimulating peristalsis. Clysodrast is contraindicated in patients under the age of 10 years and in the presence of extensive ulcerative colitis. The manufacturers of the drug state that it is important that the total dosage used in the enemas (cleansing and barium) not exceed 7.5 grams (3 packets).

[1]Welin, S.: Modern trends in diagnostic roentgenology of the colon, Brit. J. Radiol. **31:**453-464, 1958.

[2]Welin, S.: Results of the Malmo technique of colon examination, J.A.M.A. **199:**369-371, 1967.

The cleansing enemas must be administered by a specially trained person who understands the importance of cleansing the colon for this examination. The enema is given slowly under low pressure (enema container about 18 inches above the rectum), and the patient is encouraged to take and retain the full 2 liters of solution. The enema is started with the patient on his left side. He is then turned, first onto his abdomen, next on his right side, and finally on his back. One 2-liter enema is usually adequate, but the results of the evacuation are inspected and the enema is repeated if the return is not clear.

After thorough cleansing of the colon, the patient is placed on the radiographic table for the first stage of the examination.

Barium suspension

The positive contrast enema consists of a thick colloidal barium sulfate–water mixture into which has been dissolved one packet (2.5 grams) of Clysodrast per liter of barium mixture. In order to obtain optimal mucosal coating, Welin recommends the use of a heavy barium mixture, specifying that the mixture have a specific gravity of 6.5 as tested with the Phillips Ba-test Hydrometer.* The weight of the different types of barium varies considerably. For this reason, the exact barium-to-water proportions required for the mixture must be established with the preferred barium in each radiology department by testing and adjusting the mixture with the use of the Ba-test Hydrometer. It can be stated that the proportions will be in the area of three and one-half to four parts of barium to five parts of water. Welin has the enema container fitted with long tubing so that it can be hung on a pulley device mounted on the ceiling. The extreme height of the container provides enough pressure to make the thick barium mixture flow.

Stage one of examination

With the patient placed in the prone position to prevent possible ileal leak, the radiologist fills the colon up to the splenic flexure, after which one conventional film is taken, a right lateral projection of the barium-filled rectum. The patient is then sent to the lavatory to evacuate. After this, if he feels the need to do so, he is allowed to lie down and rest for awhile.

Stage two of examination

When the patient is returned to the examining table, the enema nozzle is inserted, and the patient is again turned to the prone position. The prone position not only prevents ileal leak with resultant opacification and overlap of the small intestine on the rectosigmoid area, but it also aids in adequate drainage of excess barium from the rectum.

The radiologist allows the barium mixture to run up to the middle of the sigmoid colon, slightly farther if the sigmoid is long. The patient is then turned onto his right side, and air is instilled with a hand-blower such as the Higginson or Webber insufflation devices. The air forces

*Phillips Medical Systems, Inc., 5932 East 10th St., Indianapolis, Ind. 46219.

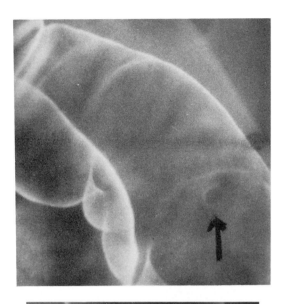

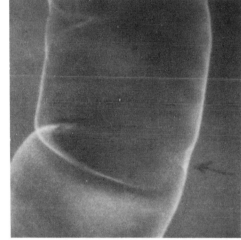

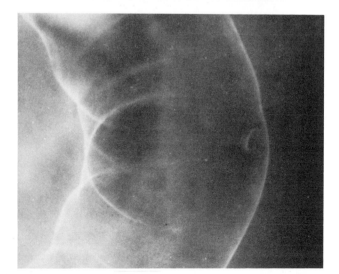

Protuberant polyp shown, from above downward, en face, profile, and oblique.

Radiographs and diagnostic information courtesy Dr. Sölve Welin.

LARGE INTESTINE—cont'd

Welin technique for double-contrast enemas—cont'd

Stage two of examination—cont'd

the barium along, distributing it throughout the colon, and the patient is turned as required for even coating of the entire colon. Spot films are made as indicated. If barium has flowed back into the rectum, it is drained out through the enema nozzle into a kidney basin placed between the thighs. More air is then instilled. Welin stresses the importance of instilling enough air to obtain proper distention of the colon, from 1,800 to 2,000 cc. or more.

When sufficient distention of the colon has been obtained, conventional films are taken in the following sequence: first, on 14″ × 17″ films and all to include the rectum, direct posteroanterior projection, left prone oblique projection, and right prone oblique projection and next a right lateral projection of the rectum on a 10″ × 12″ film. The patient is then turned to the supine position for a direct anteroposterior projection, a supine left oblique projection, and a supine right oblique projection on 14″ × 17″ films and all to include the upper colon and its flexures. These studies are followed by right and left lateral decubitus projections, both to include the rectum. Finally, the patient is placed in the erect position for posteroanterior and right and left oblique projections of the transverse colon and the splenic and hepatic flexures. The films are immediately processed and submitted to the examining radiologist.

In order to obtain the finest possible detail, Welin recommends that the films be taken at a 1.5-meter (60-inch) target-film distance, with 90 to 100 kilovolts, 200 to 300 milliamperes, and a small focal spot.

When any considerable amount of this work must be performed, a specially designed cleansing room setup such as the one described by Welin[1] is a necessity.

The eleven films shown on the three following pages represent a full set of double-contrast studies on a normal colon, and are presented here through the courtesy of Dr. Sölve Welin.

[1]Welin, S.: Modern trends in diagnostic roentgenology of the colon, Brit. J. Radiol. **31:**453-464, 1958.

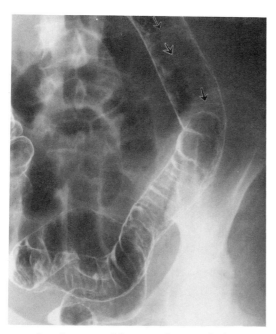

Granulomatous colitis, new pathognomonic sign.

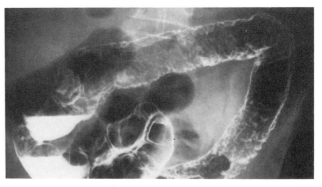

Granulomatous colitis, cobblestone.

Radiographs and clinical information courtesy Dr. Sölve Welin.

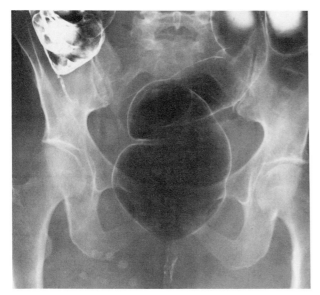

Direct posteroanterior projection.

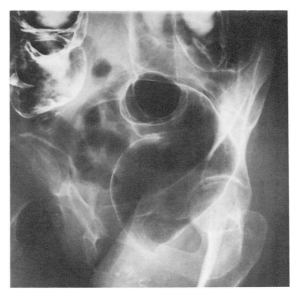

Prone oblique rectum, left side down.

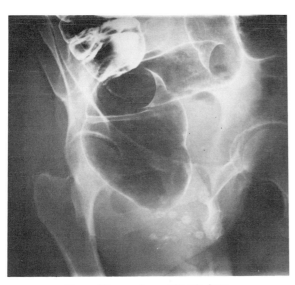

Prone oblique rectum, right side down.

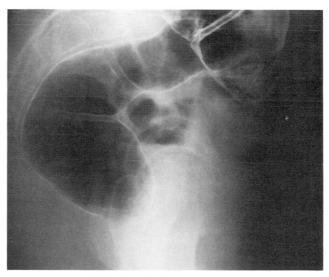

Right lateral projection of rectum.

Radiographs and clinical information courtesy Dr. Sölve Welin.

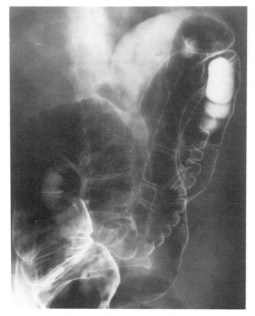

Supine oblique, left side down.

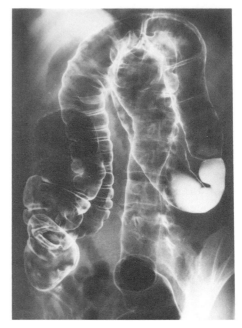

Supine oblique, right side down.

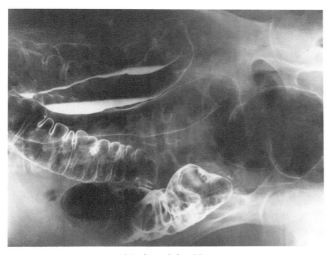

Right lateral decubitus.

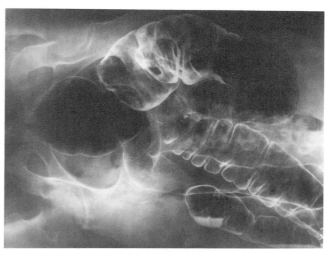

Left lateral decubitus.

Radiographs and clinical information courtesy Dr. Solve Welin.

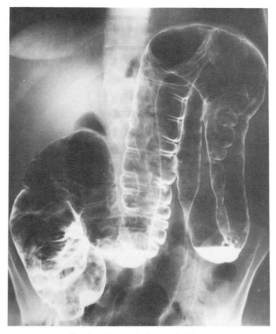

Erect posteroanterior projection.

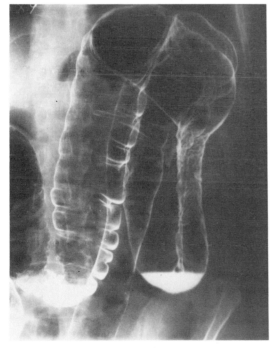

Erect oblique of splenic flexure.

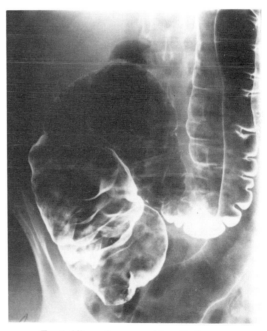

Erect oblique of cecum and hepatic flexure.

Radiographs and clinical information courtesy Dr. Sölve Welin.

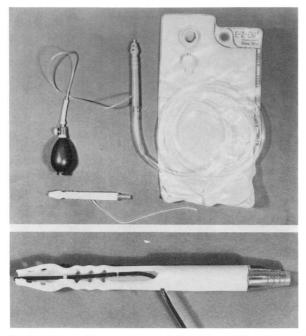

The closed-system plastic enema bag and the Miller air tip allow complete control of barium, air, and rectal drainage at any point in the examination. The air tube extends to the end of the enema nozzle so that the instillation of air does not force residual barium in the tubing into the rectum. The lower part of the illustration is an enlarged view of a section of the Miller tip. The air tube was filled with ink to show its position in the enema tip.

Courtesy Dr. Roscoe E. Miller.

MILLER MODIFICATION OF THE WELIN DOUBLE-CONTRAST ENEMA TECHNIQUE

Miller[1-3] uses the Welin technique in cases of rectal bleeding, carcinoma, and polyps and in all excessively obese patients. He has made the following modifications in the technique for use in his department:

1. He performs a single-stage examination with the use of the closed-system, disposable enema bag, which he equips with an air rectal tip that he designed.

2. He administers two laxative drugs, one that acts primarily on the small intestine and one that acts primarily on the colon.

3. He uses Clysodrast in the cleansing enema only when considerable barium remains from a previous gastro-intestinal series and in patients in the 60- to 70-year-old age group.

4. He uses a combination of two brands of barium sulfate. He recommends the use of a barium sulfate suspension (a single brand or a combination of two brands) that will adhere well and will not bubble or flake out. He reports that this factor varies according to the calcium and other dissolved material in the local water supply, so that tests must be made in each locality to find the correct mixture. He further recommends that the water be taken from the cold water tap in hospitals where softeners are added to the hot water supply and that a few drops of simethicone (Mylicon*) be added to the suspension to counteract foaming where the water supply is very soft.

Miller's formula calls for two and one-half parts of Intropaque and one part of Barosperse to enough water (about five parts) to bring the suspension to a 65% weight/volume mixture that tests 6.5 on the Ba-test Hydrometer. He reports that the mixture is about as thick as heavy whipping cream. The thick mixture must be squeezed through large-bore tubing (3⁄8 inch internal diameter) with manual pressure on the plastic bag. Miller also uses an alternate contrast medium consisting of one gallon of Novopaque† to one-half gallon of Liquipake.‡ These liquid preparations are simply poured into a larger container, mixed together, and are then ready for use. He states that this barium mixture provides excellent coating of the mucosa and that it eliminates any problem with local water supply as well as the bother of mixing dry ingredients.

[1]Dr. Roscoe E. Miller: Personal communication.

[2]Miller, R. E.: Examination of the rectum. In Detection of colon lesions, Chicago, 1973, American College of Radiology, pp. 162-171.

[3]Miller, R. E.: The barium enema as a cancer detection procedure: its use and abuse. In Radiologic and other biophysical methods in tumor diagnosis, Chicago, 1974, Year Book Medical Publishers, Inc.

*Stuart Pharmaceuticals, Wilmington, Del. 19889.

†Picker X-ray Corporation, Cleveland, Ohio 44143.

‡General Electric Corporation, Milwaukee, Wisc. 53201.

Preliminary preparation

When possible, the patient is placed on a restricted diet for two or three days preceding the examination, on a low residue diet for one or two days, and on a nonresidue liquid intake on the day prior to the examination. Sugar can be used in strained fruit juices and in coffee or tea. No milk product is permitted.

The patient is encouraged to drink water freely during the afternoon and evening prior to the examination, a full glass every hour for six to eight hours, to aid in flushing the bowel. If no medical contraindication exists, 2 ounces of castor oil are administered at noon or shortly thereafter, and this drug is followed with 2½ ounces of extract of senna fruit (X-Prep liquid*) at 6:00 P.M. In the presence of diabetes, Miller replaces one of these purgatives with 10 ounces of magnesium citrate or by 20 grams of magnesium sulfate.

On the morning of the examination no breakfast is permitted. On arrival in the radiology department, a cleansing enema consisting of a full 2,000 ml. (2 quarts) of lukewarm water is administered by a specially trained person on the staff of the radiology department. The patient is allowed a full thirty minutes for evacuation.

Ten minutes before the examination the patient is given an intramuscular injection of 2 mg. of glucagon. This drug relaxes the bowel so that it can be adequately distended with air with little or no discomfort to the patient. Miller reports that glucagon is a more effective intestinal relaxant than atropine and that, unlike atropine, glucagon can be given in the presence of glaucoma.

Single-stage examination

The rectal tip is inserted, and the patient then turned to the prone position. The prone position is used to prevent the possibility of barium entering the small intestine before the initial five films of the rectum and rectosigmoid area can be obtained.

Manual pressure is applied on the plastic bag to move the thick barium suspension, which is allowed to flow to

*Gray Pharmaceutical Co., Yonkers, N. Y. 10701.

the splenic flexure. The enema bag is then quickly lowered to the floor, and the barium contained in the rectum is drained back into the bag. If necessary, air is instilled in the rectum to aid in draining it of all excess barium so that only a thin coating remains. Air, 1,800 to 2,000 cc. or more, is then instilled through the air tip with a hand inflation bulb. The air forces the remaining barium forward, and by angling the table and by having the patient rotate under radioscopic control, an even distribution of the barium is obtained throughout the colon. Spot films are made as indicated during radioscopy.

When the rectum is seen to contain no excess barium and the entire colon is well distended, conventional films are obtained. Since the first five films are taken to demonstrate the rectum and the rectosigmoid area, the films should be placed so that the lower margin of the film is at the level of the transverse gluteal fold. Miller recommends that all oblique positions of the colon be taken at a 20-degree body rotation, stating that greater degrees of rotation result in too much superimposition of the bowel loops. For the lateral view of the rectum the patient is turned onto his right side to keep the barium contained in the cecum in its dependent portion with the air uppermost, thus to prevent barium from leaking through the ileocecal valve. The films are taken in the following sequence: first, on 14″ × 17″ films, prone angled projection (central ray 30 degrees toward the feet), direct posteroanterior projection, prone 20 degrees left oblique, prone 20 degrees right oblique, and then a right lateral projection of the rectum on a 10″ × 12″ film. The patient is then turned to the supine position for filming of the upper colon and its flexures in a direct anteroposterior projection, a supine 20 degree left oblique, and a supine 20 degree right oblique. Following these films, right and left lateral decubitus projections are taken, both to include the rectum. When indicated, the Chassard-Lapiné position is used for an axial view of the rectum and rectosigmoid area. After the conventional filming, the patient is placed in the erect position for four full-sized spot films of the splenic flexure, transverse colon, hepatic flexure, and cecum.

The conduct of the single stage closed system double contrast examination

Filling the colon with barium

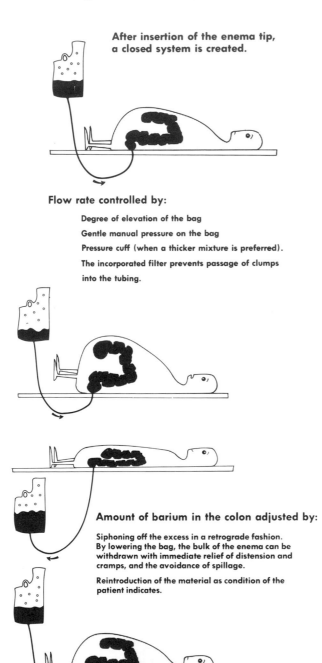

After insertion of the enema tip, a closed system is created.

Flow rate controlled by:

Degree of elevation of the bag

Gentle manual pressure on the bag

Pressure cuff (when a thicker mixture is preferred).

The incorporated filter prevents passage of clumps into the tubing.

Amount of barium in the colon adjusted by:

Siphoning off the excess in a retrograde fashion. By lowering the bag, the bulk of the enema can be withdrawn with immediate relief of distension and cramps, and the avoidance of spillage.

Reintroduction of the material as condition of the patient indicates.

Filming of the filled colon.

Drawings and legends courtesy Dr. Rubem Pochaczevsky.

LARGE INTESTINE—cont'd
Examination procedure in diagnostic enema studies

DISPOSABLE BARIUM ENEMA APPARATUS

The development of the closed-system, disposable barium enema kit[1] represents, for the technologist, one of the greatest procedural improvements to date in radiologic examinations of the large bowel. The sealed bag of this apparatus, by forming a closed system when the rectal tube is inserted, permits siphonage without concern about contamination or about fouling the air of the tightly closed radioscopic room. Because the entire apparatus is disposable (plastic bag, tubing, and rectal tube), the danger of inadequate sterilization[2-5] is eliminated. After being used, the bag and tubing are drained into a toilet, wrapped in newspaper, and discarded in a lined disposal can or in an incinerator. The technologist is thus relieved of the time-consuming sterilization procedure, including the unpleasant preliminary washing of such offensively contaminated equipment.

The disposable enema kit may include the barium sulfate preparation, prepackaged in the plastic bag and ready for mixing. The manufacturer offers several standard barium formulas, or will formulate the barium preparation to the specifications of the radiologist when prepackaging is desired. The bag has a capacity of 3 quarts (3,000 ml.) when fully distended and has graduated markings on its side so that uniform suspensions can be prepared and routinely duplicated with accuracy. A filter may be incorporated within the bag to prevent the passage of any unmixed lumps of barium. The tubing is 6 feet in length. The plastic rectal tubes, available in several sizes, are soft and flexible. A gum-rubber faucet-to-tubing adapter is supplied to facilitate retrograde filling of the sealed bag, unless a top-fill bag having a snap cap or a screw cap is used.

[1]Meyers, P. H., Nice, C. M., Mouton, R., and Stern, H. S.: Controlled standardization in examination of the colon, Southern Med. J. **57**:1429-1431, 1964.

[2]Meyers, P. H.: Contamination of barium enema apparatus during its use, J.A.M.A. **173**:1589-1590, 1960.

[3]Meyers, P. H., and Richards, M.: Transmission of polio virus vaccine by contaminated barium enema with resultant antibody rise, Amer. J. Roentgen. **91**:864-865, 1964.

[4]Steinbach, H. L., Rousseau, R., McCormack, K. R., and Jawetz, E.: Transmission of enteric pathogens by barium enemas, J.A.M.A. **174**:1207-1208, 1960.

[5]Dreyfuss, J. R., Robbins, L. L., and Murphy, J. T.: Disposable plastic unit for barium enema examination, Radiology **77**:834-835, 1961.

DISPOSABLE BARIUM ENEMA APPARATUS—cont'd

A smooth suspension is quickly and cleanly mixed in the plastic bag. After removing the kit from its individual plastic wrapper, uncoil the tubing and relieve any kink. Lay the bag on a flat surface and connect the tubing to the hopper faucet with the gum-rubber adapter. Add enough *hot* water to thoroughly wet the barium preparation. Shake the bag vigorously for about thirty seconds to obtain a smooth suspension of colloidal barium; kneading is necessary to mix some of the suspended preparations. Add cold or lukewarm water to obtain the desired temperature and volume. Disconnect the tubing, press the bag to remove air and any excess water, clamp the tubing with a hemostat, and then shake and knead the mixture again. The kit is now ready for use.

When a single-stage double-contrast study[1] is to be made, the specified volume of air or carbon dioxide is introduced into the bag through the tubing. The gaseous medium rises to occupy the space above the opaque medium. Upon completion of the barium enema filming, the opaque mixture is siphoned back by lowering the bag, the extent of evacuation being controlled radioscopically. After the postevacuation film has been taken, the bag is suspended in the inverted position so that the tubing exit is above the fluid contents of the bag. The colon is then insufflated by gently pressing the bag to displace the gaseous medium; this also is done under radioscopic observation. Upon completion of the film studies, the gas can be siphoned back into the bag.

[1]Pochaczevsky, R., and Sherman, R. S.: A new technique for the roentgenologic examination of the colon, Amer. J. Roentgen. **89**:787-796, 1963.

Passive, controlled evacuation is effected by lowering the bag.

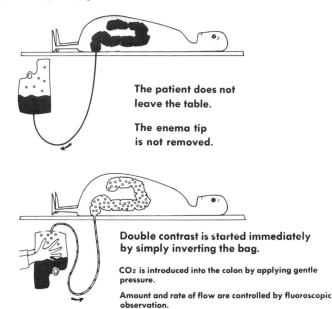

The patient does not leave the table.

The enema tip is not removed.

Double contrast is started immediately by simply inverting the bag.

CO2 is introduced into the colon by applying gentle pressure.

Amount and rate of flow are controlled by fluoroscopic observation.

Examination complete. Closed system has not been broken. Entire examination is performed in a single stage.

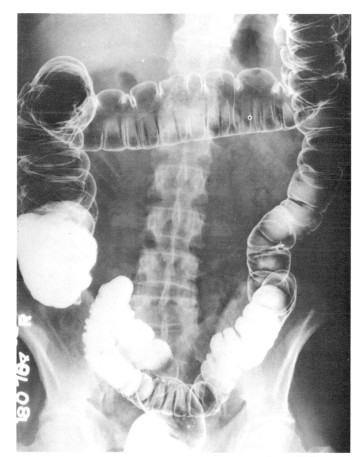

Courtesy Dr. Rubem Pochaczevsky.

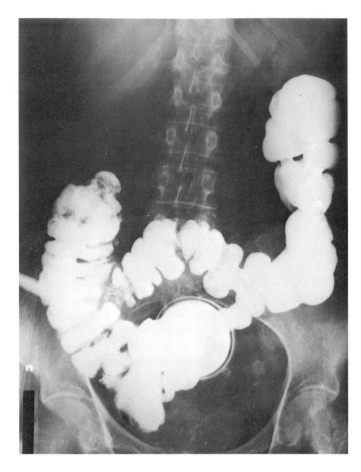

LARGE INTESTINE—cont'd
Diagnostic enema studies via colostomies

Enterostomy (Gr. *enteron*, intestine + *stoma*, opening) is the general term applied to the surgical procedure of forming an artificial opening into the intestine, usually through the abdominal wall, and to the resultant fecal passage. The regional terms are *colostomy*, *cecostomy*, *ileostomy*, and *jejunostomy*.

The colon is the most frequent site of pathology and, therefore, of operation. Loop colostomy is sometimes performed to divert the fecal column, either temporarily or permanently, from areas of diverticulitis or ulcerative colitis. Most colostomies, however, are performed because of tumors of the lower bowel and rectum. When a tumor is present, the lower carcinomatous part of the bowel is resected and the end of the remaining part of the bowel is then brought to the surface through the abdominal wall. This passage, or stoma, has no sphincter. By a more recent surgical procedure, known as perineal colostomy or proctosigmoidectomy with "pull through," the end of the remaining part of the colon is brought out at the natural location. The anal canal is saved when possible, but there is usually little sphincter control.

Colostomy patients must wear some form of protective dressing—a colostomy pad or pouch—until they can, by diet and daily irrigation, regulate evacuation to a once-a-day schedule. Before leaving the hospital, the patient is taught how to regulate his diet, irrigate the bowel by way of the colostomy, and care for the skin around the stoma.

PREPARATION OF INTESTINAL TRACT

Postoperative contrast enema studies are performed at suitable intervals to determine the efficacy of treatment in cases of diverticulitis and ulcerative colitis, and to detect any new or recurrent lesion in the patient who had a tumor. The demonstration of polyps or other intraluminal lesions depends upon adequate cleansing of the bowel, which is as important in the presence of colostomy as otherwise. Unless contraindicated, the usual preparation with castor oil or another, comparable cathartic is given on the evening preceding the examination, and an irrigation is given on the morning of the examination. In the presence of diarrhea, or if a cathartic is contraindicated, irrigation the night before and again on the morning of the examination may be sufficient.

COLOSTOMY ENEMA EQUIPMENT

While all equipment must be scrupulously clean, and nondisposable items must be sterilized after each use, sterile technique is not required because the stoma is part of the intestinal tract. Except for a suitable device to prevent stomal leakage of the contrast material, the equipment employed in the presence of a colostomy is the same as that used in routine contrast enema studies. The same barium sulfate formula is used, and gas studies are made. The opaque and double-contrast studies can be performed in a single-stage examination with the use of a disposable enema kit such as that described on the two preceding pages.

Without the use of some device to prevent spillage, the contrast enema may, due to the absence of sphincter control, escape through the colostomy almost as rapidly

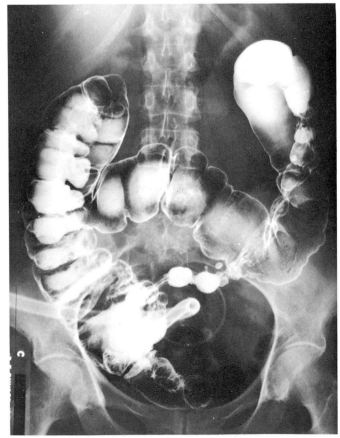

Opaque and double-contrast studies by way of abdominal colostomy.
Radiographs courtesy Dr. Ruth E. Snyder.

as it is injected. This would result in unsatisfactory filling of the bowel as well as in obscuring shadows cast by barium soilage of the abdominal wall and the examining table. Abdominal stomas must be effectively occluded for studies made by retrograde injection, and leakage around the stomal catheter must be prevented for studies made by injection into either an abdominal or a perineal colostomy. Numerous devices have been described for this purpose.

Pendergrass and Cooper[1] suggested a simple and effective method for occlusion of abdominal stomas in retrograde studies. This method utilizes a rubber bulb of the type used in Asepto irrigation syringes, which are available in a variety of sizes. The neck of a bulb of the correct size is inserted into the stoma, and the bulb is then strapped down firmly with long strips of adhesive tape extending across the abdomen.

Robin,[2] with the use of the same type of rubber bulb described above and a somewhat thinner barium sulfate mixture, administered enemas through the colostomy. For this method, the bulb is placed and strapped in position, and a 15-gauge needle is inserted into the bulb and then connected to the tubing of the usual enema container. For the patient with a double-barrel colostomy, Robin used two bulbs, one inserted into each stoma. The enema tubing is bifurcated a few feet from the end by a Y-shaped connector, and each tubing arm is then connected to a needle inserted into the respective bulb.

Another method of administering enemas through the colostomy utilizes a solid but soft rubber ball through which a rectal catheter has been inserted. The rubber ball may be held firmly in place by the patient during radioscopy and by adhesive or other strapping tightened across the abdomen for filming.

Land[3] described a practical, effective, and readily available device that can be quickly fabricated by cutting off the tip of an infant feeding nipple and inserting a soft rubber catheter through the enlarged hole. The tube and nipple are inserted within the colostomy opening, and the patient then places his fingers on the flat edge of the nipple to hold it firmly against the stoma during radioscopy and until it can be strapped in position for filming.

Burhenne[4] wrote an excellent and well-illustrated description of a wide variety of colostomy enema devices. He prefers to administer diagnostic enemas with the use of the tips and adhesive disks designed for the patient's use in irrigating his colostomy. The Laird tip* comes in four sizes to accommodate the usual sizes of colostomy stomas. These tips have a flange to prevent them from slipping through the colostomy opening. An adhesive disk (Stomaseal†) is placed over the flange to minimize reflux soilage. The enema tubing is attached directly to the tip, which the patient holds in position to prevent the weight of the tubing from displacing it to an angled position. In addition to keeping a set of Laird tips on hand, Burhenne recommends that the patient be asked to bring his own irrigation device with him.

[1]Pendergrass, R. C., and Cooper, F. W., Jr.: Simple method for study of the colon in the presence of a colostomy, Amer. J. Roentgen. **52**:563, 1944.

[2]Robin, P. A.: A method for barium enema examination of the patient with a colostomy, Amer. J. Roentgen. **55**:782-783, 1946.

[3]Land, R. E.: Colostomy enema; description of a catheter-nipple device, Radiology **100**:36, 1971.

[4]Burhenne, H. J.: Technique of colostomy examination, Radiology **97**:183-185, 1970

*John F. Greer Co., P.O. Box 2898, Oakland, Calif. 94618.

†3-M Co., 15 Henderson Drive, West Caldwell, N. J. 07006.

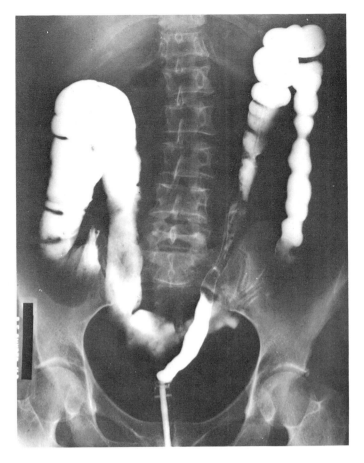

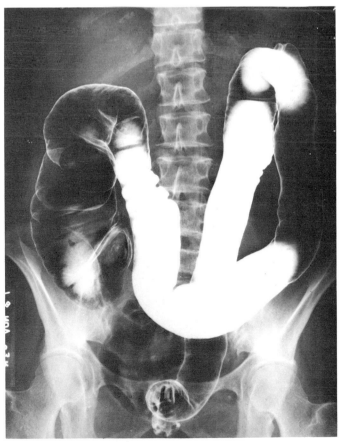

Opaque and double-contrast studies by way of perineal colostomy.

Radiographs courtesy Dr. Ruth E. Snyder.

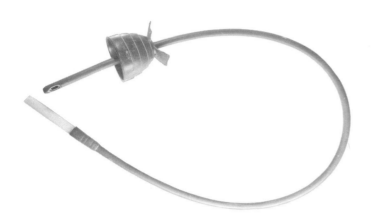

Plastic eggcup device. Loaned for photography.

Courtesy Dr. Ruth E. Snyder.

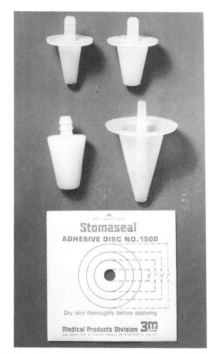

Laird colostomy irrigation tips and Stomaseal discs.

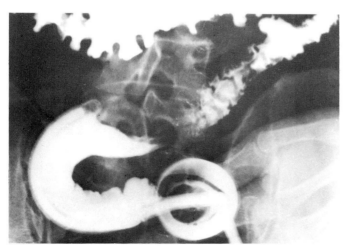

Spot-film study.

Courtesy Dr. Ruth E. Snyder.

LARGE INTESTINE—cont'd
Diagnostic enema studies via colostomies—cont'd
COLOSTOMY ENEMA EQUIPMENT—cont'd

Retention catheters are widely used in colostomy examinations. Some radiologists use them alone, and others insert them through some device to prevent slipping and to collect leakage, such as the enterostomy bag described by Cross.[1] Colostomy stomas are fragile and thus are subject to perforation by any undue pressure or trauma. Perforations have occurred at the insertion of an inflated bulb into a blind pouch and from overdistention of the stoma. Snyder and Sherman[2] state that, for these reasons, they believe that no inflated balloon should be used in colostomies, either abdominal or perineal.

Snyder and Sherman use a colostomy device consisting of half of a plastic eggcup and a soft-rubber rectal catheter. A hole is drilled into the center of the eggcup for the transmission of the catheter, which is passed through the stoma for 4 to 6 inches. This is done by the radiologist or by the patient if he is accustomed to inserting a catheter into his stoma for irrigations and knows by feel when he has it properly seated in the lumen of the gut. The eggcup fits over the protruding stoma and is held firmly against the skin by the patient during radioscopy. The eggcup may be held firmly in place by the patient during radioscopy, and by adhesive or another suitable strapping during filming. A large hand towel, twice folded lengthwise, and placed across the stomal device and held by the patient at the sides of his abdomen serves this purpose well. The tubing of the enema container is connected to the stomal catheter or tube, and the examination is carried out in the usual manner.

Snyder and Sherman, with the use of disposable enema kits with carbon dioxide in the bag, perform single-stage double-contrast studies on all their colostomy patients. For evacuation by way of an abdominal stoma, the patient sits on the side of the examining table, leans forward, and drains the barium mixture through the tubing. They recommend that massage be used to aid evacuation and, if there is little tendency to emptying, that a small amount of gas be injected to stimulate the process. When a sufficient amount of the barium mixture has been passed, the patient is readjusted in the supine position, the disposable bag is inverted, and the gas is gently forced into the bowel until the cecum is well filled. Radiographic studies, including an erect film for the delineation of the hepatic and splenic flexures, are then taken in the usual manner.

[1]Cross, F. S.: A new method for obtaining barium enemas in colostomy patients, Surgery **30**:460-464, 1951.
[2]Snyder, Ruth E., and Sherman, Robert S.: Personal communication.

Snyder and Sherman recommend that the same caution with the catheter and cup or sponge device be used in administering enemas by way of perineal colostomies, and that patients be examined in the prone position, where better filling may be obtained. The radiologist here adjusts the stomal device so that the patient can hold it firmly in position between the buttocks.

PREPARATION OF PATIENT

If the patient uses any special dressing, a colostomy pouch, or a stomal seal, he should be advised to bring a change for use after the examination. When fecal emission is such that a pouch is required, the patient should be given a suitable dressing to place over the stoma after he has removed the device.

It is desirable to clothe the patient in a kimono type of gown, with the opening in front or back, according to the location of the colostomy. The patient is placed on the examining table in the supine position if he has an abdominal colostomy, and in the prone position if he has a perineal colostomy.

Before taking the preliminary film, the technologist, wearing clean rubber or disposable plastic gloves to protect his hands from possible soilage when there is stomal emission, should remove any dressings and discard them in newspaper wrapping. The skin around the stoma should be cleansed with cotton balls or disposable wipes soaked in alcohol, or in benzene for the removal of zinc oxide ointment. Cotton balls or tissue wipes are used in preference to gauze swabs because the latter are harsh and may irritate the skin. When adhesive strips are to be applied across the abdomen to secure the colostomy device in position, the areas to be strapped should be shaved of any hair, and oily perspiration secretions should be removed with alcohol. A gauze dressing should be placed over the stoma to absorb any seepage until the radiologist is ready to start the examination. The stomal catheter or tube should be well lubricated (but not excessively so) with a water-soluble lubricant such as K-Y jelly. The insertion of the catheter must be performed by the radiologist or the patient, never by the technologist.[1,2]

[1]Spiro, R. H., and Hertz, R. E.: Colostomy perforation, Surgery 60:590-597, 1966.
[2]Becker, M. H., Genieser, N. B., and Clark, H.: Perforation of colon during barium enema, New York J. Med. 67:278-282, 1967.

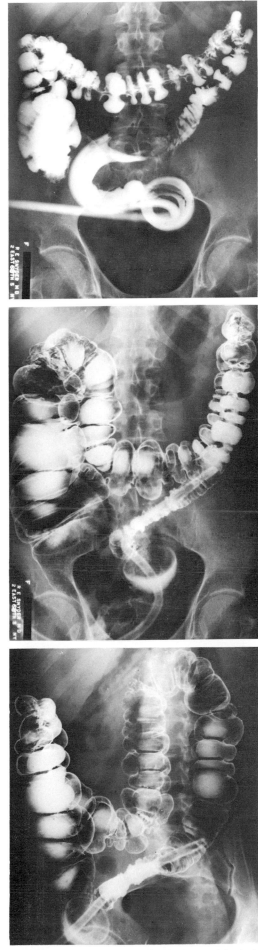

Opaque and double-contrast studies on a patient having an abdominal colostomy.

Radiographs courtesy Dr. Ruth E. Snyder.

761

Anatomy and positioning of the urinary system

Urinary system

The urinary system comprises (1) a pair of glandular organs, the *kidneys*, which function to remove waste materials from the blood and to eliminate the waste in the urine which they form and excrete to the extent of about 3 pints per day, and (2) a series of musculomembranous excretory ducts, or canals, which transport the urine to the exterior. The excretory ducts consist of (1) a variable number of beginning stems called the calyces and an expanded portion called the renal pelvis, which together are known as the pelvicalyceal system, (2) a pair of long tubes, one extending from the pelvis of each kidney, which are called the *ureters*, (3) a saclike portion, the *urinary bladder*, which serves as a reservoir, and (4) a third and smaller tubular portion, the *urethra*, which conveys the urine to the exterior.

The *suprarenal*, or *adrenal*, *glands* have no functional relationship with the urinary system. They are included in this chapter because of their anatomic location, for which they are called suprarenal glands. Each adrenal gland, two in number, consists of a small, flattened body composed of an internal, medullary portion and an outer, cortical portion. The adrenal glands are ductless.

Each is enclosed in a fibrous sheath and is situated, one on each side, in the retroperitoneal tissue in close contact with the fatty capsule overlying the medial and superior aspects of the upper pole of the kidney. The adrenals furnish important secretions—epinephrine, which is secreted by the medulla, and the cortical hormones, which are secreted by the cortex. These glands are subject to malfunction and to a number of diseases. They are not usually demonstrable on plain films but are clearly delineated in the gaseous field furnished by retroperitoneal insufflation. The adrenal circulation is demonstrable by selective catheterization of an adrenal artery or vein in angiographic procedures.

The kidneys are bean-shaped bodies, the lateral border of each organ being convex and the medial border being concave, and they present slightly convex anterior and posterior surfaces. They are arbitrarily divided into upper and lower extremities, which are more commonly referred to as upper and lower poles. The kidneys measure approximately 4½ inches in length, 2 to 3 inches in width, and about 1¼ inches in thickness. The left kidney usually is slightly longer and narrower than the right.

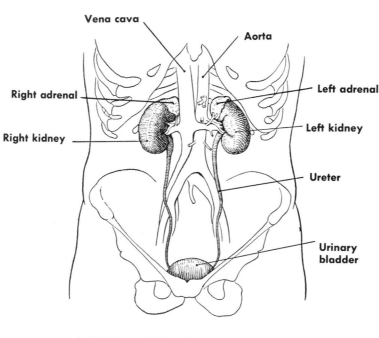

ANTERIOR ASPECT OF URINARY SYSTEM IN RELATION TO SURROUNDING STRUCTURES

The kidneys are situated behind the peritoneum and are in contact with the posterior wall of the abdominal cavity, one kidney lying on each side of, and in the same coronal plane with, the upper lumbar vertebrae. They lie in an oblique plane from above downward, forward, and lateralward, the forward slant following the curve of the last thoracic vertebra and the upper three lumbar vertebrae. The kidneys normally extend from the level of the upper border of the twelfth thoracic vertebra to the level of the transverse processes of the third lumbar vertebra in patients of average build; they are somewhat higher in patients of hypersthenic habitus and somewhat lower in those of asthenic habitus. Because of the large space occupied by the liver, the right kidney is a little lower in position than the left. Each kidney is embedded in a mass of fatty tissue called the adipose capsule, and the whole is enveloped in a sheath of fascia, which is attached to the diaphragm, the lumbar vertebrae, the peritoneum, and other adjacent structures. The kidneys are supported in a fairly fixed position, partially through the fascial attachments and partially by the surrounding organs. They have a respiratory excursion of approximately 1 inch and normally drop no more than 2 inches in the change from the supine to the erect position.

The concave medial border of each kidney presents a longitudinal slit, or hilus, for transmission of the blood and lymphatic vessels, the nerves, and the ureter. The hilus expands into the body of the gland to form a central cavity called the renal sinus. The kidney is composed of an outer, cortical substance and an inner, medullary substance (illustrated in the coronal section on the following page) and is covered by a thin layer of fibrous tissue, which is prolonged inward to line the renal sinus.

The medullary substance is composed mainly of the collecting tubules, which gives it a striated appearance, and it consists of eight to fifteen cone-shaped segments called the renal pyramids. The segments arise in the cortical substance and converge toward the renal sinus, where the apex of each pyramid is received into a beginning stem of a calyx. The more compact cortical substance lies between the periphery of the organ and the bases of the medullary segments and extends inward between the pyramids to the renal sinus.

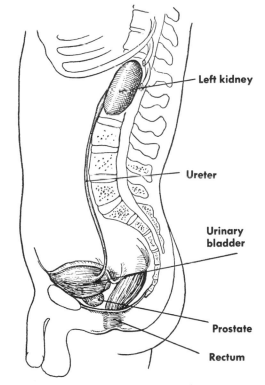

LATERAL ASPECT OF URINARY SYSTEM IN RELATION TO SURROUNDING STRUCTURES

The essential microscopic components of the parenchyma of the kidney are called the *nephron*, formerly called the renal corpuscles, and the uriniferous tubules. The proximal nephron consists of a double-walled membranous sac, called the capsule of Bowman, and a cluster of blood capillaries, called the glomerulus, which is invaginated into the capsule. The glomerulus is formed by a minute branch of the renal artery entering the capsule and dividing into capillaries, which then turn back and, as they ascend, unite to form a single vessel leaving the capsule. The vessel entering the capsule is called the afferent artery, and the one leaving is called the efferent artery. After leaving the corpuscles, the efferent arteries pass on to form the capillary networks that communicate with the renal veins.

The thin inner wall of the capsule is closely adherent to the capillary coils and is separated by a comparatively wide space from the outer layer, which is continuous with the beginning of a renal tubule. The glomerulus serves as a filter for the blood, permitting water and finely dissolved substances to pass through the walls of the capillaries into the capsule. This fluid is called the glomerular filtrate. The change from filtrate to urine is due in part to the water and the usable dissolved substances being absorbed by the epithelial lining of the tubules.

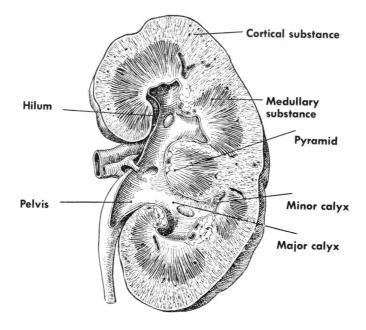

Cortical substance

Hilum

Medullary substance

Pyramid

Pelvis

Minor calyx

Major calyx

CORONAL SECTION OF KIDNEY

Each renal tubule arises from a glomerular capsule in the cortex of the kidney and then travels a circuitous path through the cortical and medullary substances, becoming in turn the proximal convoluted tubule, the descending and ascending limbs of the loop of Henle, and the distal convoluted tubule. The latter opens into a straight, or collecting, tubule that begins in the cortex. The collecting tubules converge toward the renal pelvis and unite along their course so that each group within the pyramid forms a central tubule that opens at the apex and drains its tributaries into the calyx.

The calyces are cup-shaped stems arising from the sides of the apices of the renal pyramids, each calyx enclosing one or more apices, so that there are usually fewer calyces than pyramids. The beginning stems are called the minor calyces, numbering from seven to twelve, and they unite to form two to five larger tubes called the major calyces or infundibula. The infundibula unite to form the expanded, funnel-shaped renal pelvis. The wide upper portion of the renal pelvis lies within the renal sinus, while its tapering lower part passes through the hilus to become continuous with the ureter.

The ureter is 10 to 12 inches in length. It descends behind the peritoneum and in front of the psoas muscle and the transverse processes of the lumbar vertebrae, passes downward and backward in front of the sacral ala, and then curves forward and medialward to enter the posterolateral surface of the urinary bladder. The ureters convey the urine from the renal pelves to the bladder by slow, rhythmic contractions.

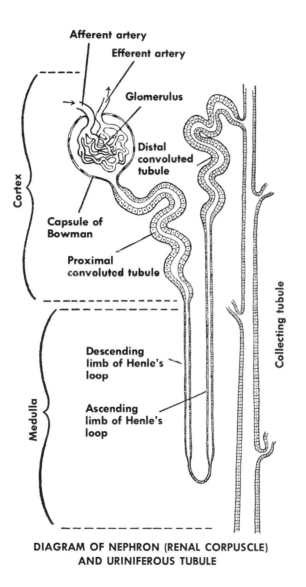

DIAGRAM OF NEPHRON (RENAL CORPUSCLE) AND URINIFEROUS TUBULE

767

The *urinary bladder* is a musculomembranous sac that serves as a reservoir for urine. It is situated immediately behind and above the symphysis pubis, and its fundus (the lower posterior part of the viscus) is in relation to the rectal ampulla in the male and to the uterus and the upper part of the vaginal canal in the female. The bladder varies in size, shape, and position according to the amount of its content, being approximately tetrahedral in shape and situated entirely within the pelvic cavity when empty. As it fills, the viscus gradually assumes an oval shape while expanding upward and forward into the abdominal cavity.

The ureters enter the wall of the bladder at the lateral margins of the upper part of its base, or fundus, and pass obliquely through the wall to their respective internal orifices. These two openings are about 1 inch apart when the viscus is empty and about 2 inches apart when it is distended, being an equal distance from the internal urethral orifice, which is placed at the lowest part, called the neck, of the bladder. The triangular area between the three orifices is called the trigone. The mucosa over the trigone is always smooth, whereas the remainder of the lining is thrown into folds when the viscus is empty.

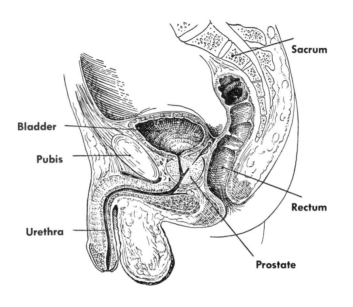

MIDSAGITTAL SECTION THROUGH MALE PELVIS

768

The *urethra*, which serves to convey the urine to the exterior, is a narrow musculomembranous canal with a sphincter type of muscle at the base of the bladder. It arises at the internal urethral orifice in the urinary bladder and extends for a distance of about 1½ inches in the female, and 7 to 8 inches in the male.

The female urethra passes along the thick anterior wall of the vagina to the external urethral orifice, which is located in the vestibule about 1 inch anterior to the vaginal opening. The male urethra extends from the bladder to the end of the penis and is divided into prostatic, membranous, and cavernous portions. The prostatic portion is about 1 inch in length, reaches from the bladder to the floor of the pelvis, and is completely surrounded by the prostate. The membranous portion of the canal passes through the pelvic floor; it is slightly constricted, and is about ½ inch long. The cavernous portion passes through the shaft of the penis, extending from the floor of the pelvis to the external urethral orifice. The membranous and cavernous parts of the male urethra also serve as the excretory canal of the reproductive system.

The *prostate* is a small, glandular body surrounding the proximal part of the male urethra, and is situated just behind the lower portion of the pubic symphysis. It is conical in shape, its base is attached to the inferior surface of the urinary bladder, and its apex is in contact with the floor of the pelvis. It measures about 1½ inches transversely and ¾ inch anteroposteriorly at its base and is approximately 1 inch in length.

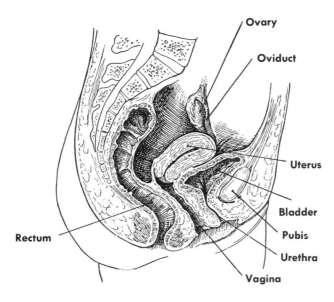

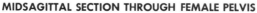

MIDSAGITTAL SECTION THROUGH FEMALE PELVIS

Radiography of the urinary system

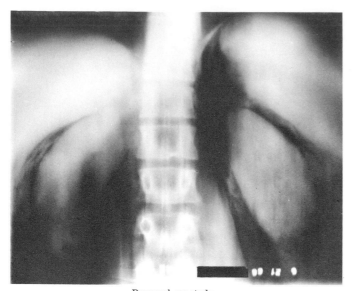

Presacral gas study.

Courtesy Dr. Joshua A. Becker.

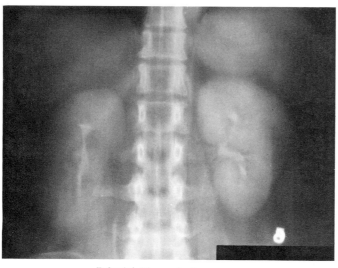

Bolus injection nephrotomogram.

Courtesy Dr. John A. Evans.

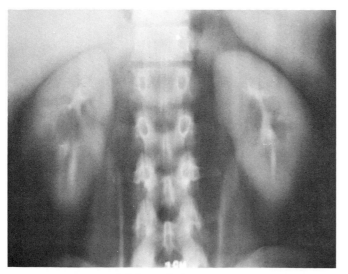

Infusion nephrotomogram.

Courtesy Dr. Joshua A. Becker.

Radiography of the urinary system comprises numerous specialized procedures, each of which requires the use of an artificial contrast medium, and each of which was evolved to serve a specific purpose. The specialized procedures are preceded by a plain or scout film study of the abdominopelvic areas for the detection of any abnormality demonstrable by this means. The preliminary examination may consist of no more than a supine film of the abdomen. When indicated, oblique and/or lateral projections are taken to localize calcareous shadows and tumor masses, and an erect study may be made to demonstrate the mobility of the kidneys.

The position and mobility of the kidneys, and usually their size and shape, can be demonstrated on plain films when the intestinal content is not too heavy. This is possible because of the contrast furnished by the radiolucent fatty capsule surrounding them. Visualization of the thin-walled drainage or collecting system (the calyces and pelves, the ureters, the urinary bladder, and the urethra) requires that the canals be filled with a contrast medium. The urinary bladder is outlined when it is filled with urine, but it is not adequately demonstrated. The ureters and the urethra are not distinguishable on plain films.

In order to outline clearly the surfaces of the kidneys and the adrenal glands, and to detect the reason for any displacement or deformity in the shadow of the kidneys (displacement or deformity may be caused by a space-occupying lesion of an adjacent organ), *retroperitoneal gas insufflation* is employed. The gaseous medium is usually introduced by way of the presacral retroperitoneal space.

Presacral retroperitoneal pneumoradiography is used with selected patients in conjunction with intravenous and retrograde opaque-contrast procedures in order to obtain dual-contrast studies.

For the delineation and differentiation of cysts and tumor masses situated within the kidney substance, the renal parenchyma is opacified by an intravenously introduced, organic, iodinated contrast medium and is then radiographed by tomographic sectioning. The contrast solution may be introduced into the vein by rapid injection or by infusion. These procedures are respectively called *bolus injection nephrotomography* and *infusion nephrotomography*. In another method of investigating cysts and tumor masses of the renal parenchyma, a long needle is inserted through the flank into the cyst or tumor for direct injection of the contrast medium. This procedure is called *percutaneous renal puncture*.

Investigations of the blood vessels of the kidneys and of the adrenal glands are performed by angiographic procedures, which are described in the discussion of the circulatory system.

NOTE: *Double-contrast study.* The radiologic procedure in which the inner walls of hollow organs, and of capsuled joint structures, are examined by introducing two contrast agents, one positive and one negative, within the lumen of the hollow structure or within the capsule of the joint under investigation.

Dual-contrast study. The radiologic procedure in which the inner and outer walls of a hollow organ, or of the outer contour of a relatively solid organ and of the walls of its inner passages, are simultaneously delineated by establishing pneumoperitoneum or pneumoretroperitoneum and then introducing a suitable contrast medium into the hollow portion of the structure under investigation.

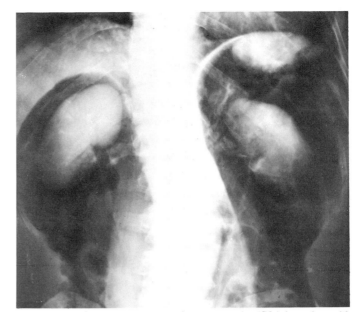

Intravenous pyelography and presacral pneumography (CO_2) in patient with left adrenal adenoma.

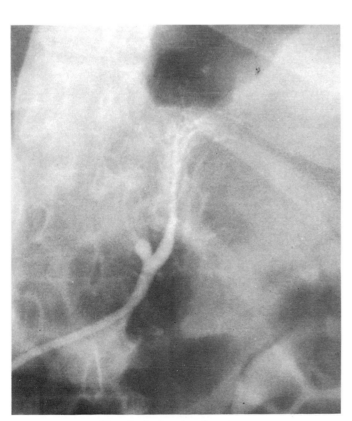

Normal selective adrenal venogram.

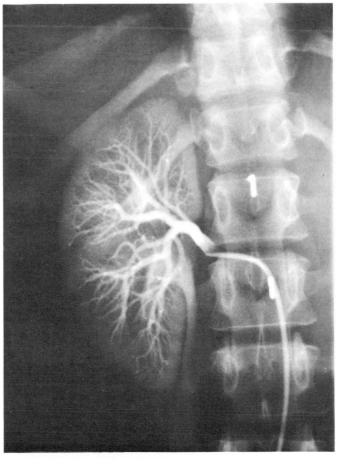

Normal selective renal arteriogram.

All radiographs and diagnostic information courtesy Dr. Joshua A. Becker.

771

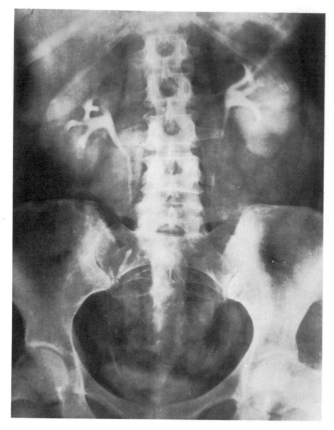

Excretion pyelogram.

Radiologic investigations of the renal drainage, or collecting, system are performed by various procedures classified under the general term *urography*. This term embraces two routinely employed methods of filling the urinary canals with a contrast medium. The first and most frequently employed is the physiologic method, in which the contrast agent may be administered intravenously, intramuscularly, or subcutaneously. This method is called *excretory, excretion*, or *descending urography*. The second is the instrumental method, called *retrograde* or *ascending urography*. The contrast medium is introduced directly into the canals by means of catheterization—ureteral catheterization for contrast filling of the upper urinary tracts, and urethral catheterization for the lower tracts. Cystoscopy is required in order to localize the vesicoureteral orifices for the passage of ureteral catheters. In selected patients, a contrast solution is introduced directly into the pelvicalyceal system by means of percutaneous puncture of the renal pelvis. This method is called *percutaneous antegrade urography*.

Investigations of the lower urinary tract—the bladder, the lower ureters, and the urethra—are usually made by the retrograde method, which requires no instrumentation beyond the passage of a urethral catheter. However, investigations may also be made by the physiologic method. These examinations are usually denoted by the general term *cystography*, a procedure understood to include inspection of the lower ureters (*cystoureterography*) and of the urethra (*cystourethrography*).

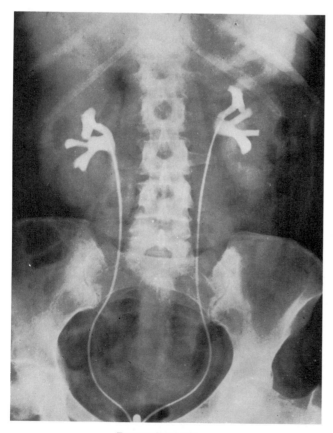

Retrograde pyelogram.
Radiographs courtesy Dr. Oswald S. Lowsley.

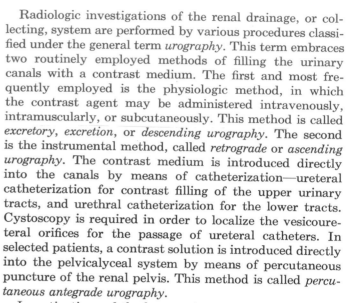

The excretion method of urography is employed in examinations of the upper urinary tracts of infants and children, and is generally considered to be the method of choice for adults unless there is definite indication for the use of the retrograde method. While the contrast solution may be administered intramuscularly or subcutaneously, with the possible exception of infants and children, the intravenous route is generally employed. For this reason, the excretion method is commonly referred to as intravenous urography or, simply, I.V.U. (formerly I.V.P.). Once the opaque substance enters the bloodstream by any one of these routes, it is conveyed to the renal glomeruli and is discharged into the capsules with the glomerular filtrate, which is excreted as urine. With the reabsorption of water, the contrast material becomes sufficiently concentrated to render the urinary canals radiopaque. The urinary bladder is well outlined by this method, and satisfactory voiding urethrograms may be obtained

Retrograde urographic examinations of the upper urinary tracts are primarily urologic procedures, and the catheterization and contrast filling of the urinary canals are performed by the attending urologist in conjunction with his physical or endoscopic examination. This method enables the urologist to take catheterized specimens of urine directly from each renal pelvis, and because the canals can be fully distended by direct injection of the contrast agent, it sometimes gives more information regarding the anatomy of the different parts of the collecting system than is always possible by the excretion method. In this procedure an evaluation of kidney function depends upon an intravenously administered dye substance to stain the urine subsequently trickling through the respective ureteral catheters. Both methods of examination are occasionally required for a complete urologic study.

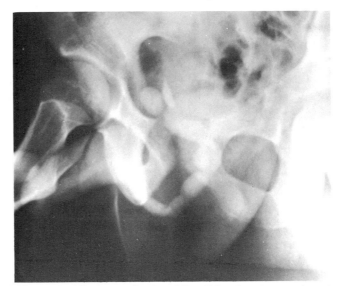

Voiding study following routine dose I.V.U. Dilatation of proximal urethra secondary to urethral stricture.

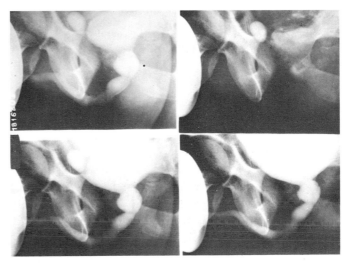

Voiding studies of above patient following infusion nephrourography. Note increase in opacification by this method.

Radiographs and diagnostic information courtesy Dr. Joshua A. Becker.

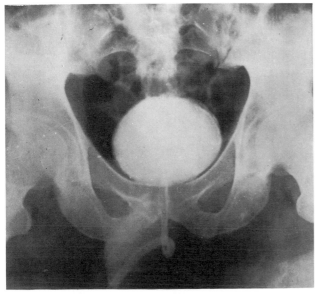

Cystogram.

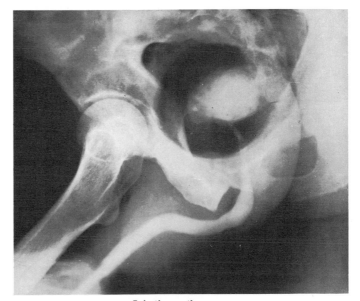

Injection urethrogram.

Radiographs courtesy Dr. Oswald S. Lowsley.

773

CONTRAST MEDIA IN UROGRAPHY

Retrograde urography began in 1904, when, by the introduction of air into the urinary bladder, the first step was made toward the development of an artificial contrast medium for the demonstration of the urinary canals. Air is still used as the contrast agent for the demonstration of intraluminal lesions of the bladder (the method is called *pneumocystography*); and in order to obtain a double-contrast study, air is frequently injected after the mucosa of the bladder has been coated with an opaque substance.

In 1906, retrograde urography as well as cystography was performed with the first opaque medium, a colloidal silver preparation that is no longer used. Silver iodide, which is a nontoxic inorganic compound, was introduced in 1911. Colloidal solutions of silver iodide were used in examinations of the bladder and urethra but were not introduced into the renal pelves or ureters because of the tendency of the medium to precipitate out and to coat the mucosa with floccules, which were difficult to eliminate. Sodium iodide and sodium bromide, also inorganic compounds, came into use for retrograde urography in 1918. The bromides and iodides are no longer in general use for examinations of the renal pelves and ureters because

they irritate the mucosa and frequently cause the patient considerable discomfort. For economic reasons, since a large quantity of solution is required to fill the urinary bladder, solutions of chemically pure sodium iodide in concentrations of 5% to 20% are used extensively in cystography. By irrigating the bladder immediately following exposure of the cystograms, the urologist is able to reduce irritation of the mucosa to a minimum, so that the patient suffers little or no discomfort from the use of the sodium iodide. A 15% solution of iodohippurate sodium (Hippuran) is also used for cystographic and urethrographic studies, although a more viscous medium, such as acetrizoate sodium (Thixokon), Rayopak, or Skiodan viscous, is usually used for urethrography.

The first organic contrast compound for use in urography, an iodine pyridine derivative, was introduced by Swick[1] in 1929. There are now available a number of iodinated organic compounds for use in urography. Because they are nonirritating, the organic media are widely used in the retrograde method, but they must be diluted to reduce opacification. A gaseous medium is sometimes used in investigations of the upper urinary canals.

[1]Swick, M.: Darstellung der Niere und Harnwege im Röntgenbild durch intravenöse Einbringung eines neuen Kontraststoffes des Uroselectans, Klin. Wchnschr. 8:2087-2089, 1929. Abstr.: Amer. J. Roentgen. 23:686-687, 1930.

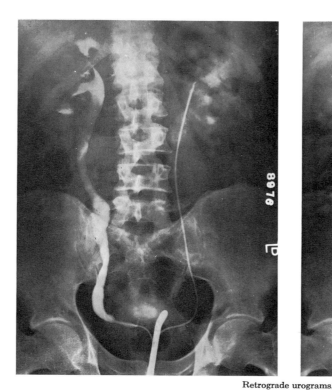
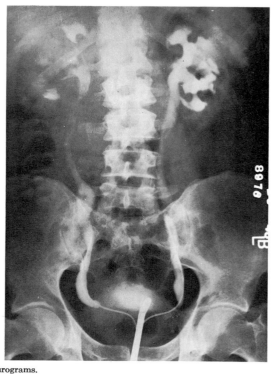

Retrograde urograms.

Courtesy Dr. Marcy L. Sussman.

774

Excretory urography was first reported by Rowntree, Sutherland, Osborne, and Scholl, in 1923.[1] These investigators employed a 10% solution of chemically pure sodium iodide as the contrast medium. This agent was excreted too slowly to give a satisfactory demonstration of the renal pelves and ureters, and it also proved to be too toxic for functional distribution. Early in 1929, Roseno and Jepkins[2] introduced a compound in which they combined sodium iodide with urea. The latter constituent, which is one of the nitrogenous substances removed from the blood and eliminated by the kidneys, served to accelerate excretion and thus to quickly fill the renal pelves with opacified urine. While satisfactory renal shadows were obtained with this compound, the patients experienced considerable distress as a result of its toxicity. It was later in the same year, 1929, when Swick developed the organic compound mentioned above (Uroselectan), which

[1]Rowntree, L. G., Sutherland, C. G., Osborne, E. D., and Scholl, A. J., Jr.: Roentgenography of the urinary tract during excretion of sodium iodide, J.A.M.A. 8:368-373, 1923.
[2]Roseno, A., and Jepkins, H.: Intravenous pyelography, Fortschr. Roentgenstr. 39:859-863, 1929. Abstr.: Amer. J. Roentgen. 22:685-686, 1929.

had an iodine content of 42%. The present-day contrast media for excretory urography are the result of extensive research by many investigators. They are available under various trade names in concentrations ranging from about 50% to 70%. Sterile solutions of the media are supplied in dose-size ampules.

Untoward side reactions to iodinated media

The iodinated organic preparations that are compounded for urologic examinations are of low toxicity, with the result that untoward side reactions are usually mild and of short duration. The characteristic reactions are a feeling of warmth, flushing, and sometimes a few urticarial patches. There is an occasional reaction of nausea, vomiting, and edema of the respiratory mucous membrane. Severe and serious reactions occur only rarely, but since they are an ever-present possibility, the radiologist checks the clinical history of each patient, has the patient kept under observation for any sign of systemic reaction, and has full emergency equipment at hand.

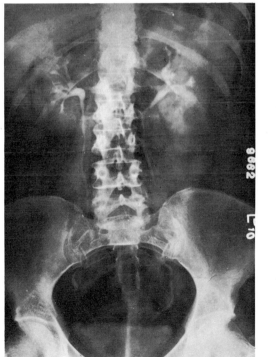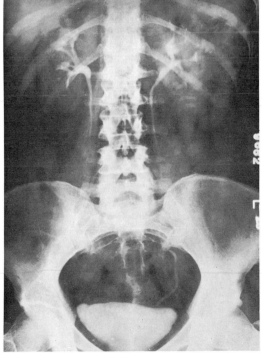

Excretory urograms.

Courtesy Dr. Marcy L. Sussman.

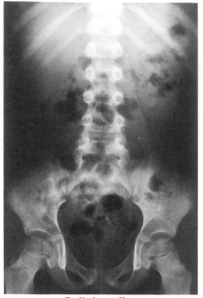

Preliminary film.

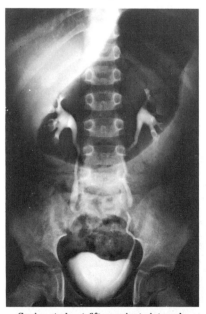

Supine study at fifteen-minute interval.

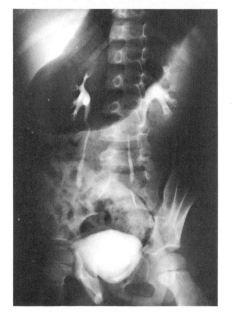

One of the oblique studies made at fifteen-minute interval.

Radiographs courtesy Dr. David L. Bloom.

PREPARATION OF INTESTINAL TRACT

While unobstructed visualization of the urinary tracts requires that the intestinal tract be free of gas and solid fecal material, preparation is not attempted in infants and children, and whether any cleansing measure is possible in adults depends, as always, on the condition of the patient. Gas (particularly swallowed air, which is quickly dispersed through the small bowel) rather than fecal material is usually the offender in these patients. Adult patients should be advised to try to refrain from unnecessary swallowing before and during the examination,[1] and every effort should be made to pacify infants and young children to prevent crying. Colonic gas can usually be eliminated by passing a soft-rubber rectal catheter well into the rectum (6 to 8 inches) and then having the patient lie on his right side. The distal end of the flatus tube should be immersed in a basin of deodorant solution. A flatus tube is also used to clear the rectum of gas before cystography.

Hope[2] recommends that infants and children be given a carbonated soft drink to distend the stomach with gas. By this maneuver, the gas-containing intestinal loops are usually pushed downward, and the upper urinary tracts, particularly the left, are then clearly visualized through the negative shadow of the gas-filled stomach. Hope states that the aerated drink must be given in an amount adequate to fully inflate the stomach; at least 2 ounces are required for a newborn infant, and a full 12 ounces are required for a child 7 or 8 years of age. In conjunction with the carbonated drink, Hope uses a highly concentrated contrast medium.

Berdon and Baker,[3,4] of Babies Hospital, Columbia-Presbyterian Medical Center, New York City, state that the prone position resolves the problem of obscuring gas shadows in a majority of patients. The need to inflate the stomach with either air alone or with air as part of an aerated drink is eliminated. By exerting pressure on the abdomen, the prone position shifts the gas laterally away from the pelvicalyceal structures. Gas contained in the antral end of the stomach is displaced into its fundic portion, that in the transverse colon shifts into the ascending and descending segments, and that in the sigmoid colon shifts into the descending colon and rectum. Berdon and Baker say that the prone position occasionally fails to produce the desired result in small infants when the small bowel is dilated. It was found that gastric inflation also fails in these patients because the dilated small bowel merely elevates the gas-filled stomach and thus does not improve visualization. They recommend that this group of infants be examined after the intestinal gas has passed.

[1]Magnusson, W.: On meteorism in pyelography and on the passage of gas through the small intestine, Acta Radiol. **12**:552-561, 1931.

[2]Hope, J. W., and Campoy, F.: The use of carbonated beverages in pediatric excretory urography, Radiology **64**:66-71, 1955.

[3]Berdon, W. E., and Baker, D. H.: Personal communication.

[4]Berdon, W. E., Baker, D. H. and Leonidas, J.: Prone radiography in intravenous pyelography in infants and children, Amer. J. Roentgen. **103**:444-455, 1968.

Geraghty[1] advocates the use of the prone position for the displacement of gas shadows in excretory urographic studies of adults as well as of infants and children. Geraghty administers no preliminary preparation of the intestinal tract, nor does he restrict diet or fluid intake. After the patient has emptied his bladder, he is placed on the examining table in the prone position. A scout film is taken ten minutes later. If the intestinal tract is found to be essentially free of gas, the contrast medium is administered. If it is not sufficiently free of gas, the patient is given one or two cupfuls, according to his capacity, of unsweetened tea at a temperature cool enough to permit rapid drinking. When possible, the tea is given through a drinking tube while the patient maintains the prone position. If the patient must sit up to drink the tea, he is replaced in the prone position immediately after drinking. A second scout film is taken ten minutes later. Geraghty states that this procedure usually clears the gas or reduces the fractions in the small bowel and transverse colon enough to permit satisfactory visualization of the urinary tracts.

The contrast medium may be injected when the patient is in the prone position, or he may be turned onto his right side for injection into the extended right arm and then readjusted in the prone position for the usual interval studies. Additional compression of the lower ureters can be easily applied by adjusting a radioparent pad under the suprapubic region. A small pillow or other soft support should be placed under the knees, and a sandbag should be placed under the ankles.

To minimize the danger of metastases in patients being investigated for intra-abdominal neoplasm, especially infants and children, Geraghty cautions against pressure on the abdomen, either by the prone position or by a compression band.

[1]Geraghty, J. A.: An approach to the problem of intestinal gas in diagnostic radiology, Brit. J. Radiol. **39**:42-46, 1966.

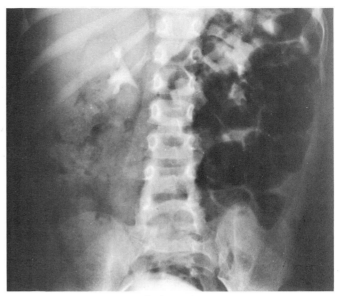

Supine study.

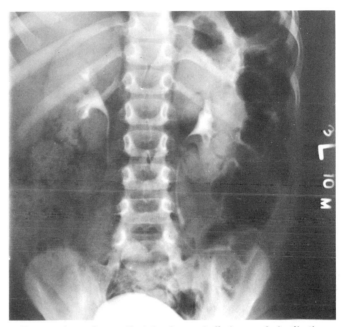

Prone study on above patient showing markedly improved visualization.

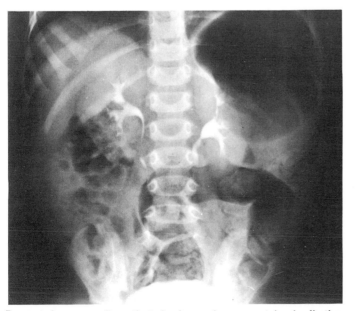

Prone study on opposite patient showing no improvement in visualization.

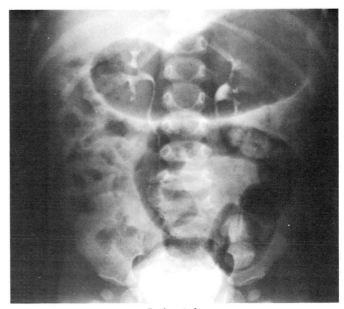

Supine study.

Radiographs courtesy Dr. Walter E. Berdon and Dr. David H. Baker.

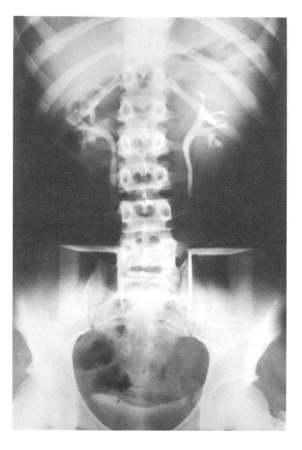

PREPARATION OF INTESTINAL TRACT—cont'd

There is wide variation in medical opinion with regard to preparative measures. With modifications as required, the following procedure seems to be in general use:

1. When time permits, a low-residue diet for one or two days to prevent gas formation due to excessive fermentation of the intestinal contents.

2. A light evening meal (sometimes withheld).

3. When indicated by costive bowel action, a nongas-forming cathartic such as castor oil or licorice powder the evening before the examination.

4. A light breakfast is permitted by some radiologists; it is given without a beverage when routine excretory urography is to follow, and possibly when infusion urography and nephrotomography are to follow.

5. A cleansing enema about thirty minutes before the examination. For information regarding the use of hydrogen peroxide (H_2O_2) enemas for the elimination of gas, see page 736.

6. The withholding of fluids for a minimum of twelve hours preceding excretory urography. When fluids are not withheld, the medium is excreted at a faster rate and is therefore diluted in a larger volume of urine. The resultant opacification of the collecting canals is not so dense as that obtained when the patient is partially dehydrated.

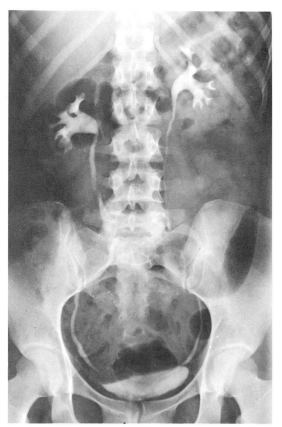

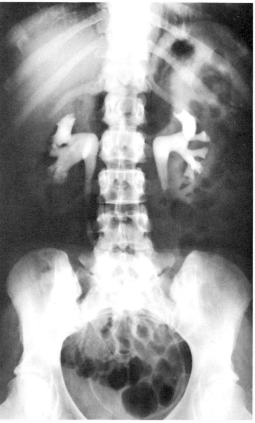

Excretion pyelographic studies.

Radiographs courtesy Dr. Alex Norman.

778

7. In preparation for retrograde urography, the patient is required to force water (four or five glassfuls) for several hours before the examination. This is done to ensure excretion of urine in an amount sufficient for bilateral catheterized specimens and renal function tests.

Outpatients should be given explicit directions, preferably typed or mimeographed, covering any order that the radiologist has given pertaining to diet, fluid intake, cathartic, or other medication. The patient should also be given a suitable explanation for each preparative measure in order to ensure his cooperation.

EQUIPMENT

Retrograde urographic procedures requiring cystoscopy are carried out on a combination cystoscopic-radiographic unit. Any standard radiographic table equipped with a Potter-Bucky diaphragm is suitable for routine excretory urography and for most retrograde studies of the bladder and urethra. The cystoscopic unit is also used for these procedures, but for the patient's comfort, it is desirable that it have an extensible leg rest.

For infusion nephrourography it is necessary to use a table that is equipped with tomographic apparatus. Tomography is also employed in routine excretory urography, particularly when the intestinal content is heavy.

FILM QUALITY AND EXPOSURE TECHNIQUE

Urograms should have the same contrast and density and the same degree of soft-tissue detail as plain films of the abdomen. The films must show a sharply defined outline of the kidneys, the lower border of the liver, and the lateral margin of the psoas muscles. The amount of bone detail visible in these studies varies according to the thickness of the abdomen. All other factors remaining the same, it is frequently necessary to convert the foundation milliampere-second factor to a high-current, short-exposure-time combination in order to obviate motion.

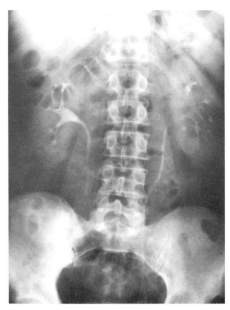

Routine excretory pyelogram by stationary projection.

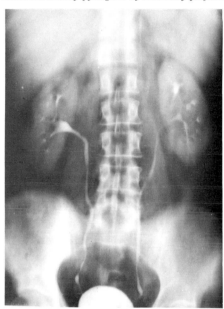

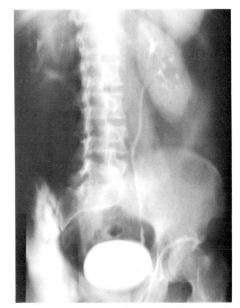

Frontal and oblique tomograms of above patient. Note elimination of gas shadows.

Radiographs courtesy Dr. Robert L. Pinck.

779

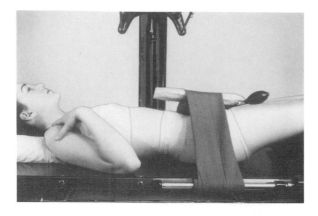

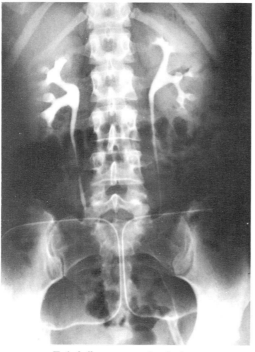

Twin-balloon compression device.

Courtesy Dr. Joshua A. Becker.

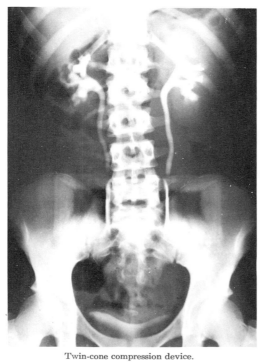

Twin-cone compression device.

Courtesy Dr. Alex Norman.

MOTION CONTROL

An immobilization band is not applied over the abdomen in urographic examinations because the resultant pressure might interfere with the passage of fluid through the ureters and might also cause distortion of the canals. This means that the elimination of motion in urographic examinations depends upon securing the full cooperation of the patient and upon the speed of the exposure.

The examination procedure should be explained to the adult patient so that he will be prepared for any transitory distress caused by the injection of the contrast solution or by the cystoscopic procedure, and he should be assured that everything possible will be done for his comfort. Much of the success of these examinations depends upon the ability of the technologist to gain the confidence of the patients, and upon his ability to convert the exposure factors to meet the requirements of the individual patient.

URETERIC COMPRESSION

In excretory urography, compression is applied over the lower ends of the ureters. This is done to retard the flow of the opacified urine into the bladder and thus ensure adequate filling of the renal pelves and calyces. A small, fully inflated, gum-rubber balloon may be used for this purpose. It is placed so that the pressure over the lower ends of the ureters is centralized about 2 inches above the upper border of the pubic symphysis, and as much pressure as the patient can comfortably tolerate is then applied with the immobilization band. The disadvantage of this device is that the immobilization band, being attached to the table, does not permit rotation of the patient for oblique studies.

Ureteric compression devices of the belt type are now available. In addition to permitting oblique studies while maintaining ureteric compression, these belt devices have twin balloons or twin cones that are spaced so that the pressure is centered directly over each ureter. The belt is adjusted to center the balloons or cones just below the level of the umbilicus. According to the preference of the radiologist, the compression device is applied upon completion of the injection of the contrast material or immediately after the five-minute postinjection film. Following satisfactory studies of the upper urinary tracts, compression is released to permit contrast filling of the lower ureters and the bladder. Because of the amount of pressure applied in this procedure, the pressure should be released slowly when the compression device is removed to avoid the possibility of visceral rupture.

Some radiologists recommend lowering the head end of the table approximately 15 degrees immediately after the injection of the contrast medium to further retard the emptying of the pelvicalyceal system.

RESPIRATION

For the purpose of comparison, all exposures are made at the end of the same phase of breathing—at the end of exhalation unless otherwise requested by the radiologist or urologist. Since the respiratory excursion of the kidneys varies from ½ to 1½ inches, it is occasionally possible to differentiate renal from other shadows by making an exposure at a different phase of arrested respiration. When an exposure is made at other than the respiratory phase usually employed, the film should be so marked.

After being carefully instructed, the patient should be required to rehearse the breathing procedure until he is able not only to suspend respiration at the correct phase but to relax completely.

PRELIMINARY EXAMINATION

A preliminary examination of the abdomen is made before a specialized investigation of the urinary tracts is conducted. This examination sometimes reveals extrarenal lesions that are responsible for the symptoms attributed to the urinary tracts and thereby renders the urographic procedure unnecessary. An erect anteroposterior projection may be made at this time to demonstrate the mobility of the kidneys. An oblique and/or lateral cross-table projection may be required to localize a tumor mass or to differentiate renal stones from gallstones or calcified mesenteric nodes.

The scout film, an anteroposterior projection with the patient recumbent, demonstrates the contour of the kidneys and their location in the supine position, and reveals the presence of any renal or other calculi. This film also serves to check the preparation of the gastrointestinal tract and to enable the technologist to make any necessary alteration in the exposure factors.

In order to overcome the forward slant of the kidneys—to place their long axis as nearly parallel with the plane of the film as possible—the lumbar curve must be reduced by elevating the patient's shoulders and knees enough to place his back in contact with the table. No other alteration in the routine procedure that is employed for plain films of the abdomen is required.

RADIATION PROTECTION

It is taken for granted that every filter slot is equipped with a minimum of 2 mm. of aluminum and that, within the limits of the apparatus, a low-dosage exposure technique is employed. It is then the duty of the technologist to apply a gonadal shield if it will not overlap the area under investigation, to restrict radiation to the area of interest by close collimation, and to do his work so carefully that repeat exposures will not be necessary.

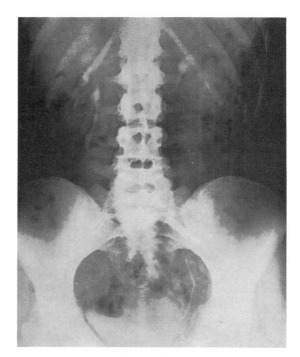

Supine position.

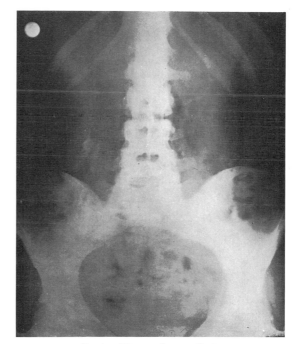

Erect position on above patient.

Radiographs courtesy J. Bentley Squier Urological Clinic, Columbia-Presbyterian Medical Center, New York City.

781

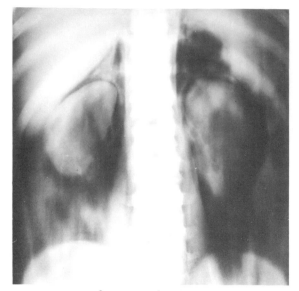

6 cm. pneumotomogram.

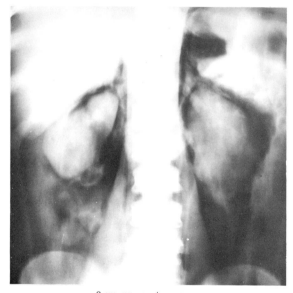

8 cm. pneumotomogram.

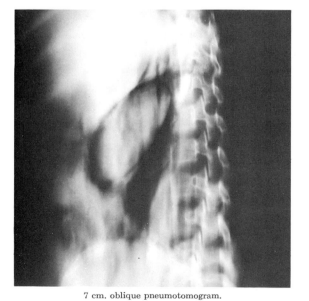

7 cm. oblique pneumotomogram.

Radiographs courtesy Dr. Joshua A. Becker.

KIDNEYS AND ADRENALS

Retroperitoneal pneumoradiography

Retroperitoneal pneumoradiography and *pneumoretroperitoneum* are terms used to denote radiologic examinations of the surfaces of the retroperitoneal structures by means of a gaseous contrast medium. Two injection techniques are employed for the introduction of the gas. In one, *presacral pneumoradiography*, the patient is placed in the knee-chest position, and after surgical cleansing and draping of the puncture area, the needle is inserted through the skin midway between the anus and the tip of the coccyx and advanced into the loose areolar tissue in the presacral retroperitoneal space between the rectum and the sacrum. By this route the gas ascends through the tissue planes and diffuses around the upper retroperitoneal structures of both sides. This injection technique was introduced by Ruiz Rivas.[1,2] In the other method, called *perirenal pneumoradiography* or *perirenal gas insufflation*, the gas is injected directly into the perirenal space by percutaneous puncture through the adjacent flank. This method, introduced by Carelli,[3] requires bilateral injections when both sides are to be examined and, usually, a general anesthetic. For these reasons, the perirenal method is not so widely used as the presacral method.

Retroperitoneal pneumoradiography is utilized in the investigation of the kidney surfaces, particularly to detect the reason for any displacement of, or deformity in, a renal shadow that might be due to a space-occupying lesion of an adjacent organ. It is also used to examine the adrenal glands. The adrenals do not have sufficient physical density to be readily distinguishable on plain films but are well defined on pneumoradiograms.

[1]Ruiz Rivas, M.: Diagnóstico radiológico; el neumorrionon; técnica original, Arch. Espan. Urol. 4:228-233, 1948.

[2]Ruiz Rivas, M.: Generalized subserous emphysema through a single puncture, Amer. J. Roentgen. 64:723-734, 1950.

[3]Carelli, H. H., and Sordelli, E.: Un nuevo procedimiento par explorar el rinon, Rev. Asoc. Med. Argent. 34:424, 1921.

The gaseous medium employed may be either air, oxygen, or carbon dioxide. The subsequent filming time depends upon the absorption characteristics of the medium. Absorption of the nitrogen of air takes several days, oxygen absorption requires several hours, and carbon dioxide is absorbed rapidly.

After receiving an injection by the presacral route, the patient is placed in the erect position when possible and, depending upon his condition, is requested to walk about to aid in distributing the gas about the adrenals and the kidneys. Proper distribution of the medium is determined by radioscopy or by a scout film.

Pneumograms of the adrenal glands are made in frontal and both oblique projections, with the patient erect or recumbent, as desired. Decubitus projections may be made for further delineation of the kidneys. Pneumotomographic studies are utilized where the equipment is available. For dual-contrast studies in selected patients, intravenous or retrograde urography is performed immediately following the initial pneumoradiograms.

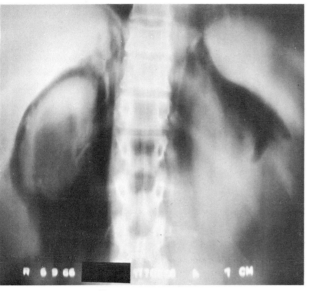

7 cm. pneumotomogram.

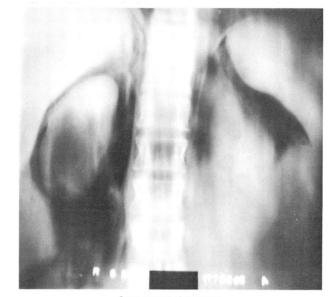

8 cm. pneumotomogram.

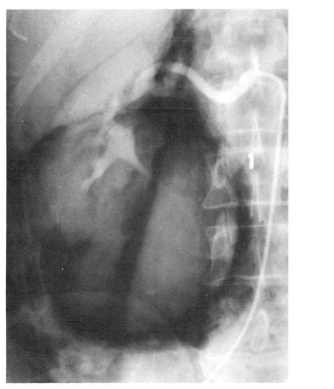

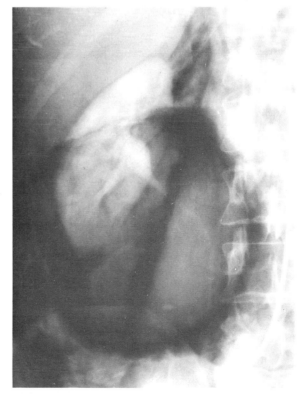

Selective renal arteriograms after presacral gas insufflation (O₂) showing large renal cyst.

Radiographs and diagnostic information courtesy Dr. Joshua A. Becker.

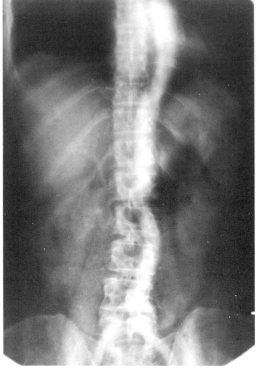

Aortogram.

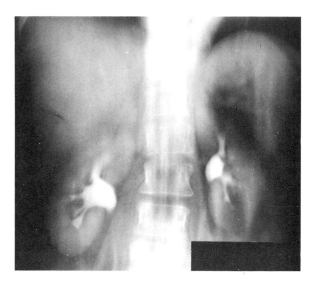

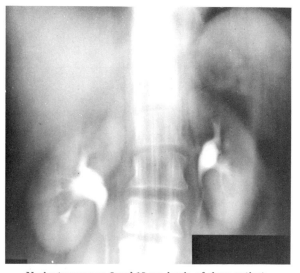

Nephrotomograms, 9 and 10 cm. levels, of above patient.

Radiographs courtesy Dr. John A. Evans.

RENAL PARENCHYMA

Bolus injection nephrotomography

Bolus injection nephrotomography is the radiologic procedure in which tomography is utilized in combination with the rapid-injection method of intravenous nephrography.[1] Evans and associates,[2,3] who introduced nephrotomography, found that, by the use of sectional rather than stationary projections, not only could intestinal-content shadows be eliminated but small intrarenal lesions could be more clearly defined.

This examination is performed by a procedure similar to the Robb-Steinberg method of angiocardiography, in that (1) the arm-to-tongue circulation time of dehydrocholic acid (Decholin) is determined so that the contrast studies can be timed to coincide with the filling of the renal vessels, and (2) a large bolus of highly concentrated, iodinated contrast solution is rapidly injected into the venous bloodstream by way of a large-bore needle inserted into an antecubital vein. This method of introducing the contrast medium usually provides visualization of the abdominal aorta and renal arteries as well as of the renal parenchyma. By this rapid-injection technique, the renal blood vessels and corticomedullary structures are opacified only during the brief passage of the jet of contrast material. This requires that the filming procedure, from the exposure of the arteriogram to the completion of the nephrotomograms, be carried out as quickly as possible. Skilled teamwork and technical accuracy are essential to high-quality studies.

The patient is adjusted in the supine position on a table equipped with tomographic apparatus. Scout sectional films are made to establish the exposure technique and to determine the optimal level for the contrast tomographic studies. A scout film of the abdomen is then made to establish the desired exposure technique for the first contrast study—a stationary projection of the opacified abdominal aorta and renal arteries.

Before starting the examination, the radiologist explains the procedure to the patient and rehearses it with him so that, knowing what sensations to expect, he will be better able to cooperate for the film studies.

Following the determination of the circulation time of Decholin, and prior to injection of the highly concentrated contrast agent, Evans[2] administers a smaller dose of a contrast medium of standard concentration for the purposes of reinforcing parenchymal opacification and of opacifying the pelvicalyceal system for simultaneous visualization.

[1]Weens, H. S., Olnick, H. M., James, D. F., and Warren, J. V.: Intravenous nephrography; a method of roentgen visualization of the kidney, Amer. J. Roentgen. 65:411-414, 1951.

[2]Evans, John A., Dubilier, W. J., and Monteith, J. C.: Nephrotomography, Amer. J. Roentgen. 71:213-223, 1954.

[3]Evans, John A.: Nephrotomography in the investigation of renal masses, Radiology 69:684-689, 1957.

Postinjection filming consists of one stationary projection of the abdomen during the arterial phase of opacification, and of multiple sectional projections of the upper abdomen during the nephrographic phase. From the beginning of the rapid injection of the highly concentrated contrast medium, the predetermined circulation time is clocked with a stopwatch, and at the proper signal, a two- to three-second exposure is made. Evans[1] states that the prolonged exposure time of two or three seconds is designed to capture the opacified abdominal aorta and renal arteries and that it enhances the chances of obtaining a satisfactory aortogram. Immediately following the arterial phase, the renal parenchyma becomes opacified, producing the nephrographic phase. It is during this phase that tomography is used (hence the term *nephrotomography*).

PERCUTANEOUS RENAL PUNCTURE

Percutaneous renal puncture, introduced by Lindblom,[2,3] is another radiologic procedure used in the investigation of renal masses; specifically, it is used to differentiate cysts and tumors of the renal parenchyma. The patient is placed in the prone position on a radioscopic-radiographic table equipped with tomographic apparatus, and preliminary films are made. These examinations can, with few exceptions, be performed with suitable sedation and local anesthesia, so that the patient is usually able to cooperate for film studies. Under strict aseptic conditions, and under radioscopic guidance, a long needle is inserted through the flank into the renal cyst. After aspirating fluid for culture and microscopic study, the radiologist injects an iodinated organic solution for sectional and/or stationary film studies.

By a similar procedure, the renal pelvis is entered percutaneously for direct contrast filling of the pelvicalyceal system in selected patients with hydronephrosis.[4-6] This procedure, called *percutaneous antegrade pyelography*[6] to distinguish it from the retrograde method of direct pelvicalyceal filling, is usually restricted to the investigation of patients with large hydronephrosis, and to patients with suspected hydronephrosis for which conclusive information could not be gained by either excretory or retrograde urography.

[1]Evans, John A.: Personal communication.

[2]Lindblom, K.: Percutaneous puncture of renal cysts and tumors, Acta Radiol. **27**:66-72, 1946.

[3]Lindblom, K.: Diagnostic kidney puncture in cysts and tumors, Amer. J. Roentgen. **68**:209-215, 1952.

[4]Wickbom, I.: Pyelography after direct puncture of the renal pelvis, Acta Radiol. **41**:505-512, 1954.

[5]Weens, H. S., and Florence, T. J.: The diagnosis of hydronephrosis by percutaneous renal puncture, J. Urol. **72**:589-595, 1954.

[6]Casey, W. C., and Goodwin, W. E.: Percutaneous antegrade pyelography and hydronephrosis, J. Urol. **74**:164-173, 1955.

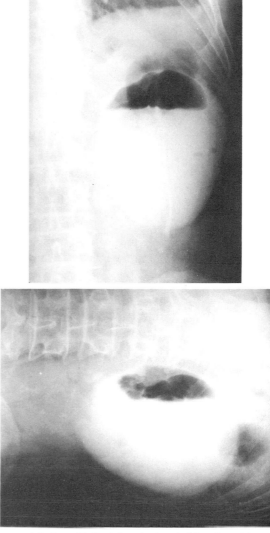

Percutaneous injection of iodinated contrast material and gas into renal cyst. Note fluid level in erect and decubitus projections.

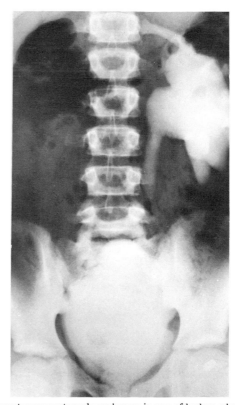

Percutaneous antegrade pyelogram in case of hydronephrosis.

Radiographs and diagnostic information courtesy Dr. Joshua A. Becker.

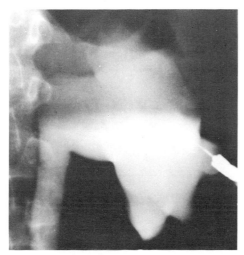

Spot-film study of opposite patient.

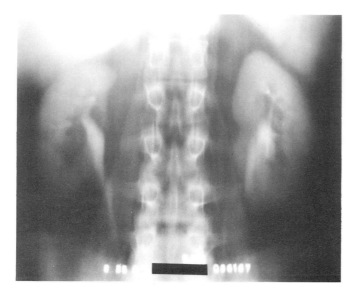

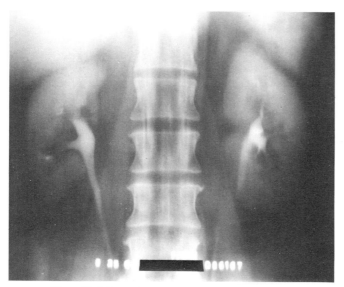

Normal infusion nephrotomograms, 9 and 11 cm. level.

Radiographs and diagnostic information courtesy Dr. Joshua A. Becker.

RENAL PARENCHYMA—cont'd

Infusion nephrotomography and nephrourography

Infusion nephrotomography and nephrourography were introduced by Schencker.[1] This method of administering the contrast medium provides opacification of the renal parenchyma as well as of the renal drainage canals and thus embraces both nephrography and urography. With several exceptions, the examination is performed by a procedure somewhat similar to that used for routine intravenous urography. The infusion procedure differs from the routine procedure in that (1) the patient is not necessarily dehydrated, (2) the contrast medium is introduced into the venous bloodstream by infusion rather than by injection,* and (3) both nephrotomographic and nephrourographic studies are made.

PREPARATION OF PATIENT

While fluids are not necessarily withheld, it has been found that partial dehydration provides more intense opacification of the drainage canals. When preparation of the intestinal tract is possible, the patient may be placed on a low-residue diet for one or two days, a non-gas-forming cathartic may be given on the preceding evening, and a cleansing enema may be given on the morning of the examination. For information regarding the use of hydrogen peroxide (H_2O_2) enemas for the elimination of colonic gas, see page 736.

PREPARATION OF CONTRAST SOLUTION

A large volume of an organic iodinated contrast medium of standard concentration is in current use for this procedure. In each case, the exact amount of the medium is based on the patient's body weight (usually 1 ml. per pound is used). The contrast medium is transferred to a sterile infusion bottle and then is diluted with an equal volume of sterile distilled water or other specified diluent. Because of the possibility of contamination in transferring a sterile fluid from one container to another, the preparation of the infusion apparatus and solution must be performed by a qualified person.

[1]Schencker, B.: Drip infusion pyelography; indications and applications in urologic roentgen diagnosis, Radiology 83:12-21, 1964.

*An injection is forced into a vessel (or organ), whereas an infusion flows in by gravity.

EXAMINATION PROCEDURE

The patient is placed in the supine position on a table equipped with tomographic apparatus. A scout film of the abdomen is made to establish the exposure technique for the nephrourograms. Scout sectional films are made to establish the exposure technique and to determine the level for the nephrotomograms.

The infusion is made through an 18-gauge needle, which is inserted into an antecubital vein just as for routine intravenous urography. The infusion flask is hung on a standard, and the contrast solution is allowed to flow through the needle without restraint; the infusion usually takes no more than six or seven minutes.

Opacification of the renal substance (referred to as the nephrographic phase) generally reaches optimum density at the end of the infusion, at which time nephrotomograms are made. In certain instances, the radiologist may have sectional studies made during the infusion. In addition to frontal plane sections, oblique and/or lateral sectional studies are made as indicated.

Timed from the beginning of the infusion, conventional studies of the urinary canals are usually made at ten- twenty- and thirty-minute intervals. Delayed urograms are taken as required. Studies of the urinary bladder and voiding urethrograms may be made.

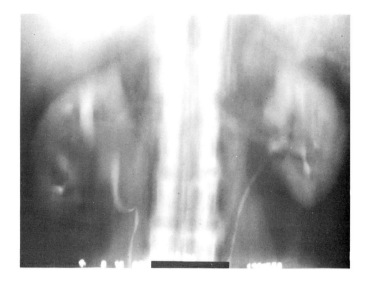

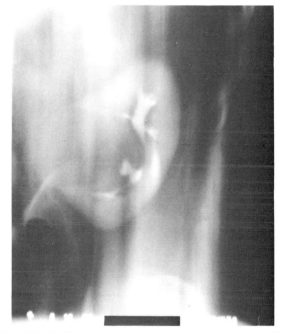

Frontal and lateral infusion nephrotomograms demonstrating a parapelvic cyst.
Radiographs and diagnostic information courtesy Dr. Joshua A. Becker.

EXCRETORY UROGRAPHY

The excretory, or excretion, method of urography is often referred to as *descending* urography to distinguish it from the *ascending*, or retrograde, method of introducing the contrast medium into the canals. The route by which the contrast solution is administered (intravenous, intramuscular, subcutaneous) is specified. In general practice, the term pyelography is still used more frequently than the term urography, but it is understood to include an examination of the bladder as well as of the kidneys and the ureters, and, when indicated, voiding studies of the urethra. The intravenous method is the one that is most frequently used and the one that gives the most satisfactory results. There is a variation in the time intervals between the injection of the contrast substance and the exposure of the series of radiographs, but the examination procedure is otherwise the same, irrespective of the route by which the contrast agent is administered.

Intravenous urography (I.V.U.)

For the patient's comfort as well as to obviate delays during the examination, all preparations for the examination procedure should be made before the patient is placed on the table for the preliminary film. In addition to the identification and side marker, a time-interval marker is required for each postinjection study. Body-position markers (supine, prone, erect or semi-erect, Trendelenburg, decubitus) should also be ready for use. An ample supply of films of each size should be at hand. Some radiologists have excretory pyelograms (upper urinary tracts) made on $10'' \times 12''$ or $11'' \times 14''$ films placed crosswise. These studies are more often made on $14'' \times 17''$ films placed lengthwise. The erect study is made on a $14'' \times 17''$ film because it is taken to demonstrate the mobility of the kidneys as well as to outline the lower ureters and bladder. With the use of a polygraph, four voiding urethrograms may be made on one $11'' \times 14''$ film. Studies of the bladder after voiding are usually taken on $10'' \times 12''$ films.

The emergency cart should be fully equipped and conveniently placed. The instrument layout for the injection of the contrast agent should be arranged on a small, movable table or an instrument cart. The usual sterile items used are a 30 or 50 ml. syringe and intravenous needles of the specified size, hypodermic syringes and needles, gauze or cotton sponges soaked in alcohol, and a forceps. Disposable syringes and needles, sterilized and packaged in plastic kits, are available in standard sizes and are widely used in this procedure. The nonsterile items required are an ampule file, a tourniquet, a small waste basin, an emesis basin and disposable wipes, one or two ampules of the contrast medium, and a small prepared dressing for application to the puncture site. The contrast solution is warmed to body temperature by placing the ampule in a basin of warm water. A folded towel or a small pillow should be ready for placement under the elbow to relieve pressure during the injection. It is also well to have a towel and, unless there is cold running water in the room, a basin of ice water; for five or ten minutes following the injection of the contrast agent, many patients experience a sensation of intense heat, which can be relieved somewhat by placing a cold, wet towel on the forehead or throat.

Immediately before being placed on the examining table, the patient is always required to empty the bladder completely. This is done to obviate the possibility of rupture of a distended bladder when ureteric compression is applied as well as to prevent dilution of the opacified urine when it enters the bladder.

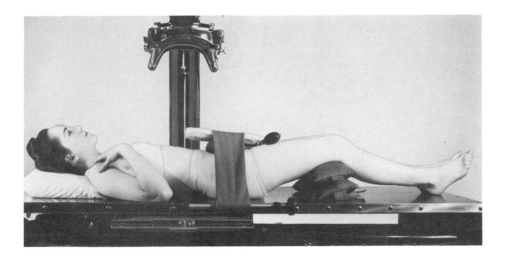

The patient is placed on the table in the supine position and is adjusted to center the median sagittal plane of the body to the midline of the table. The footboard should be attached in preparation for the erect or semi-erect ureterogram. If the head end of the table is to be lowered further to enhance pelvicalyceal filling, the shoulder support should be attached and adjusted to the patient's height. To place the long axis of the kidneys as nearly parallel as possible with the plane of the film for the pyelograms, the head and shoulders are elevated on one or two pillows, and the knees are then flexed enough to place the back in contact with the table. A folded sheet or other radioparent pad should be placed under the pelvis to relieve painful pressure when the immobilization band is to be used to apply ureteric compression. When a belt type of device is to be used for this purpose, it should be placed so that it is ready for immediate application at the specified time.

The technologist should prepare for the first postinjection film before calling the radiologist to inject the contrast medium. Place the cassette in the Potter-Bucky tray and the identification, side, and time-interval markers in position, and make any change in centering or exposure technique indicated by the scout film. Have the folded towel or other suitable pad and the tourniquet ready for placement under the selected elbow, and since the contrast medium is injected slowly, have a stool ready for the physician's use. If trained in aseptic technique, the technologist should load the contrast-medium syringe.

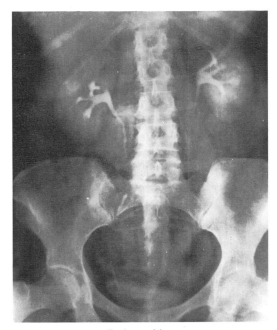

Supine position.

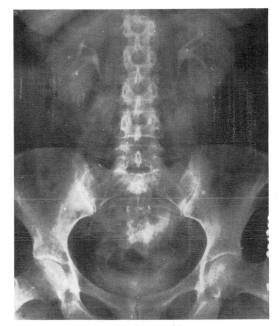

Trendelenburg position.

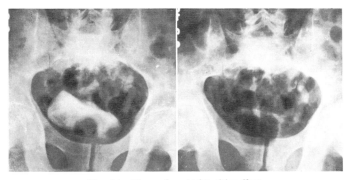

Premicturition and postmicturition films.

Courtesy Dr. William H. Shehadi.

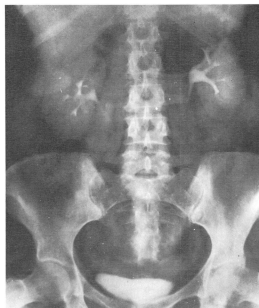

789

Semi-erect position. Note mobility of kidneys.

Radiographs courtesy Dr. Oswald S. Lowsley.

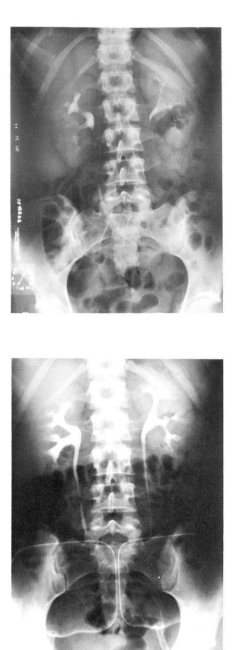

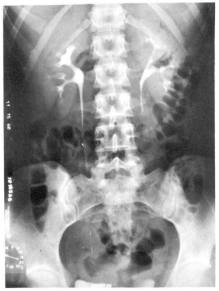

Radiographs courtesy Dr. Joshua A. Becker.

INTRAVENOUS UROGRAPHY—cont'd

According to the preference of the examining radiologist, 30 to 60 ml. of the contrast medium is administered to patients of average size who are 14 years of age or over. The dosage administered to infants and children is regulated according to age.

The radiologist slowly injects the contrast solution (this usually requires from four to six minutes), and film studies are then made at specified intervals from the time of the completion of the injection. Depending on whether the patient is partially dehydrated and on the speed of the injection, the contrast agent normally begins to appear in the pelvicalyceal system in two to eight minutes, the greatest concentration usually occurring in fifteen to twenty minutes. As soon as each film is exposed, it is immediately processed and presented to the radiologist so that he can determine, according to the kidney function of the individual patient, the time intervals at which the most intense shadows will be obtained.

In the most frequently recommended procedures for intravenous urography, anteroposterior urograms are made at five-, ten-, and twenty-minute postinjection intervals. Oblique studies are usually obtained at the fifteen- or twenty-minute interval; ureteric compression is maintained for these when a belt type of device is employed. Unless delayed studies are indicated by diminished renal function, the compression device is removed after the twenty- or twenty-five–minute urogram, and the patient may then be turned for a postero-anterior projection. Handel and Schwartz[1] and Elkin[2] recommend the prone position for the demonstration of the ureteropelvic region and for filling the obstructed ureter in the presence of hydronephrosis. As pointed out by Handel and Schwartz, the ureters fill better in the prone position because it reverses the curve of their downward course. The kidneys are situated obliquely, slanting forward in the transverse plane, so that the opacified urine tends to collect in, and distend, the dependent part of the pelvicalyceal system; thus, the more posteriorly placed, upper calyces fill more readily in the supine position, and the forward, lower parts of the calyces and renal pelvis fill more easily in the prone position.

Immediately after the last urogram, the patient is adjusted in an erect or semi-erect position for an anteroposterior projection to demonstrate the opacified bladder and the mobility of the kidneys. Unless further study of the bladder is indicated or voiding urethrograms are to be made, the patient is sent to the lavatory. A pos-micturition film of the bladder area is taken to detect, by the presence of residual urine, such conditions as small tumor masses or, in the case of the male patient, enlargement of the prostate gland.

Braasch and Emmett[3] recommend that the central ray be angled 5 degrees toward the head on supine urograms in order to project the costochondral shadows above those of the kidneys. They further recommend that the central ray be angled 5 degrees toward the feet on supine cystograms to project the shadow of the pubic symphysis distal to the bladder neck and vesicourethral junction.

Rolleston and Reay[4] recommend a cross-table lateral projection for the demonstration of the ureteropelvic junction in the presence of hydronephrosis; the patient is placed in the supine or prone position, as required. Cook and Associates[5] use cross-table lateral projections to determine whether an extrarenal mass in the flank is intraperitoneal or extraperitoneal, and they state that the cross-table lateral is an easy way to screen both kidneys and ureters for any abnormal anterior displacement.

Oblique and direct lateral projections are used to demonstrate such conditions as rotation or pressure displacement of a kidney and to

[1]Handel, J., and Schwartz, S.: Value of the prone position for filling the obstructed ureter in the presence of hydronephrosis, Radiology **71**:102-103, 1958.

[2]Elkin, M.: The prone position in intravenous urography for study of the upper urinary tract, Radiology **76**:961-967, 1961.

[3]Braasch, W. F., and Emmett, J. L.: Clinical urology, Philadelphia, 1951, W. B. Saunders Co.

[4]Rolleston, G. L., and Reay, E. R.: The pelvi-ureteric junction, Brit. J. Radiol. **30**:617-625, 1957.

[5]Cook, I. K., Keats, T. E., and Seale, D. L.: Determination of the normal position of the upper urinary tract in the lateral abdominal urogram, Radiology **99**:499-502, 1971.

localize calcareous shadows and tumor masses.

An anteroposterior projection with the head end of the table lowered 15 or 20 degrees and with the central ray directed vertically is sometimes employed to demonstrate the lower ends of the ureters. In this angled position, the weight of the contained fluid stretches the bladder fundus cranialward, giving an unobstructed view of the lower ureters and the vesicoureteral orifice areas.

For the investigation of bladder lesions by the excretion method of urography, Elkin[1] recommends right-angle views (frontal and cross-table lateral) in which the bladder wall that is under inspection is placed in the dependent position; that is, to place the posterior bladder wall in the dependent position, the patient should be supine, and to place the anterior wall in the dependent position, he should be prone. Elkin states that the dependent bladder wall stretches under the weight of the contained fluid and that it becomes more densely opacified because the absence of peristaltic activity of the bladder musculature permits the heavy, opacified urine to settle below the lighter-weight, nonopacified urine. As elsewhere, space-occupying intraluminal lesions cause filling defects that are more readily identified when they are in a dependent position and when they are projected in profile.

Urea washout test

The urea washout test[2,3] is used to assess urinary output in cases of renovascular hypertension. The test consists of administering a rapid (fifteen-minute) intravenous infusion of 40 grams of urea dissolved in 500 ml. of physiologic saline solution immediately after intravenous urography. The urea induces increased urinary output and thereby demonstrates whether the washout time of the contrast material is equal on the two sides. Using the

last (fifteen- or eighteen-minute) urogram as a baseline study, films are exposed at three-minute intervals during and after the urea infusion until the contrast medium is uniformly washed out or until a definite delay in washout time on one side is demonstrated.

The patient is then rehydrated with an intravenous infusion of 500 ml. of physiologic saline solution and an equal volume of water by mouth.

[1]Elkin, M.: Supine and prone positions in intravenous urography for diagnosis of bladder lesions, Radiology 78:904-913, 1962.

[2]Amplatz, K.: Two radiographic tests for assessment of renovascular hypertension, Radiology 79:807-815, 1962.

[3]Remmers, A. R., Schreiber, M. H., Smith, G. H., Canales, C. D., and Sarles, H. E.: The pyelogram urea washout test in the evaluation of renovascular hypertension, Amer. J. Roentgen. 107:750-755, 1969.

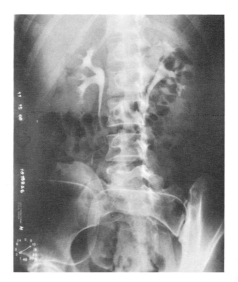

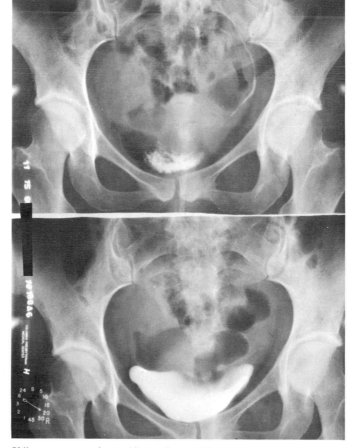

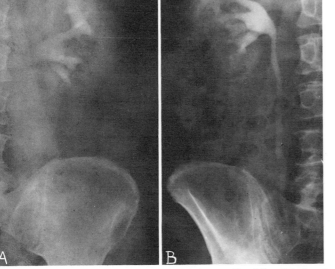

A, Supine study; right urinary tract outlined normally, left pelvicalyceal system opacified, but ureter did not. B, Prone study taken about three minutes later; note excellent opacification of entire left urinary tract.

Courtesy Dr. William H. Shehadi.

Oblique urogram and prevoiding and postvoiding cystograms of patient shown on opposite page.

Courtesy Dr. Joshua A. Becker.

RETROGRADE UROGRAPHY

Pelvicalyceal system and ureters

Retrograde urography requires that the ureters be catheterized so that a contrast agent can be injected directly into the pelvicalyceal system. Retrograde urography is classified, as are all examinations requiring instrumentation, as an operative procedure. This combined urologic-radiologic examination is carried out under careful aseptic conditions by the attending urologist with the assistance of a nurse and a technologist. The examination is performed in a specially equipped cystoscopic-radiographic examining room which, because of the collaborative nature of these examinations, may be located in either the urology department or the radiology department. The nurse is responsible for the preparation of the instruments, the care and draping of the patient, and the adjustment of waterproof sheeting for the protection of the examining table. One of the duties of the technologist is to see that the overhead parts of the radiographic equipment are at all times free of dust for the protection of the operative field and the sterile layout.

The patient is placed on the cystoscopic table, and his knees are flexed over the stirrups of the adjustable leg supports; this is a modified lithotomy position, the true lithotomy position requiring acute flexion of the hips and knees. Before the filming procedure, the technologist should rehearse the breathing procedure with the patient and should check his position on the table. The kidneys and the full extent of the ureters in patients of average height are included on a 14″ × 17″ film when the third lumbar vertebra, which usually corresponds with the level of the iliac crests, is centered to the Potter-Bucky diaphragm. The elevation of the thighs usually reduces the lumbar curve; if not, the pillow may be readjusted under the head and shoulders so that the back is in contact with the table. Smooth out any folds in the sheet under the patient. Most cystoscopic-radiographic tables are equipped with an adjustable leg rest to permit extension of the patient's legs for certain film studies. It is desirable to have a mobile unit and a stationary grid or grid-front cassettes nearby in case cross-table projections are indicated.

Catheterization of the ureters is performed through a ureterocystoscope, which is a cystoscope with an arrangement that aids insertion of the catheters into the vesicoureteral orifices. After the endoscopic examination, the urologist passes a ureteral catheter well into one or each ureter, and leaving the catheters in position, he usually withdraws the cystoscope. After taking two catheterized specimens of urine from each kidney for laboratory tests— one specimen for culture and one for microscopic examination—the urologist makes a kidney function test. For this test, usually referred to as the P.S.P. estimation, phenolsulfonphthalein or indigo carmine is injected intravenously, and the function of each kidney is then determined by the time required for the dye substance to appear in the urine as it trickles through the respective catheters.

Immediately following the P.S.P. injection, the technologist should recheck the position of the patient and make the preliminary film, if it has not been made previously, so that it will be ready for inspection by the time the kidney function test has been completed. The urologist will then be ready to inject the contrast medium and to proceed with the urographic examination. When a bilateral examination is to be performed, both sides are filled simultaneously in order to avoid subjecting the patient to unnecessary radiation exposure. Additional studies in which one side only is refilled may then be made as indicated.

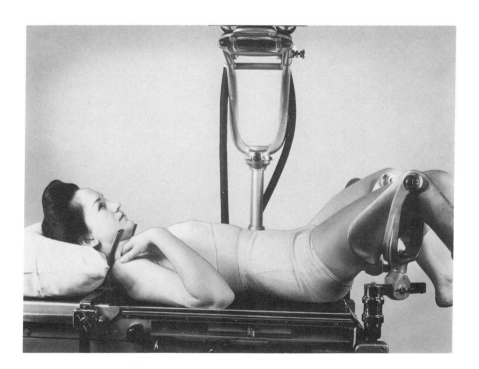

The routine retrograde urographic series usually consists of three films: the preliminary radiograph showing the ureteral catheters in position, the pyelogram, and the ureterogram. Some urologists recommend that the head of the table be lowered 10 to 15 degrees for the pyelogram in order to prevent the contrast solution from escaping into the ureters. Other urologists recommend that pressure on the syringe be maintained during the pyelographic exposure in order to ensure complete filling of the pelvicalyceal system. The head of the table is usually elevated 35 or 40 degrees for the ureterogram in order to demonstrate any tortuosity of the ureters as well as the mobility of the kidneys.

From 3 to 5 ml. of solution will fill the average normal renal pelvis; however, a larger quantity is required when the structure is dilated. The best index of complete filling, and the one most frequently employed, is an indication from the patient as soon as he feels a sense of fullness in his back.

When both sides are to be filled, the urologist, with the aid of his nurse assistant, injects the contrast solution through the catheters in an amount sufficient to fill the renal pelves and calyces. At the physician's signal, the patient is instructed to suspend respiration at the end of exhalation, and the exposure for the pyelogram is then made.

Following the pyelographic exposure, the cassette is quickly changed and the head of the table is elevated in preparation for the ureterogram. The penetration should be increased approximately 6 kilovolts for the ureterogram to allow for the increased thickness of the abdomen in the semi-erect position. For this exposure, the patient is instructed to inhale deeply and then to suspend respiration at the end of full exhalation. Simultaneously with the breathing procedure, the catheters are slowly withdrawn to the lower ends of the ureters as the contrast solution is being injected into the canals. At a signal from the urologist, the ureterographic exposure is made.

It is sometimes necessary to make stereoscopic and serial exposures. Right and/or left oblique views are frequently required. Occasionally a lateral view, with the patient turned onto the affected side, is taken to demonstrate anterior displacement of a kidney or ureter and to delineate a perinephritic abscess. Cross-table lateral projections, with the patient supine or prone as required, are used to demonstrate the ureteropelvic region in patients with hydronephrosis. To differentiate between a ureteral calculus and a calculus-like shadow lying along the course of a ureter, it is sometimes necessary to make a double exposure with a ureteral catheter in situ. The first exposure is made with the x-ray tube centered in the usual manner, and the second exposure is made with the tube shifted laterally 2 or 3 inches away from the side of interest; the normal exposure time is reduced by one-third. When the calcification is within the ureter, its shadow shifts with that of the opaque catheter; otherwise, the two shadows are projected some distance apart. The use of the "shift technique" in urography was first described by Kretschmer,[1] who accredited the suggestion for this application of the method to Earl Ball.

[1]Kretschmer, H. L.: A new procedure for the localization of ureteral stone, Surg. Gynec. Obstet. 27:472-474, 1918.

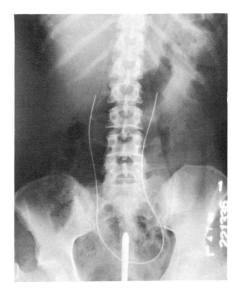

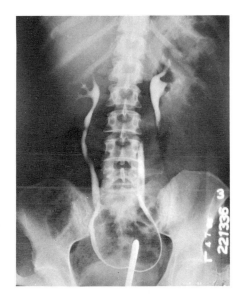

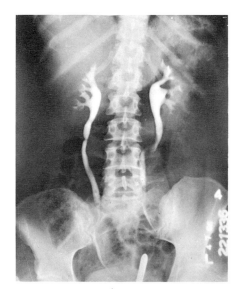

Radiographs courtesy Dr. Robert L. Pinck.

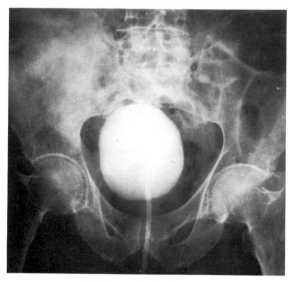

Positive contrast cystogram.

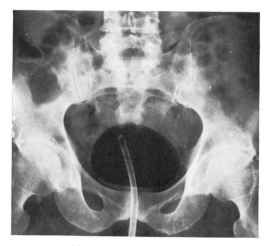

Negative contrast cystogram.

Radiographs courtesy Dr. Marcy L. Sussman.

RETROGRADE UROGRAPHY—cont'd

Urinary bladder, lower ureters, urethra, and prostate

With few exceptions radiologic examinations of the lower urinary tracts are performed with the retrograde method of introducing the contrast material. These examinations are denoted, according to the specific purpose of the investigation, by the terms *cystography, cystoureterography, cystourethrography,* and *prostatography.* More often they are denoted by the general term cystography. Cystoscopy is not a required preliminary to retrograde contrast filling of the lower urinary canals, but when both examinations are indicated, they are usually performed in a single-stage procedure to spare the patient preparation and instrumentation for separate examinations. When cystoscopy is not indicated, these examinations are best carried out on an all-purpose radiographic table unless the combination table is equipped with an extensible leg rest.

CONTRAST MEDIA

The contrast agents currently employed for positive contrast studies of the lower urinary tracts are solutions of chemically pure sodium iodide in concentrations of 5% to 20%, a 15% solution of iodohippurate sodium (Hippuran), or a dilute solution of one of the iodinated organic compounds used for intravenous urography. A water-soluble, viscous agent, such as Rayopak or Skiodan viscous, is used in urethrography, and as the coating agent for double-contrast studies of the bladder. An iodized oil with low specific gravity, so that it will float on the aqueous contents of the bladder, currently Lipiodol ascendant, 10%, is used in conjunction with a water-soluble, iodinated medium in the standardized gravity method of cystography.

The gaseous medium used for negative contrast studies and for double-contrast studies of the bladder may be oxygen, carbon dioxide, or, more commonly, room air.

The reader is referred to the paper by Lang[1] for an excellently detailed description of the use of barium sulfate as the opaque medium in double-contrast studies of the bladder in selected cases.

CONTRAST INJECTION TECHNIQUE

For retrograde cystography, cystoureterography, and voiding cystourethrography, the contrast material is introduced into the bladder by injection or infusion through a catheter passed into position by way of the urethral canal. A small, disposable Foley catheter is used to occlude the vesicourethral orifice in the examination of infants and children and may be used in the examination of adults when interval studies are to be made for the detection of delayed ureteral reflux. Studies are made during voiding for the delineation of the urethral canal and for the detection of ureteral reflux, which may occur only during micturition. When urethral studies are to be made during the injection of contrast material, a soft-rubber urethral-orifice acorn is fitted directly onto a contrast-loaded syringe for female patients and, usually, onto a cannula that is attached to a clamp device for male patients.

[1]Lang, E. K.: Double-contrast, gas-barium cystography in the assessment of diverticula of the bladder, Amer. J. Roentgen. **107:**769-775, 1969.

INJECTION EQUIPMENT

These examinations are carried out under careful aseptic conditions. Infants and children, and usually adult patients, are catheterized before they are brought to the radiology department. When the patient is to be catheterized by the radiologist, a sterile catheterization tray, set up to his specifications, must either be prepared or obtained from the central surgical supply room. The tray will include several urethral catheters of the specified size and type, lubricant jelly, gloves or finger cots, an antiseptic solution such as boric acid, large cotton balls, a forceps for cleansing the meatus and surrounding area, and gauze swabs or cotton balls soaked in 70% alcohol for cleansing the end of the catheter before injecting the contrast medium. The nonsterile items consist of a catheter clamp, a waste receptacle, a large basin or other container when the bladder has not been previously emptied, and the flask or other container of sterile contrast medium. Because of the danger of contamination in transferring a sterile liquid from one container to another, dilute contrast solutions must be prepared by a qualified person.

PRELIMINARY PREPARATIONS

The examining table must be protected from urine soilage with the use of radioparent plastic sheeting and with disposable underpadding such as Chux, which has a waterproof backing. In addition to a suitable receptacle, correctly arranged, disposable padding does much to reduce soilage during voiding studies and, consequently, eliminates the need for extensive cleaning between patients. The room should be aired as often as possible, and a spray deodorant should be used after each patient. Lysol spray disinfectant, which has a clean, nonmedicinal, and nonperfumed scent, is excellent for this purpose.

The outpatient, just a few minutes before time for the examination, is conducted to a lavatory, given supplies for perineal care, and instructed to empty the bladder completely. Then the patient is placed on the examination table for the catheterization procedure.

Patients are usually tense, chiefly because of embarrassment. It is important that they be given as much privacy as possible. The examining room door should be kept closed, and only the required personnel should be present during the examination. The patient should be properly draped and should be covered according to room temperature.

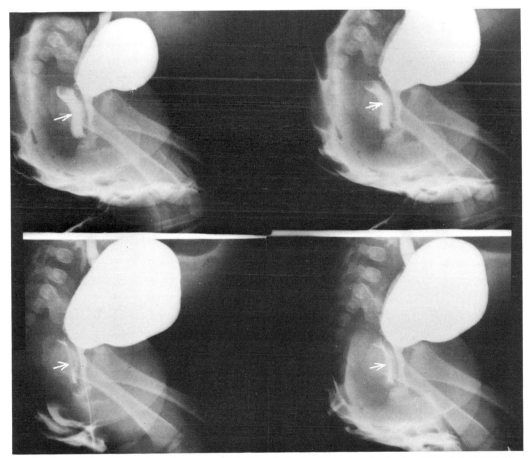

Serial (polygraphic) voiding cystourethrograms of infant female having bilateral ureteral reflux. Urethra is normal. Vaginal reflux (arrows) is normal finding.

Radiographs and diagnostic information courtesy Dr. Walter E. Berdon and Dr. David H. Baker.

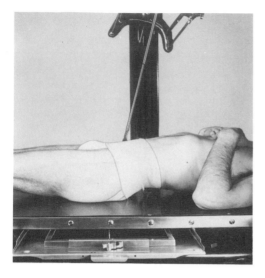

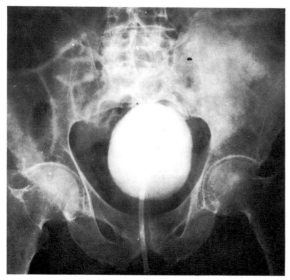

Positive contrast cystogram.

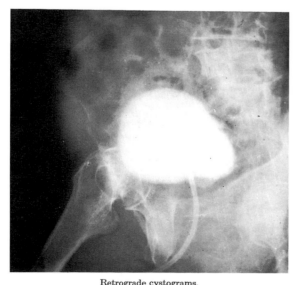

Retrograde cystograms.

Courtesy Dr. Marcy L. Sussman.

RETROGRADE CYSTOGRAPHY

Contrast injection method

With the urethral catheter in place, the patient is adjusted in the supine position for a preliminary film and for the first cystogram. Cystograms of adult patients are usually taken on $10'' \times 12''$ films that are placed lengthwise. This size of film is centered at the level of the soft tissue depression just above the most prominent point of the greater trochanters. This centering coincides with the mid-area of the filled bladder of average size. Therefore, a 12-inch film will include the region of the lower end of the ureters for the demonstration of any evidence of ureteral reflux, and it will include the prostate and proximal part of the male urethra. Large films should be nearby for use when ureteral reflux is shown. With the use of a polygraph, four serial studies can be made on one film. Some radiologists have these studies made during the filling of the bladder as well as during voiding.

After inspecting the preliminary film, the radiologist unclamps the catheter and drains the bladder in preparation for the introduction of the contrast material. This may be an iodinated solution for positive contrast studies, a gas for negative contrast studies, or a combination of an iodinated medium and a gas for double-contrast studies. Following the introduction of the contrast agent or agents, the physician clamps the catheter and tapes it to the thigh to prevent its displacement during position changes.

The initial cystographic filming generally consists of four projections—anteroposterior, right and left oblique, and direct lateral. Further studies, including voiding cystourethrograms, are made as indicated.

POSITIONING OF PATIENT

1. For anteroposterior projections of the bladder and the proximal part of the urethra, it is desirable to have the patient's legs extended so that the lumbosacral spine is arched enough to tilt the anterior pelvic bones downward. In this position, the shadow of the pubic bones can more easily be projected below that of the bladder neck and proximal urethra. A 5-degree caudal angulation of the central ray is usually sufficient. When there is loss of the normal lumbar lordosis, the pelvis is tilted forward and upward, so that it is necessary to use a 15- or 20-degree caudal angulation for these patients.

2. For oblique cystograms the patient is rotated 40 to 60 degrees, according to the preference of the examining physician. The patient is then adjusted so that the dependent pubic arch is aligned over the midline of the table. The uppermost thigh must be extended and abducted enough to prevent its superimposition on the bladder area. Usually, the central ray is directed vertically for these studies, although an angle of 10 degrees toward the feet is sometimes recommended.

3. For posteroanterior projections of the bladder and the upper part of the urethra, the central ray is directed through the region of the bladder neck at an angle of 10 to 15 degrees toward the head. It enters about 1 inch distal to the tip of the coccyx and exits a little above the upper border of the pubic symphysis. This position, usually with a 20- to 25-degree cranial angulation of the central ray, is used to project the shadow of the prostate above that of the pubes.

4. Both frontal positions (supine and prone), usually with the central ray directed vertically, are used in gas and double-contrast studies. It is necessary to use both positions because the uppermost bladder wall is the one delineated in these studies.

5. Lateral views, taken with the central ray directed either vertically or horizontally as indicated, are used for the demonstration of the anterior and posterior bladder walls and the base of the bladder.

6. The Chassard-Lapiné position (page 745), sometimes called the "squat shot," is used to obtain an axial view of the posterior surface of the bladder and of the lower end of the ureters when they are opacified.

7. An anteroposterior projection of the lower end of the opacified ureters can be obtained by lowering the head end of the table 15 to 20 degrees to permit the filled bladder to stretch upward, where it will not superimpose the ureters. The central ray is directed vertically.

These views of the bladder are also employed when it is opacified by the excretion method of urography.

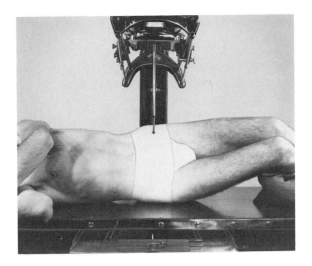

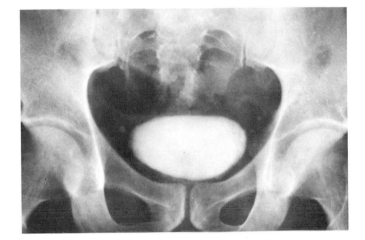

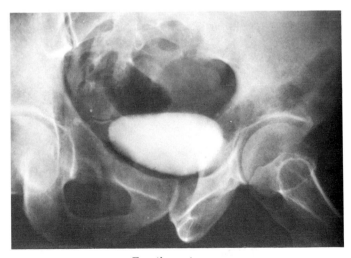

Excretion cystograms.

Radiographs courtesy Dr. Joshua A. Becker.

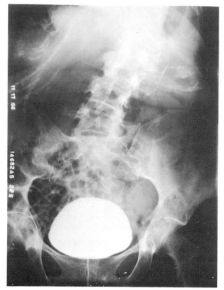

Immediate study after introduction of 225 ml. of contrast solution. Delayed study showed no ureteral reflux.

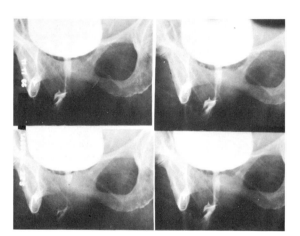

Voiding cystourethrograms.

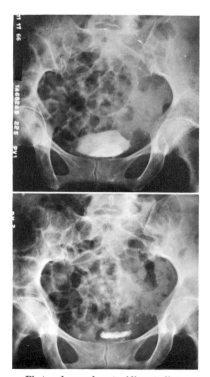

First and second postvoiding studies.
Radiographs courtesy Dr. Joshua A. Becker.

RETROGRADE CYSTOGRAPHY—cont'd

Contrast infusion method

In this method of cystography, which was developed by Dean and associates,[1] the contrast solution is introduced into the bladder with infusion apparatus by controlled gravity at a standard pressure. These physicians state that unless the contrast medium is introduced into the bladder with identical pressure and by the same technique in each examination, pretreatment and posttreatment studies cannot be reliably compared, and that valid comparison of these studies is important for the evaluation of progress of patients with impaired renal drainage, particularly infants and children with dilated urinary tracts. Because triple voiding, with a film study after each attempt, may be required for complete urinary evacuation in cases of impaired urinary drainage, this method is frequently referred to as "triple voiding cystography."

CONTRAST MEDIA

The contrast solution recommended by Dean and associates consists of two 30 ml. ampules of Hypaque, 50%, mixed with 200 ml. of sterile isotonic saline solution, to which they add an antibiotic (500 mg. of neomycin). The saline solution is available in 250 ml. disposable flasks, and 50 ml. of the solution are discarded before the contrast agent is added. Some radiologists use a commercially prepared contrast solution. The one currently available is supplied in 250 ml. disposable flasks (Cystokon).

When kept in the bladder for delayed studies, water-soluble contrast media undergo some degree of dilution as urine trickles down from the upper urinary tracts. Depending on the degree of dilution, retention of a small amount of one of these agents may not be discernible for the detection of partial impairment of bladder efficiency. To obviate this possibility, 5 ml. of Lipiodol ascendant, 10%, may be injected through the urethral catheter just before it is attached to the infusion tubing. This lightweight, iodinated oil floats on the surface of the bladder contents, so that it is voided last. Because water and oil are immiscible, any urinary retention is clearly visible.

INFUSION EQUIPMENT

The items required for the introduction of the contrast material are (1) an intravenous standard, (2) a flask of sterile contrast solution, (3) sterile, disposable plastic tubing with a threaded cap at one end for attachment to the infusion flask (Venopak), (4) sterile adapter for connecting the tubing to the urethral catheter, (5) when requested, a 5 ml. ampule of Lipiodol ascendant, 10%, and a sterile 5 ml. syringe for injecting it into the catheter, and (6) sterile gauze swabs or cotton balls and an antiseptic solution for cleaning the end of the urethral catheter before the introduction of the contrast agent or agents.

[1]Dean, A. L., Jr., Lattimer, J. K., and McCoy, C. B.: The standardized Columbia University cystogram, J. Urol. **78:**662-668, 1955.

EXAMINATION PROCEDURE

With the urethral catheter in place, the patient is adjusted in the supine position for a preliminary film of the abdomen. After inspecting this study, the radiologist unclamps the urethral catheter and drains the bladder. The flask of contrast solution is hung on a standard adjusted to hold it exactly 24 inches (60 cm.) above the patient's symphysis pubis. The pressure of flow obtained at this height was standardized because it was found that higher pressures may cause kidney pain in the presence of ureteral reflux and that lower pressures may result in inadequate filling. A little of the contrast solution is run through the infusion tubing to free it of air, and after the injection of the oily medium (when this is to be used), the tubing is connected to the cleaned end of the urethral catheter. The screw clamp is then adjusted to fill the bladder slowly, at the rate of 120 drops per minute. When an infant is undergoing the procedure, he is given a bottle of formula to pacify him during the filling of the bladder.

With the use of a polygraph, four interval studies of the bladder may be made on one film during the filling. When the inflow ceases, the catheter is clamped off, and a film bearing a marker indicating the number of milliliters introduced and large enough to include the entire abdomen is exposed. Unless this film shows bilateral ureteral reflux, the catheter is left in position and a later film, bearing a marker indicating the retention time (usually thirty minutes), is taken for the detection of delayed reflux. The radiologist inspects the films as they are processed, varies the routine procedure, and orders additional views as they are indicated.

Upon completion of the initial phase of the examination, voiding and/or postvoiding studies are made in accordance with the findings.

1. In the absence of ureteral reflux, the catheter is removed, and studies are made during voiding for the detection of reflux that may occur only during micturition. For these studies, the male patient is turned to an oblique position, with the penis overlying the soft tissues of the thigh. The female patient may be kept in the supine position or may be turned to an oblique or a lateral position, as directed by the radiologist. When this voiding does not result in complete urinary evacuation, a film is taken after each of one or two further voidings, for which the ambulatory patient is sent to a lavatory.

2. When ureteral reflux occurs during the filling of the bladder, the presence of retention, or "trapping," in the ureters and the time required for complete urinary evacuation are investigated with postvoiding studies. The infant's bladder is drained through the urethral catheter. A film is then taken, and if ureteral "trapping" is present, further studies are made until complete evacuation has occurred.

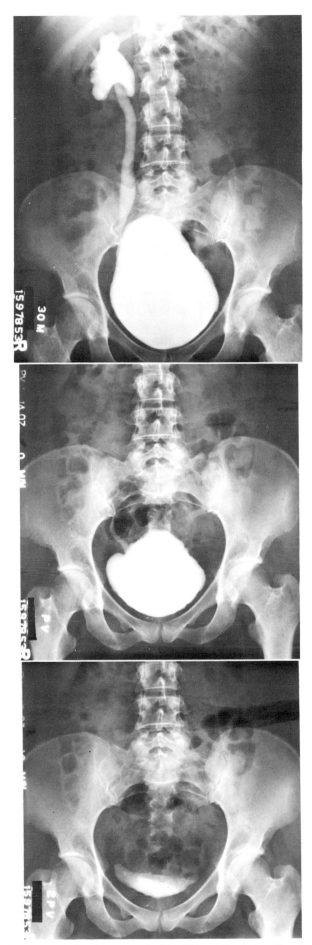

Right ureterovesical reflux seen at bladder filling. After first voiding there is poor emptying of bladder; second attempt shows almost complete emptying.

Radiographs and diagnostic information courtesy Dr. Joshua A. Becker.

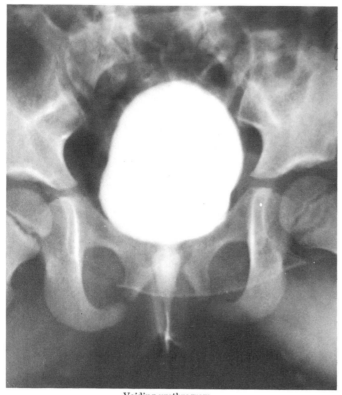

Voiding urethrogram.

Courtesy Dr. William B. Seaman.

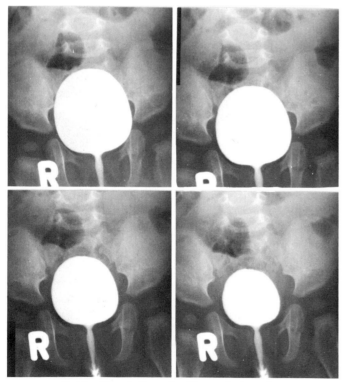

Serial voiding studies made with use of polygraph.

Courtesy Dr. Walter E. Berdon and Dr. David H. Baker.

FEMALE CYSTOURETHROGRAPHY

Contrast injection method

The female urethra averages 3½ cm. in length. Its opening into the bladder is situated at the level of the upper border of the pubic symphysis, from whence the vessel slants obliquely downward and forward to its termination in the vestibule of the vulva, about 1 inch anterior to the vaginal orifice. The female urethra is subject to such conditions as tumors, abscesses, diverticula, dilatation, strictures, and, due to some abnormality, to urinary incontinence during the stress of increased intra-abdominal pressure such as occurs on sneezing or coughing. In the investigation of abnormalities other than stress incontinence, contrast studies are made during the injection of the contrast medium and/or during voiding.

Usually, cystourethrography is preceded by an endoscopic examination. For this reason, it is usually carried out by the attending urologist or gynecologist with the assistance of a nurse and a technologist.

Following the physical examination, the cystoscope is removed and a catheter is inserted into the bladder so that the bladder can be drained just before the injection of the contrast solution. The patient is then adjusted in the supine position at a point on the combination table that will permit the films (8″ × 10″ or 10″ × 12″ placed lengthwise) to be centered at the level of the upper border of the symphysis pubis.

After inspecting the preliminary film, the physician drains the bladder and withdraws the catheter. The physician uses a syringe fitted with a blunt-nosed, soft-rubber acorn, which he holds firmly against the urethral orifice to prevent reflux as he injects the contrast solution during the exposure of the film or films. In addition to the frontal view, oblique studies may be made. For the latter, the patient is rotated 35 to 40 degrees so that the urethra is posterior to the pubic symphysis. The uppermost thigh must be extended and abducted enough to prevent overlapping.

The physician fills the bladder for each voiding study to be made. For a frontal view, the patient may be maintained in the horizontal position, or the head end of the table may be elevated enough to place the patient in a semi-seated position. A lateral voiding study of the female vesicourethral canal may be made with the patient recumbent, or she may be seated laterally on a commode type of chair or stool before a vertical grid. In either case, the film is centered at the level of the upper border of the symphysis pubis, as for frontal and oblique studies.

Metallic bead chain method

The metallic bead chain method of investigating anatomic abnormalities responsible for stress incontinence in women was described by Stevens and Smith[1] in 1937 and by numerous other persons more recently. This method is employed to delineate anatomic changes that occur in the shape and position of the bladder floor, in the posterior urethrovesical angle, in the position of the proximal urethral orifice, and in the angle of inclination of the urethral axis under the stress of increased intra-abdominal pressure as exerted by the Valsalva maneuver. Comparison studies, which are made with the patient standing at rest and during straining, are taken in frontal and lateral directions

For this examination, the physician extends a flexible metallic bead chain through the urethral canal. The proximal portion of the chain rests within the bladder, and the distal end is taped to the thigh. In order to demonstrate the length of the urethra, a small metal marker is attached with a piece of masking tape to the vaginal mucosa just lateral to the urethral orifice. After the instillation of the metallic chain, a catheter is passed into the bladder, its content is drained, 60 ml. of an opaque contrast solution are injected, and then the catheter is removed for the filming procedure.

Barnes[2] performed this examination with the patient in a recumbent oblique position, obtaining one rest film and one stress film. Hodgkinson and associates[3] recommend that the erect position be used in order to utilize gravity and thus to simulate normal bodily activity. These physicians obtain two sets of films, frontal and lateral projections, and they specify that the rest studies must be exposed before the stress studies because the bladder does not immediately return to its normal resting position after straining. Calatroni and associates[4] advocate serial (polygraphic) studies during straining so that different degrees of stress can be demonstrated.

After the instillation of the metallic chain and the contrast solution, the patient usually must be transported to the main radiology department for erect films. The examining room should be prepared in advance so that these uncomfortable patients can be given immediate attention. Waterproof sheeting should be placed on the floor in front of the vertical grid in case of leakage during the stress studies. These patients must be given kindly reassurance and must be examined behind closed doors. Klawon[5] found that these patients can be relieved of the fear of involuntary voiding and thus willingly apply full pressure during the stress studies, by the simple act of placing a folded towel or a disposable pad between the thighs before the stress films are taken.

The film size and centering point is the same as for other female cystourethrograms.

NOTE: Hoffman and Ulrich[6] perform this examination with the use of a contrast medium made up of equal parts of sterile micro-disperse barium sulfate and sterile physiologic saline solution. They state that the dense barium mixture delineates the base of the bladder more clearly in the lateral projections.

[1]Stevens, W. E., and Smith, S. P.: Roentgenological examination of the female urethra, J. Urol. **37**:194-201, 1937.
[2]Barnes, A. C.: A method for evaluating the stress of urinary incontinence, Amer. J. Obstet. Gynec. **40**:381-390, 1940.
[3]Hodgkinson, C. P., Doub, H. P., and Kelly, W. T.: Urethrocystograms: metallic bead chain technique, Clin. Obstet. Gynec. **1**:668-677, 1958.
[4]Calatroni, C. J., Poliaka, A., and Kohana, A.: A roentgenologic study of stress incontinence in women, Amer. J. Obstet. Gynec. **83**:649-656, 1962.
[5]Klawon, Sister M. M.: Urethrocystography and urinary stress incontinence in women, Radiol. Techn. **39**:353-358, 1968.
[6]Hoffman, J., and Ulrich, J.: Cystourethrography and female urinary stress incontinence, Acta Radiol. [Diagn.] **4**:1-13, 1966.

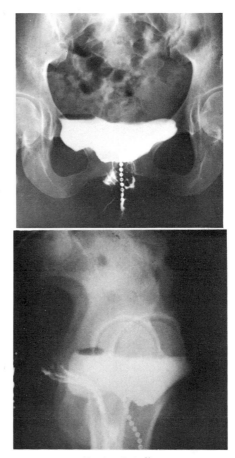

Erect rest studies.

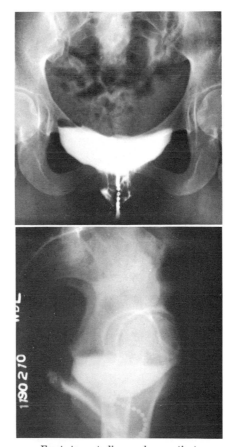

Erect stress studies on above patient.
Radiographs courtesy Dr. Howard P. Doub.

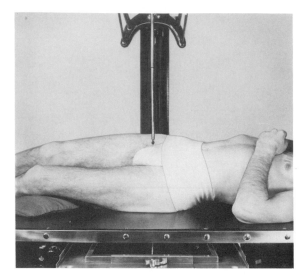

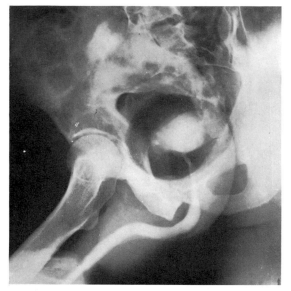

Study during injection.

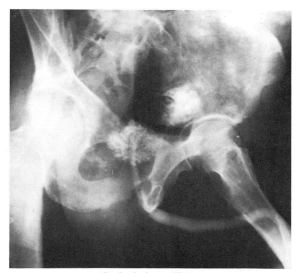

Study during voiding.

Radiographs courtesy Dr. Oswald S. Lowsley.

MALE CYSTOURETHROGRAPHY

Male cystourethrography may be preceded by an endoscopic examination, following which the bladder is catheterized so that it can be drained just before the injection of the contrast material. This may be one of the viscous contrast agents such as Thixokon, or it may be one of the water-soluble, iodinated solutions.

Cystourethrograms of adult male patients are taken on 10″ × 12″ films placed lengthwise. The patient is adjusted on the combination table so that the films can be centered at the level of the upper border of the pubic symphysis. This centering coincides with the root of the penis, and a 12-inch film will include both the bladder and the external urethral orifice.

After inspecting the preliminary film, the physician drains the bladder and withdraws the catheter. The patient is then adjusted in an oblique position. The aim is to adjust the degree of body rotation so that the bladder neck and the entire urethra are delineated as free of bony superimposition as possible. By rotating the body 35 to 40 degrees and then adjusting it so that the elevated pubis is centered to the midline of the table, the superimposed pubic and ischial rami of the dependent side and the body of the elevated pubis usually are projected well anterior to the bladder neck, the proximal part of the urethra, and the prostate. The dependent knee is flexed only slightly so as to keep the soft tissues on the medial side of the thigh as near to the center as possible. The elevated thigh is extended and retracted enough to prevent overlapping.

With the patient correctly placed, the physician inserts the contrast-loaded urethral syringe or the nozzle of a device such as the Brodney clamp into the urethral orifice. He then extends the penis along the soft tissues of the medial side of the dependent thigh in order to obtain a uniform density of both the deep and the cavernous portions of the urethral canal. At a signal from the physician, the patient is instructed to hold still, and while the injection of the contrast material is continued to ensure filling of the entire urethra, the exposure is made. The bladder may then be filled with a contrast material so that a voiding study can be made. This is usually done without changing the patient's position. When a standing-erect voiding study is required, the patient is adjusted before a vertical grid and is supplied with a urinal.

Anatomy and positioning of the male reproductive system

Male reproductive system

The male genital system consists of (1) a pair of *gonads*, or *testes*, that produce the germ cells, or spermatozoa, (2) two excretory channels, the *seminal ducts*, one leading from each testis, and through which the spermatozoa pass from the gonad to the prostatic portion of the thenceforward commonly shared urethral canal, and (3) a *prostate gland* and a pair of *bulbourethral glands* that produce secretions which, along the path, are added to the secretions of the testes and the ductal mucosa to constitute the final production, the seminal fluid.

The *seminal ducts* present anatomic variations along their course that necessitate individual description; the several portions of each duct are called the *epididymis*, the *ductus deferens* or *vas deferens*, the *seminal vesicle*, and the *ejaculatory duct*. The penis, the scrotum, and the structures enclosed by the scrotal sac (the testes, the epididymides, part of the vasa deferens, and the spermatic cords) are called the external genital organs.

The *testes* (or testicles) are ovoid bodies averaging 1½ inches in length and about 1 inch in both width and depth.

Each testis is divided into 200 to 300 partial compartments, each compartment housing one or more of the convoluted, seed-producing tubules, which constitute the glandular substance of the testis. These seminiferous tubules converge toward the dorsum of the testis (this part of the gland is called the mediastinum testis), where they empty into a network of tubules, the rete testis. These tubules, in turn, converge and unite to form some 15 to 20 tubules that emerge from the testis to enter the head of the epididymis.

The *epididymis* is an oblong structure; its larger upper part is called the head, and its distal part is called the tail. It is attached to the upper and lateroposterior aspects of the testicle. The ductules leading out of the testicle enter the head of the epididymis to become continuous with the coiled and convoluted ductules that make up this structure. As they pass downward, the ductules progressively unite to form the main duct, which is continuous with the ductus deferens.

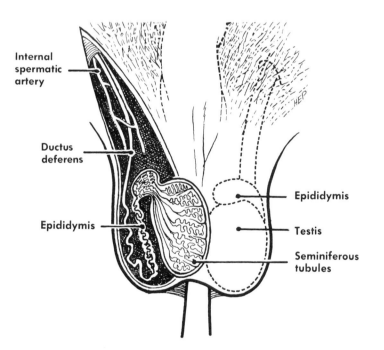

Internal spermatic artery

Ductus deferens

Epididymis

Epididymis

Testis

Seminiferous tubules

The *ductus deferens* is 16 to 18 inches in length, and only its first part is tortuous, or convoluted. It extends from the tail of the epididymis to the posteroinferior surface of the urinary bladder. From its beginning, it ascends along the medial side of the epididymis on the posterior surface of the testis to join the other constituents of the spermatic cord, with which it emerges from the scrotal sac, to pass into the pelvic cavity through the inguinal canal. The deferent duct separates from the spermatic cord and passes downward through the pelvis, over the bladder just medial to the ureter, and then downward along the upper border of the adjacent seminal vesicle. Near its termination, the duct expands into an ampulla for the storage of seminal fluid, and then ends by uniting with the duct of the seminal vesicle.

The *seminal vesicle* is a sacculated structure about 2 inches in length. It is situated obliquely on the lateroposterior surface of the bladder, where, from the level of the ureterocystic junction, it slants downward and medialward to the base of the prostate. The ampulla of the deferent duct lies along the upper border of the seminal vesicle.

The *ejaculatory duct* is formed by the union of the ductus deferens and the duct of the seminal vesicle. It averages about ½ inch in length and is situated behind the neck of the bladder. The two ejaculatory ducts enter the base of the prostate and, passing obliquely downward through the substance of the gland, open into the urethra at the lateral margins of the prostatic utricle.

The *prostate gland* is a somewhat cone-shaped body, the upper part of which is known as the base of the gland and the lower part as the apex. The gland averages 1¼ inches from base to apex, and somewhat more across its base. It encircles the proximal portion of the male urethra and, extending from the bladder neck to the pelvic floor, lies about 1 inch posterior to the lower two-thirds of the pubic symphysis and in front of the rectal ampulla. The prostate is composed of muscular and glandular tissue. Its ducts open into the prostatic portion of the urethra.

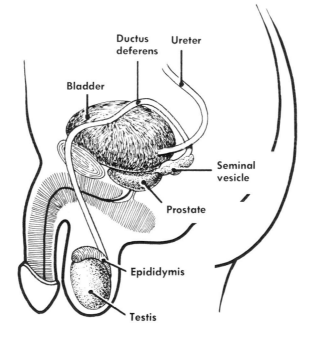

Radiography of the male reproductive system

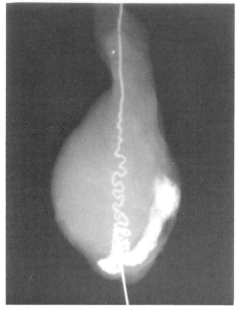

Normal epididymis showing origin of vas deferens. Needle is at epididymovasal kink, which can be palpated.

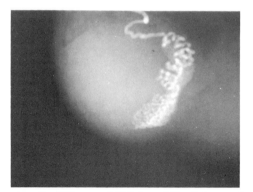

Possible covering of epididymovasal kink by epididymis in one plane demonstrates need for making several radiographs at different angles.

Seminal ducts

Radiologic examinations of the seminal ducts[1-3] are performed in the investigation of various genitourinary abnormalities, such as cysts, abscesses, tumors, inflammation, and sterility. The regional terms applied to these examinations are *vesiculography* and *epididymography*, and when combined, *epididymovesiculography*.

The contrast medium employed for these procedures is one of the water-soluble, iodinated compounds used for intravenous urography. Air is sometimes injected into each scrotal sac in order to improve contrast in the non-screen studies of the extrapelvic structures.

The seminal vesicles are sometimes opacified directly by urethroscopic catheterization of the ejaculatory ducts. More frequently, the entire duct system is inspected by introducing the contrast solution into the canals by way of the deferent ducts. This requires that small bilateral incisions be made in the upper part of the scrotum for the exposure and identification of these ducts. The needle that is used for the injection of the contrast medium is inserted into the duct in the direction of the portion of the tract under investigation—distally for the study of the extrapelvic ducts and then cranially for the study of the intrapelvic ducts.

[1]Boreau, J., Jagailloux, S., Vasselle, B., and Hermann, P.: Epididymography, Med. Radiogr. Photogr. **29**:63-66, 1953.

[2]Boreau, Jacques: L'étude radiologique des voies séminales normales et pathologiques, Paris, 1953, Masson & Cie.

[3]Vasselle, B.: Étude radiologique des voies séminales de l'homme, Paris, 1953, Thesis.

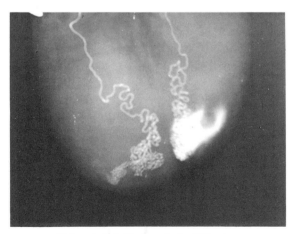

Tuberculosis (cold abscess) of epididymis.

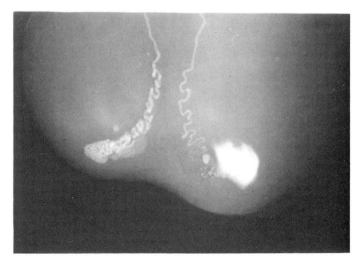

Epididymal abscess observed during acute orchitis (third relapse). Note atrophy of epididymovasal kink.

Radiographs and diagnostic information courtesy Dr. Jacques Boreau.

Radiologic examinations of the seminal ducts are performed in a minor-surgery operating room, with the patient under general anesthesia. This requires the use of a mobile radiographic unit, preferably of high-current capacity (200 to 300 milliamperes), and a portable Potter-Bucky diaphragm. The exposure technique should be established for both the extrapelvic and intrapelvic areas with preliminary films.

A nonscreen exposure technique is used for the delineation of the extrapelvic structures. For these studies, Boreau and associates[1] recommend the use of a fine-grained industrial film, a short focal-film distance (60 cm.), and 60 kilovolts at the milliampere-second factor required for the individual patient. The examining urologist places the film holder and adjusts the position of the testicles for the desired views of the ducts.

A grid technique is used for the demonstration of the intrapelvic ducts. Anteroposterior and oblique projections are made on 8″ × 10″ or 10″ × 12″ films that are placed lengthwise and centered at the level of the upper border of the symphysis pubis. Mazurek[2] recommends the Chassard-Lapiné projection for the demonstration of the seminal vesicles. Boreau[3] reversed this projection to adapt it to the anesthetized patient. In the Boreau position, which he calls the *perineosacral view*, the patient's thighs are flexed on the abdomen (page 249, Volume I), and the central ray is centered to the perineum midway between the root of the scrotum and the anus at an angle of 20 degrees toward the head.

[1]Boreau, J., Jagailloux, S., Vasselle, B., and Hermann, P.: Epididymography, Med. Radiogr. Photogr. 29:63-66, 1953.
[2]Mazurek, L. J.: Examen radiologique des voies séminales en incidence dorsosacrale, Ann. Radiol. 7:69-72, 1964. (In French.) Abstr.: Radiology 83:753, 1964.
[3]Boreau, J.: Images of the seminal tracts, New York, 1974, S. Karger.

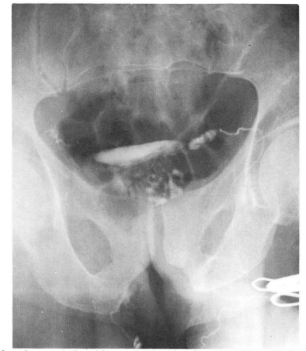

Tuberculous seminal vesicle associated with deferentitis with small abscesses, ampulitis, and considerable vesiculitis on left.

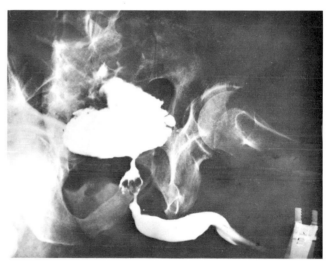

Beginning (budding) metastasis of crista urethralis discovered two years after prostatectomy for cancer of prostate.

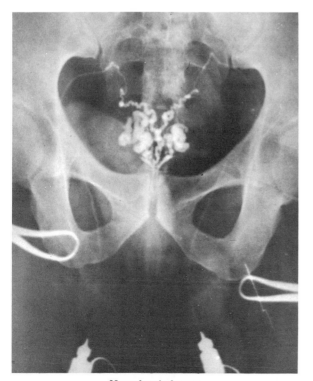

Normal vesiculogram.

Courtesy Dr. David L. Benninghoff.

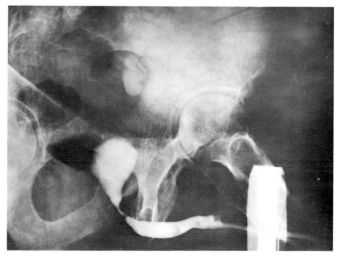

Cavity of residual abscess of prostate.

Radiographs and diagnostic information courtesy Dr. B. Vasselle.

807

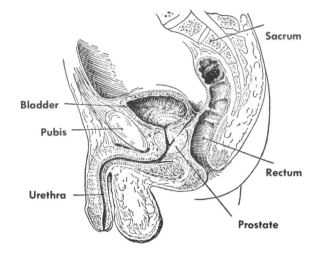

MIDSAGITTAL SECTION THROUGH MALE PELVIS

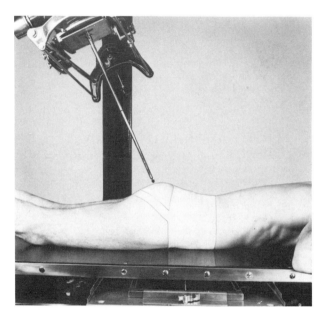

Prostate gland

Prostatography is a term applied to radiologic investigation of the prostate gland by either plain film studies or by cystographic or vesiculographic procedures.

The normal prostate is not radiographically demonstrable. Plain film studies are made for the detection of calcareous deposits and, as shown by urinary retention, of prostatic enlargement. Other known or suspected abnormalities of the gland are investigated by cystourethrographic or vesiculographic procedures. Sugiura and Hasegawa[1] reported a method of contrast prostatography wherein a water-soluble contrast medium is injected directly into the prostate by way of the rectal wall. These authors describe the technique in detail in their paper.

The preparation of the patient for plain film studies usually consists of evacuating the lower bowel with a cleansing enema and requesting the patient to empty his bladder immediately before the examination.

The supine position may be employed, with the central ray directed to a point about 1 inch above the pubic symphysis at a caudal angulation of 15 degrees. The prone position is preferable because it places the prostate closer to the film and the sacrococcygeal vertebrae farther from the film, where their shadows can be projected above the region of the prostate.

With the patient in the prone position, the median sagittal plane of the body is centered to the midline of the table. An 8″ × 10″ or 10″ × 12″ film is placed lengthwise in the grid tray and is centered approximately 2 inches above the pubic symphysis. The central ray is directed through the region of the anus at an angle of 20 to 25 degrees toward the head in order to project the shadow of the prostate above that of the pubic arch.

[1]Sugiura, H., and Hasegawa, S.: Clinical evaluation of transrectal prostatography, Amer. J. Roentgen. 111:157-164, 1971.

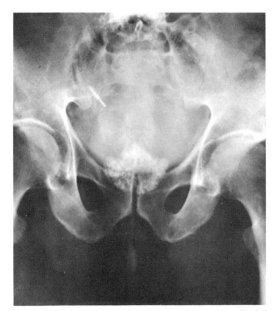

Plain film study showing prostatic enlargement with extensive glandular calcification.

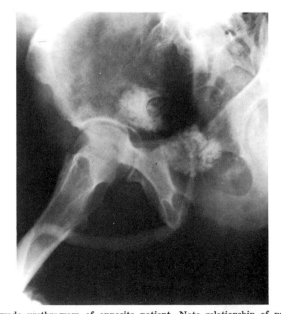

Retrograde urethrogram of opposite patient. Note relationship of proximal urethra to prostate gland.

Radiographs and diagnostic information courtesy Dr. Oswald S. Lowsley.

Anatomy and positioning of the breast

Breast

Revised and expanded by
Barbara M. Curcio, R.T.
Associate Professor of Radiologic Technology
College of Health and Allied Health Professions
University of Oklahoma Health Sciences Center, Oklahoma City

ANATOMY OF THE BREAST

The breasts, or mammae, are lobulated, glandular structures situated, one on each side, within the superficial fascia of the anterolateral surface of the thorax of both males and females. In the male, the breasts are rudimentary and functionless. The male breast is subject to neoplasms and other conditions that require radiologic investigation although such conditions in the male are not common. In the female, the breasts function as accessory glands of the reproductive system, their purpose being to secrete milk for the nourishment of the newborn infant.

The female breast is usually hemispherical in shape, its size varying considerably in different individuals, at different age periods, with the menstrual cycle, and with lactation. The posterior surface of the mammary gland overlies the pectoralis major and serratus anterior muscles, and its base normally extends from the second or third rib downward to the sixth or seventh rib, and from near the lateral margin of the sternum outward to the anterior axillary plane. Projecting from the upper lateral side of its base, the gland presents a large process that extends into the axillary fossa and is known as the axillary prolongation, or axillary "tail," of the breast. This is shown in the left drawing below and, extending upward from the body of the gland with its milk ducts filled, in the dual-contrast radiographic study on page 812. The breast tapers forward from its base and ends in a papilla, or nipple, where its ducts open. The nipple is surrounded by a circular area of pigmented skin called the areola. The breasts are supported in position by suspensory ligaments attached to the skin.

The adult female breast consists of 15 to 20 lobes, each of which comprises numerous lobules. The lobules are composed of dense glandular tissue and are held together by connective tissue and blood vessels and by lactiferous ductules, which unite to form a main duct leading from the lobe to the nipple. The lobes are covered and are loosely connected together by fibrous tissue, and the intervals between the lobes are occupied by fatty tissue. A layer of fatty tissue, the thickness of which determines the size of the breast, envelopes the gland except in the area immediately under the nipple and the areola.

The lymphatic vessels of the mammary glands are drained by the axillary lymph nodes. A variable number of large lymph nodes (12 to 30 or more) are situated in the axilla. This region may be radiographed during examinations of the breasts.

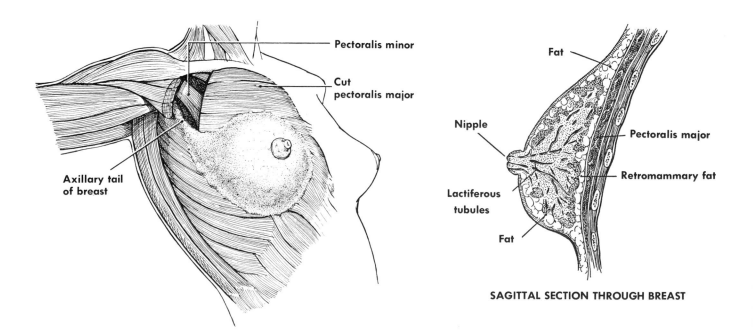

SAGITTAL SECTION THROUGH BREAST

Tissue variations

Because of the similarity in the physical density and radiation absorption characteristics of the firm glandular and connective tissues constituting the mammary gland, the intrastructural contrast required for satisfactory tissue differentiation depends in large measure upon the amount of fatty, comparatively radioparent tissue occupying the perimammary and interlobar spaces.

Because of immature development of the glandular elements, the young breast is composed largely of connective tissue, and it usually has only a small amount of fat, with the result that it casts a homogeneous radiographic shadow that shows little or no tissue differentiation. The immature breast is normally pyramidal in shape, and the tissues are firm to the touch. Due to the combination of scant fatty tissue in the retromammary space and the firm tone of the suspensory ligaments, the breast is held in close contact with the chest wall. This, coupled with the convexity of the thoracic cage, makes it difficult, if not impossible, to project all of the young breast onto the film. I found that a central ray angulation of 5 degrees toward the chest wall usually projects all of the small, firm breast onto the film. This type of breast, usually referred to as the adolescent breast, requires a comparatively heavy exposure for optimal penetration of the compact tissues; the exposure should be two to three times heavier than that required for a mature, normally fatty breast of equal tissue thickness. The large, pyramid-shaped breast presents acute changes in thickness from apex to base, which may necessitate two exposures for satisfactory visualization of both the basilar and the apical portions.

The average mature breast of the patient who is 30 to 45 years of age varies in shape from hemispherical to conical; the tissues are soft to the touch, and there is usually enough fatty infiltration to afford excellent intrastructural detail. After menopause the glandular elements undergo gradual senile atrophy, the tone of the suspensory tissues deteriorates so that the breast becomes pendulous, and unless considerable fatty tissue is present, it becomes wrinkled and flabby.

External factors can also profoundly affect breast density. Major external factors are artificial menopause as a result of oopherectomy and/or hysterectomy and the ingestion of hormones, particularly anovulatory (birth control) drugs. In each of these situations normal involution of glandular components is interrupted or altered, and the expected age- and parity-related variations of tissue density cannot be relied on. Anovulatory drugs almost always produce engorgement of glandular elements of the breast similar to that found in pregnancy, and the breasts exhibit the marked increase in density associated with that state. Similarly, artificial menopause may retard or arrest the expected involutional process of breast tissue components. In these patients, despite advancing age, the breast may retain the admixture of glandular elements, connective tissue, and fat that was present at the time of surgical menopause.

In approaching breast radiography, the student must keep in mind that the most important factor in adjusting the exposure technique to the individual patient is an accurate evaluation of the firmness, that is, of the radiation-absorption characteristics, of the tissues composing the breast. Age and parity serve to classify the breast as having immature or mature development or senile atrophy of the glandular elements. Proficiency in judging the many anatomic and physiologic variations within each classification of breasts depends on an understanding of the relationship of age and parity to breast density, the normal involutional cycle of the breast, and the effect of various external factors on the normal cycle. Critical observation and an acute sense of touch, developed through careful training and experience, also aid in the selection of optimal exposure factors.

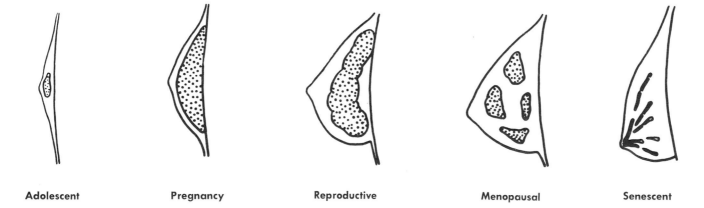

| Adolescent | Pregnancy | Reproductive | Menopausal | Senescent |

Diagrammatic profile drawings of the mammary gland illustrating the most likely variation and distribution of radiographic density related to normal life cycle from adolescence to senescence. Density is represented by the shaded areas. This normal sequence may be altered by external factors described in the text.

811

MAMMOGRAPHY

Radiologic examinations of the mammary glands and ducts are denoted by the terms *mammography* (L. *mamma*, breast) and *mastography* (Gr. *mastos*, breast). The breasts are examined with the use of a specialized soft-tissue technique, and when indicated, individual milk ducts are investigated by means of filling the lumina with a water-soluble, iodinated contrast medium.

Soft tissue radiography of the breasts was described by Salomon[1] in 1913, but for many years it was a seldom-used method of diagnosing breast lesions. This was because the exposure techniques, not being specialized to the delineation of the delicate breast structures, failed to provide reliable diagnostic information. Therefore, the breasts were examined with the use of subcutaneously injected gas and/or by filling the ducts with an iodinated oil. Because of the unpleasant side effects of these contrast agents, they are no longer employed. The two examples of these early techniques (shown below) are retained for historical interest and further illustration of the anatomy of the breast.

Present-day breast radiology is the result of intensive research by many investigators into (1) the development of exposure techniques that can be relied upon to produce diagnostically acceptable films, (2) the study of the radiographic appearance of normal breast tissues and the study of the changes characterizing different pathologic lesions, and (3) the establishment of criteria whereby early cancers and even precancerous signs can be recognized. The history of this radiologic specialty has been excellently outlined by Gershon-Cohen.[2]

Mammography is now widely used in the investigation of breast symptoms to detect the nature and extent of the condition that is causing the symptoms, to differentiate between benign and malignant neoplasms, and, accordingly, to determine the course of treatment. Gershon-

Cohen and Berger[3] stated that early diagnosis is the most important function of breast radiography—that once a cancer has reached the palpable stage, the chances of cure are seriously diminished.

Since mammography can identify tiny malignant lesions in the breast before they are palpable, it contributes significantly to a reduction in the mortality statistics of breast cancer. Strax and associates[4] report a one-third reduction in the mortality rate due to breast cancer in a mass screening program covering a period of ten years. Their work supports an earlier study by Gershon-Cohen and associates[5] in which 1,300 asymptomatic women received biennial mammography examinations to detect early unsuspected cancer. The technique is now widely used for the evaluation of symptomatic breasts as well as a screening device for early detection of malignancy in asymptomatic breasts.[6]

Exposure techniques

The detection of an abnormal condition always depends on clear delineation of the tissues constituting the part, and no region requires a more highly specialized exposure technique for such delineation than does the breast.

Although most mammography is performed with suitably modified conventional equipment, in late 1960 and early 1970 specialized mammography units and tubes, which collectively are termed *mammography systems*, were developed to overcome some of the basic problems in technique that have plagued mammography from its genesis as a diagnostic procedure. These problems relate to the great variability in size and density of the breast and the need to provide a diagnostic image of maximum contrast and detail. Exposure techniques, positioning,

[1]Salomon, A: Beiträge zur Pathologie und Klinik der Mammakarzinome, Arch. Klin. Chir. **101**:573-668, 1913.

[2]Gershon-Cohen, J.: Breast roentgenology, Amer. J. Roentgen. **86**:879-883, 1961.

[3]Gershon-Cohen, J., and Berger, S. M.: Mastography, Radiol. Clin. N. Amer. 1:115-143, 1963.

[4]Strax, P., Venet, L., and Shapiro, S.: Value of mammography in reduction of mortality from breast cancer in mass screening, Amer. J. Roentgen. **117**:686-689, 1973.

[5]Gershon-Cohen, J., Ingleby, H., and others: Mammographic screening for breast cancer: results of a ten-year survey, Radiology 88:663-667, 1967.

[6]Demonstration Projects for Early Detection of Breast Cancer in Major Institutions in the United States, initiated 1973 and jointly sponsored by the National Cancer Institute and the American Cancer Society, Bethesda, Md. 20014.

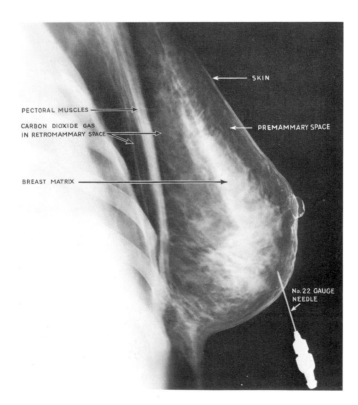

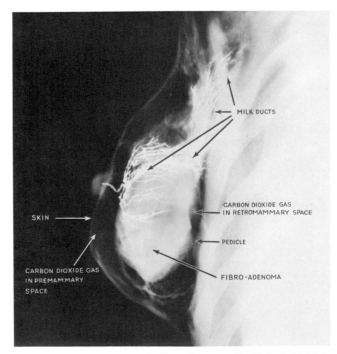

Radiographs courtesy Dr. N. Frederick Hicken.

and the special features of these systems, are described later in this discussion. The exposure factors and techniques utilized with conventional radiographic equipment will be considered first.

Radiologists tested many soft tissue techniques before the establishment of the several now in general use. Gershon-Cohen[1,2] advocates the use of a no-screen medical film with which the milliampere-second factor is varied from 100 to 400, according to the tissue composition and thickness of the breast. Egan[3,4] advocates the use of the Kodak M industrial film. The emulsion of this film is finely grained, and it has a long scale of gray tones, both highly desirable characteristics; however, it has low radiation sensitivity, so that an exposure of 1,800 milliampere-seconds is required for each projection. Many radiologists are using a faster industrial film that produces excellent results with an average exposure of 600 milliampere-seconds.[5]

Direct exposure film is generally used. Both medical nonscreen film and a wide range of industrial films of varying sensitivity, which can be manually or automatically processed, are available for mammography. A vacuum-sealed screen and film combination, specifically designed for mammography, is also available.[6] Although the use of intensifying screens in mammography has previously resulted in a lack of detail and a prohibitive hazard of screen artifacts, the vacuum-sealed method is reported to eliminate these problems while significantly reducing exposure to the patient.[7]

With conventional equipment, all these techniques require that the x-ray transformer deliver energies in the 20- to 36-kilovolt range at a specified current setting. It is also necessary to reduce the added filtration to no more than 0.5 mm. of aluminum over that which is inherent in the tube. This amount of added filtration is considered adequate for the low energies employed in mammography. The focal spot utilized should be as small as possible consistent with the current employed.

In the techniques in which a short focal-film distance is used, accurate centering of the beam of radiation necessitates the use of special mammography cones. These have one flat side with a semielliptical cutout at the distal end so that they may be adjusted over the breast in close approximation to the chest wall; this side of the cone is lined with lead for the protection of the adjacent intrathoracic structures. Mammography cones are available in several lengths and in sizes suitable for use with small, average, and large breasts. A 4″ × 12″ extension cone is advocated by Egan for use in techniques in which a longer focal-film distance is used.

A foundation exposure technique is developed for the average patient in each of the three main types of female breast (immature, mature, atrophic) and for the male breast. The variable factor or factors of the technique (kilovoltage, milliamperage, distance, or combination thereof) are then adjusted as required for individual patients in each classification. The technologist must be familiar with the preferred technique of the examining radiologist and should keep in mind the basic considerations that apply to the selection of technical factors in any of the imaging methods in mammography.

The quality of the radiation produced by the x-ray tube in use and the quantity of the resultant radiation necessary to obtain optimal penetration of the part are prime considerations. Radiation exposure to the patient per film is a critical factor if mammography is to be employed for

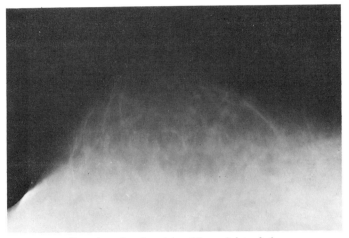

Dense immature breast (age 16 years), lateral view.

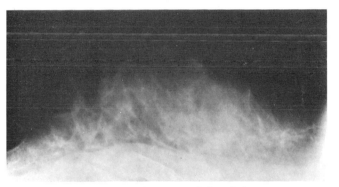

Mature breast (age 34 years), lateral view.

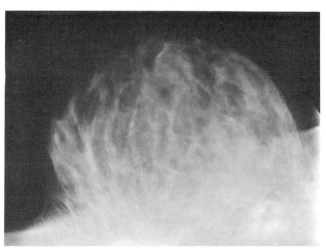

Breast in premenopause stage (age 45 years), lateral view.

Radiographs courtesy Dr. J. Gershon-Cohen.

[1]Gershon-Cohen, J.: Breast roentgenology, Amer. J. Roentgen. 86:879-883, 1961.
[2]Gershon-Cohen, J.: Mammography; some remarks on techniques, Radiol. Clin. N. Amer. 3:389-401, 1965.
[3]Egan, R. L.: Experience with mammography in a tumor institution, Radiology 75:894-900, 1960.
[4]Egan, R. L.: The technical aspects of mammography, Med. Radiogr. Photogr. 42:2-5, 1966.
[5]Siler, W. M., Snyder, R. E., Garrett, R., McLaughlin, J. S., and Sherman, R. S.: The development and use of mammographic technique, Amer. J. Roentgen. 91:910-918, 1964.
[6]Lo-dose Mammography System, E. I. DuPont de Nemours & Co., Wilmington, Del.
[7]Ostrum, B. J., Becker, W., and Isard, H. J.: Low-dose mammography, Radiology 109:323-326, 1973.

MAMMOGRAPHY—cont'd
Exposure technique—cont'd

regular, interval checkups, rather than for a single examination.[1-3] Low kilovoltage is essential, and the kilovolt range most compatible with the film utilized should be employed. No-screen medical film provides optimum contrast at 25 to 30 kilovolts, but finer-grain industrial emulsions respond best to the 30- to 36-kilovolt range. The length of exposure should be as brief as possible to eliminate the possibility of patient motion. Finally, all the legitimate variables of equipment and films must be explored and weighed, always keeping in mind that the prime objective is to obtain maximum diagnostic information with the lowest possible radiation exposure, and the least amount of discomfort, to the patient.

[1]Gilbertson, J. D., Randall, M. G., and Fingerhut, A. G.: Evaluation of roentgen exposure in mammography. Part I. Six views, Radiology 95:383-394, 1970.
[2]Gurley, L., and Harwood, S.: A practical technique for baseline mammography, Radiol. Techn. 44:138-145, 1972.
[3]Ostrum, B. J., Becker, W., and Isard, H. J.: Low-dose mammography, Radiology 109:323-326, 1973.

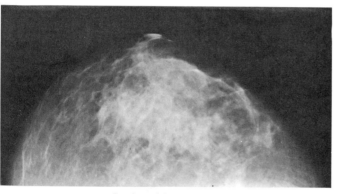

Craniocaudal projection.

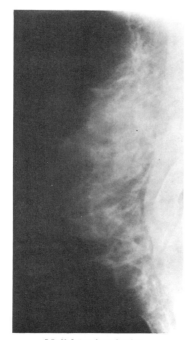

Mediolateral projection.
Radiographs courtesy Dr. J. Gershon-Cohen.

Examination procedures

The patient is clothed in an open-front gown. The breast must be bared for the examination because the low kilovoltages employed in these techniques would record the slightest wrinkle in any cloth covering.

During his physical examination of the breasts, the radiologist may attach a small lead shot over any palpable mass or area of suspicion with a tab of radioparent tape or an adhesive substance such as Elmer's glue. The lead marker identifies the area on the resultant radiographs, and it also aids the technologist in taking localized studies and/or supplemental views to delineate the area or areas to better advantage. The physician may attach a line of lead pellets along old scars to aid in his evaluation of the resultant underlying structural distortions. After each position adjustment and with care not to alter the placement of the pellet, the technologist should, if necessary, carefully ease any tabs to release puckering of the skin that may have occurred in changing the position of the breast.

The breasts, both male and female, are routinely examined in right-angle positions, craniocaudal and mediolateral. It is essential that all the glandular elements be visualized, in both planes if possible. When a large breast is examined, it is necessary to take additional projections that are centered to the upper, outer portion of the breast. A simultaneous bilateral, craniocaudal projection of the medial aspect of the breasts is obtained by centering the film and central ray midway between the breasts. Both breasts are examined for comparison, and a study of each axilla may be made for the detection of metastatic involvement of the axillary lymph nodes.

In addition to the basic right-angle views, localized studies are made of tumor-bearing portions of the breast or those suspected of such, with the area of interest in close contact with the film. This may require no more than a reversal of the right-angle projections—that is, a lateromedial projection for lesions located in a medial quadrant, and a caudocranial projection for lesions located in an upper quadrant of the breast. For the latter projection, the cone is directed upward; its orifice is covered with radioparent plastic wrap, which when held tautly in place with elastic bands, serves to support the breast in position.

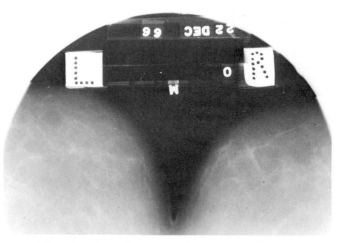

Bilateral craniocaudal projection of medial aspect of breasts.
Courtesy Dr. Ruth E. Snyder.

For tangential projections of tumor-bearing areas, the breast is adjusted so that the lesion is placed as nearly at right angles to the film as possible. The central ray is then directed at right angles to the lesion. These views, of necessity, are varied to meet the requirements of the individual patient.

Localized studies of tumor-bearing or suspected portions of the breast may also be made with a spot cone and compression technique. Spot-coning of suspected lesions has long been recommended by both Gershon-Cohen and Egan as a means for more accurate delineation of such areas. With conventional equipment, spot films are usually made with a cone of the smallest diameter possible. To provide compression during spot-coning, Styrofoam, Lucite, or other suitable radioparent material may be placed on the breast and in contact with the distal end of the cone. The cone is then gently pressed against the compressing material to reduce tissue thickness. This technique displaces superimposed glandular and fibrous tissue from the area under study, affording better evaluation of a suspected lesion.[1] Some physicians find it preferable to have a faint outline of the entire breast projected on the same film as the spot view of suspected pathology. This may be accomplished by first making a short "flash exposure" of the entire breast contour. Without changing the position of the breast, the small-diameter extension

[1]Minagi, H., Tennant, J. C., and Youker, J. E.: Coning and breast compression: an aid in mammographic diagnosis, Radiology 91:379-381, 1968.

cone is then positioned over the area of suspicion, the compression applied, and the spot film made.[2] Special mammographic units designed to provide maximal, uniform compression of the entire breast are described on pages 820 to 823.

Milk ducts. An opaque medium is utilized in the investigation of otherwise undemonstrable exudative lesions of the lactiferous ducts. An organic, water-soluble, iodinated medium is employed for this purpose.[3,4] The few items that are needed for the injection are a sterile hypodermic syringe fitted with a 30-gauge needle having a specially prepared smooth, round tip; a skin-cleansing agent such as 70% alcohol; a jar of sterile gauze squares or cotton balls; a waste basin; and a 1 ml. ampule of the specified contrast agent.

After cleansing the nipple and identifying the discharging duct, the radiologist inserts the round-tipped needle into the orifice of the duct for the injection of the contrast solution. In order to prevent unnecessary discomfort and possible extravasation, he terminates the injection as soon as the patient experiences a sense of fullness, a maximum of 1 ml. of the medium being employed. Immediate contrast studies are made in the craniocaudal and lateral directions. The exposure factors are the same as those used for the initial soft tissue films. Absorption of the contrast medium is verified with a follow-up study, usually after an interval of approximately thirty minutes.

Stevens[2] advocates a modified sialography injection technique for contrast mammography of the lactiferous ducts. Suture material is inserted into the discharging duct, over which a specially flared catheter is then passed. Injection of the contrast material is made via the catheter.

[2]Stevens, G. M.: Variations and supplementary techniques in mammography, Oncology 23:120-125, 1969.
[3]Funderburk, W. W., Syphax, B., and Smith, C. W.: Contrast mammography in breast discharge, Surg. Gynec. Obstet. 119:276-280, 1964.
[4]Funderburk, W. W., Syphax, B., and Ruguero, W.: The value of contrast medium injection in locating lesions of the breast causing discharge, with particular reference to duct papillomas, J. Nat. Med. Ass. 56:127-132, 1964.

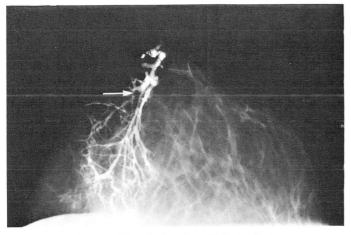

Craniocaudal projection of opacified milk ducts.

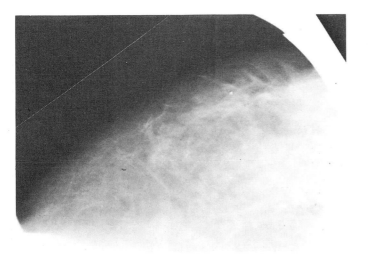

Localized craniocaudal projection of tumor.

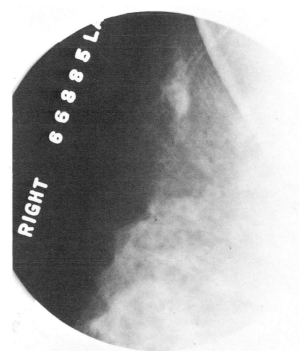

Localized mediolateral projection of tumor.

Radiographs and diagnostic information courtesy Dr. J. Gershon-Cohen.

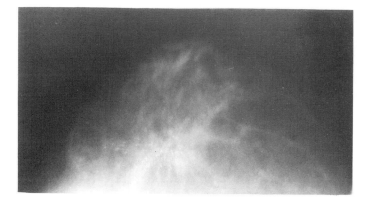

MAMMOGRAPHY—cont'd
Routine positions

For each of the basic right-angle projections, the breast must be firmly supported and adjusted so that the nipple is directed straight forward in an exact profile position. Firm support is utilized to compress the adjacent surface of the breast. This tends to spread the breast, so that the tissue thickness is equalized by distributing it more evenly over the film and so that better separation of the glandular elements is achieved. It also aids in profiling the nipple and in smoothing any wrinkling or puckering of the skin. Exact positioning of the breast must be performed consistently so that any lesion can be accurately localized in the respective quadrant of the gland and valid comparison can be made between periodic examinations.

The similarity in the contour of the breast in the craniocaudal and lateral projections makes it important that the identification marker be placed in an exact position. The identification marker should be placed along the upper border of the breast for lateral projections and along the lateral border of the breast for axial projections. The marker should be placed so that its face is up and it reads toward the axilla.

The special mammography cone is centered over the breast, with the flat side in contact with the chest just above the base of the breast. The focal-film distance varies according to the size of the breast. The extension cone is centered over the breast, and then the focal-film distance is adjusted so that the beam of radiation extends about ¾ inch beyond the periphery of the breast.

After the tissue thickness is measured, the cone is centered, and the exposure factors are adjusted. The position of the breast should be rechecked before the exposure is made.

Respiration is suspended for all exposures. It is also important that the patient be rested and calm in order to prevent acceleration of the heartbeat and thereby minimize motion resulting from pulsations.

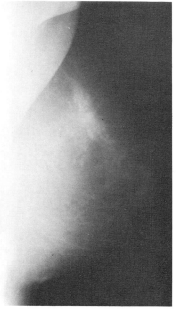

Typical infiltrating duct carcinoma with noncircumscribed tumor mass and calcifications.

Typical infiltrating duct carcinoma with noncircumscribed tumor mass and calcifications.

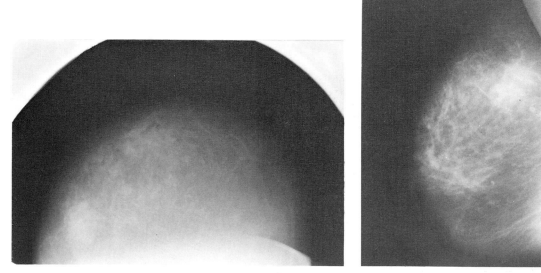

Noncircumscribed mass without calcifications but diagnostic for malignant tumor.

Radiographs and diagnostic information courtesy Dr. Ruth E. Snyder.

816

CRANIOCAUDAL PROJECTION

The positioning of the breast for this view is facilitated by the use of a height-adjustable mammography stand. Its film platform must be radiation-proof to protect the patient's gonads from the vertically directed beam of radiation.

The patient is placed in the erect position, either seated or standing, and the film platform is then adjusted to the approximate height required. About ¾ inch of the film should be curved over the edge of the platform so that it will fit snugly against the chest wall for the inclusion of as much of the base of the breast as possible. This requires the use of a flexible film holder.

With the film holder correctly placed, the breast is extended over it, and then the height of the platform is adjusted to support the breast as firmly as is consistent with comfort. The patient must sit or stand erect to prevent superimposition of the clavicular shadow. The patient is asked to grasp the stand and to keep the film platform pressed firmly against the body. Place the fingers of both hands transversely under the patient's breast, and with a gentle outward movement smooth out any wrinkling of the skin. Adjust the breast so that the nipple is placed in exact profile.

When an adjustable stand is not available, the patient may be seated at the end of the radiographic table. The gonads must be protected with a sheet of leaded rubber. The film is elevated to the correct height on wooden or foam-rubber blocks, which must be immobilized in position to prevent slipping. The breast is positioned as described above.

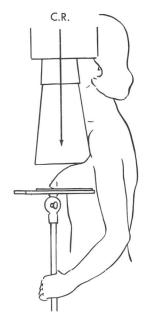

Positioning for routine craniocaudal projection.

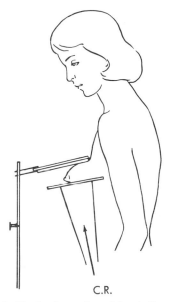

Positioning for caudocranial projection.

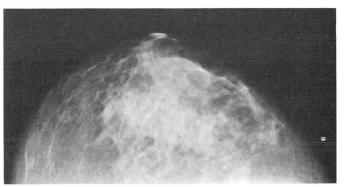

Routine craniocaudal projection.

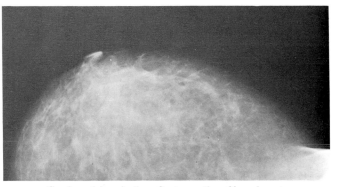

Craniocaudal projection of outer portion of large breast.

Radiographs courtesy Dr. J. Gershon-Cohen.

817

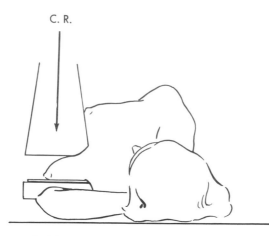

Positioning for routine mediolateral projection.

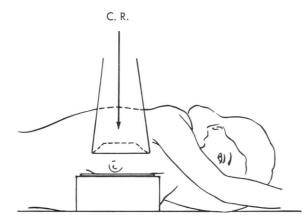

Positioning for lateromedial projection.

MAMMOGRAPHY—cont'd
Routine positions—cont'd
MEDIOLATERAL PROJECTION

The patient is placed in a semilateral position, on the side being examined. The arm is adjusted at right angles to the body.

Wooden or foam-rubber blocks or sandbags are used to elevate the film holder so that the breast is supported firmly. To ensure inclusion of all of the base of the breast, about 1 inch of the film is adjusted to project over the edge of the support so that it can curve in close contact with the chest wall. With the film placed correctly on the support, it is then placed well under the breast to include a portion of the rib cage.

The rotation of the patient's body is adjusted so that the nipple is placed in exact profile, and any wrinkling of the skin on the underside of the breast is then smoothed out. When the breasts are pendulous, the patient is asked to hold the opposite breast in a retracted position.

In the routine mediolateral projection shown below, note the small, spiculated density (arrow) representing a tumor. This is visualized to better advantage in the adjacent axillary "tail" projection and in the right-angle spot studies shown on the opposite page.

NOTE: A pendent lateral position of the breast, wherein the patient leans over a vertically placed film holder to allow the gland to gravitate well away from the chest wall for a cross-table projection, was described by Gershon-Cohen[1] in 1937 and more recently by others.[2,3]

[1]Gershon-Cohen, J.: Cradle for the roentgen x-ray of the female breast, Radiology **28**:234-236, 1937.
[2]Lasky, H. J.: A new mamographic technic, Radiology **91**:381-382, 1968.
[3]Jabczenski, M. A.: Pendent mammography: a new approach to an old technique, J. Canad. Ass. Radiol. **21**:43-45, 1970.

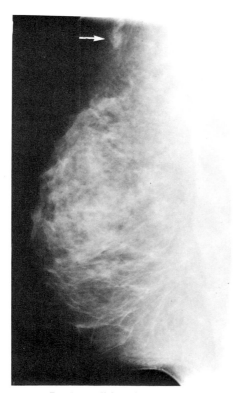

Routine mediolateral projection.

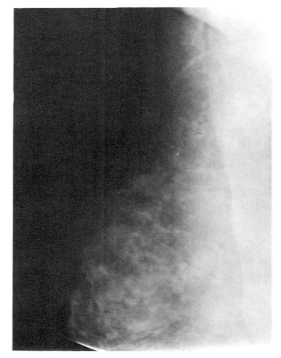

Mediolateral projection centered over axillary prolongation.

Radiographs and diagnostic information courtesy Dr. J. Gershon-Cohen.

818

AXILLARY PROJECTION

The axillary projection is used for the demonstration of the axillary prolongation, or "tail," of the breast as well as for the demonstration of the axillary lymph nodes.

From the supine position, the patient is turned 30 to 35 degrees toward the side being examined. The arm is adjusted at, or slightly above, the right-angle position, as preferred by the examining radiologist.

The film holder, usually 8″×10″, is placed lengthwise directly on the table and is centered about 2 inches distal to the apex of the axillary fossa. The breast is allowed to hang unsupported. Using a standard cone of the correct diameter, direct the central ray vertically to the midpoint of the film.

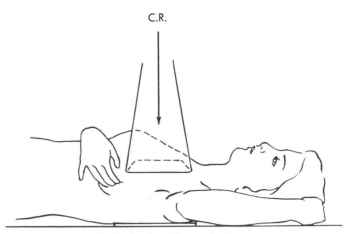

Positioning for axillary projection.

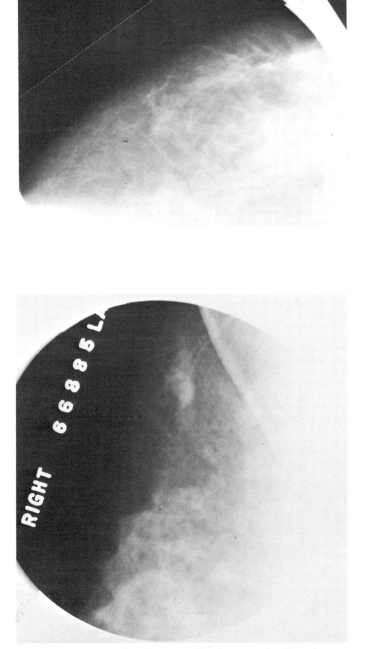

Craniocaudal and mediolateral spot studies of tumor of patient shown on opposite page.

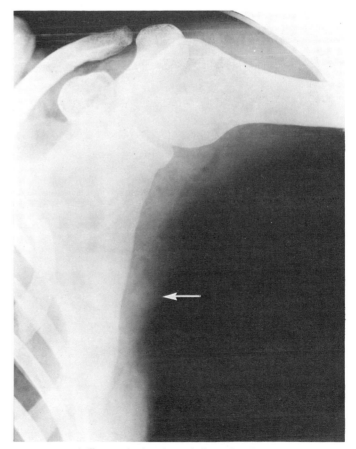

Axillary projection. Arrow indicates lymph node.

Radiographs and diagnostic information courtesy Dr. J. Gershon-Cohen.

819

SPECIALIZED MAMMOGRAPHY SYSTEMS

General features

Specialized mammography systems[1] were developed to overcome basic problems in mammography related to the variation in the size and density of the mammary gland and to meet the need for diagnostic imaging of maximum contrast and definition. These specialized units vary somewhat in the details of their structure and circuitry, but the rationale and objective of each is similar. Molybdenum target material is utilized to produce an x-ray beam of optimum energy and wavelength for visualizing breast structures. Compression systems are built into the units to improve detail and definition of breast structures by maximal, uniform compression of the breast. These units have been designed to be compact in size, and they provide for examining the patient in the seated position for all views of the breast. The prototype for these machines is generally considered to be the Senographe.

Although the diagnostic, technical, and radiobiologic ramifications of these specialized mammography systems are still under discussion and trial,[2,3] the equipment is utilized by many mammography experts. Gershon-Cohen and associates[4] report that the Senographe produces films of superior definition and detail.

[1]Senographe, CGR Medical Corp., Baltimore, Md.; Mammorex Breast X-ray System, Picker Corp., Cleveland, Ohio; MMX Mammographic X-Ray System, General Electric Corp., Milwaukee, Wisc.; Gemini Mammographic System, Litton Medical Systems, Des Plaines, Ill.

[2]Rini, J., Horowitz, A., Balter, S., and Watson, R.: A comparison of tungsten and molybdenum as target material for mammographic x-ray tubes, Radiology 106:657-661, 1973.

[3]Palmer, R. C., Egan, R. L., and others: Absorbed dose in mammography using three tungsten and three molybdenum target tubes, Radiology 101:697-699, 1971.

[4]Gershon-Cohen, J., Hermel, M. B., and Birsner, J. W.: Advances in mammographic technique, Amer. J. Roentgen. 108:424-427, 1970.

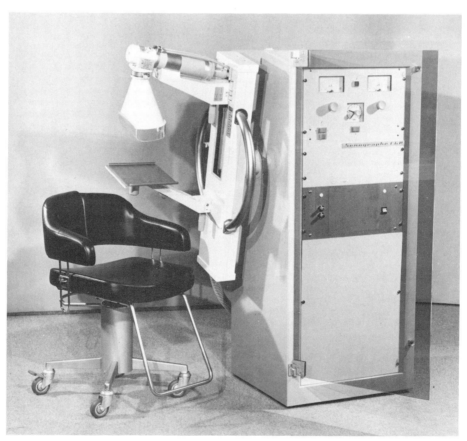

CGR Senographe.

Courtesy CGR Medical Corp., Baltimore, Md.

Molybdenum target tubes produce an x-ray beam with a longer wave-edge length of K-radiation, which is ideally suited for soft tissue radiography. The mammography systems also feature exceedingly fine focal spots, so that they produce maximum detail. The Senographe has a water-cooled, fixed molybdenum anode tube, with the target at the end, rather than in the middle of the tube. Mammography systems of conventional construction have rotating molybdenum anode tubes.

All these units provide the low kilovoltage range necessary for mammography. The Senographe, because of the unique construction of its tube, utilizes from 30 to 40 milliamperes. Other units provide from 250 to 400 milliamperes. The MMX Mammographic X-Ray System also provides a phototiming device. The average length of exposure varies with the thickness of the breast tissue and with the type of film employed. Since maximum compression is utilized, breast thickness is markedly reduced. Both industrial and nonscreen medical film may be used with these units. Manual processing is recommended, but it is not mandatory.

Flared mammography cones of various sizes are utilized in the mammographic systems. Cylinder spot cones are also available. In the Senographe compression material is attached to the distal end of the cones. In the other units compression is aided by an adjustable compression plate attached to the film-holding tray so that compression may be applied to both sides of the breast.

The specialized systems are extremely mobile, and they are designed to permit radiography of the patient in the seated position for all views of the breast and axilla. However, with the patient in the seated position the chest wall or retromammary space is not visualized in the lateral view. In the opinion of many physicians this is a serious drawback because it may lead to failure to identify a deeply seated tumor. These examiners state that visualization of the chest wall is required to assure complete visualization of all of the breast tissue. Others regard the increased convenience, speed, and smaller space required for these units to be important advantages, particularly when large numbers of patients are to be radiographed. Some examiners have the mediolateral view of the breast made in the conventional lateral recumbent position. By removing the film-holding assembly, the tube may be used over the radiographic table to accomplish this.

Although there are variations from unit to unit, the Senographe demonstrates the positioning technique that is required with most of the specialized mammography units.

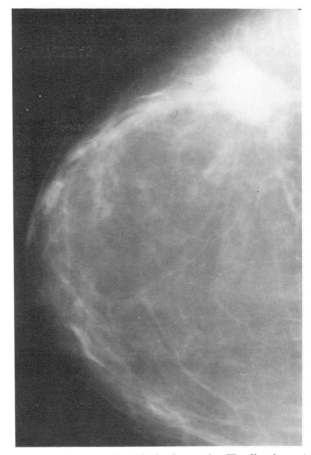

Craniocaudal projection made with the Senographe. The film demonstrates excellent contrast and detail. The fibrous infiltrative "tails" of the tumor are extremely well identified.

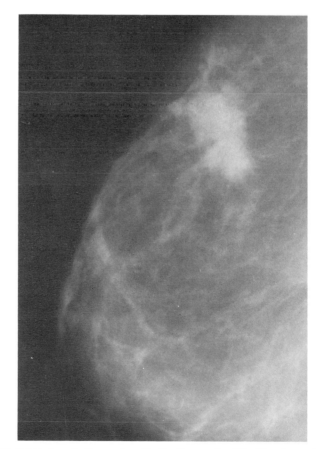

Mediolateral projection made with the Senographe. The film demonstrates excellent contrast and detail due to maximal compression and the quality of the x-ray beam produced with a molybdenum anode tube. Positioning in the erect position rarely makes possible the visualization of the chest wall or retromammary line. A large scirrhous carcinoma is present in the breast.

Above films (taken by Patricia Lewicki, R.T.) and diagnostic information courtesy Department of Radiology, University of Chicago Hospitals and Clinics.

SPECIALIZED MAMMOGRAPHY SYSTEMS—
cont'd

Positioning techniques

CRANIOCAUDAL PROJECTION

The patient is seated on an adjustable stool facing the film holder, which is adjusted at a height sufficient for the breast to lie comfortably on the film. The breast is placed on the film and centered with the nipple in profile. A contoured cone of the size required to completely cover the breast is selected and placed in the cone mounting bracket. The cone is brought down to just below the shoulder level,

the position of the breast is checked, and the patient is asked to grip the ring of the positioning assembly. After informing the patient that compression of the breast will be initiated, the technologist brings the cone into contact with the breast and slowly applies compression. As further compression is applied, the patient is asked to indicate when compression becomes uncomfortable. Compression is adequate when palpation of the patient's breast reveals tenseness of the breast tissue and firmness of the skin. When full compression is accomplished, the patient is instructed to suspend breathing, and the exposure is made.

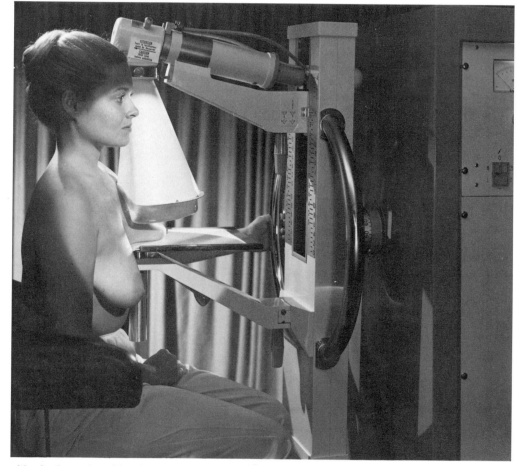

Patient in position for the craniocaudal projection utilizing a specialized mammography system.

Courtesy CGR Medical Corp., Baltimore, Md.

MEDIOLATERAL PROJECTION

The mediolateral position is one of the most difficult positions to execute with the patient in the seated position. The positioning assembly is rotated 90 degrees, with the cone on the medial side of the breast. A 30-degree wedged sponge may be used to support the film against the film holder on the lateral side of the breast. The patient should be obliqued slightly to bring the nipple into profile. The cone is brought into position covering the breast. After rechecking the patient's position to ascertain complete coverage of the breast including the axillary tail, compression is applied, and the degree of compression is checked by palpating the skin as described earlier.

LATEROMEDIAL PROJECTION

The lateromedial position is accomplished by rotating the positioning assembly 90 degrees, with the tube on the lateral side of the breast. The film holder should be at the sternal line between the two breasts. The breast is placed in close proximity to the film holder, and the height of the stool is adjusted to the degree necessary to cover the breast completely by the cone. If the breast is pendulous, it must be supported by the technologist while bringing the cone into contact, and enough pressure must be ap-

plied to support the breast in the desired position. The patient is requested to place the hand of the side under study on her head. The opposite hand is placed on the positioning ring. The patient is now rotated toward the film and the cone is brought in contact with the breast. The rotation should place the nipple in profile and bring the base of the breast into the field. Compression is again applied by bringing the cone into contact with the breast, and slowly increased until the breast tissue is firm to palpation.

Additional views may be taken of a tumor or specific area of interest with a cylinder localizer cone. Axillary projections are also possible with these units. Should it be necessary, the entire tube and film-holding assembly may be rotated to obtain a caudiocranial projection. This projection places the film at the superior aspect of the breast and the tube under its inferior aspect. It is also possible to do conventional lateral views with the patient positioned in the lateral recumbent position on the radiographic table. The film-holder assembly may be removed by moving it to the right or left. With the film supported by a sponge or block, full compression should be utilized, and the patient positioned in the conventional manner for the lateral view of the breast.

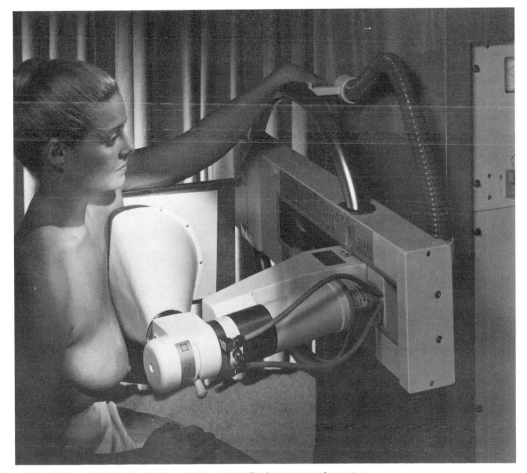

Patient in position for the mediolateral projection utilizing a specialized mammography system.

Courtesy CGR Medical Corp., Baltimore, Md.

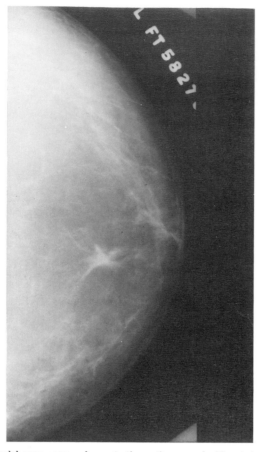

Craniocaudal mammogram demonstrating a tiny nonpalpable scirrhous carcinoma. Excision was guided by the localization drawing technique described in the text.

SUPPLEMENTAL PROCEDURES

Radiographic preoperative localization of nonpalpable tumors

When routine mammography identifies a nonpalpable tumor, the surgeon must rely solely on localization provided by the radiographs to determine the excision site for biopsy. It thus becomes the prime responsibility of the radiology team to provide accurate localization information. The method utilized must be precise and definitive, allowing the surgeon to remove a minimal amount of tissue from the suspected area for microscopy.

The method of preoperative localization described by Simon and associates[1] utilizes a minor surgical maneuver in which, under radiographic guidance, a 20-gauge needle is inserted into the breast and a mixture of 0.1 ml. of methiodized oil and an equal amount of Evans blue is injected at the site of the lesion. To verify the placement of the needle at the precise site of the lesion, additional radiographs and image intensification radioscopy may be necessary, and the needle may have to be repositioned before the injection. This method deposits the blue dye at the site of the tumor, which may then be identified by the surgeon during exploration of the breast at surgery.

A more widely used method of radiographic preoperative localization is that reported by Berger and associates.[2] This method provides the surgeon with an anatomic drawing of the breast showing the location of the tumor. The drawing is made from the original right-angle mammograms, and accuracy depends on precise mammographic technique.

[1]Simon, N., Lesnick, G. J., Lerer, W. N., and Bachman, A. L.: Roentgenographic localization of small lesions of the breast by the spot method, Surg. Gynec. Obstet. 134:572-574, 1972.

[2]Berger, S. M., Curcio, B., Gershon-Cohen, J., and Isard, H.: Mammographic localization of unsuspected breast cancer, Amer. J. Roentgen. 96:1046-1052, 1966.

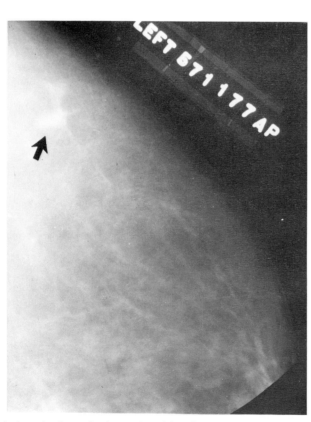

Spot view of a breast in the craniocaudal projection demonstrating a small tumor (arrow) that was nonpalpable and clinically asymptomatic. Excision and microscopy were aided by the localization technique described. A small carcinoma was found at biopsy.

Radiographs and diagnostic information courtesy Dr. J. Gershon-Cohen.

824

TECHNIQUE USED TO MAKE LOCALIZATION DRAWING

The two basic mammography views (lateral and craniocaudal) used in all breast radiography will suffice, provided that the breast and nipple have been profiled in each film. Also, the markers must clearly identify the axillary pole of the breast in each film, since this serves as a primary point of reference in transposition of the lesion site to the subsequent drawing. A base line is drawn from the nipple to the base of the breast on each radiograph. The suspicious area is circled on each film, including an additional perimeter of 0.5 cm. of breast tissue to allow for minute projection variations. With the use of a horizontally placed illuminator, the midnipple lines drawn on the films are aligned with the corresponding transverse and vertical midnipple lines of a standard anatomic diagram of the breast. The axillary poles of the breast identified on the film are kept in proper alignment with the drawing. Transposition of the tumor location from the films to the drawing is then made. The lateral film establishes the relative location of the lesion superiorly or inferiorly to the transverse midnipple line. The craniocaudal film identifies the medial or lateral relationship of the lesion to the vertical midnipple line. A final diagram is then prepared from this preliminary drawing. The final diagram should include precise measurements of the tumor from each midnipple line, one quadrant of the breast and the axilla should be clearly identified, and the approximate measurement indicated of the depth of the suspected lesion from the skin. The depth measurement is expressed as a minimum to maximum depth and may be obtained from the radiographs in each projection. It is also helpful to show the triangular wedge of breast tissue within which the tumor lies, as shown in the drawing on this page. A note must be included advising the surgeon of the necessity to position the patient for surgery so that the transverse and vertical midnipple lines of the breast simulate those shown in the drawing, that is, perpendicular to each other and bisecting at the nipple. Because of the pendant position of the breast in the supine position, this positioning maneuver is essential for maximum accuracy in using the drawing. Localization diagrams are virtually always successful,[1] provided that the original mammograms are made with the breast in true profile, the transposition is executed with care and precision, and the patient is positioned correctly for surgery.

[1]Curcio, B.: Technique for radiographic localization of non-palpable breast tumors, Radiol. Techn. **42**:155-160, 1970.

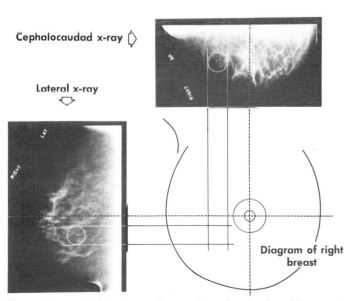

Transposition method for breast diagram shows line drawing of breast and adjacent radiographs in position for transposition.

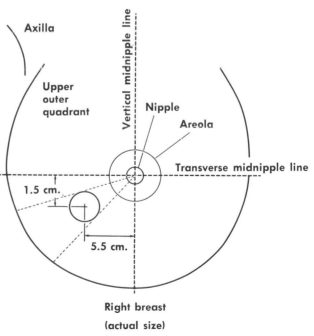

Final localization diagram. The heavily circled area within the lower outer quadrant identifies the site of a suspected malignancy.

Above illustrations and legends courtesy Dr. S. M. Berger.

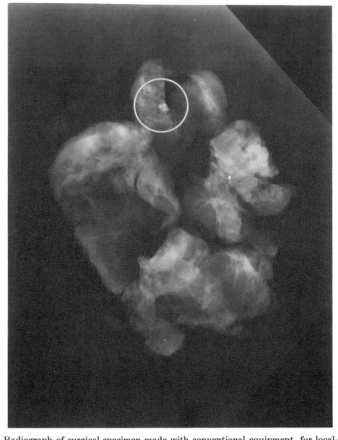

Radiograph of surgical specimen made with conventional equipment, for localization of area for microscopy in otherwise unremarkable tissue. Technical factors utilized were approximately 10% of those required for original mammogram. Permanent sections revealed tiny intraductal cancer.

Radiograph and diagnostic information courtesy Dr. S. M. Berger.

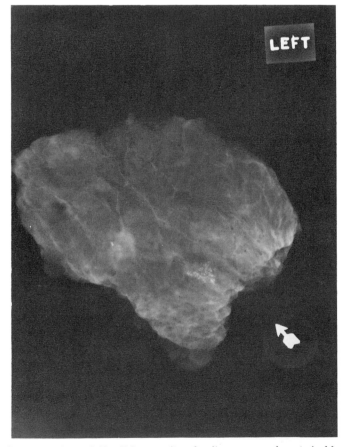

Specimen radiograph identifying two sites of malignancy, one characterized by punctate calcification (arrow). Guided microscopy confirmed two areas of malignancy as shown.

Radiograph and diagnostic information courtesy Dr. J. Gershon-Cohen.

SUPPLEMENTAL PROCEDURES—cont'd

Breast specimen radiography

Of equal importance with accurate preoperative localization of the site for excision is the need to provide immediate postoperative radiographs to confirm removal of the suspected lesion and to identify in the gross specimen the area for microscopy by the pathologist. This procedure is extremely important because tumors may be only millimeters in size or characterized merely by tissue irregularity or the presence of minute calcifications, and thus the removed tissue may be unremarkable to palpation and visual inspection by the pathologist.

If specimen radiography is to be done as an immediate postexcision procedure while the patient is kept under anesthesia, all due speed is imperative. Thus the details of film type, technical factors, and procedure of handling must be established beforehand. The cooperation of radiologist, technologist, surgeon, and pathologist is also a necessity.

Radiographic units specifically designed for gross and microscopic tissue sections are in use. Wallace[1] reports the use of such an instrument to identify calcification in breast tissue as an immediate postoperative procedure and as a survey technique in otherwise unremarkable breast tissue. Although special units have great utility in correlative mammographic and microscopy studies, acceptable specimen radiography may also be obtained with conventional equipment.[2]

When conventional equipment is used, technical factors vary between 10% and 25% of the original mammography technique, depending on the thickness of the biopsy specimen. Extremely fine grain films may be utilized, since exposure to the patient and longer exposure times, which would be prohibitive in terms of patient motion, are not factors.

[1]Wallace, T.: Radiographic identification of calcifications in breast specimens, Radiol. Techn. 40:211-215, 1969.

[2]Curcio, B.: Technique for radiographic localization of non-palpable breast tumors, Radiol. Techn. 42:155-160, 1970.

METHOD FOR POSTOPERATIVE
BREAST SPECIMEN RADIOGRAPHY

The removed tissue is brought directly from the operating room to the radiology department where the technologist has the radiographic equipment ready and the necessary ancillary supplies at hand. Since the patient remains under anesthesia, maximum speed is essential. The specimen is placed on a piece of waxed paper and positioned on the film. Surgical gloves should be worn, since some handling of the specimen is required to arrange it in as flat a position as possible before filming. This placement eliminates superimposition of structures and provides maximum stability of the tissue as it is moved from film to film via the waxed paper vehicle. An identifying marker is taped to the waxed paper and included in the exposure field of the subsequent radiographs. At least two films using different exposure techniques should be made, but for maximum speed, the first should be processed as the second is made. The specimen and marker are maintained unchanged in position and are moved from film to film on the waxed paper. After filming, the specimen is transferred (still on the waxed paper) to a piece of cardboard or other suitable firm support material and covered with wet gauze. The radiologist immediately inspects the film and advises the surgeon of the results of the excision. The specimen, on its cardboard support, and the radiograph are taken immediately to the pathology laboratory. Since the tissue and identifying marker have been maintained in the exact position in which they were filmed, the marker can be used as a reference point to identify the exact area in the gross specimen for immediate palpation, inspection, and frozen section microscopy. The procedure, if well planned and executed, need add only a few minutes to the total time required for the biopsy.

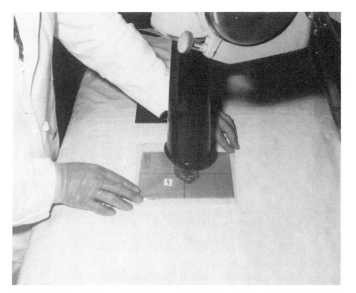

Breast tissue specimen positioned on waxed paper and suitably labeled for filming.

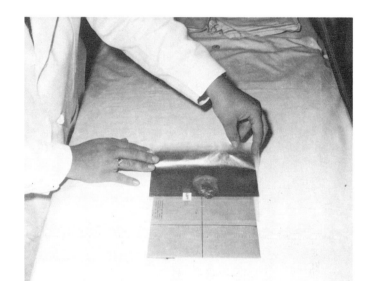

Transferral of breast tissue specimen to cardboard support via the waxed paper vehicle. This maneuver is done without changing the position of the tissue or marker.

827

Anatomy and positioning of the female reproductive system

Female reproductive system

The female reproductive system consists of an internal and an external group of organs, the two groups being connected by the vaginal canal. The anatomy of the external genitalia will not be considered since these structures do not require radiographic demonstration. The internal genital organs consist of the *gonads*, or *ovaries*, which are two glandular bodies homologous with the testes in the male, and of a system of canals made up of the *uterine tubes*, the *uterus*, and the *vagina*.

The ovaries are small, glandular organs with an internal secretion that controls the menstrual cycle and an external secretion containing the *ova*, or female reproductive cells. The ovaries are approximately almond-shaped and measure about 1 inch in width, ½ inch in thickness, and 1½ inches in length. The ovaries lie, one on each side, below and behind the uterine tube and near the lateral wall of the pelvis, being attached to the posterior surface of the broad ligament of the uterus by the mesovarium. The ovaries have no direct connection with

the uterine tubes: the ovum is extruded through the wall of the ovary into the pelvic cavity, whence it is wafted toward the tubal canal by the current set up in the peritoneal fluid by the cilia on the fringed end of the tube.

The ovary is composed of a core of vascular tissue, the medulla, by which it is attached to the mesovarium, and of an outer, or cortical, portion of glandular tissue. The cortex contains ovarian vesicles, or ovisacs, in all stages of development, and each vesicle contains one ovum. A fully developed ovisac is about ½ inch in diameter, and is referred to as a graafian follicle. As the minute ovum matures, the size of the follicle and its fluid content increase, so that the wall of the sac approaches the surface of the ovary and in time ruptures, liberating the ovum and the follicular fluid into the peritoneal cavity. The extrusion of an ovum by the rupture of a follicle is called ovulation, and the process occurs once during each menstrual cycle.

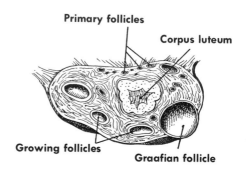

SECTION OF OVARY

The two *uterine tubes*, also called *fallopian tubes* and *oviducts*, serve to collect ova liberated by the ovaries and to convey the cells to the uterine cavity. Each tube is 3 to 5 inches in length. It arises from the superior angle, or cornu, of the uterus, passes lateralward through the upper margin of the broad ligament, forms an arch above the ovary, and opens into the peritoneal cavity. The tube is of small diameter at its uterine end, which opens into the cavity of the uterus by a minute orifice. It gradually broadens toward its ovarian extremity and terminates in a series of irregular, prolonged processes called the fimbriae. One of the fimbriae, termed the ovarian fimbria, is longer than the other processes and is attached either to or near the ovary.

The mucosal lining of the oviduct is ciliated and is arranged in folds that increase in number and complexity as they approach the fimbriated extremity of the tube. The cilia of the fimbriae draw the liberated ovum into the tube, which then conveys it to the uterine cavity by peristaltic movements. The passage of the ovum through the tube is believed to require several days, fertilization of the cell occurring in the outer part of the tube, whence it normally migrates to the uterus.

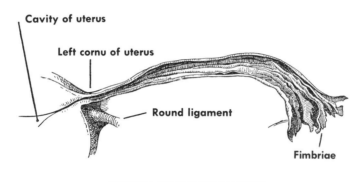

Cavity of uterus

Left cornu of uterus

Round ligament

Fimbriae

SECTION OF FALLOPIAN TUBE

The *uterus* is essentially a muscular organ. Its chief functions are to receive and retain the fertilized ovum until it develops into a mature fetus, and finally to expel the fetus during parturition.

The uterus consists of an upper, expanded portion called the *body*, and a lower, cylindrical portion called the *cervix* or *neck*. The organ is more or less pear-shaped, being somewhat flattened anteroposteriorly, and presents a *superior angle*, or *cornu*, on each side of the upper part of its body where the uterine tube enters. The rounded part of the body lying above the cornua is called the *fundus*. The nulliparous uterus is approximately 3 inches in length, almost one-half of which represents the length of the cervix. The body is about 1 inch in thickness and 2 inches in width between the cornua, its widest part. The cervix is approximately ¾ inch in diameter. During pregnancy the body of the uterus gradually expands into the abdominal cavity, reaching the epigastric region in the eighth month. Following parturition, the organ shrinks to almost its original size but presents characteristic changes in shape.

The uterus is situated in the central part of the pelvic cavity, lying behind and above the urinary bladder and in front of the rectal ampulla. Its long axis, which is slightly concave anteriorly, is directed downward and backward at a near right angle to the axis of the vaginal canal, into which the lower end of the cervix projects. The free, anterior surface of the organ rests on the urinary bladder, and its posterior surface is in apposition with the rectal ampulla and the sigmoid colon. The uterus is supported in position by ligaments attached to the surrounding structures and to the lateral walls of the pelvis, the most important of the supports being the broad and the round ligaments. The broad ligaments, one on each side, pass lateralward from the uterus to the pelvic wall and floor and thus divide the pelvic cavity into anterior and posterior compartments. The body of the uterus is freely movable, bending backward or forward on the less movable cervix when the urinary bladder or the rectum becomes distended.

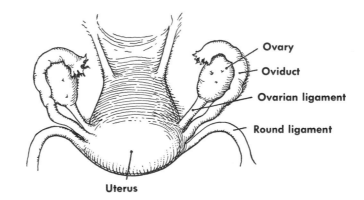

SUPEROPOSTERIOR VIEW OF UTERUS, OVARIES, AND OVIDUCTS

The cavity of the body of the uterus, the uterine cavity proper, is triangular in shape when viewed in a frontal plane. In the nongravid state, the anterior and posterior walls of the cavity are in contact, so that the space is more potential than real. The canal of the cervix is dilated in the center and constricted at each extremity; its upper orifice is called the internal os, and its lower orifice is called the external os. The latter orifice is bounded by two thick, prominent lips that are normally in contact with the posterior wall of the proximal end of the vaginal canal.

The mucosal lining of the uterine cavity is called the *endometrium*. It undergoes cyclic changes, called the menstrual cycle, at about four-week intervals from puberty to menopause. The endometrium is prepared during each premenstrual period for the implantation and nutrition of the fertilized ovum. If fertilization has not occurred, the menstrual flow of blood and of necrosed particles of uterine mucosa ensues. If fertilization has taken place, the premenstrual histologic changes continue, and the thickened endometrium is then called the *decidua*.

The *vagina* is a muscular canal lying posterior to the urinary bladder and the urethra and anterior to the rectum. Averaging about 3 inches in length, it extends downward and forward from the uterus to the vulva, where it opens to the exterior. The proximal portion of the vagina encircles the uterine cervix and is known as the vaginal fornix. The fornix is shallow anteriorly but gradually deepens to form a pouch, or cul-de-sac, posteriorly, where it is in close proximity to the peritoneal cavity. Pelvic endoscopy (culdoscopy) is performed by posterior fornix puncture, and peritoneal gas insufflation may be performed by this route. The space between the labia minora is known as the vaginal vestibule, and in it are situated the vaginal introitus, or orifice, and the urethral meatus.

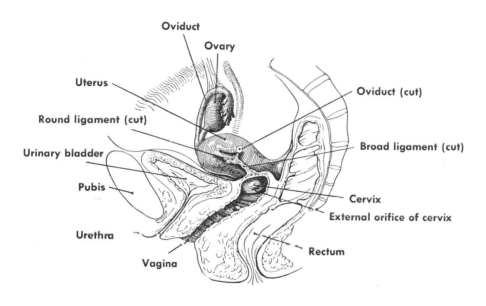

**SAGITTAL SECTION SHOWING RELATION OF
INTERNAL GENITALIA TO SURROUNDING STRUCTURES**

833

The fertilized ovum is passed from the oviduct into the uterine cavity, where it adheres to, and becomes embedded in, the decidua; this process is called *implantation*. During this period, which requires about two weeks, the growing ovum is chiefly concerned with the establishment of its nutritive and protective covering, the *chorion* and the *amnion*. The cells of the developing egg separate into an outer layer, from which the chorion is formed, and a central cell mass, from which the amnion and the embryo are formed. As the chorion develops, it forms (1) the outer layer of the protective membranes enclosing the embryo and (2) the embryonic portion of the placenta, by which the umbilical cord is attached to the uterus and through which food is supplied to, and waste is removed from, the fetus. The deep, or maternal, portion of the placenta is formed by the decidua underlying the growing ovum. The portion of the decidua covering the ovum and separating it from the cavity of the uterus is pushed before the growing embryo, eventually obliterating the uterine cavity by fusing with the decidua on the opposite wall. The amnion, also called the bag of waters, forms the inner layer of the fetal membranes and contains amniotic fluid in which the fetus floats. The decidua is expelled with the fetal membranes and the placenta at parturition; these structures constitute the afterbirth. A new endometrium is regenerated.

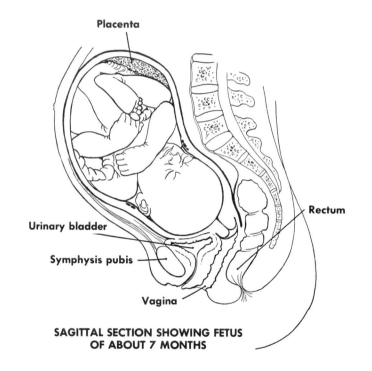

**SAGITTAL SECTION SHOWING FETUS
OF ABOUT 7 MONTHS**

After the preliminaries of the implantation have been completed, about three weeks after the fertilization of the ovum, the embryo begins to appear. The developing egg is referred to as an ovum during the process of implantation; as an embryo for the succeeding six weeks while the different organs are being formed; and as a fetus from the beginning of the third month, when it assumes a human appearance, until the birth of the baby.

The ovum usually becomes embedded near the fundic end of the uterine cavity, most frequently on the anterior or posterior wall. Implantation occasionally occurs so low, however, that the fully developed placenta encroaches upon or obstructs the cervical canal. This condition results in a premature separation of the placenta, which is termed *placenta previa*.

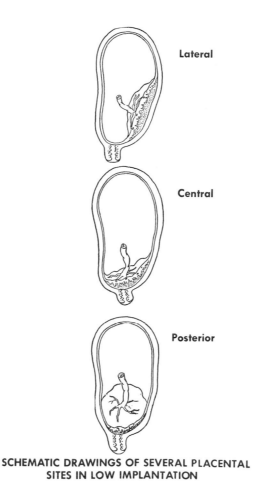

Lateral

Central

Posterior

SCHEMATIC DRAWINGS OF SEVERAL PLACENTAL
SITES IN LOW IMPLANTATION

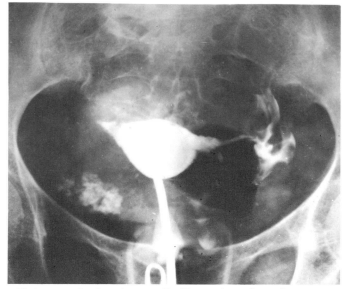

Hysterogram showing submucous fibroid occupying entire uterine cavity.
Radiograph and diagnostic information courtesy Dr. Richard H. Marshak.

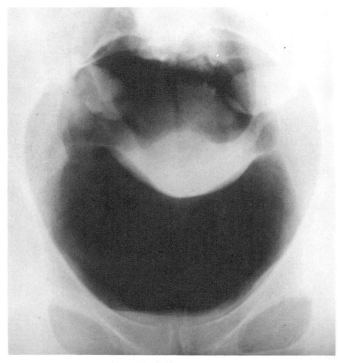

Normal pelvic pneumogram.
Radiograph and diagnostic information courtesy Dr. Emil Schulz.

NONGRAVID FEMALE PATIENT

Radiologic investigations of gynecologic abnormalities in nongravid females are denoted by the terms *hysterosalpingography*, *pelvic pneumography*, and *vaginography*. Each of these procedures requires the use of a contrast medium, and each is carried out under careful aseptic conditions.

Hysterosalpingography is employed to determine the size, shape, and position of the uterus and oviducts, to delineate such lesions as polyps, submucous tumor masses, and fistulous tracts, and to investigate the patency of the oviducts in cases of sterility. *Pelvic pneumography* is performed for the purpose of delineating the outer surfaces of the uterus and the adnexa uteri for the detection of abnormalities that alter the normal contour and/or position of these structures. *Vaginography* is performed in the investigation of congenital abnormalities, of vaginal fistulas, and of other pathologic conditions of the vagina.

CONTRAST MEDIA

Various opaque media are employed in examinations of the female genital passages. The iodinated organic preparations compounded for intravenous urography are widely used for both hysterosalpingography and vaginography. Some physicians prefer the iodinated oils for the former procedure, and a thin barium sulfate mixture is used for the demonstration of fistulous communications between the vagina and the intestine. Nitrous oxide and carbon dioxide are the gaseous agents most frequently used for peritoneal insufflation. The reasons for the use of these two gases are that they are nonirritating and they are more rapidly absorbed than other gases.

PREPARATION OF INTESTINAL TRACT

Preparation of the intestinal tract for any one of these examinations usually consists of the following: (1) administering a nongas-forming cathartic on the preceding evening if the bowel action is costive, (2) instructing the patient to take cleansing enemas until the return flow is clear an hour or so before reporting for the examination (this is followed up with further irrigation, as indicated by the preliminary film), and (3) withholding the preceding meal.

APPOINTMENT DATE AND CARE OF PATIENT

Gynecologic examinations are scheduled for the seventh or eighth day after the cessation of menstruation. This is the interval during which the endometrium is least congested, and more important, it is a few days before ovulation normally occurs, so that there is no danger of irradiating a recently fertilized ovum.

The relatively minor instrumentation required for the introduction of the contrast medium in these examinations does not normally necessitate either hospital admission or premedication. Some patients do experience unpleasant but transitory aftereffects, however, and the radiology department should have facilities for outpatients to rest in the recumbent position for an hour or so before returning home.

The patient is requested to empty her bladder completely immediately before the examination. This is to obviate pressure displacement of, and superimposition on, the pelvic genitalia. For all except those having pneumography by abdominal-wall puncture, a vaginal irrigation is administered just before the examination. At this time, the patient should be given the necessary supplies and instructed to cleanse the perineal region.

FILM QUALITY

The quality of positive-contrast studies should approximate that of films exposed for the bony parts of the region. Negative-contrast studies require an exposure reduction of approximately half of the milliampere-second factor required for the bony parts.

RADIATION PROTECTION

In order to deliver the least possible radiation to the gonads, the physician restricts radioscopy and/or filming to the minimum required for a satisfactory examination. Other important measures are adequate filtration of soft radiation, the use of low-dosage exposure techniques, and careful work to obviate the need for repeat exposures.

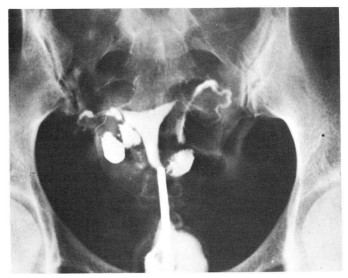

Hysterosalpingography revealed bilateral hydrosalpinx. Uterine cavity is normal.
Radiograph and diagnostic information courtesy Dr. Richard H. Marshak.

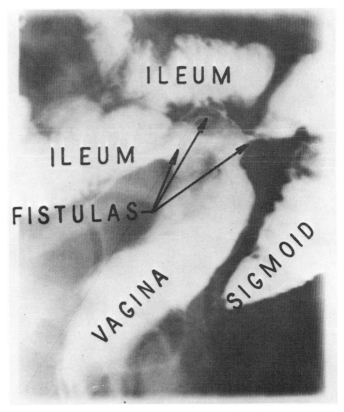

Vaginogram showing three enterovaginal fistulas.
Radiograph and diagnostic information courtesy Dr. Roger W. Lambie.

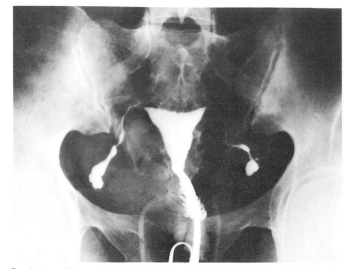

Cervical canal is seen to be dilated and serrated (chronic endocervicitis). Uterine cavity is normal. There is minimal bilateral hydrosalpinx.

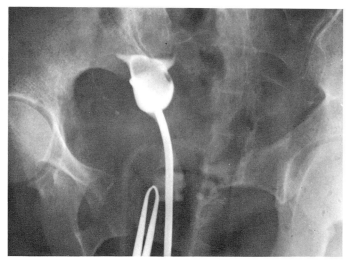

Hysterography revealed a submucous fibroid.

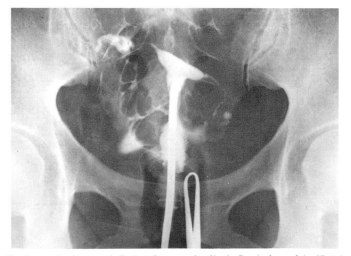

Uterine cavity is normal. Both tubes are visualized. Cervical canal is dilated and serrated.

Radiographs and diagnostic information courtesy Dr. Richard H. Marshak.

NONGRAVID FEMALE PATIENT—cont'd

Uterus and oviducts

Radiologic investigations of the nongravid uterus and the adnexa uteri may be divided into two main examination procedures: (1) *hysterosalpingography*, in which, by uterine cannulation, a radiopaque contrast medium is introduced for the delineation of the uterine cavity and the lumen of the tubal passages, and (2) *pelvic pneumography*, in which, usually by abdominal wall puncture, a gaseous medium is introduced into the peritoneal cavity for the delineation of the external contours of the uterus, the oviducts, and the ovaries.

The supine body position, which best delineates the uterine cavity and the lumen of the oviducts, is at variance with the prone Trendelenburg position, which is required for the delineation of the gas-enveloped outer contours of these structures and the ovaries. Because of this, hysterosalpingography and pelvic pneumography are combined in selected cases only. The gaseous medium is then injected first.

Hysterosalpingography

Hysterosalpingography is usually performed with the patient adjusted on a combination cystoscopic-radiographic table, and the examination is carried out by the attending gynecologist with the assistance of a nurse and a radiologic technologist. In many institutions and offices this procedure is carried out by the radiologist with image intensification equipment and may be recorded with spot films or with video tape.

Following irrigation of the vaginal canal, complete emptying of the bladder, and perineal cleansing, the patient is placed on the examining table and adjusted in the cystoscopic position, with her knees flexed over the leg rests. When the combination table is used, the patient's position must be adjusted so as to permit the films to be centered to a point 2 inches proximal to the pubic symphysis; 10″ × 12″ films are used for all studies, and are placed lengthwise.

Following inspection of the preliminary film, and with a vaginal speculum in position, the physician inserts a uterine cannula through the cervical canal, fits the attached rubber plug, or acorn, firmly against the external cervical os, applies counterpressure with a tenaculum to prevent reflux of the contrast medium, and then withdraws the speculum unless it is radioparent. Either an opaque or a gaseous medium may now be introduced via the cannula into the uterine cavity, from whence it will flow through patent fallopian tubes and "spill" into the peritoneal cavity. Patency of the oviducts can be determined by transuterine gas insufflation (Rubin's test), but the length, position, and course of the ducts can be demonstrated only by opacifying the lumina.

When an iodinated oil is used, it is warmed to body temperature so that it will flow more freely. This contrast medium is usually followed up with a twenty-four–hour study to detect the extent of delayed peritoneal spill. The free-flowing iodinated organic solutions are usually used at room temperature. These agents pass through patent oviducts quickly, and the resultant peritoneal spill is absorbed and eliminated by way of the urinary system, usually within two hours or less.

For Rubin's test, carbon dioxide is introduced under controlled pressure with a specially designed pressometer apparatus that registers the pressure and the volume of gas being injected. The tube of the device is attached to the uterine cannula with a Luer connector, and the gas pressure, as registered by the manometer, indicates full or partial patency or occlusion of the oviducts. When the passages are found to be patent, the physician may allow a sufficient volume of the gas to flow into the peritoneal cavity for dual-contrast studies. When this is done, the patient is turned to the prone position, and the head end of the table is lowered for the injection of the opaque medium and the filming procedure. More frequently, only an opaque medium is used.

The opaque medium may be injected with a pressometer or with a Luer syringe. Intrauterine pressure is maintained for the film studies by closing the cannular valve, thus protecting the physician's hands from radiation exposure. In order to prevent excessive peritoneal spillage, the opaque medium, in the absence of radioscopy, is introduced in two to four fractional doses, each of which is followed by a film study to determine whether the filling is adequate as shown by the peritoneal spill.

The filming may consist of no more than a single anteroposterior projection taken at the end of each fractional injection. Other views (oblique, axial, lateral, and angled projections) are taken as indicated by some abnormality not otherwise well shown.

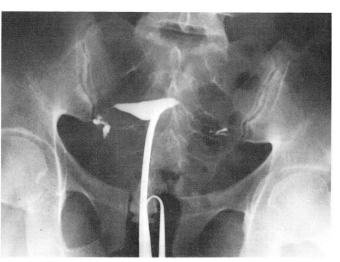

Hysterosalpingography reveals normal uterus and tubes.

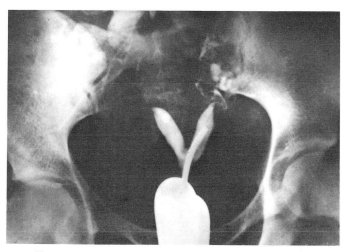

Hysterography reveals uterine cavity to be bicornuate in outline.

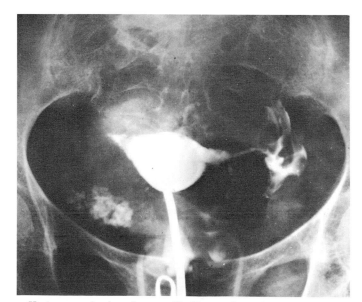

Hysterogram showing submucous fibroid occupying entire uterine cavity.
Radiographs and diagnostic information courtesy Dr. Richard H. Marshak.

839

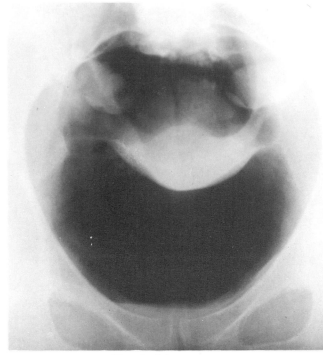

Normal pelvic pneumogram.

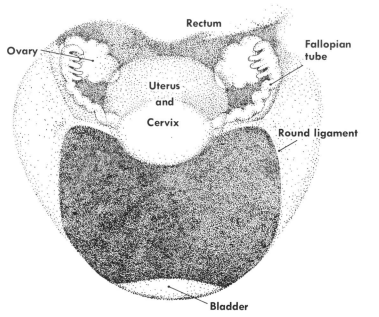

Drawing of above pneumogram.
Illustrations and diagnostic information courtesy Dr. Emil Schulz.

NONGRAVID FEMALE PATIENT—cont'd

Pelvic pneumography

Pelvic pneumography, gynecography, and *pangynecography* are terms used to denote radiologic examinations of the female pelvic organs by means of intraperitoneal gas insufflation. This procedure is used in the investigation of numerous gynecologic conditions, and it does not usually require hospital admission.

Pelvic pneumography is also used in conjunction with pelvic angiography[1] and with hysterosalpingography[2] in the investigation of gynecologic abnormalities.

PREPARATION OF EXAMINING ROOM

The examining room should be prepared in advance, and every item needed or likely to be needed should be at hand. An ample supply of 10" × 12" films, the size usually used for both the preliminary film and the contrast studies, should be conveniently placed, and several 14" × 17" films should be readily available in case they are needed.

Several types of apparatus suitable for introducing the gas are in use. One of the most convenient is a flowmeter attached to the tank of gas, which is usually nitrous oxide.

The following sterile items, including those used in the Schulz-Rosen procedure,[3] in which the gas is removed after the examination, are required for the injection: (1) hypodermic syringes and needles, (2) a selection of spinal puncture needles of the specified gauge and length, each fitted with a stylet, (3) a small hemostat, (4) medicine glasses, (5) sponges soaked in alcohol, (6) two fenestrated sheets or four towels and towel clips, (7) two sections of latex tubing, each about 2 feet in length, and a Y-shaped glass connector, (8) a one-way stopcock with syringe adaptor, and (9) surgical gloves. The nonsterile items consist of a vial of sterile local anesthetic solution, a small flask of sterile isotonic saline solution or sterile water, a waste basin, and a small prepared dressing.

[1]Rådberg, C., and Wickbom, I.: Pelvic angiography and pneumoperitoneum in the diagnosis of gynecologic lesions, Acta Radiol. [Diagn.] 6:133-144, 1967.

[2]Stern, W. Z., and Wilson, L.: Pelvic pneumography with simultaneous hysterosalpingography, Radiology 96:87-92, 1970.

[3]Schulz, Emil, and Rosen, S. W.: Gynecography: technique and interpretation, Amer. J. Roentgen. 86:866-878, 1961.

PRELIMINARY FILM

The patient is requested to empty her bladder completely just before being placed on the table for a scout film. This film is taken to check the bowel content, to determine whether further irrigation is necessary to cleanse the lower bowel, and to establish the desired film density for the contrast studies. The optimum film density for the gas studies is usually obtained by reducing the milliampere-second factor to half that required to delineate the bony structures of the region in the absence of pneumoperitoneum. The kilovoltage and focal-film distance factors are not changed.

The patient is adjusted in the prone position, and the shoulder support and footboard are adjusted to her height. Her feet may be secured to the footboard with a boot and strap arrangement or by broad adhesive straps applied as for leg traction to give her a greater sense of security when the table is acutely angled. The preliminary film is taken with the table angled to the full Trendelenburg (45-degree) position, and with the central ray directed to the region of the coccyx, either vertically or at a specified caudal angle.

Depending upon the time lapse between the initial voiding and the injection procedure, the patient may be returned to the lavatory to again empty her bladder immediately before the examination.

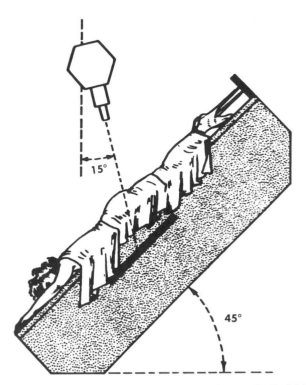

Courtesy Dr. Emil Schulz.

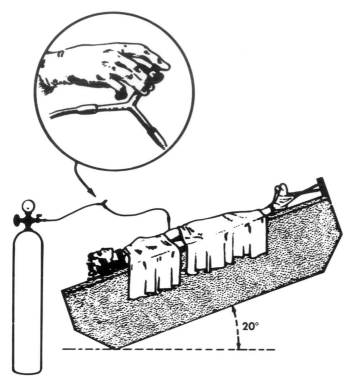

Positioning of patient during establishment of pneumoperitoneum (note glass connector valve arrangement).

NONGRAVID FEMALE PATIENT—cont'd
Pelvic pneumography—cont'd
EXAMINATION PROCEDURE

The patient is adjusted in the supine position for the injection procedure. After the skin has been cleansed and the abdomen has been draped, the radiologist infuses the tissues about the selected puncture site with a topical anesthetic solution. He then inserts a spinal puncture needle of the required length, advances it into the peritoneal cavity, and secures it in position with a hemostat. Schulz and Rosen[1] recommend that the head end of the table be lowered 20 to 25 degrees for the introduction of the gas. They state that this precaution prevents abdominal discomfort and shoulder pain resulting from subdiaphragmatic gas accumulation, and that the patient should experience nothing more than a sense of increasing abdominal fullness.

The two sections of latex tubing are connected by the glass Y tube, and one free end of the tubing is attached to the flowmeter of the gas tank and the other end to the stopcock. The physician then checks the system for leaks, flushes it with gas, presets the rate of flow, connects the stopcock to the puncture needle, and opens it to the gas line. When a scout film is required during the insufflation of the gas, a $14'' \times 17''$ film is used and the central ray is directed at right angles to the plane of the film.

When the desired volume of gas has been introduced, the stopcock is closed, the needle is removed, and a small prepared dressing is placed over the puncture site. The patient is then turned and adjusted in the prone position, and the table is angled to the full Trendelenburg position for filming. The gravitational effects of this angulation of the patient's body are that the intestinal loops move cranialward out of the pelvis, and that the gas then rises to fill the cavity and to envelope the uterus and adnexal organs.

[1]Schulz, E., and Rosen, S. W.: Gynecography: technique and interpretation, Amer. J. Roentgen. **86**:866-878, 1961.

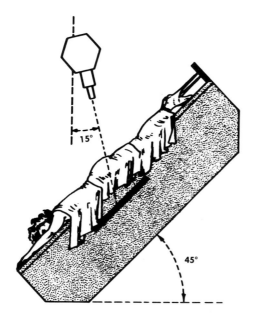

Positioning of patient and equipment during roentgenography.

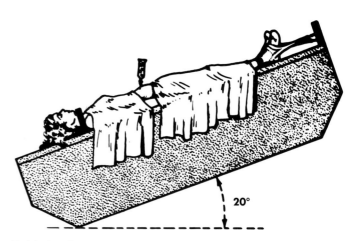

Positioning of patient during removal of gas from peritoneal cavity (note gas bubbling through fluid in syringe).

Drawings and legends courtesy Dr. Emil Schulz.

842

For all posteroanterior and oblique projections, the central ray is directed through the region of the coccyx to the midpoint of the film. The initial posteroanterior projection may be made with the central ray directed vertically or with a specified caudal angulation of the central ray, as directed by the radiologist. Schulz and Rosen[1] recommend a 15-degree caudal angulation of the central ray; this angulation added to the angulation of the patient's body, results in a 60-degree pelvic-inlet view. Stevens and associates[2] obtain a stereoscopic pair by having one film taken with a 10-degree caudal angulation of the central ray and a second film taken with a 20-degree caudal angulation.

With the table maintained in the Trendelenburg position, oblique studies are made with the patient rotated about 30 degrees from the prone position, and lateral studies are made by cross-table projection.

After satisfactory contrast studies are obtained, the peritoneal cavity may be deflated. For this procedure, the table angulation is reduced to the 20- to 25-degree, head-down position, and the patient is then turned to the supine position. Peritoneal puncture is repeated through the previously anesthetized site. A syringe loaded with 1 ml. of sterile saline solution or sterile water is attached to the needle and the plunger is withdrawn. When the escaping gas ceases to bubble through the liquid, the needle is removed and the puncture site is dressed.

While rest is usually not necessary, the patient may wish to rest in the recumbent position for an hour or so before returning home.

[1]Schulz, Emil, and Rosen, S. W.: Gynecography: technique and interpretation, Amer. J. Roentgen. **86**:866-878, 1961.
[2]Stevens, G. M., Weigen, J. F., and Lee, R. S.: Pelvic pneumography, Med. Radiogr. Photogr. **42**:82-127, 1966.

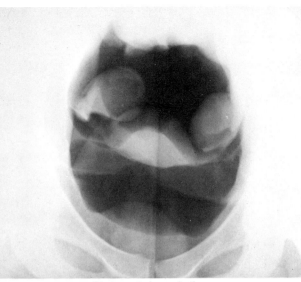

Posteroanterior projection.

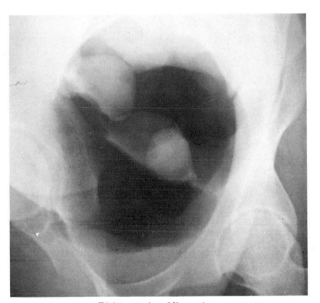

Right anterior oblique view.

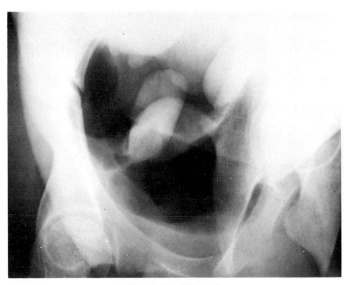

Left anterior oblique view.

Above studies demonstrate large, thick ovaries and a relatively small uterine fundus in a patient with Stein-Leventhal syndrome. Note smooth bladder anteriorly, collapsed rectosigmoid colon posteriorly, cervical shadow superimposed upon the fundus shadow, and sharp delineation of fallopian tubes. In the oblique studies, note shift of ovaries with shift of patient.

Posteroanterior projection showing excellent visualization of enlarged ovaries and of the uterus in another patient with Stein-Leventhal syndrome. Note fimbriated ends of fallopian tubes.

Radiographs and diagnostic information courtesy Dr. Emil Schulz.

843

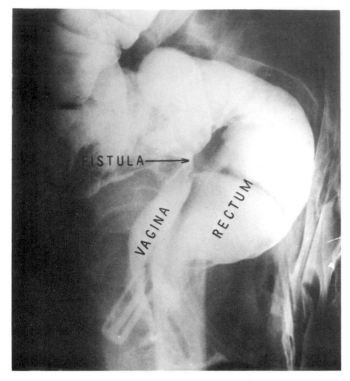

Direct lateral colon study showing fistulous communication between sigmoid and vagina.

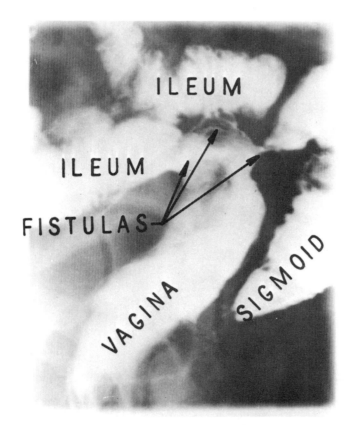

Oblique spot vaginogram on above patient showing sigmoid fistula and two fistulas to ileum.

NONGRAVID FEMALE PATIENT—cont'd
Vaginography

As noted in the introduction to the discussion of the nongravid female patient, vaginography is used in the investigation of congenital malformations and such pathologic conditions as vesicovaginal and enterovaginal fistulas. The examination is performed by introducing a contrast medium into the vaginal canal. Lambie and associates[1] recommend the use of a thin barium sulfate mixture for the investigation of fistulous communications with the intestine. At the end of the examination, the patient is instructed to expel as much of the barium mixture as possible, and the canal is then cleansed by vaginal irrigation. For the investigation of other conditions, Coe[2] advocates the use of an iodinated organic compound (any one of those used for intravenous urography).

In the presence of abnormalities other than fistulous communications between the vagina and the intestinal tract, the equipment required for the introduction of the contrast medium must be sterile. For the investigation of enterovaginal fistulas, the equipment must be scrupulously clean (medically aseptic) and must be washed and sterilized after each use.

A rectal retention tube of the Bardex type is employed for the introduction of the contrast medium, so that the moderately inflated balloon can be used to prevent reflux. By one method, the radiologist inserts only the tip of the tube into the vaginal orifice. The patient is then requested to extend her thighs and to hold them in close approximation so as to keep the inflated balloon pressed firmly against the vaginal introitus. By another method, the tube is inserted far enough to place the deflated balloon within the distal end of the vagina, and the bag is then inflated under radioscopic observation. The barium mixture is introduced with the usual enema equipment. The water-soluble medium is injected with a syringe.

[1]Lambie, R. W., Rubin, S., and Dann, D. S.: Demonstration of fistulas by vaginography, Amer. J. Roentgen. **90:**717-720, 1963.
[2]Coe, Fred O.: Vaginography, Amer. J. Roentgen. **90:**721-722, 1963.

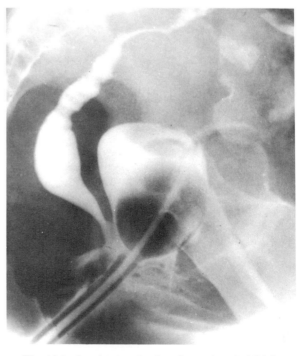

Direct lateral vaginogram showing a low rectovaginal fistula.

Radiographs and diagnostic information courtesy Dr. Roger W. Lambie.

Vaginography is carried out on a combination radioscopic-radiographic table. The contrast medium is injected under radioscopic control and spot films are exposed as indicated during the filling.

These examinations are preceded by vaginal irrigation, complete emptying of the bladder, and perineal cleansing. The patient is then adjusted in the supine position for a preliminary film. This study and the following vaginograms are taken with the central ray directed vertically to the midpoint of the film; for localized studies, centering is at the level of the upper border of the pubic symphysis.

In preparation for the introduction of the retention tube, the patient is instructed to flex her hips and knees to a modified lithotomy position. Suitable disposable padding is adjusted under the buttocks. Following the insertion of the retention tube the patient is asked to extend her legs. In order to prevent strain and to ensure a firm grip on the externally placed balloon, the patient should cross her ankles.

In each examination, the radiographic views required are determined by the radiologist according to his radioscopic findings. Lambie[1] has found that low rectovaginal fistulas are best shown in the direct lateral view and that communications with the sigmoid and/or ileum are shown to best advantage in oblique views, although they are usually demonstrated in lateral views. Lambie stated that he has found a direct anteroposterior projection to be of particular value in only one examination. This film and Lambie's diagnosis appear below.

[1]Lambie, Roger W.: Personal communication.

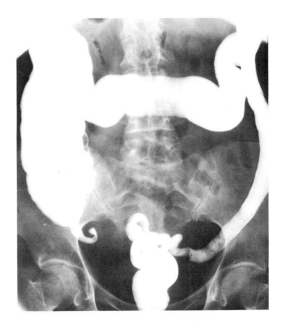

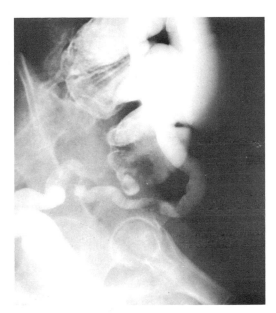

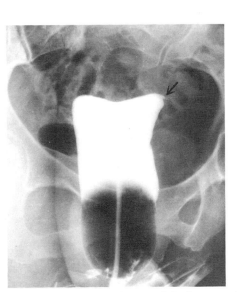

Direct anteroposterior vaginogram showing a small fistulous tract (arrow) projecting directly lateralward from apex of vagina and ending in an abscess.

Radiographs and diagnostic information courtesy Dr. Roger W. Lambie.

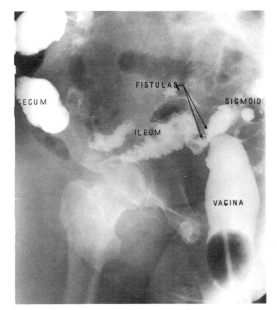

Oblique vaginogram showing fistulas to ileum and sigmoid. These were not shown on above colon studies of this patient.

845

GRAVID FEMALE PATIENT

Radiologic examinations of the gravid uterus are performed in the investigation of various obstetric complications. These examinations may be grouped under three general headings, as follows:

1. *Fetography*, which is the demonstration of the fetus in utero. Because of the danger of radiation-induced fetal malformations, this method of examination is avoided if at all possible until after the eighteenth week of gestation. Fetography is employed to detect suspected abnormalities of development, to confirm suspected fetal death, to determine the presentation and position of the fetus, and to determine whether the pregnancy is single or multiple.

2. *Placentography*, in which the walls of the uterus are investigated to locate the site of the placenta in cases of suspected placenta previa. When the placenta is not visualized in the fundus or upper uterine segment by soft tissue techniques, the lower segment may be investigated by introducing air or an opaque contrast solution into the urinary bladder for the delineation of the anterior and lateral aspects of the uterus, and by introducing air into the rectum for the delineation of the posterior aspect. Contrast studies are made with the patient standing erect. Other methods of placental localization include (1) arteriographic placentography, (2) intravenous placentography, (3) amniography, in which a water-soluble iodinated medium is injected into the amnion, (4) isotope placentography (page 970), (5) ultrasonography, and (6) thermography (pages 946 to 959). The last two methods involve no irradiation of the fetus and the maternal gonads and are used in preference to any of the other methods when the equipment is available.

3. *Roentgen pelvimetry* and *fetal cephalometry* (also called roentgen pelvicephalometry and cephalopelvimetry, and pelviradiography). This examination is performed for the purpose of demonstrating the architecture of the maternal pelvis and of comparing the size of the fetal head with the size of maternal bony pelvic outlet, in order to determine whether the pelvic diameters are adequate for normal parturition or will necessitate delivery by cesarean section. While there are many excellent methods and combinations of methods employed in roentgen pelvimetry and fetal cephalometry, space permits the inclusion in this text of the body positions and pertinent technical factors of only a few methods. (See the papers by the respective originators, listed in the bibliography, for a detailed study of the various methods.)

RADIATION PROTECTION

Radiologic examinations of pregnant patients are performed only when information is required that cannot otherwise be obtained.[1] In addition to the danger of genetic changes that may result from reproductive-cell irradiation, there is the danger of radiation-induced malformations of the developing individual. Radiation for any purpose, especially during the first trimester of gestation, is avoided whenever possible, and any examination involving the abdominopelvic region is restricted to the absolute minimum number of views required to obtain the necessary information. The technologist's responsibility, as always, is to carry out his work carefully and thoughtfully to obviate the need for repeat exposures.

EQUIPMENT

A comparatively high milliampere-second factor is required in many of these examinations in order to obtain sufficient contrast, and it is imperative that a short exposure time be used in order to overcome movement of the fetus. The generator and the x-ray tube should be capable of a high-current output—at least 200 milliamperes.

The special accessory equipment required for several of the pelvimetric methods is adaptable to any all-purpose radiographic table. A tilt table or a vertical Potter-Bucky diaphragm is required for certain examinations. The Potter-Bucky diaphragm or a stationary grid is used in all instances, and should be supplemented with close collimation or a cone of the smallest size feasible.

FILM QUALITY

The demonstration of soft tissue structures in the abdominopelvic region in the presence of amniotic fluid requires a highly selective exposure technique. Roentgenograms of the uterine wall for the localization of the placenta should show a wealth of detail in the soft parts and comparatively little detail in the osseous parts. For the production of these radiographs, the following requirements must be met:

1. Secondary radiation must be reduced to a minimum through the use of intensifying screens, the Potter-Bucky diaphragm, and close collimation or the smallest cone possible.

2. The structures must not be overpenetrated. This necessitates the use of a high milliampere-second factor with a relatively low kilovoltage, the ratio between the two factors depending upon the wave form of the unit.

3. Light, chemical, and age fog must be eliminated by using fresh films, by handling them in a light-tight room, and by processing them in fresh solutions, preferably at a temperature of not more than 68° F.

[1]Schwartz, G. S.: Radiation hazards to the human fetus in present-day society: Should a pregnant woman be subjected to a diagnostic x-ray procedure? Bull. N. Y. Acad. Med. 44:388-399, 1968. Abstr.: Amer. J. Roentgen. 103:962, 1968.

The frontal placentogram presents few difficulties, but because of the great difference in thickness between the base and the apex of the approximately cone-shaped abdomen, the lateral view requires graded filtration in order to demonstrate both the anterior and the posterior walls of the uterus on one film without having to use a strong spotlight to inspect the overexposed anterior wall. Rossi and associates[1] recommend the use of three films in the cassette. The top (or bottom) film delineates the posterior uterine wall and the spine and bony pelvis, while the middle film outlines the anterior uterine wall. The third film (either front or back) may be used repeatedly to block fluorescence of the adjacent screen. Vaughan and associates[2] designed a graded metal filter that covers all of the exposure field except the dense pelvic portion. With the use of this filter and a heavy exposure, it is possible to produce a fairly uniform density throughout the roentgenogram, so that both the upper and the lower segments of the uterus can be visualized in most instances without a spotlight. This filter is mounted in a large cone in such a way that it can be flipped to the correct position for the exposure of either a right or a left lateral view. Cahoon[3] perfected a formula for a wedge-shaped, opaque plastic filter which produces excellent results and is suitable for use on all patients regardless of size. This filter is easily made of inexpensive materials, and it lasts indefinitely. (See Cahoon's book for full details on the construction and use of the opaque plastic filter.)

The quality of fetograms and of pelvimetric studies should approximate as closely as possible the quality of films exposed for the vertebrae and pelvis of the nongravid patient. It is not reasonable, however, to expect the same degree of contrast. The thickness and composition of the pregnant abdomen, the presence of amniotic fluid, and the movements of the fetus all combine to make it difficult to obtain good roentgenograms during the third trimester of pregnancy, except with the use of equipment having a high kilovoltage output.

PREPARATION OF PATIENT

While it is desirable to clear the large bowel of gas and fecal material with a cleansing enema shortly before any one of these examinations, preliminary preparation of the patient depends entirely upon her condition and is under no circumstance administered without the express permission of the attending obstetrician. The patient is requested to completely empty her bladder immediately before the examination. This is particularly important when the erect position is being used because the filled bladder prevents the fetus from descending to the most dependent portion of the uterine cavity.

CARE OF PATIENT

All preparations for the examination should be made before the patient is placed on the radiographic table, and every item needed or likely to be needed should be at hand. The technologist should make every effort to position advanced obstetric patients carefully and to relieve strain insofar as it is possible, and remembering that at best these patients are uncomfortable, he should work quickly but not hurriedly. All preliminary adjustments for each view should be made before the patient is positioned so that she will not be required to maintain a strained position longer than is strictly necessary.

Patients who are in labor and those who are bleeding from a placental separation must be treated as emergencies and must be under the constant observation of a nurse from the obstetric division.

RESPIRATION

A change in the oxygen content of the maternal blood causes the fetus to react quickly by movement. For this reason, the patient should be required to rehearse the breathing procedure to be used before she is placed on the examining table, so that she will be able to follow instructions without practice for the exposures.

Hubeny and Delano[1] recommend that just before the suspension of respiration for the exposure, the mother's blood be hyperaerated by having her inhale deeply several times and then suspend respiration on the inhalation phase. Cameron[2] points out a second advantage in suspending respiration on the inhalation phase when the patient is laterally recumbent for placentography. She stated that in this position the maneuver draws the distal portion of the uterus forward, placing its long axis in a more horizontal plane, and thus permits better visualization of a posteroinferiorly placed placenta.

[1]Rossi, P., Rizzi, J., and De Santis, V.: Simultaneous lateral placentography, Radiology 74:298-299, 1960.

[2]Vaughan, C. E., Weaver, R. T., and Adamson, D. L.: Roentgenographic visualization of the placenta, utilizing the plastic filter, Canad. Med. Ass. J. 46:314-321, 1942.

[3]Cahoon, John B.: Formulating x-ray techniques, ed. 6, Durham, N. C., 1965, Duke University Press.

[1]Hubeny, M. J., and Delano, P. J.: A plea for the more frequent use of the lateral roentgenogram in the diagnosis of pregnancy, Radiology 32:546-549, 1939.

[2]Cameron, M. F.: Placentography, Canad. Xray News Letter 5:2-4, 1949.

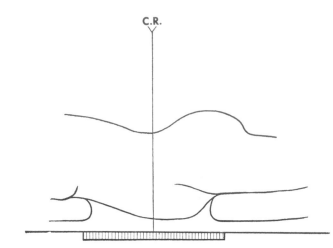

C.R.

FETOGRAPHY
Posteroanterior projection
Anteroposterior view

Fetography is employed to determine the age, position, and presentation of the fetus, and to detect a multiple pregnancy and such conditions as developmental anomalies, fetal death, and hydramnios.

The patient is asked to empty her bladder immediately before the examination. This allows the fetal head to descend to its lowest position, and it also prevents secondary radiation from the urine.

Film: $14'' \times 17''$ placed lengthwise for all views.

Position of patient

For the frontal projection of the abdomen the patient is adjusted in the prone position whenever possible, so that the fetus is closer to the film. For anteroposterior and lateral projections the patient is adjusted as for placentography (described on pages 850 and 851). An oblique view is sometimes required fully to demonstrate developmental abnormalities. For this view, the patient is rotated to the right or left, as indicated by the frontal view.

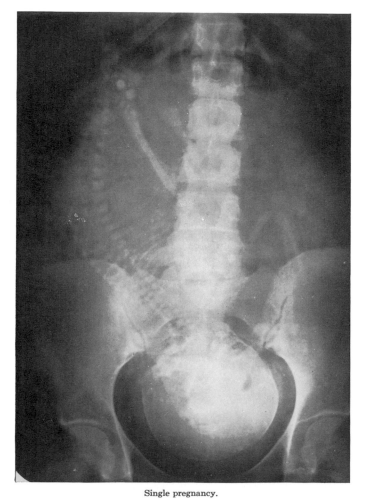

Single pregnancy.

Courtesy Dr. Benjamin Blechman.

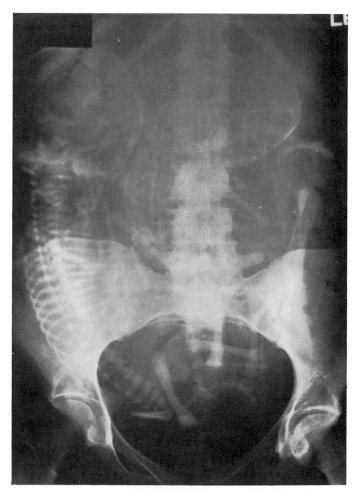

Twin pregnancy.

Courtesy W. Wm. Pollino.

FETOGRAPHY
Posteroanterior projection
Anteroposterior view—cont'd

Position of part

In preparation for adjusting the patient in the prone position, pillows or foam-rubber supports are placed on the table to elevate the thorax and pelvis. This prevents undue pressure on the abdomen and aids in adjusting the body in a direct posteroanterior position. Center the median sagittal plane of the body to the midline of the table. Have the patient flex her elbows and adjust her arms in a comfortable position. The head should rest on the chin to prevent rotation of the spine. Support the ankles on sandbags to relieve pressure on the toes.

With the cassette in the Potter-Bucky tray, adjust its position so that the entire uterus is included; the lower border of the film usually reaches to the tip of the coccyx.

The compression band is not employed. After ascertaining from the patient that the fetus is quiet, instruct her to breathe deeply several times and then to suspend respiration at the end of inhalation for the exposure.

CENTRAL RAY

Direct the central ray vertically to the midpoint of the film.

NOTE: When radiography of an early pregnancy is requested, the examination is usually restricted to one film. After emptying her bladder, the patient is placed on the table in the prone position. The central ray is directed through the region of the anus to the center of a 10″ × 12″ film at an angle of 25 to 30 degrees toward the head. This angulation is used to project the sacral shadow above that of the uterus.

If pregnancy exists and is not too early, the calcified portions of the fetal skeleton will be shown. Ossification of certain parts of the fetal skeleton commences in the eighth or ninth week but is not advanced enough for radiographic demonstration before the thirteenth or fourteenth week. Most of the fetal bones are visible by the seventeenth or eighteenth week.

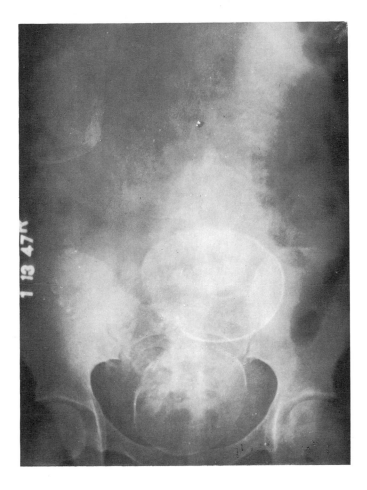

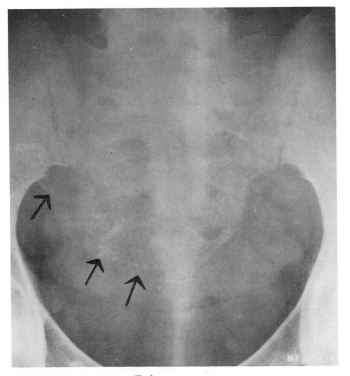

Early pregnancy.

Courtesy Dr. Marcy L. Sussman.

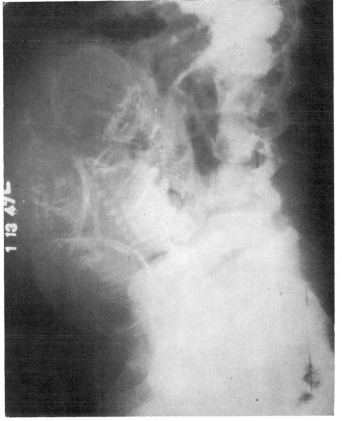

Frontal and lateral views of triplet pregnancy.

Courtesy Dr. William H. Shehadi.

849

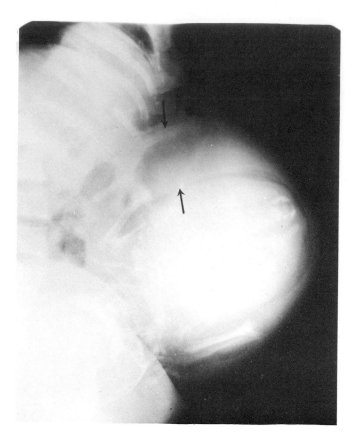

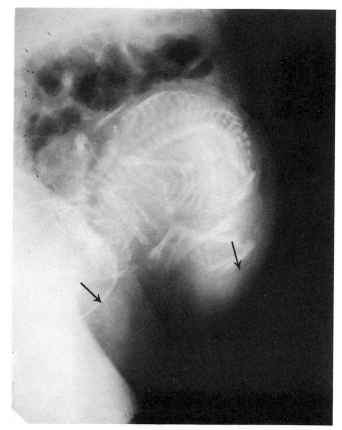

Placentograms courtesy John B. Cahoon, R.T.

PLACENTOGRAPHY

Lateral projection

Placentography is employed for the purpose of determining the site of placental implantation in cases of suspected placenta previa. The upper segment of the pregnant uterus extends well above the bony pelvis and can thus be examined by a plain film study. The placenta is most frequently implanted largely or entirely on the anterior or posterior uterine wall; implantation on the lateral wall is an uncommon finding. Therefore, a lateral view is taken and inspected, and only when it fails to reveal the location of the placenta is the anteroposterior projection employed.

The radiopaque plastic filter described by Cahoon[1] for lateral placentograms produces excellent results on these studies.

Film: $14'' \times 17''$ lengthwise.

Position of patient

For the demonstration of the upper segment of the uterine wall and for fetography, the patient is adjusted in a lateral recumbent position. A coronal plane passing midway between the anterior axillary line and the anterior surface of the abdomen is centered to the midline of the table.

Position of part

A radioparent support should be adjusted under the distended abdomen so that the abdomen is elevated to the lateral position. A sandbag placed under the dependent knee prevents forward rotation of the pelvis. The body is adjusted in an exact lateral position.

With the cassette in the grid tray, the film is centered at the level of the apex of the curve of the abdomen.

After ascertaining from the patient that the fetus is quiet, instruct her to breathe deeply several times and then to suspend respiration at the end of inhalation.

Central ray

The central ray is directed vertically to the midpoint of the film.

[1]Cahoon, John B.: Formulating x-ray techniques, ed. 6, Durham, N. C., 1965, Duke University Press.

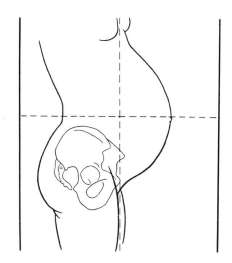

PLACENTOGRAPHY
Anteroposterior projection
Posteroanterior view

Film: 14″ × 17″ lengthwise.

Position of patient

The patient is adjusted in the supine position for the demonstration of the lateral walls of the upper segment of the pregnant uterus, and for fetography when the patient cannot be adjusted in the prone position.

Position of part

Center the median sagittal plane of the body to the midline of the table. A small pillow or sandbags should be placed under the knees to relieve strain, and another pillow or other sandbags should be placed under the ankles.

With the cassette in the grid tray, center the film at the level of the apex of the abdominal curve.

After ascertaining from the patient that the fetus is quiet, instruct her to take several deep breaths and then to suspend respiration at the end of inhalation for the exposure.

Central ray

The central ray is directed vertically to the midpoint of the film.

NOTE: By means of catheterization, air or an opaque contrast solution is introduced into the urinary bladder for the delineation of the anteroinferior and lateral walls of the *lower uterine segment.* The contrast studies are made with the patient standing erect to permit the fetal head to descend to the lowest position possible. In the absence of placenta previa, the head will lie in close approximation to the upper border of the filled bladder. Air is sometimes injected into the rectum for the delineation of the posterior wall of the lower uterine segment.

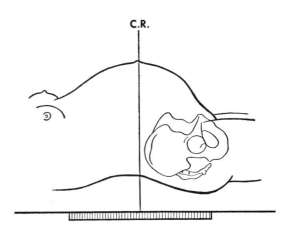

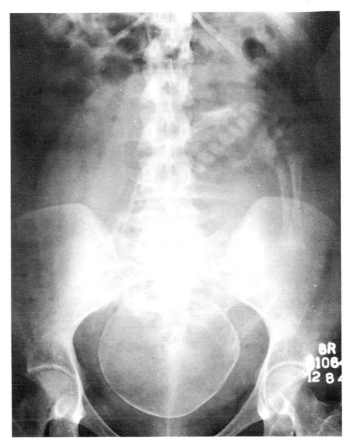

Placentogram showing left lateral wall implantation.

Courtesy John B. Cahoon, R.T.

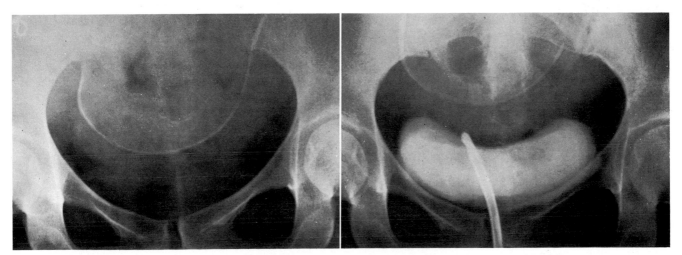

Radiographs showing central placenta previa.　　　*Courtesy Dr. William H. Shehadi.*

851

ROENTGEN PELVIMETRY

Thoms method

In the Thoms method of pelvic mensuration, two views are required—a lateral view and an inlet view. Both views are made at a focal-film distance of 36 inches. Thoms and Wilson[1] recommend that the same fixed distance be used in order to maintain relative size values of the two images and in order to minimize error due to divergence of the beam of radiation.

For the lateral view the patient is placed in the erect position and a metal centimeter rule is adjusted against the sacrum within the fold of the nates.

The inlet view requires two exposures on one film. For the first exposure, the patient is placed in a semiseated position and adjusted so that the plane of the pelvic inlet closely parallels the plane of the film and the inlet-to-table-top distance is measured. For the second exposure, the patient is removed (while the film and tube remain in situ), a perforated centimeter grid is adjusted to lie in the plane formerly occupied by the pelvic inlet, and a flash exposure is then made.

With the older type of lead grid, which has pinhole perforations at 1 cm. intervals in an allover pattern, the resultant black dots represent a centimeter scale that has the same degree of magnification as the pelvic inlet, so that any desired diameter of the inlet may be read by counting the dots. In the modified lead grid the perforations are placed along one edge and are so spaced that the transverse diameters of levels other than those of the pelvic inlet may be measured. The only change in the technique of using the two grids is that, whereas the tube remains centered to the film for the older type, which has the allover pattern of perforations, it must be shifted so the focal-spot is centered over the perforated strip when the modified grid is used. The focal-film distance must not be changed in either instance.

[1]Thoms, Herbert, and Wilson, Hugh M.: The roentgenological survey of the pelvis, Yale J. Biol. Med. **13**:831-839, 1941.

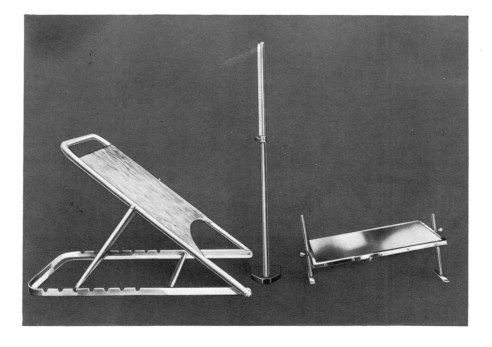

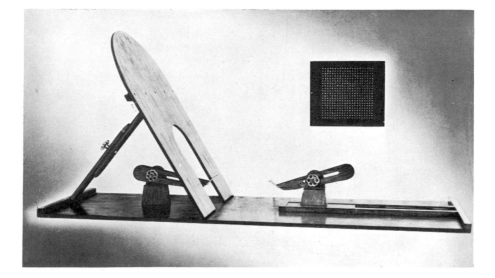

In addition to the perforated lead grid, the inlet view requires an adjustable backrest, preferably the Torpin-Thoms apparatus. This device consists of a platform upon which are mounted an adjustable backrest and two adjustable landmark indicators that also serve to support the perforated grid in the correct position for the second exposure. The posterior landmark indicator is mounted on a fixed post. The anterior indicator is attached to a post that can be moved along a channel so that, after the indicator arm has been correctly adjusted and locked, the post can be temporarily shifted while the patient is removed from the table. When the Torpin-Thoms pelvimeter is not employed, the distance between each end of the anteroposterior diameter of the pelvic inlet and the tabletop must be measured with a caliper, and the perforated grid must be adjustably mounted on two upright posts.

External landmarks for plane of pelvic inlet. The entrance to the true pelvis is called the *superior strait* or *pelvic inlet*, and is bounded by the sacral promontory, the linea terminalis, and the crests of the pubes and the symphysis. The internal anteroposterior diameter of the inlet is measured from the center of the sacral promontory to the upper posterior margin of the pubic symphysis, and is called the *internal conjugate diameter* or the *conjugata vera*. Other internal diameters of the pelvic cavity are shown in the accompanying illustrations.

The *external conjugate diameter* extends from the interspace between the spinous process of the fourth and fifth lumbar vertebrae to the top of the symphysis pubis. The posterior landmark, the interspinous space, can be palpated at the upper angle of the Michaelis rhomboid. The Michaelis rhomboid is the diamond-shaped depression overlying the lumbosacral region. It is bounded laterally by the dimples overlying the posterior superior iliac spines, above to the fifth lumbar spinous process by the lines formed by the gluteus muscles, and below by the groove at the end of the vertebral column.

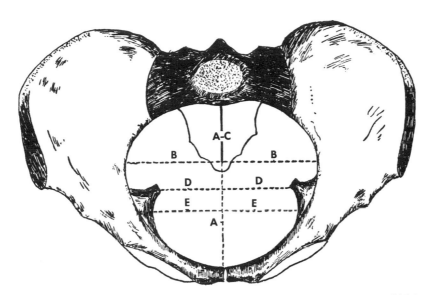

Pelvis seen from above. **A,** Anteroposterior diameter of inlet; **B,** transverse diameter of inlet; **C,** posterior sagittal diameter of inlet; **D,** interspinous or transverse diameter of midplane; **E,** widest transverse diameter of outlet.

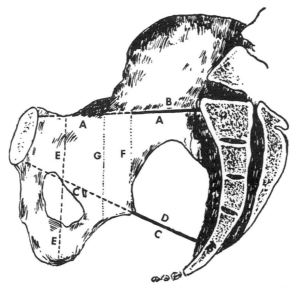

Lateral aspect of pelvis. **A,** Anteroposterior diameter of inlet; **B,** posterior sagittal diameter of inlet; **C,** anteroposterior diameter of midplane; **D,** posterior sagittal diameter of midplane.

Illustrations courtesy Dr. Herbert Thoms.

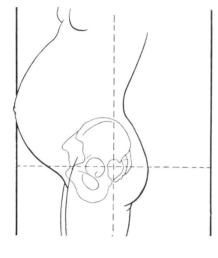

ROENTGEN PELVIMETRY
Thoms method
Lateral position

Film: $10'' \times 12''$ or $11'' \times 14''$ crosswise.

Position of patient

Have the patient wear a cotton gown open at the back. Supply her with paper or other heelless slippers.

Place the patient in front of a vertical Potter-Bucky diaphragm in either a right or a left lateral position.

Position of part

Locate by palpation, and place a mark at, a site just below a point one-third the distance from the symphysis pubis to the depression under the fifth lumbar vertebra. This mark serves as the centering point.

With the patient's adjacent hip in contact with the vertical table, have her stand straight, with the weight of the body equally distributed on the feet, and cross the forearms over the chest.

Adjust the height of the Potter-Bucky diaphragm so that the film is centered to the previously marked localization point. Align the body in a true lateral position with the method suggested by Coe.[1] Using calipers to measure the distance, adjust the position so that the midgluteal fold and the midlabial fold are equidistant from the table. Adjust the height of the upright centimeter rod and place its perforated scale against the sacrum between the folds of the nates.

Respiration is suspended for the exposure.

Central ray

Direct the central ray horizontally to the midpoint of the film; it enters the marked site overlying the middle region of the greater sciatic notches.

Structures shown

The last lumbar vertebra, the sacrum, the sacrosciatic notch, the ischial spines and tuberosities, the acetabula, and the anterior and posterior borders of the symphysis pubis. The black dots cast by the perforations of the centimeter scale are seen just posterior to the sacrum.

[1]Coe, Fred O.: Roentgenographic cephalopelvimetry, Amer. J. Roentgen. **67**:449-457, 1952.

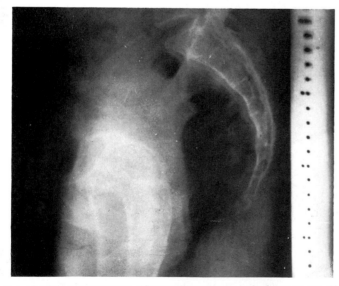

Lateral pelvic roentgenogram. "Corrected" centimeter scale shown on one side of film. All anteroposterior pelvic diameters may be measured.

Courtesy Dr. Herbert Thoms.

ROENTGEN PELVIMETRY
Thoms method
Inlet position

Film: $10'' \times 12''$ crosswise.

Position of patient

After placing the roentgen pelvimeter platform on the radiographic table, adjust the backrest at an angle of about 50 degrees and slide the anterior post well toward the foot of the platform.

Palpate the interspace between the spinous processes of the fourth and fifth lumbar vertebrae (the upper angle of the Michaelis rhomboid), mark the site, and then place the patient on the pelvimeter platform in the seated position.

Position of part

With the patient seated erect, center the median sagittal plane of her body to the midline of the platform, and have her lean against the backrest. Determine the position of the plane of the pelvic inlet and make any required adjustment in the height of the backrest. While the aim is to place the plane of the pelvic inlet as nearly parallel with the plane of the film as possible, the posterior end of the conjugate diameter may be a little higher than the anterior end; however, it is imperative that it not be lower in order to avoid distortion of the conjugata vera. With the body correctly positioned, separate the legs, place a small sandbag under each knee, and immobilize the ankles.

Adjust the posterior indicator arm so that its transverse bar rests against the marked interspinous space, and then lock it in position. Slide the anterior post into position and adjust the arm so that the transverse bar rests against the pelvis 1 cm. below the top of the pubic symphysis.

The film is centered to the pelvic cavity, about $2\frac{1}{2}$ inches posterior to the pubic symphysis.

Ascertain from the patient that the fetus is quiet, and then instruct her to suspend respiration at the end of inhalation for the exposure.

Central ray

Direct the central ray vertically in the median sagittal plane to a point 6 cm. ($2\frac{1}{2}$ inches) posterior to the pubic symphysis.

Structures shown

An axial view of the pelvic inlet, the ischial spines, and the pelvic outlet. The black dots cast by the perforated grid are seen as an allover pattern when the older grid is used, and as a narrow strip with six rows of dots near the top of the film when the modified grid is used.

NOTE: The reader is referred to Moir[1] for a detailed description of his "graph method" of interpreting the inlet view of the pelvis. He states that the cephalopelvic relationship can be quickly assessed with the use of three charts that represent the pelvis at the brim level, the ischial spine level, and the outlet level, respectively.

Diehl and Fernström[2] and de Villiers[3] describe inlet views wherein, without moving the patient or the film, a separate, closely collimated exposure is made of the lateral margin of the pelvic brim on each side. By this technique the fetal and maternal gonads receive minimum radiation exposure.

[1]Moir, J. C.: The uses and value of radiology in obstetrics. In Browne, F. J., and Browne, J. C. M.: Antenatal and postnatal care, ed. 9, London, 1960, J. & A. Churchill, pp. 389-409.

[2]Diehl, J., and Fernström, I.: Radiologic pelvimetry with special reference to widest transverse diameter of pelvic inlet, Acta Radiol. [Diagn.] 4:557-568, 1966.

[3]de Villiers, P. D.: Radiation dose with the orthometric view in x-ray pelvimetry, S. Afr. Med. J. 44:820-822, 1970.

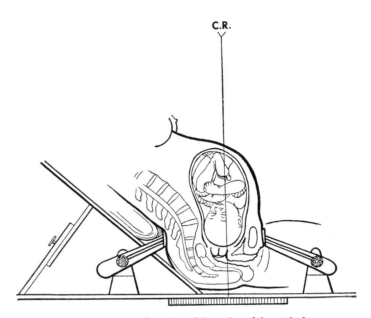

C.R.

Drawing adapted from that of the author of the method.

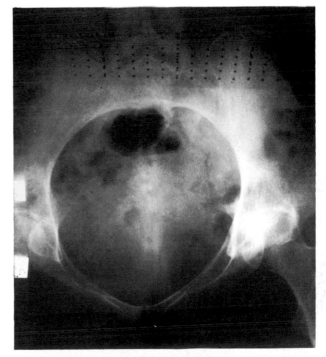

Pelvic inlet roentgenogram. Top row of dots represents "corrected" centimeters for level of pelvic inlet. Interspinous and other lower level diameters are measured by using other series of dots which are calibrated for 5, 6, 7, 8, and 9 centimeter levels below that of the inlet.

Courtesy Dr. Herbert Thoms.

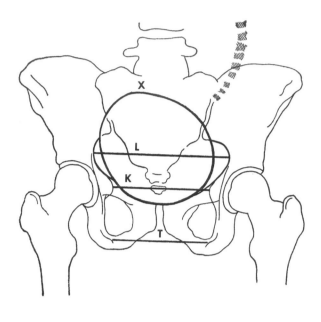

ROENTGEN PELVIMETRY AND CEPHALOMETRY

Ball method

This method requires no special apparatus or accessories in exposing the films. The examination normally consists of two views—a single or a stereoscopic anteroposterior projection, and a lateral projection. In cases of breech presentation and multiple pregnancy it is necessary to take two additional projections (anteroposterior and lateral), with the films centered at the level of the tip of the xiphoid process. The focal-film distance is optional, but it is usually 36 inches.

For roentgenographic mensuration of the fetal head and the maternal pelvis, the degree of image magnification is compensated simply by adjusting the movable arm of the calculator to the correct point on the anode-film distance scale.

This method of examination was designed by Ball for the purpose of utilizing the roentgenograms for both clinical obstetrics and roentgen anthropometry. Ball[1] states that mensuration of the roentgen image is optional, and in a majority of cases not necessary, to determine whether a disproportion exists between the fetal head and the maternal pelvis. In borderline cases, where measurements might be indicated, the author of the method advocates a comparison of the fetal head with the pelvic diameters in terms of volume and volume capacity respectively, rather than linear measurements. (See articles by Ball and Golden[2,3] for details of film analyses.)

[1]Ball, Robert P.: Personal communication.

[2]Ball, Robert P., and Golden, Ross.: Roentgenographic obstetrical pelvicephalometry in the erect posture, Amer. J. Roentgen. **49**:731-741, 1943.

[3]Ball, Robert P., and Golden, Ross.: Roentgenologic sign for detection of placenta previa, Amer. J. Obstet. Gynec. **42**:530-533, 1941.

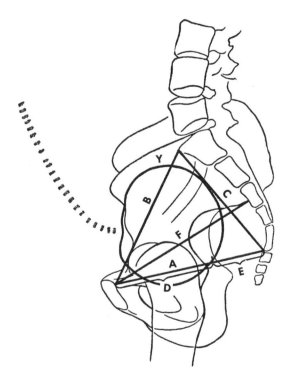

Tracings of anteroposterior and lateral roentgenograms showing usual position of term fetus in cephalic presentation at or near term. Lettered lines refer to pelvic dimensions which are used by the author of the method to analyze the pelvis.

Courtesy Dr. Robert P. Ball.

Position of patient

The patient is placed in the erect position, by preference, for both anteroposterior and lateral projections. The shoes are removed when anthropometric measurements are to be made.

Ball states that the purposes of the erect position are the following: "(1) To utilize the effect of gravity upon the fetus. In uncomplicated, normal cases the fetus will come to rest in the most dependent portion of the amniotic sac. This is well below the inlet of the pelvic brim and near the level of the ischial spines during the last two months of pregnancy. (2) To disclose any displacement of the fetus. Normally the head of the fetus is in the midsagittal and midcoronal planes of the pelvic inlet when the fetus is in cephalic presentation and the mother is standing. A displacement of the fetal head from its normal position is indicative of a mass that is preventing it from moving into the most dependent portion of the uterine cavity. This mass might be a low implantation of the placenta or a pelvic mass outside of the uterus."[1]

[1]Ball, Robert P.: Personal communication.

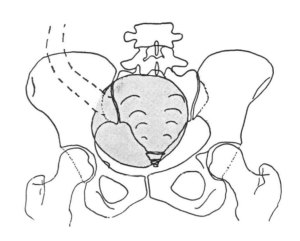

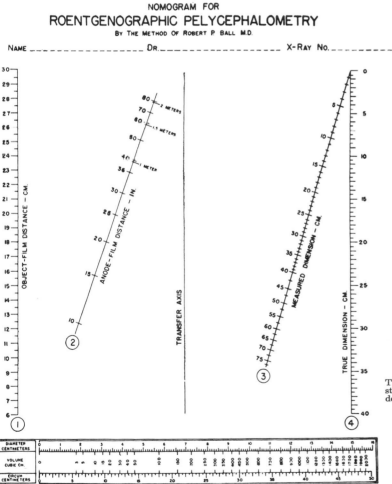

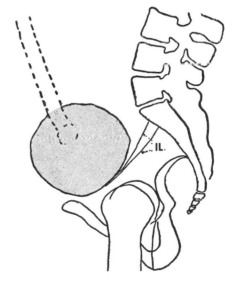

Tracings of anteroposterior and lateral placentograms (made with patient standing) showing lateral displacement of fetal head as well as its failure to descend below pelvic inlet.

Courtesy Dr. Robert P. Ball.

Nomograph (calculator) used by Dr. Ball for correcting film image magnification at any convenient anode-film distance.

Courtesy Dr. Robert P. Ball.

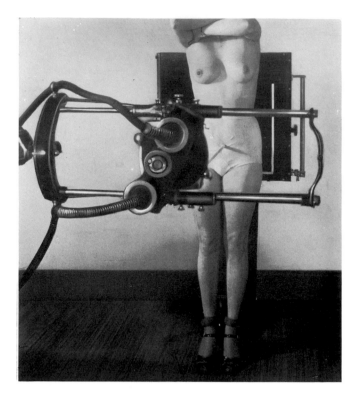

ROENTGEN PELVIMETRY AND CEPHALOMETRY

Ball method

Film: $14'' \times 17''$ placed crosswise.

Anteroposterior position

With the patient in the erect position, center the median sagittal plane of the body to the midline of the Potter-Bucky diaphragm. The film is placed crosswise to include the greater trochanters. Adjust the height of the Potter-Bucky diaphragm so that the lower border of the film will be about 1 inch below the level of the ischial tuberosities (the gluteofemoral fold is a convenient landmark).

Have the patient stand straight, with the weight of the body equally distributed on the feet, and then immobilize with a compression band applied across the pelvis at the level of the hips.

After ascertaining that the fetus is quiet, instruct the patient to suspend respiration at the end of inhalation for the exposure.

Central ray

The exposure is made with the central ray directed perpendicularly through the median sagittal plane at the level of the superior margin of the symphysis pubis.

When stereoscopic films are desired, the tube is shifted caudally for a distance of about 3 inches from the original centering point.

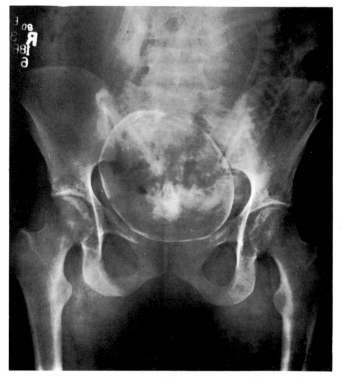

Illustrations courtesy Dr. Robert P. Ball.

858

ROENTGEN PELVIMETRY AND CEPHALOMETRY
Ball method

Film: $14'' \times 17''$ placed lengthwise.

Lateral position

From the anteroposterior position, have the patient turn 90 degrees into a true lateral position; using calipers to measure the distance, adjust the position so that the midgluteal fold and the midlabial fold are equidistant from the table. Place the film lengthwise in order to include the fundus of the uterus. The height of the Potter-Bucky diaphragm is not changed.

Adjust the position of the body so that the posterior margin of the gluteus is barely included on the lateral border of the film. This position places the hip joints slightly to one side of the midline of the Potter-Bucky diaphragm. Have the patient stand straight with the weight of the body equally distributed on the feet.

After ascertaining that the fetus is quiet, instruct the patient to suspend respiration at the end of inhalation for the exposure.

Central ray

Shift the tube laterally so that the central ray passes through the upper margin of the hip joint; it enters the body about 1 inch above the upper margin of the greater trochanter.

Ball[1] suggests that the anode end of the tube be uppermost whenever possible in order to utilize the "heel effect" by projecting the greatest concentration of radiation toward the thickest part of the pelvis.

[1]Ball, Robert P., and Golden, Ross.: Roentgenographic obstetrical pelvicephalometry in the erect posture, Amer. J. Roentgen. **49**:731-741, 1943.

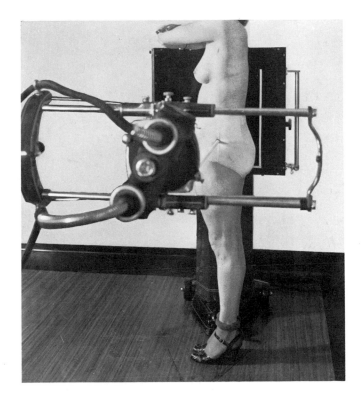

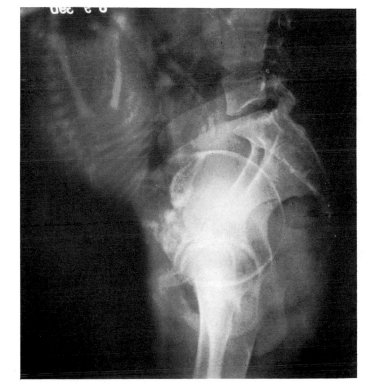

Illustrations courtesy Dr. Robert P. Ball.

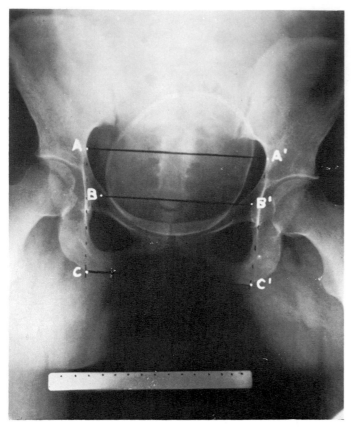

ROENTGEN PELVIMETRY

Colcher-Sussman method

Each of the two projections (anteroposterior and lateral) employed in this method of pelvimetry requires the use of the Colcher-Sussman pelvimeter. This device consists of a metal ruler perforated at centimeter intervals and mounted on a small stand in such a way that it is always parallel with the plane of the film. The ruler can be rotated in a complete circle and can be adjusted for height.

Film: $14'' \times 17''$ for each exposure.

Anteroposterior projection

Place the patient in the supine position and center the median sagittal plane of her body to the midline of the table. Flex the knees to elevate the forepelvis, and being careful to place a towel so as not to expose the patient, separate the thighs enough to permit correct placement of the pelvimeter. Immobilize the feet with sandbags.

Turn the ruler transversely and center it to the gluteal fold at the level of the ischial tuberosities. The tuberosities are easily palpable through the median part of the buttocks; if preferred, the tuberosities may be localized by placing the ruler 10 cm. below the upper border of the pubic symphysis.

The film is centered 1½ inches cephalad to the pubic symphysis. After ascertaining that the fetus is quiet, instruct the patient to suspend respiration at the end of inhalation for the exposure.

The central ray is directed perpendicularly to the midpoint of the film from any desired focal-film distance.

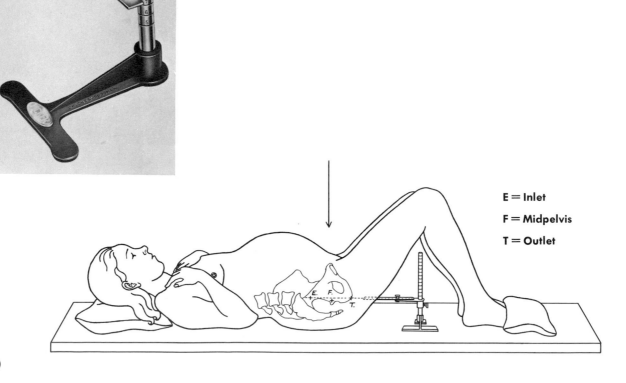

E = Inlet

F = Midpelvis

T = Outlet

ROENTGEN PELVIMETRY
Colcher-Sussman method—cont'd

Lateral projection

Ask the patient to turn to a lateral position and center the midaxillary line of the body to the midline of the table. Partially extend the thighs so they will not obscure the pubes. Place sandbags under and between the knees and ankles and immobilize the legs. Place a folded sheet or other suitable support under the lower thorax and adjust it so that the long axis of the lumbar vertebrae is parallel with the tabletop. Adjust the body in a true lateral position and have the patient grasp the side of the table for support. Check the position with calipers, and adjust the body so that the midgluteal and the midlabial folds are equidistant from the table.

Turn the ruler lengthwise and adjust its height to coincide with the median sagittal plane of the patient's body. Place the pelvimeter so that the metal ruler lies within the upper part of the gluteal fold and against the midsacrum.

Center the film at the level of the most prominent point of the greater trochanter. After ascertaining that the fetus is quiet, instruct the patient to suspend respiration at the end of inhalation for the exposure.

The central ray is directed vertically to the midpoint of the film, the focal-film distance being the same as that used for the anteroposterior projection.

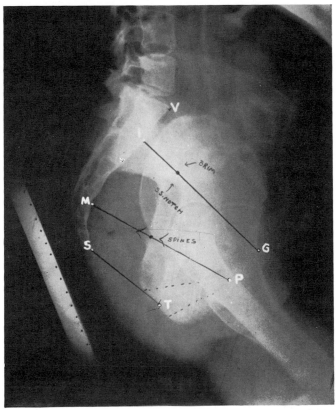

Courtesy Dr. A. E. Colcher.

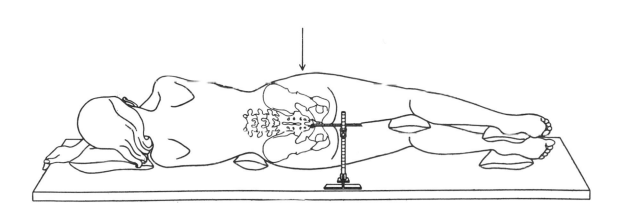

861

PELVIORADIOGRAPHY

Caldwell-Moloy method

In the Caldwell-Moloy method of pelvioradiography a complete examination requires three views of the pelvis: (1) anteroposterior stereoscopic projections for the determination of the pelvic type and the fetal-pelvic relationship, and for mensuration of the fetal head and the maternal pelvic diameters; (2) a lateral projection for the demonstration of the sacrosciatic notch, the sacrum, and the pubes, and for mensuration of the sagittal diameters; and (3) an inferosuperior anteroposterior projection for the demonstration of the subpubic arch. The authors of the method[1] state that the subpubic arch view may be omitted when the patient is in labor.

This method requires a specially constructed cassette frame and, for measurement purposes, a special marker for the anteroposterior position. A Weitzner or other roentgen centimeter ruler is recommended for the lateral projection. No special equipment is needed for the subpubic arch view.

In order to duplicate the setup of the original exposure in the stereoscope, the authors of the method devised the cassette frame to obviate error due to a shift of the film in the cassette or to a shift of the cassette in the Potter-Bucky tray. The frame is placed over the cassette and has four overlapping arrow points, one being centrally placed at each end of the frame, and two spaced at equidistant points from center on one side. The images of the arrow points are projected onto the films and, by being superimposed over corresponding lines on the viewing boxes, are used for the correct placement of the films in the precision stereoscope.

The special marker consists of two triangular pieces of lead spaced exactly nine centimeters apart and embedded in either (1) a strip of wood supported by a right-angled upright that is attached to, and slides along, the side of the table, or (2) a horseshoe-shaped piece of bakelite supported by a small metal stand that is placed on the

[1]Caldwell, W. E., Moloy, Howard C., and Swenson, Paul C.: Use of roentgen ray in obstetrics; roentgen pelvimetry and cephalometry; technique of pelvioradiography, Amer. J. Roentgen. 41:305-316, 1939.

table between the patient's thighs. The marker is adjusted immediately over, but not quite in contact with, the region of the symphysis pubis. This position of the marker, below the enlarged abdomen, is used to reduce magnified distortion of the marker images. When the films are placed in the precision stereoscope, the marker is measured in the phantom image, and if necessary, the optical system is moved forward or backward so that the distance between the marker images measures its known length. The size and shape of the fetal head and of the maternal pelvis as seen in the phantom image are then the same as in the original setup, and direct measurement of the diameters can be made.

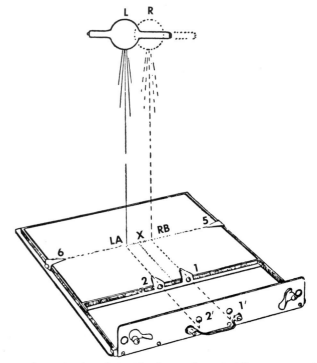

Cassette frame showing relationship of target for each shift to arrow markers around periphery. **X** = Base point. Target **R** and **L** at 25-inch target-film distance shifts along common line joining arrows **5** and **6**. For each exposure note perpendicular relationship of target along lines: **L, LA, 2, 2′,** or **R, RB, 1, 1′.**

Courtesy Dr. Howard C. Moloy.

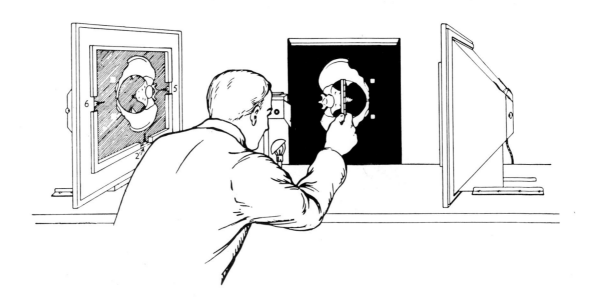

Illustration to show precision stereoscope in use. Film is placed in view box with image of arrows **5** and **6** and either **1** or **2** of illustration above superimposed over corresponding lines permanently marked on celluloid ledge of view box.

Courtesy Dr. Howard C. Moloy.

PELVIORADIOGRAPHY
Caldwell-Moloy method
Anteroposterior position

Film: $11'' \times 14''$ lengthwise for each exposure.

Position of patient

The patient is placed in the supine position, with the median sagittal plane of the body centered to the midline of the table.

Position of part

Elevate the head and shoulders on pillows, and adjust a thick radioparent pad (a roll of sheets serves the purpose well) under the lower spine to arch the back as much as possible. These supports (the pillows and pad) are used to tilt the forepelvis downward and thus place the pelvic inlet more nearly parallel with the plane of the film. Adjust and rigidly fix the marker over, but not quite in contact with, the region of the symphysis pubis.

With the cassette and cassette frame in position, center at the level of the anterior superior iliac spines. Lock the Potter-Bucky carriage securely to prevent any possibility of a shift in its position during the change of cassettes.

After ascertaining from the patient that the fetus is quiet or, if the patient is in labor, that the contraction has subsided, instruct her to suspend respiration at the end of inhalation for the exposure.

Central ray

The central ray is directed vertically from an exact focal-film distance of either 25 or 30 inches. With either focal-film distance, the tube is shifted exactly 1¼ inches cephalad and caudad from center for the two exposures. The focal-film and tube-shift distances *must* be exact.

Structures shown

A stereoscopic view of the maternal pelvis and lower abdomen and of the contained parts of the fetal skeleton.

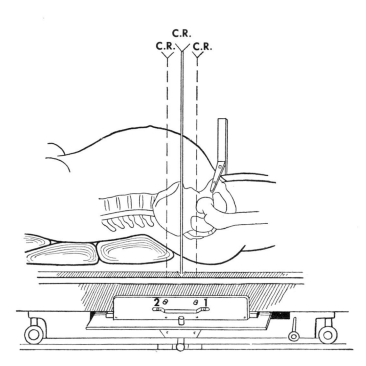

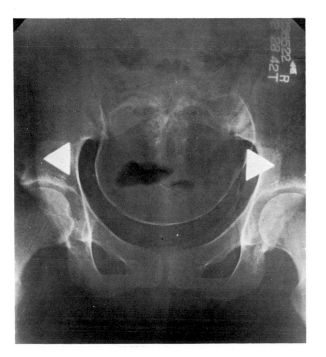

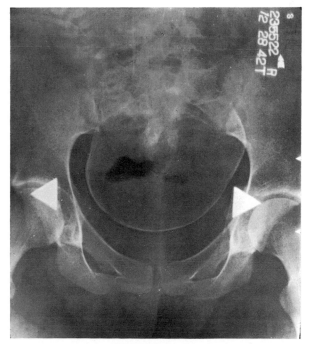

Radiographs courtesy Dr. Howard C. Moloy.

863

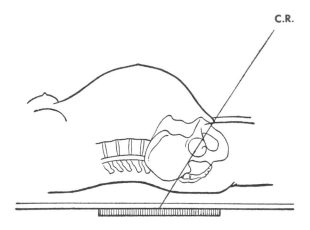

C.R.

PELVIORADIOGRAPHY
Caldwell-Moloy method
Subpubic arch position

Film: $10'' \times 12''$ crosswise.

Position of patient

This projection immediately follows the exposure of the stereoscopic pelvioradiographs and is made with the patient in the same body position, that is, supine.

Position of part

Remove the supporting pads from beneath the shoulders and back to allow the pelvis to assume its normal position, so that the pubic symphysis will be placed at a right angle, or at a near right angle, to the central ray. In subjects having an acute lumbar lordosis, the pelvis tilts downward, placing the superior strait almost parallel with the plane of the film, and placing the pubic symphysis in a nearly vertical position. In order to overcome this downward tilt, the knees should be semiflexed over a pillow or sandbags so that the symphysis is tilted backward at an angle of about 45 degrees to the vertical plane.

With the cassette in the Potter-Bucky tray, adjust its position so that the midpoint of the film will coincide with the central ray.

After ascertaining from the patient that the fetus is quiet or, if she is in labor, that the contraction has subsided, instruct her to suspend respiration at the end of inhalation for the exposure.

Central ray

Direct the central ray to the inferior border of the pubic symphysis at an angle of 45 degrees toward the head. When the inclination of the pelvis is correct, the central ray enters the upper part of the subpubic arch at right angles to the descending rami of the pubes.

Structures shown

An inferosuperior projection of the lower pelvic bones, showing the size and shape of the subpubic arch.

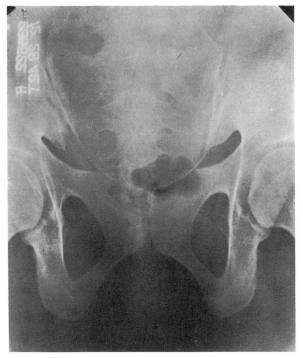

Courtesy Dr. Howard C. Moloy.

PELVIORADIOGRAPHY
Caldwell-Moloy method
Lateral projection

Film: $14'' \times 17''$ lengthwise.

Position of patient

While the patient may be examined in either the recumbent or the erect position, the erect position is preferable because it allows the fetal head to descend to its lowest position.

Position of part

For the erect position, have the patient remove her shoes. For either body position, center the posterior axillary line of the body to the midline of the table. This centering places the superimposed sacrosciatic notches over the midline of the Potter-Bucky grid; the notches lie in the coronal plane passing through the soft tissue depressions just above and behind the greater trochanter.

When the body is erect, its weight must be equally distributed on the feet. The arms may be crossed over the chest, or, preferably, an enema standard may be placed directly in front of the patient so that she can grasp it with both hands. When the patient is recumbent, place a firm pillow under the lower thorax and adjust it so that the long axis of the vertebral column is parallel with the tabletop. Have the patient grasp the side of the table for support. Extend her thighs, place small sandbags under and between her knees and ankles, and then immobilize her legs by placing sandbags against them.

Adjust the body in a true lateral position, with the midgluteal fold and the midlabial fold equidistant from the table.

Place the centimeter ruler within the gluteal fold and adjust the ruler so that it is parallel with the plane of the film.

Center the film at the level of the anterosuperior iliac spines. After ascertaining from the patient that the fetus is quiet or, if she is in labor, that the contraction has subsided, instruct her to suspend respiration at the end of inhalation for the exposure.

Central ray

Direct the central ray perpendicularly through the soft tissue depression just above and behind the adjacent greater trochanter.

Structures shown

A lateral view of the pelvis, demonstrating the sacrosciatic notches, the sacrum, and, usually, the fetal head.

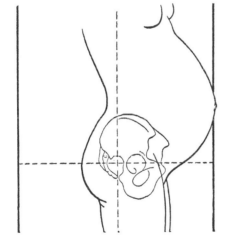

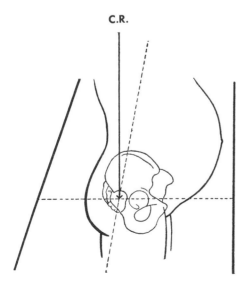

C.R.

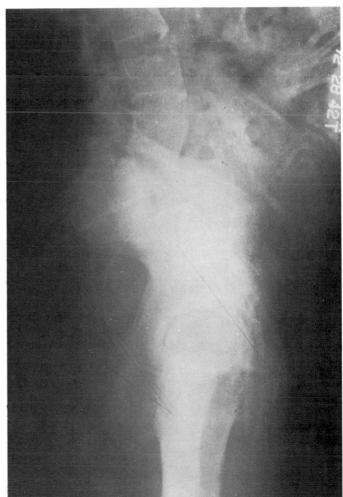

Courtesy Dr. Howard C. Moloy.

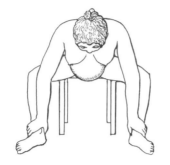

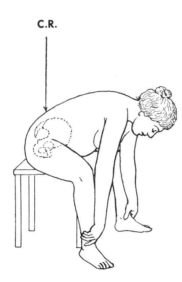

C.R.

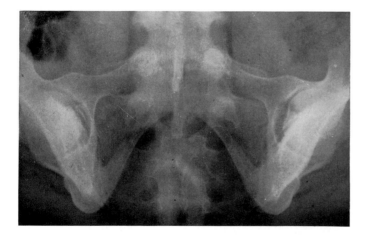

PELVIC OUTLET
Superoinferior projection
Chassard-Lapiné position

Film: $10'' \times 12''$ crosswise.

Position of patient

This projection requires that the patient be seated in an acutely flexed position. The measurements of the maternal pelvis are usually investigated in the third trimester, when the expansion of the abdomen is such that it restricts the patient's ability to assume a sharply flexed position unless so seated that she can abduct her thighs enough to accommodate the enlarged abdomen between them; the abdomen then can descend into this position without obstruction. The standard roentgenographic table is too wide to meet these requirements. The patient should be seated on a small surface at chair height—that is, on a $10'' \times 12''$ portable Potter-Bucky diaphragm or a grid-front cassette placed on a suitable stool. This arrangement enables the patient to achieve maximum abduction of her thighs and adequate flexion of her body.

Position of part

Seat the patient so that the median sagittal plane of the body is centered to the midline of the film, with the symphysis pubis approximately 2 inches posterior to the front margin of the film. Ask the patient to abduct her thighs as widely as possible. Localize the symphysis pubis, and then have her lean directly forward until the symphysis is in close contact with the cassette or diaphragm; the vertical axis of the pelvis will be tilted forward approximately 45 degrees. This position places the inferior rami of the pubes and ischia parallel with the plane of the film.

Have the patient grasp her ankles to aid in maintaining the position. Respiration is suspended for the exposure.

Central ray

Direct the central ray vertically to the median sagittal plane of the sacrum at the level of the highest (most proximal) point of the greater trochanters.

When the patient cannot be positioned so that adequate flexion of the body can be achieved, direct the central ray anteriorly at right angles to the coronal plane of the symphysis pubis.

Structures shown

A superoinferior projection showing the size and shape of the subpubic arch. Because the inferior rami of the pubes and ischia are parallel with, and in close proximity to, the film in this position, there is no distortion and little magnification of the arch.

Anatomy and positioning of the central nervous system

Central nervous system

For descriptive purposes, the central nervous system is divided into two parts: (1) the *brain*, which occupies the cranial cavity, and (2) the *spinal cord*, which is suspended within the spinal canal.

The brain is composed of an outer portion of gray matter, called the cortex, and an inner portion of white matter. The brain consists of the *cerebrum*, the *cerebellum*, the *pons varolii*, and the *medulla oblongata*, which is continuous with the spinal cord. The cerebrum composes the largest part of the brain and is referred to as the *forebrain*. The stemlike part that connects the cerebrum to the pons and the cerebellum is termed the *midbrain*. The cerebellum, the pons, and the medulla compose the *hindbrain*.

A deep cleft, called the longitudinal fissure, separates the cerebrum into right and left *hemispheres*, which are closely connected by bands of nerve fibers. The main commissure between the cerebral hemispheres is the *corpus callosum*. Each cerebral hemisphere contains a fluid-secreting cavity called a *lateral ventricle*. At their lower part, called the *diencephalon*, the cerebral hemispheres surround the *third ventricle*. The surface of the cerebral hemispheres is convoluted by many fissures and grooves that mark them into lobes and lobules.

The cerebellum, the largest part of the hindbrain, is separated from the cerebrum by a deep transverse cleft called the *transverse fissure*. The hemispheres of the cerebellum are connected by a medium constricted area called the *vermis*. The surface of the cerebellum, instead of being convoluted, as is the surface of the cerebrum, is grooved in such a way that it has a laminated appearance. The pons forms the upper part of the hindbrain, while the medulla, which extends between the pons and the spinal cord, forms the lower part.

The spinal cord is a slender, elongated structure consisting of an inner, gray, cellular substance which has the shape of the capital letter H on transverse section, and of an outer, white, fibrous substance. The cord extends from the brain, being connected to it through the medulla oblongata at the level of the foramen magnum, to the approximate level of the interspace between the first and second lumbar vertebrae. The spinal cord ends in a pointed extremity called the *medullary conus*. A delicate, fibrous strand extending from the medullary conus attaches the cord to the upper coccygeal segment. There are thirty-one pairs of spinal nerves, each arising from two roots at the sides of the spinal cord. The nerves are transmitted through the intervertebral and sacral foramina.

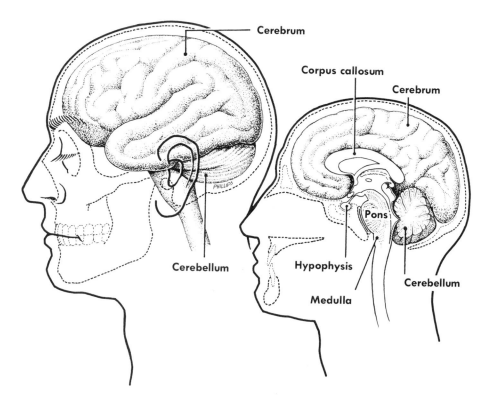

DRAWINGS SHOWING SURFACE AND MIDSECTION OF BRAIN

The brain and spinal cord are enclosed by three continuous, protective membranes called *meninges*. The inner sheath, called the *pia mater* (L. tender mother), is highly vascular and closely adherent to the underlying brain and cord structure.

The delicate central sheath is called the *arachnoid*. This membrane is separated from the pia mater by a comparatively wide space called the *subarachnoid space*, which is widened in certain areas. The areas of increased width are called *cisternae*, and the widest of these is called the *cisterna magna*. This cavity is triangular in shape and is situated at the upper, posterior part of the subarachnoid space between the base of the cerebellum and the medulla oblongata. The subarachnoid space is continuous with the ventricular system of the brain and communicates with it by way of a centrally placed opening, the *foramen of Magendie*, which is between the cisterna magna and the fourth ventricle. The ventricles of the brain and the subarachnoid space contain the *cerebrospinal fluid*. The cisterna magna is

sometimes used as a point of entry into the subarachnoid space in pneumoencephalography and in myelography.

The outermost sheath, called the *dura mater* (L. hard mother), forms the strong, fibrous covering of the brain and of the spinal cord. The dura is separated from the arachnoid by the *subdural space*, and from the vertebral periosteum by the *epidural space*. These spaces do not communicate with the ventricular system. The dura mater is composed of two layers throughout its cranial portion. The outer, or endosteal, layer lines the cranial bones, thus serving as periosteum to their inner surface. The inner, or meningeal, layer serves to protect the brain and to support blood vessels. The meningeal layer, by reduplication, also sends out four partitions for the support and protection of the various parts of the brain. The dura mater extends below the spinal cord, to the level of the second sacral segment, to enclose the spinal nerves, which are prolonged downward from the cord to their respective exits. The lower portion of the dura mater is called the *dural sac*.

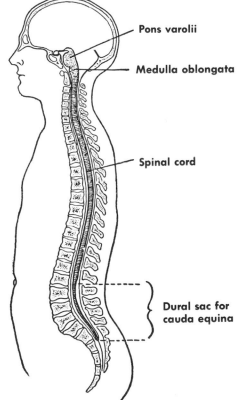

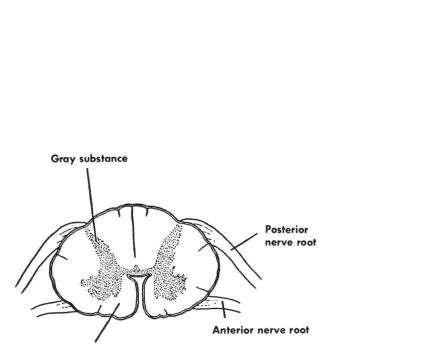

TRANSVERSE SECTION OF SPINAL CORD

SAGITTAL SECTION SHOWING SPINAL CORD

The ventricular system of the brain consists of four irregular, fluid-containing cavities that communicate with each other through connecting channels. The two upper cavities are an identical pair and are simply called *right* and *left lateral ventricles*. They are situated, one on each side of the median sagittal plane, in the lower, medial part of the corresponding hemisphere of the cerebrum. Radiographic centering for the lateral projection of these cavities is 1½ inches directly proximal to the level of the external auditory meatuses.

Each lateral ventricle consists of a central portion called the *body* of the cavity. The body is prolonged forward, backward, and downward into hornlike portions that give the ventricle an approximate U shape. The prolonged portions are known as the *anterior*, or *frontal*, the *posterior*, or *occipital*, and the *inferior*, or *temporal*, *cornua*, or *horns*. Each lateral ventricle is connected to the third ventricle by a channel called the *interventricular foramen*, or *foramen of Monro*, through which it communicates directly with the third ventricle and indirectly with the opposite lateral ventricle.

The *third ventricle* is a slitlike cavity with a somewhat quadrilateral shape. It is situated in the median sagittal plane just below the level of the bodies of the lateral ventricles. This cavity extends forward and downward from the pineal gland, which produces a recess in its posterior wall, to the optic chiasm, which produces a recess in its anterior inferior wall. Radiographic centering for the lateral projection of the third ventricle is 1 inch cranial to, and 1 inch anterior to, the external auditory meatus.

The interventricular foramina (Monro), one from each lateral ventricle, open into the upper anterior part of the third ventricle. The cavity is continuous posteroinferiorly with the fourth ventricle by a passage known as the *cerebral aqueduct*, or *aqueduct of Sylvius*.

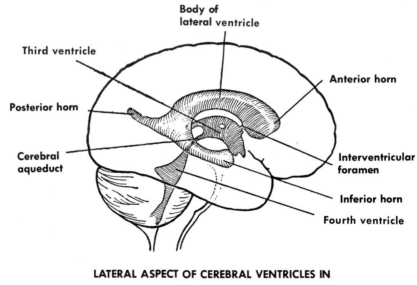

Body of lateral ventricle

Third ventricle

Anterior horn

Posterior horn

Cerebral aqueduct

Interventricular foramen

Inferior horn

Fourth ventricle

LATERAL ASPECT OF CEREBRAL VENTRICLES IN RELATION TO SURFACE OF BRAIN

The *fourth ventricle* is diamond-shaped and is the cavity of the hindbrain. It is situated in the median sagittal plane in front of the cerebellum and behind the pons varolii and the upper part of the medulla oblongata. Above, the fourth ventricle is continuous with the third ventricle by the cerebral aqueduct, and its pointed, distal end is continuous with the central canal of the medulla oblongata. A centrally placed opening, called the *foramen of Magendie*, is at the roof of the inferior portion of the ventricle. The ventricle communicates with the cisterna magna through the foramen of Magendie. Radiographic centering for lateral projections of the fourth ventricle is 1 inch directly posterior to the level of the external auditory meatuses.

The cerebrospinal fluid flows from the lateral ventricles into the third ventricle through the interventricular foramina. From the third ventricle, it passes through the cerebral aqueduct into the fourth ventricle, and from this cavity, it passes through the foramen of Magendie into the subarachnoid cisternae and channels.

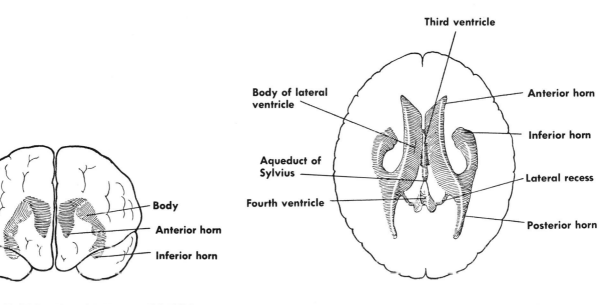

**ANTERIOR ASPECT OF LATERAL CEREBRAL VENTRICLES
IN RELATION TO SURFACE OF BRAIN**

**SUPERIOR ASPECT OF CEREBRAL VENTRICLES
IN RELATION TO SURFACE OF BRAIN**

Radiography of the central nervous system

Under central nervous system will be considered the radiologic procedures that are required for the investigation of (1) the ventricular cavities and subarachnoid spaces of the central nervous system by *cerebral pneumography* and *myelography*, (2) the nucleus pulposus of the intervertebral disks by *diskography*, and (3) the blood vessels of the brain by *cerebral angiography*.

CEREBRAL PNEUMOGRAPHY

Cerebral pneumography is a general term applied to the radiologic examination of the brain by means of the introduction of a gaseous medium into the ventricular system. Because of the radiographic homogeneity of the brain substance and fluid-containing channels, noncalcified lesions of the intracranial structures cannot be satisfactorily demonstrated without the use of a contrast medium. A gaseous medium—air, oxygen, or carbon dioxide—is generally used for this purpose in preference to radiopaque media because the gases produce less irritation in the ventricular system and because they are readily absorbable in the subarachnoid spaces. Some examiners advocate the use of a positive-contrast medium (Pantopaque) for investigations of the third ventricle and posterior fossa. This medium may be introduced by lumbar puncture,[1] or by selective ventricular cannulation through a burr hole in the cranium.[2-5]

[1]Stitt, H. L., Dunbar, H. S., Schick, R. W., and Dunn, A. A.: Pontocerebellar cisternography, Radiology **90**:942-945, 1968.

[2]Siqueira, E. B., Bucy, P. C., and Cannon, A. H.: Positive contrast ventriculography, cisternography and myelography, Amer. J. Roentgen. **104**:132-138, 1968.

[3]Wilkinson, H. A.: Selective third ventricular catheterization for Pantopaque ventriculography, Amer. J. Roentgen. **105**:348-351, 1969.

[4]Picaza, J. A., Hunter, S. E., and Cannon, B. W.: Axial ventriculography, J. Neurosurg. **33**:297-303, 1970.

[5]Lang, E. K., and Russell, J. R.: Pantopaque ventriculography; demonstration and assessment of the third ventricle and posterior fossa, J. Neurosurg. **32**:5-15, 1970.

The nonabsorbable oily contrast medium is removed by lumbar puncture.

Cerebral pneumography is employed to demonstrate space-occupying, intracranial lesions as shown by filling defects or deformations in the shadow outline of the gas-filled, ventricular system or of the subarachnoid cisternae and channels. *Pneumoventriculography* and *pneumoencephalography* are the two specific terms used respectively to denote the direct and the indirect routes of injection. These terms also indicate the extent of structural delineation obtained by each injection route. Direct injection of the gas into the central ventricular system delineates only the inner, or ventricular, surfaces of the brain, while indirect introduction of the gas by way of the subarachnoid route delineates the subarachnoid spaces of the brain as well as its ventricular system. Each procedure has specific indications and contraindications, so that the injection route is determined according to the type and location of the intracranial disorder. Cerebral pneumography was first performed by Dandy,[6,7] who introduced the method of pneumoventriculography in 1918 and of pneumoencephalography in 1919.

In pneumoencephalography, the medium is injected into the subarachnoid space by spinal puncture. The gas rises from the point of injection, and part of it enters the central ventricular system through the foramen of Magendie and part of it passes around the surface of the brain through the subarachnoid pathways. In pneumoventriculography, the gas is injected directly into the central ventricular system of the brain by trephination of the calvarium for

[6]Dandy, Walter E.: Ventriculography following the injection of air into the cerebral ventricles, Ann. Surg. **68**:5-11, 1918.

[7]Dandy, Walter E.: Roentgenography of the brain after the injection of air into the spinal canal, Ann. Surg. **70**:397-403, 1919.

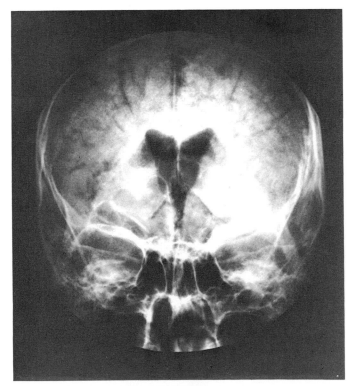

Pneumoencephalogram.

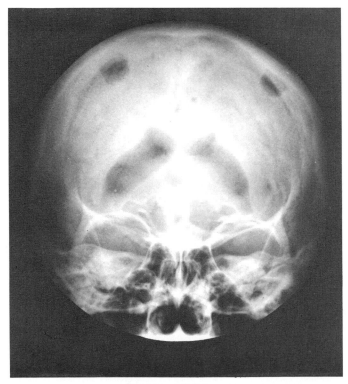

Pneumoventriculogram.

Radiographs courtesy Dr. Ernest H. Wood.

872

the introduction of a needle into one or both lateral ventricles. By this method of injection, all of the gas remains within the ventricular system for some time. Thus, because of the point of injection of the gas, the encephalographic method delineates the cortical surfaces of the brain and the subarachnoid cisternae as well as the ventricular system, whereas the ventriculographic method demonstrates only the ventricular system.

INJECTION PROCEDURES

The preparation of the patient for pneumoventriculography is an operating room procedure. Except in the case of infants, in whom the needle is introduced into the ventricular system through the open anterior fontanel or through an open suture, the neurosurgeon makes one or two small trephine openings in the calvarium, usually one on each side of the median sagittal plane in line with the oc-

cipital horns of the lateral ventricles. He then inserts a needle through the burr hole and passes it through the brain substance and into the respective lateral ventricle. After the injection of the desired amount of gas by a balanced exchange of cerebral fluid and gas, the incisions are closed and dressed, and the patient is transported to the radiology department, ready for filming.

The preparation of the patient for pneumoencephalography consists of a spinal puncture, which is usually performed in the radiology department. Whenever possible, the patient is placed in the seated-erect position before a vertical grid for the spinal puncture, the introduction of the gas, and the initial filming. Unless a chair of special construction is available, the patient is seated astride an ordinary straight-backed chair, with his upper forehead resting against the grid front.

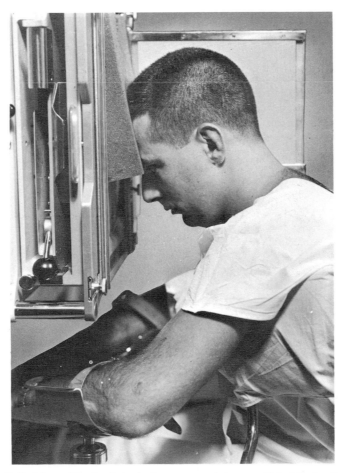

Patient in position for first set of pneumoencephalograms. Note lateral grid-cassette holder.

CEREBRAL PNEUMOGRAPHY—cont'd

INJECTION PROCEDURES—cont'd

While encephalographic injection techniques vary, the method of exchanging a large volume of cerebrospinal fluid and gas preceding the initial filming has generally been replaced by the fractional injection technique. In the latter method, a much smaller total amount of gas is used, and the initial films are taken after each of several small injections. These films delineate the fourth ventricle, the cerebral aqueduct, and the basal cisternae. Following these studies, an additional injection is made so that the lateral ventricles will be filled adequately. Regardless of the method of injection, the ventricular cavities are never fully drained and insufflated; thus it is necessary to redistribute the fluid and air posturally in order to delineate the different portions of the ventricles.

SPINAL PUNCTURE

Spinal puncture is the general term applied to the surgical procedure in which a long, hollow needle is introduced into the subarachnoid space in order to withdraw cerebrospinal fluid (for this purpose, the procedure is referred to as a *spinal tap*), or in order to inject a medicinal substance. Spinal taps are performed to obtain fluid specimens for diagnostic purposes and to relieve increased intracranial pressure by the withdrawal of fluid. Spinal punctures are also performed for the purpose of injecting therapeutic substances, spinal anesthetics, and, of interest to our specialty, contrast agents for radiologic investigations of brain and cord lesions.

For the injection of a contrast medium, the entrance is sometimes made into the cisterna magna (the procedure is called a *cisternal puncture*) or, more frequently, into the lower canal between the third and fourth lumbar spinous processes (the procedure is called a *lumbar puncture*), but the canal may be entered at other levels. Preceding a cisternal injection, the puncture site must be shaved; this is usually done before the patient is brought to the radiology department.

In order to prevent the possibility of meningeal infection, spinal punctures are carried out under rigid aseptic technique. However, the procedure is comparatively simple, so that once the sterile equipment is exposed and ready for the physician's use, he does not require the assistance of a nurse.

The following *sterile items* are required for this procedure: (1) surgical gloves, and a mask and gown for the surgeon (both of the latter are often omitted), (2) a fenestrated sheet or towels and towel clips for draping the patient, (3) a hypodermic syringe and needles for the injection of the local anesthetic solution, (4) a selection of spinal puncture needles, each with a close-fitting stylet, (5) syringes for the withdrawal of spinal fluid and for the injection of the contrast medium, (6) medicine glasses, (7) gauze squares and cotton balls, and (8) sponge forceps.

The following *nonsterile items* are used: (1) an antiseptic solution for cleansing the skin, (2) a vial of the specified local anesthetic solution, (3) a waste basin, (4) contrast medium, if one other than air is to be used, and (5) a small prepared dressing for application to the puncture site after the removal of the needle.

When a spinal tap has not been previously performed, the following items will be needed: (1) a manometer for measuring the cerebrospinal fluid pressure, (2) a sterile adapter or a sterile 6-inch length of rubber tubing with an inserted glass connector and adapters at each end, and (3) sterile test tubes for collecting fluid specimens.

The sterile tray may be obtained from the respective nursing staff or from the central sterile supply room. Otherwise, it must be prepared by a qualified member of the technological staff.

PATIENT CARE

Whenever possible, these patients are examined under suitable sedation and local anesthesia so that they will be able to cooperate for the filming procedure. The patient must be moved carefully and slowly for the numerous position changes in order to prevent unnecessary discomfort, and he must be shown every consideration possible. Patients who require close observation and care should be attended by a qualified assistant so that the technologist is free to give his undivided attention to the technical aspects of the examination.

PREPARATION OF EXAMINING ROOM

The examining room should be prepared completely in advance so that the examination can be started without delay as soon as the patient is brought into the radiology department. The ventriculographic patient arrives ready for filming, but the equipment necessary for a preceding spinal puncture must be ready for the encephalographic patient.

The radiographic equipment should be checked and adjusted according to the procedure to be followed. The table and overhead equipment must be cleaned carefully. The identification markers should be prepared, and all accessories, such as cassettes, cassette holder for cross-table projections, and compression devices, should be ready. Immobilization devices serve their purpose with patients who are conscious and with those who are under general anesthesia. It is often necessary that the head be positioned accurately and held for the exposures. This requires the skill of a physician or a qualified technologist, who must be properly protected against radiation exposure.

Arrangements should be made for each set of films to be processed immediately and to be presented to the radiologist for inspection before the body position is changed for the next set of films.

EXPOSURE TECHNIQUE

For the purpose of minimizing bone detail, many radiologists recommend the use of a high-kilovoltage exposure technique for cerebral pneumography. Where this is not the practice, the exposure factors used for noncontrast studies of the cranium are used for cerebral pneumography, except that it is frequently necessary to convert the milliampere-second factor to a short-time–high-current combination in order to prevent motion.

When the patient is not able to suspend respiration for the exposures, his breathing should be watched, and the exposures should be made at the rest phase of exhalation, with the use of the shortest exposure time possible.

874

SOMERSAULT CHAIR

In addition to a number of excellently designed Potter-Bucky head units that greatly facilitate the performance of both plain and contrast cerebral procedures, several pneumographic units, either incorporating or consisting of a motor-driven somersault chair, have been developed during the past decade. The purpose of the somersault maneuvers is to ensure air-filling of the various parts of the ventricular system and subarachnoid spaces after the completion of the initial filling films.

Somersault chair apparatus ranges from highly sophisticated, commercially constructed equipment such as the Potts[1] all-purpose head unit to homemade somersault chairs such as the one described by Baker.[2] Most of the chairs can be rotated for brow-down, brow-up, and hanging-head positions, and they can be converted to a table. Two x-ray tubes and two film holders are utilized, one pair for lateral projections and one pair for frontal projections.

The patient is securely strapped into the chair in the seated position. The head is rested on the chin support, adjusted in slight flexion, and firmly immobilized. The position of the chair is then adjusted by motor control. It is brought forward or backward and raised or lowered so as to bring the patient's head, or the area of interest within the head, to a predetermined point in space, the central point of the apparatus. With the head so adjusted, it remains accurately centered to the stationary, laterally placed film and tube and to the axis of rotation of the frontal film and tube for both direct and angulated projections throughout all maneuvers of the chair. The chair can be rotated through a complete forward or backward somersault and through a small arc during an exposure to obtain a single sweep tomogram. The new modified Potts head unit incorporates biplane image-amplifier–television systems, linear tomography, and lateral movement of the chair.

The construction and use of the several types of somersault chair apparatus have been ably described elsewhere, and since a detailed description of equipment is beyond the scope of this text, interested readers are referred to the articles listed below and to others listed in the bibliography.

The type of equipment selected by the radiologist is always based on the volume of work—whether he needs sophisticated equipment to expedite handling of the work load. Where costly apparatus cannot be so justified, high-quality cerebral studies can be obtained with comparatively simple equipment.

[1]Potts, D. G.: A new universal head unit, Amer. J. Roentgen. **95**:957-961, 1965.
[2]Baker, H. L.: Pneumoencephalography; a challenge in technique, Seminars Roentgen. 5:126-137, 1970.

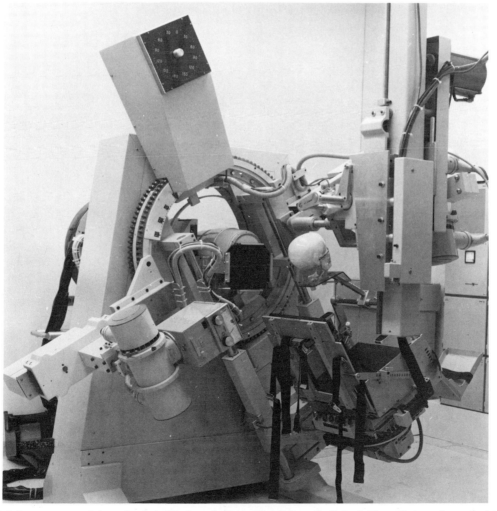

Modified "concentric" chair for pneumoencephalography. A skull is shown in the position of the patient's head. The patient may be manipulated through a forward or backward somersault with the center of the head remaining at the same point throughout the maneuver. The unit incorporates two tubes, one for frontal projections and one for lateral projections. It may be used to perform frontal or lateral linear tomography.

Photograph and legend courtesy Dr. D. Gordon Potts.

875

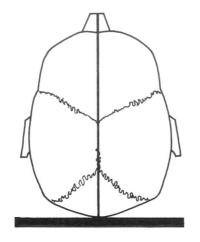

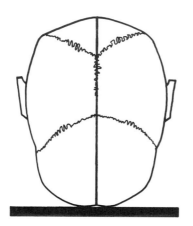

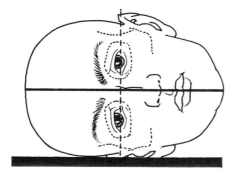

CEREBRAL PNEUMOGRAPHY—cont'd

POSITIONING OF THE HEAD

In approaching cerebral pneumography, the student must remember that the importance of accurate adjustment of the head cannot be overemphasized. Even a minimal angulation of the median sagittal plane of the head can result in enough distortion of the air shadows to obscure a space-occupying lesion that can be shown only by a midline deviation, or it can result in enough distortion of the air shadows to simulate one that does not exist. The median sagittal plane of the head must be *exactly* perpendicular to the plane of the film for frontal and basal projections, and *exactly* parallel with the plane of the film for lateral projections. Therefore, the head must be positioned accurately and immobilized rigidly.

ANGULATION OF CENTRAL RAY

The head adjustments and the central ray angulations that are used for frontal and basal projections are usually based on the *orbitomeatal line* for cerebral pneumography, and on the *infraorbitomeatal line* for cerebral angiography. Unless the head can be adjusted so that the specified localization line is placed at right angles to the plane of the film, or at the specified angle to the film, the difference must be determined, and then the central ray angulation must be adjusted accordingly. A few examples of such adjustments are shown in the illustrations below.

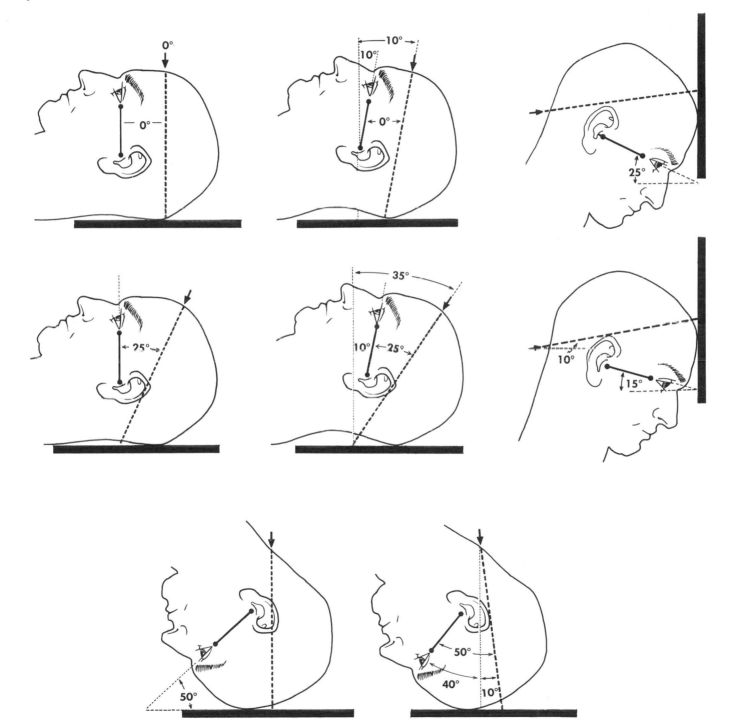

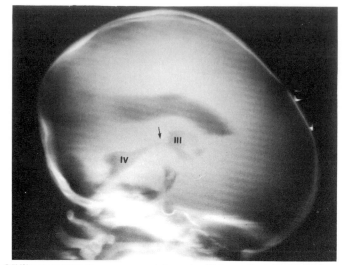

Midline tomogram in pneumoencephalography. Note excellent detail of cisterna magna, fourth ventricle (IV), aqueductus (arrow), posterior third ventricle (III), and interpeduncular cistern.

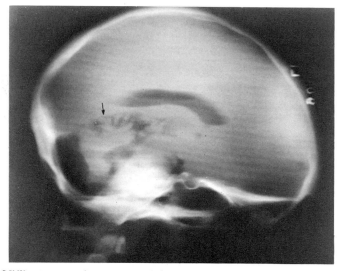

Midline tomogram in pneumoencephalography. In addition to structures visualized in above film, note air outlining the cerebellar folia (arrow).

Radiographs and diagnostic information courtesy Dr. K. Y. Chynn.

CEREBRAL PNEUMOGRAPHY—cont'd

ANGULATION OF CENTRAL RAY—cont'd

The adjustment of the patient's head, the angulation of the central ray, and the number and sequence of the projections that are used in cerebral pneumography vary according to the area under investigation and to the radiologist's findings as the examination proceeds. In the usual routine procedure, a minimum of one pair of right-angle views (frontal and lateral) is made in the erect position and one pair in each of the basic recumbent positions (supine, prone, and right and left lateral). Half-axial projections (25- to 30-degree caudal and cranial central ray angulations) are taken in each of the frontal positions. Each pair, or set, of these studies is made without changing the position of the patient's head in order to avoid altering the air-fluid distribution. Other positions that are employed are a horizontal lateral projection, with the head in extension from the supine position, and a horizontal lateral and a vertical projection, with the head in flexion from the prone position. The head is lowered over the end of the table for these studies. Except for the erect studies, which may not be made, the views that are employed in pneumoventriculography are the same as those that are employed in pneumoencephalography.

Any one or more of the basic positions may be projected stereoscopically. The supplemental positions are usually projected in single plane. Without special equipment, the horizontally projected studies are made with grid-front cassettes or a stationary grid.

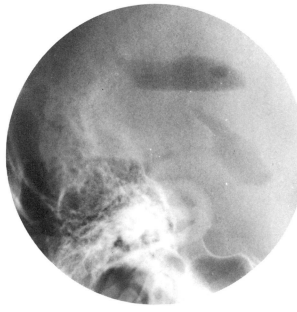

Stationary exposure, fourth ventricle.

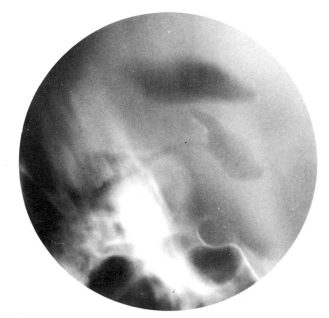

Autotomogram of opposite patient. Compare visualization of fourth ventricle.

Radiographs courtesy Dr. John A. Goree.

AUTOTOMOGRAPHY

Tomography, or if the necessary equipment is not available, autotomography,[1] is employed in pneumoencephalography. In the fractional injection method, a lateral autotomogram may be made for the demonstration of the fourth ventricle, the aqueduct of Sylvius, and the basal cisternae while the patient is seated with his head resting against the grid-front in the original position. This is done immediately following the initial postero-anterior and lateral projections.

The autotomographic maneuver consists of having the patient rock his head gently to-and-fro through an approximate 10-degree arc, as if signifying "no," during an exposure of from one to two and one-half seconds. With the forehead acting as the central axis, the practically stationary midline structures are clearly delineated, while the laterally placed, moving petrosae are blurred. Autotomography may also be employed for the delineation of the antero-inferior portion of the third ventricle. This study is made with the head extended over the end of the table from the supine position, and with the central ray directed horizontally.

Johnston and associates[2] suggest that the ears be taped forward for lateral projections of the fourth ventricle and the cerebral aqueduct. After the exposure of the initial set of erect films, and with the patient's head maintained in the original flexed position, Johnston obtains an oblique lateral projection in which the occiput is turned 7 to 10 degrees away from the film.

[1]Ziedses des Plantes, B. G.: Examen du troisième et du quatrième ventricule au moyen de petites quantités d'air, Acta Radiol. **34**:399-407, 1950.
[2]Johnston, J. D. H., Alexander, G. H., and Rosomoff, H. L.: A simplified method for the pneumoencephalographic demonstration of the fourth ventricle and aqueduct of Sylvius, J. Neurosurg. **20**:81-83, 1963.

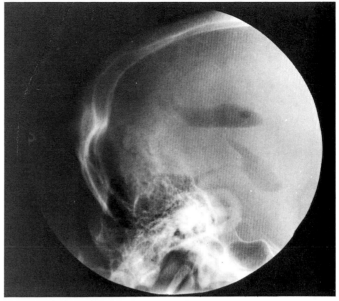

Stationary exposure, fourth ventricle.

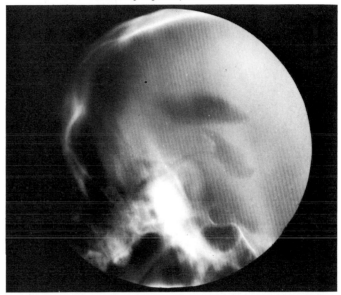

Autotomogram of above patient.

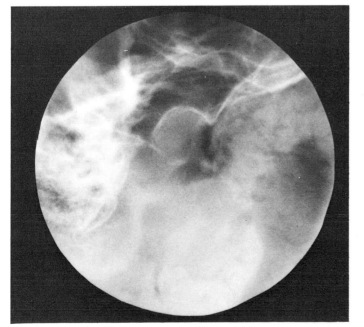

Stationary exposure, third ventricle.

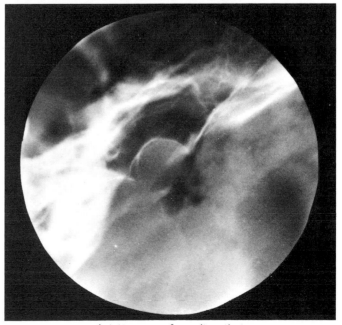

Autotomogram of opposite patient.

Radiographs courtesy Dr. John A. Goree.

879

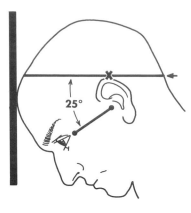

PNEUMOENCEPHALOGRAPHY
First set of upright studies in the fractional injection method

The first set of upright fractional pneumoencephalograms is made after the initial injection of gas. These studies delineate the fourth ventricle, the aqueduct of Sylvius, the cisterna magna, and the vallecula of the cerebellum. Preceding the injection, the patient's head is positioned and immobilized. Cross-table lateral and posteroanterior projections of the above structures are made without altering the position of the head. The illustrated head position shows the orbitomeatal line at an angle of 25 degrees, open forward, to the horizontal plane, but some examiners employ a greater angulation.

1. The initial study, a soft tissue lateral projection of the foramen magnum, is made with the central ray directed through the region of the mastoid process.

2. The lateral studies of the fourth ventricle, both still and autotomographic, are made with the central ray directed to a point just above the auricle. (See radiographs on pages 878 and 879.)

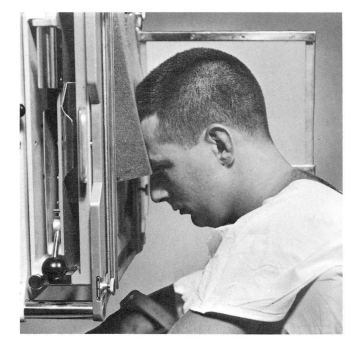

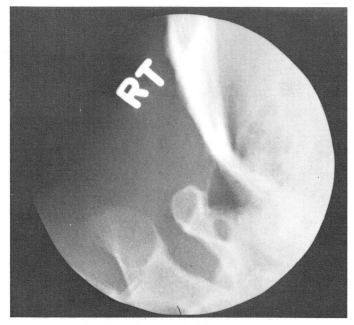

Coned, soft tissue lateral of foramen magnum.

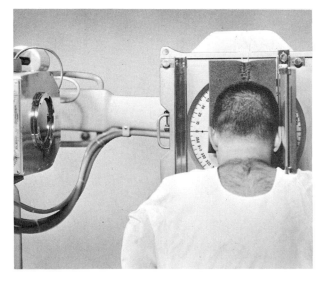

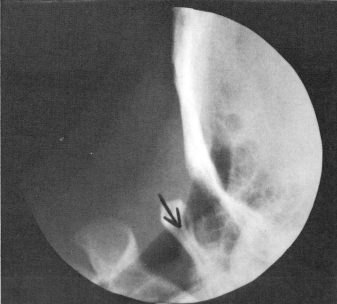

As above, on patient having herniated cerebellar tonsil (arrow) from brain tumor.

Radiographs and diagnostic information courtesy Dr. John A. Goree.

Posteroanterior projections of the fourth ventricle, and of the fourth ventricle and the vallecula, are made with the central ray directed through the head just above the level of the auricles.

1. For a supraorbital view of the fourth ventricle, the central ray is angled caudally so that it is parallel with the supraorbitomeatal line.

2. For direct posteroanterior delineation of the fourth ventricle and the vallecula, the central ray is directed horizontally.

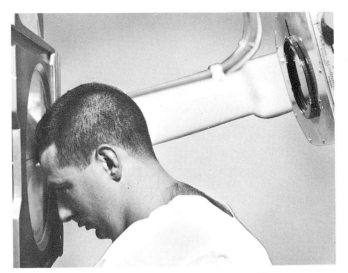

Central ray parallel with supraorbitomeatal line.

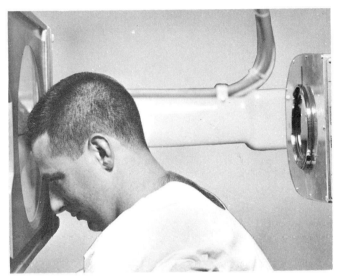

Central ray horizontal.

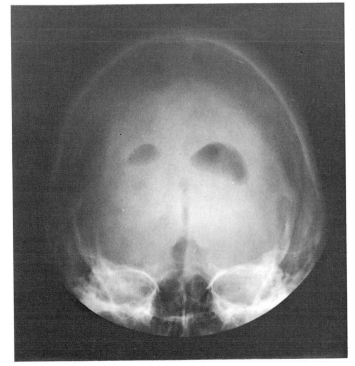

Posteroanterior supraorbital projection of fourth ventricle.

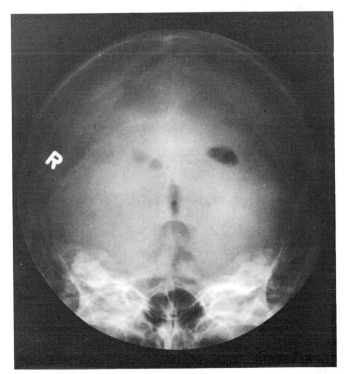

Direct posteroanterior projection of fourth ventricle and vallecula.

Radiographs courtesy Dr. John A. Goree.

881

PNEUMOENCEPHALOGRAPHY—cont'd
Second set of upright studies in the fractional injection method

For the demonstration of the basal cisterns, the patient's head is extended while a second injection of gas is given. The head is then readjusted and immobilized in the original, angled position for two posteroanterior projections, after which it is positioned for the lateral study.

1. The first posteroanterior cisternal projection is made with the central ray passing through the head just above the level of the auricles at a cranial angle of 5 degrees.

2. The second posteroanterior projection is made with the central ray directed as above but at a cranial angle of 15 degrees.

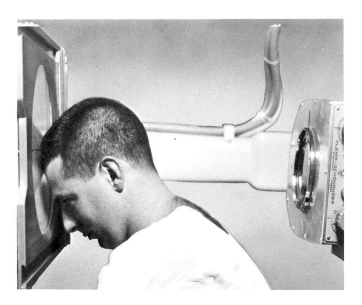

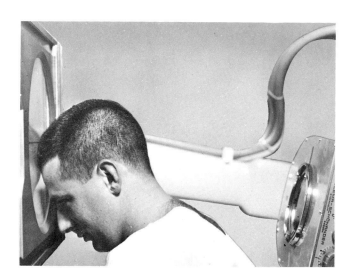

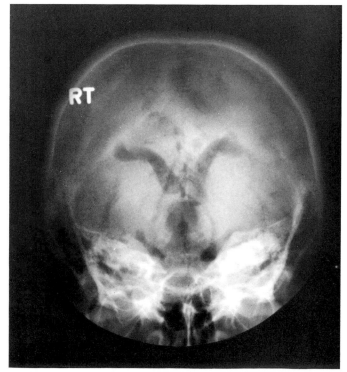

Central ray angled 5 degrees cranially.

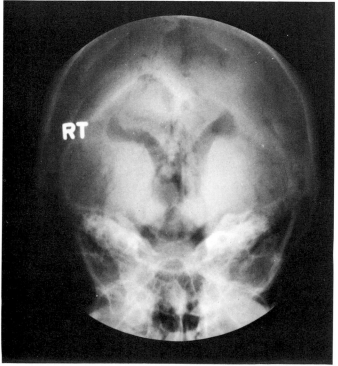

Central ray angled 15 degrees cranially.

Radiographs courtesy Dr. John A. Goree.

For lateral delineation of the basal cisterns, the head is adjusted so that the orbitomeatal line is horizontal. The central ray is directed through the sella turcica, a point ¾ inch anterior to, and ¾ inch above, the external auditory meatus.

This head position is sometimes used for the demonstration of the roofs of the lateral and third ventricles. For this purpose, the centering is just above the auricles.

Following satisfactory delineation of the basal cisterns, sufficient gas is injected for the demonstration of the third and lateral ventricles. The spinal puncture needle is then removed, and the patient is placed in the recumbent position.

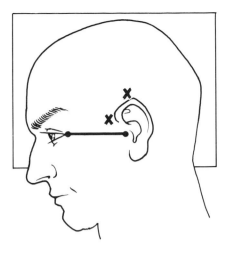

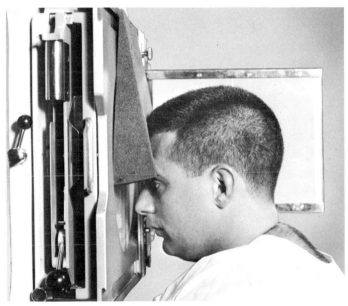

Head in neutral position (orbitomeatal line horizontal).

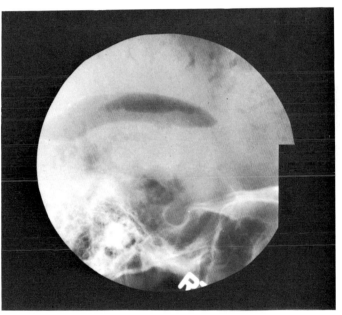

Coned lateral projection of basal cisterns.

Courtesy Dr. John A. Goree.

883

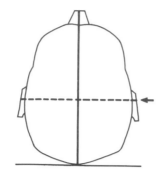

PNEUMOENCEPHALOGRAPHY AND PNEUMOVENTRICULOGRAPHY

Brow-up position

The brow-up position is used to permit the gas to rise into the frontal and temporal horns of the lateral ventricles, and into the anterior portion of the third ventricle.

The patient's head is rested on a radioparent support to center it to the vertically placed grid-cassette holder for cross-table lateral projections. The head is adjusted so that the orbitomeatal line is vertical and is then immobilized.

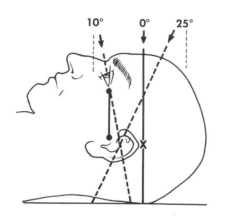

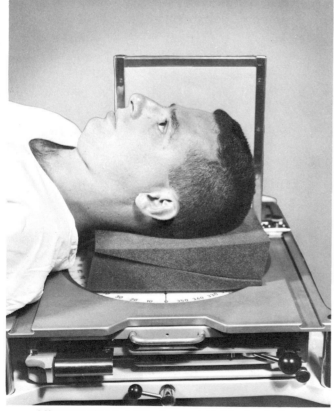

Adjustment of head and film for cross-table lateral projection.

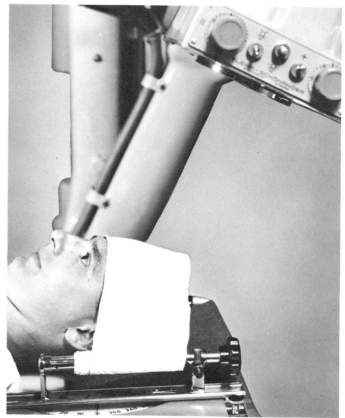

Adjustment of head and tube for half-axial projection.

The usual frontal views that are taken in this position are (1) a 10-degree cranial angulation, with the central ray directed through the center of the orbits, for the demonstration of the temporal horns through the orbital shadows, and (2) a 25- to 30-degree caudal angulation (basic half-axial anteroposterior projection), with the central ray entering at the hairline. A direct anteroposterior projection, with the central ray entering at the midpoint between the supraorbital ridge and the hairline, is sometimes taken.

In addition to the basic cross-table lateral projection, for which the central ray is directed to a point just cranial to the auricle, a lateral autotomogram may be taken for better delineation of the third ventricle. For the latter study, the central ray is directed to a point 1 inch anterior, and 1 inch cranial, to the external auditory meatus.

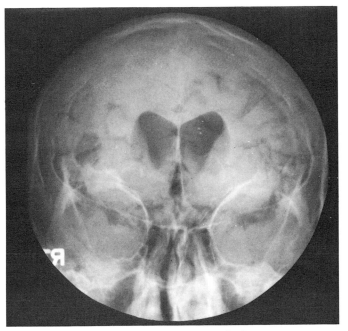

Transorbital anteroposterior projection.

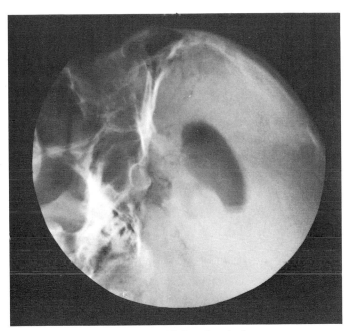

Brow-up cross-table lateral projection.

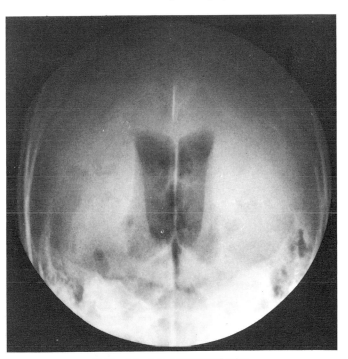

Half-axial anteroposterior projection.

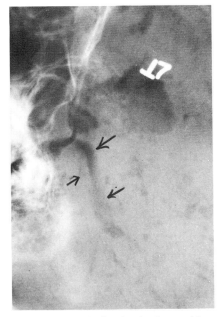

Brow-up lateral projection showing temporal horn.

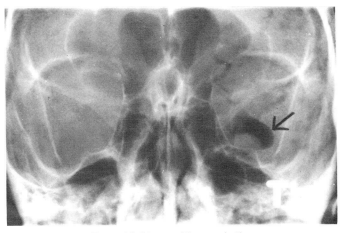

Transorbital temporal horn projection.

Radiographs courtesy Dr. John A. Goree.

885

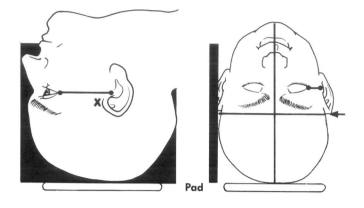

PNEUMOENCEPHALOGRAPHY AND PNEUMOVENTRICULOGRAPHY—cont'd
Lateral projection with head in extension

The purpose of this position, sometimes called the supine "hanging-head" position, is the delineation of the anteroinferior portion of the third ventricle.

The patient's head is extended from the supine position and is rested on a soft pad that is placed on a suitable support. The head is adjusted so that the orbitomeatal line is as nearly horizontal as possible, and so that the median sagittal plane is parallel with the plane of the vertically placed grid-front cassette.

The central ray is directed horizontally and is centered at the approximate level of the sella turcica, a point ¾ inch anterior, and ¾ inch cranial, to the external auditory meatus.

A lateral autotomogram may be taken with the patient in this position.

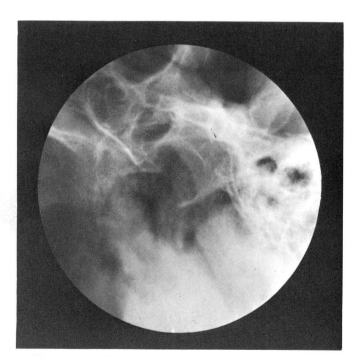

Conventional stationary projection.

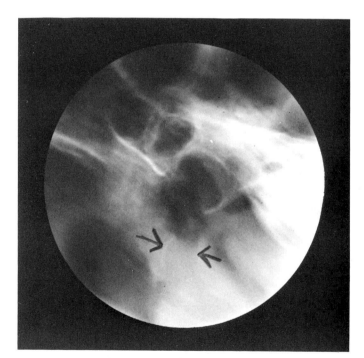

Autotomogram of opposite patient.

Radiographs courtesy Dr. John A. Goree.

886

Brow-down position

In the prone, or brow-down, position, the gas rises to fill the occipital horns of the lateral ventricles, the posterior portion of the third ventricle, and the fourth ventricle.

The patient's head is elevated on a radioparent support so that it is centered to the vertically placed grid-front cassette for lateral projections. The head is adjusted so that its median sagittal plane and the orbitomeatal line are vertical.

The usual studies made in this position consist of (1) a direct posteroanterior projection, with the central ray entering 2 inches cranial to the external auditory meatus, (2) a 25- to 30-degree, cranially inclined angulation (reverse half-axial projection), with the central ray entering at the external occipital protuberance, and (3) a cross-table lateral projection, with the central ray entering just cranial to the auricle. Satisfactory filling of the fourth ventricle by the ventricular injection method sometimes requires that the head be strongly flexed from the prone position. A horizontal lateral projection is made, and usually is referred to as the prone "hanging head" position.

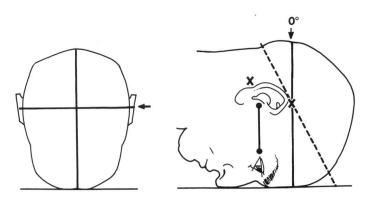

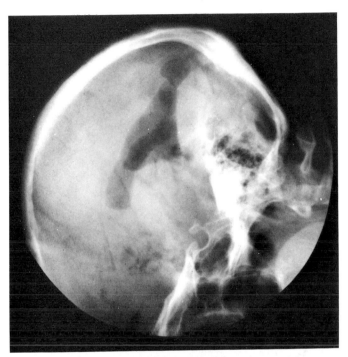

Brow-down lateral projection.

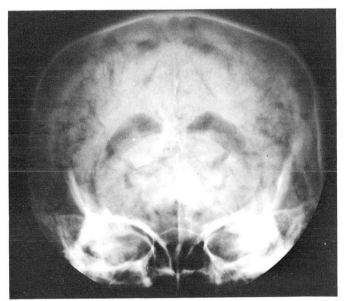

Direct or supraorbital posteroanterior projection.

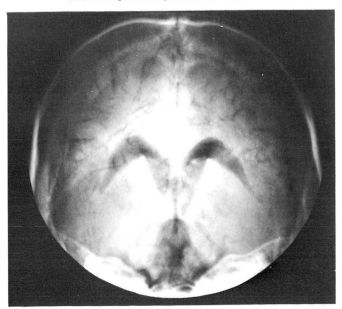

Reverse half-axial projection.

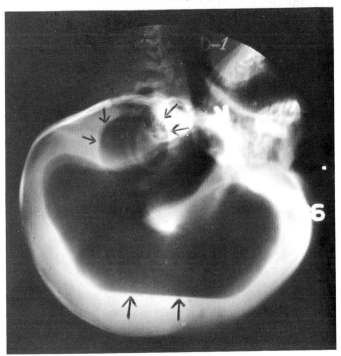

Prone hanging-head pneumoventriculogram showing an outlet obstruction to fourth ventricle (upper arrows). Note air-fluid level in lateral ventricles (lower arrows).

Radiographs and diagnostic information courtesy Dr. John A. Goree.

887

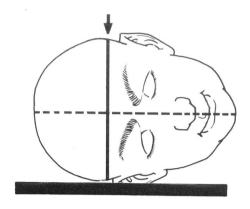

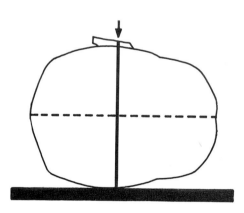

PNEUMOENCEPHALOGRAPHY AND PNEUMOVENTRICULOGRAPHY—cont'd

Recumbent lateral positions

In the lateral recumbent head position, the gas rises to fill the uppermost lateral ventricle. Both sides are examined.

The patient is rotated to a semiprone position and is adjusted so that the external auditory meatuses of the laterally placed head are over the midline of the grid. The head is adjusted so that the infraorbitomeatal line is parallel with the transverse axis of the film and so that the median sagittal plane is exactly horizontal. A suitable support is placed under the side of the jaw to prevent rotation, and the head is then immobilized.

For a single-plane projection, the central ray enters 1½ inches cranial to the external auditory meatus.

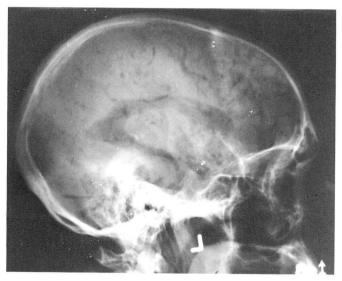

Radiograph courtesy Dr. John A. Goree.

888

MYELOGRAPHY

Myelography (Gr. *myelos* marrow; the spinal cord) is the general term applied to radiologic examinations of the central nervous system structures situated within the spinal canal. These examinations are performed by means of introducing a contrast medium into the subarachnoid space by spinal puncture. Myelography is employed for the purpose of demonstrating the site and extent of lesions of the spinal cord and nerve roots, space-occupying lesions such as cord tumors, and encroachment by posterior protrusion of herniated intervertebral disks. These lesions become evident by causing a deformity in, or by blocking the passage of, the column of contrast material. The contrast agent may be either a gaseous medium or an opaque medium, referred to specifically as *gas myelography* and *opaque myelography*. Gas myelography was first introduced by Dandy[1] in 1919, and opaque myelography was introduced by Sicard and Forestier[2] in 1922.

[1]Dandy, Walter E.: Roentgenography of the brain after the injection of air into the spinal canal, Ann. Surg. **70**:397-403, 1919.
[2]Sicard, J. A., and Forestier, J.: Méthode générale d'exploration radiologique par l'huile iodée (lipiodol) Bull. Soc. Med. Hop. Paris **46**:463-469, 1922.

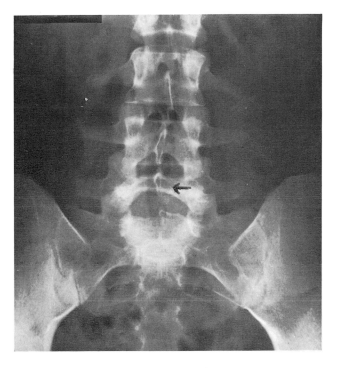

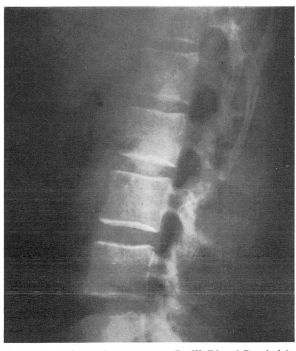

Gas myelograms courtesy Dr. W. Edward Chamberlain.

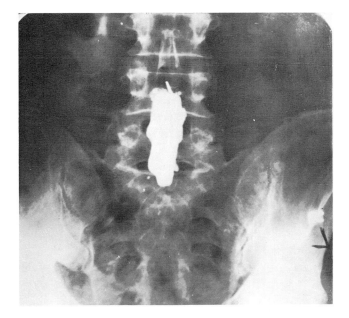

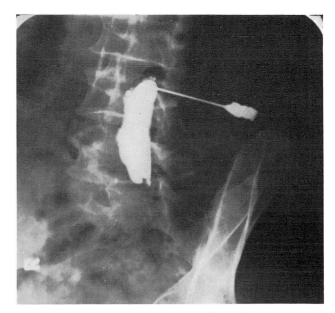

Opaque myelograms courtesy Dr. C. Wadsworth Schwartz.

MYELOGRAPHY—cont'd

CONTRAST MEDIA

Some examiners use one of the water-soluble media for opaque myelography, but an oil-based medium is more generally employed in this country. Air and oxygen (more frequently air) are the media used for gas myelography. The movement of the contrast column along the subarachnoid space depends upon gravity. Therefore, a tilting radioscopic-radiographic table with a footboard and, unless a canvas harness is used, a padded shoulder support are required. The two types of media used, due to the difference in their weight, move in opposite directions; that is, the gas rises, whereas the heavy, opaque media gravitate downward. The long axis of the body is angled accordingly.

PREPARATION OF PATIENT

Unless contraindicated, it is desirable to clear the colon for examinations involving the lumbar region of the spinal canal. The physician's orders pertaining to colonic cleansing, dietary restrictions (the preceding meal is withheld), and any necessary premedication are carried out by the respective nursing staff.

PREPARATION OF EXAMINING ROOM

One of the responsibilities of the technologic staff is the preparation of the examining room in advance of the time appointed for the arrival of the patient. The radiographic equipment should be checked, and as for every procedure involving aseptic technique, the table and overhead equipment must be carefully cleaned. The footboard should be attached, and unless a canvas harness is used, the padded shoulder support should be placed and ready for adjustment to the patient's height.

In the absence of image intensification equipment, there should be an ample supply of cassettes for spot films as well as for conventional studies. Each accessory needed or likely to be needed should be at hand. Identification markers and side markers should be ready for use. Arrangements should be made for prompt processing of the films as the examination proceeds.

The spinal puncture and the injection of the contrast medium are performed in the radiology department. This precaution is taken to eliminate the possibility of the medium entering and becoming trapped in the cerebral ventricles, and in the case of oil myelography, to prevent fragmentation or globulation of the medium as a result of moving the patient. The sterile tray and the nonsterile items required for the spinal puncture and the injection of the contrast medium (page 874) should be ready for convenient placement.

Shapiro,[1] and Wendth and Moriarty[2] suggest that a sterile plastic tubing about 16 inches long be used to connect the syringe to the needle for the withdrawal of the oily contrast medium under radioscopic control. The tubing allows the examiner to keep his hands well outside the field of radiation.

[1]Shapiro, R.: Myelography, ed. 2, Chicago, 1968, Yearbook Medical Publishers, Inc.
[2]Wendth, A. J., and Moriarty, D. J.: A simplified method for the rapid removal of myelographic contrast agent, Radiology 93:1092, 1969.

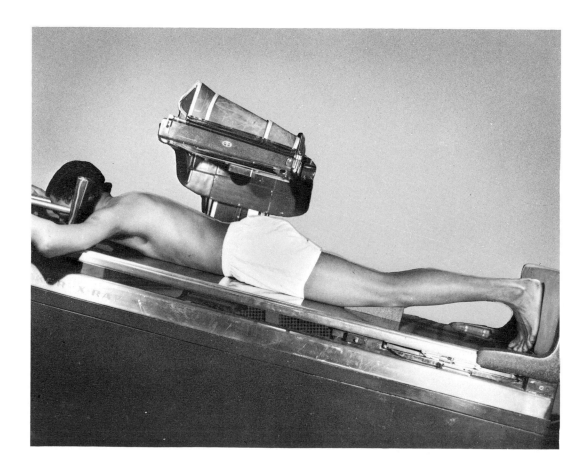

EXAMINATION PROCEDURE

The mechanical details of the myelographic procedure should be explained to the patient before the examination in order to alleviate any apprehension and to prevent alarm at unexpected maneuvers during the procedure. Where image intensification equipment is not available, the patient should be told that the room must be darkened during radioscopy. He should be told why there must be repeated and acute changes in the angulation of the examining table, and why his head must be maintained in a fully extended position when the table is tilted to the Trendelenburg position. The patient must be assured of his safety when the table is acutely angled, and he must be assured that everything possible will be done to spare him unnecessary discomfort. As in every examination, full attention to the patient, together with a pleasant expression and a calm manner, will do much to reassure the patient.

Some radiologists prefer to have the patient placed on the table in the prone position for the spinal puncture. Others have the patient adjusted in the lateral position with the spine flexed, in order to widen the interspinous spaces for easier introduction of the needle.

The physician usually withdraws spinal fluid and injects the contrast medium in equal units of exchange, particularly where a large amount of gas is to be injected. After the injection has been completed, the traveling of the contrast column is observed radioscopically, and the direction of its flow is controlled by varying the angulation of the table. Spot studies, still and/or cineradiographic, are taken at the level of any blockage of, or distortion in, the outline of the contrast column. Conventional radiographic studies, with the central ray directed vertically or horizontally as indicated, are taken as directed by the radiologist. Cross-table projections are made with grid-front cassettes or a stationary grid, and they should be closely coned.

The position of the patient's head must be guarded as the contrast column nears the cervical area to prevent it from passing on into the cerebral ventricles. Strong extension of the head compresses the cisterna magna and thus prevents further ascent of the medium. Because the cisterna magna is situated posteriorly, neither forward nor lateral flexion of the head will compress the cisternal cavity. Unless the patient is fully conscious and able to follow instructions, a nurse or a second technologist should be present to hold the patient's head as needed; this assistant must be protected by a lead apron and lead gloves.

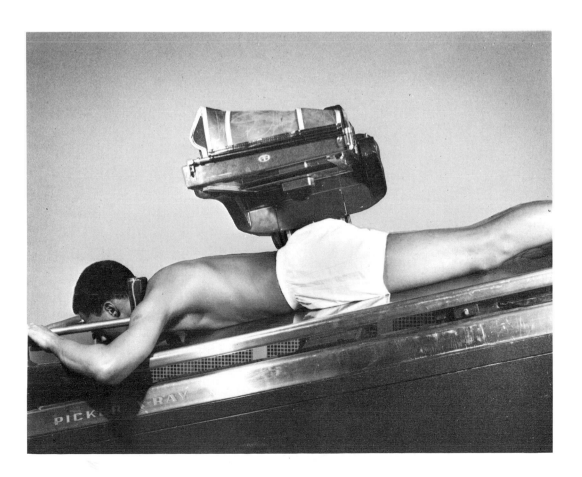

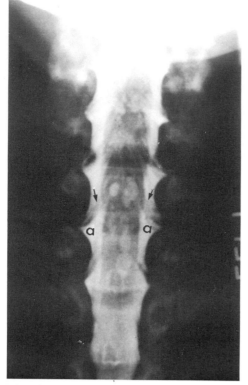

Normal cervical myelogram showing symmetrical nerve roots (arrows) and axillary pouches (**a a**) on both sides, as well as spinal cord.

OPAQUE MYELOGRAPHY

The lumbar region is the usual site of spinal puncture in opaque myelography, although the cisterna magna and a slightly lower area between the atlas and axis are other sites sometimes used.

Lumbar puncture is usually performed between the third and the fourth lumbar vertebrae, with the patient positioned according to the preference of the examining physician. The patient may be placed in the prone position, which he maintains, or he may be adjusted in the lateral position with the spine flexed for the insertion of the needle, and then turned to the prone position for the examination. The lumbar-puncture needle is left in situ for later aspiration of the opaque medium. The needle must be covered with a sterile towel and then protected from accidental bumping by adjusting the height of the radioscopic screen and securing it in position with the stop-lock device.

For *cisternal* or *cervical puncture* the patient is placed in the lateral position and asked to draw his knees up somewhat and fold his arms over his chest. The head is then elevated to spine level to place the external occipital protuberance in line with the spinous processes. It is supported, flexed well forward, on a firm pillow or folded sheets. With the puncture needle in position, the head end of the table is elevated enough to prevent leakage of the heavy, opaque medium into the ventricular system of the brain. After the needle has been removed and the puncture site has been dressed, the head is fully extended to compress the cisternal cavity. The table is then leveled and the patient is turned to the prone position or, less frequently, to the supine position for the examination.

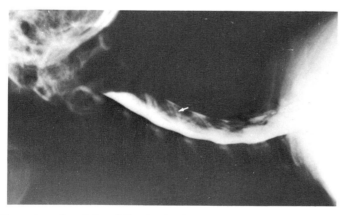

Prone shoot-through lateral film showing dentate ligament and posterior nerve roots (arrow).

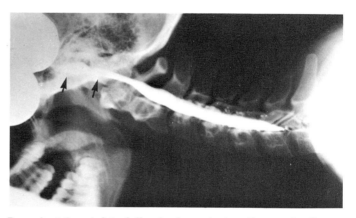

Prone shoot-through lateral film showing contrast medium passing foramen magnum and lying against lower clivus (arrows).

Radiographs and diagnostic information courtesy Dr. K. Y. Chynn.

Unlike gaseous media, opaque myelographic media are not readily absorbed; therefore, as much of the medium as possible is removed upon completion of the filming. When the injection is made by cisternal or cervical puncture, the needle must be removed for the examination. Withdrawal of the medium in this case requires a second spinal puncture, this time in the lumbar region, where the physician can pool it under the point of the needle for aspiration with a syringe.

NOTE: When the routine myelograms fail to show satisfactory filling of the root sleeves, the radiologist may attempt to fill them with the Queckenstedt[1] maneuver. This maneuver is performed by placing the hands on the neck and briefly (for four to five seconds) compressing the jugular veins. Pressure on the jugular veins causes a rapid rise in the pressure of the cerebrospinal fluid. Gilland and associates[2] report that the maneuver results in an average 38% increase in the diameter of the caudal sac and improved visualization of the root sleeves. Chin and Anderson[3] state that because of possible adverse effects, they never subject a patient with suspected intracranial disease or spinal block to jugular compression. When it is not contraindicated, they perform the Queckenstedt maneuver under radioscopic observation immediately before the removal of the contrast medium. With the patient prone and the table horizontal, the patient is instructed to breathe normally while brisk, bilateral jugular compression is performed, and one spot film is obtained when caudal distention is at the maximum.

[1]Queckenstedt, H.: Zur Diagnose der Rückenmarkskompression, Deutsche Z. Nervenheilk. **55**:325-333, 1916.

[2]Gilland, O., Chin, F., Anderson, W. B., and Nelson, J. R.: A cinemyelographic study of cerebrospinal fluid dynamics, Amer. J. Roentgen. **106**:369-375, 1969.

[3]Chin, F. K., and Anderson, W. B.: Improvement of root-sleeve filling in lumbar myelography with oil-soluble media, Radiology **96**:668-669, 1970.

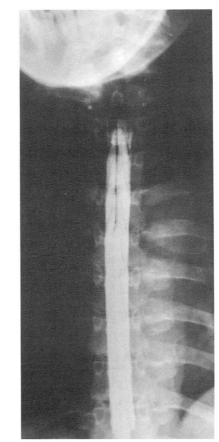

Thoracic myelogram taken in supine position showing anterior spinal vessels and thoracic nerve roots. 15 ml. of Pantopaque were used.

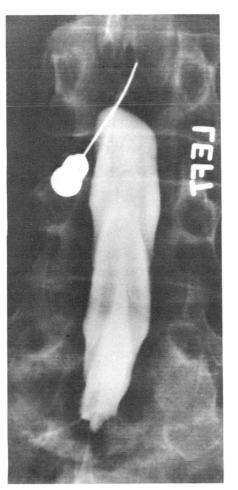

Frontal view of lumbar myelogram showing symmetrical axillary pouches and corresponding nerve roots.

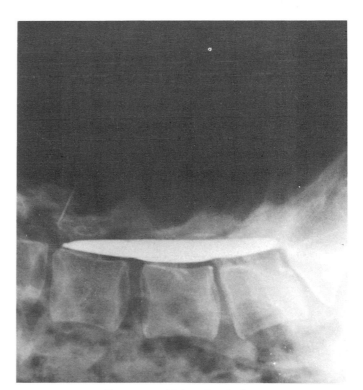

Prone cross-table lateral projection.

Radiographs and diagnostic information courtesy Dr. K. Y. Chynn.

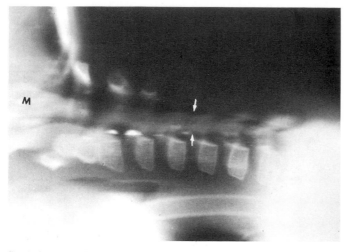

Cervical air myelography. Lateral tomogram showing clear delineation of anterior and posterior aspects (arrows) of cervical spinal cord extending through foramen magnum to medulla oblongata (**M**).

Courtesy Dr. K. Y. Chynn.

GAS MYELOGRAPHY

In the usual gas myelographic procedure the medium is introduced by way of lumbar puncture. According to the preference of the examining physician, the patient is adjusted in the prone position, or in the lateral position with the spine flexed. With the puncture needle in position, the head end of the table is lowered for the injection of the gas. This angulation of the long axis of the patient's body is made to hold the gaseous medium in the distal canal until the radiologist can direct and observe its passage along the subarachnoid space under radioscopy. When the desired amount of gas has been injected, the needle is removed and the puncture site is dressed. Because gaseous media are readily absorbable, no attempt is made to remove the medium after the examination.

By another injection method, the subarachnoid space of the spinal canal is fully drained and distended with gas, and it is then examined by a combination of conventional and tomographic studies. For this procedure the patient is placed on a tilting tomographic table, and the canal is entered by cisternal puncture. With the needle in position, the head end of the table is lowered, and equal fractional exchanges of spinal fluid and gas are made until no more fluid drains through the needle. After the injection of the desired amount of gas, and while maintaining the patient in the angled position, conventional and tomographic films are taken of the area under investigation. Because of the curve of the lumbar spine, sectional studies of the lower spine are made with the patient in the lateral and/or nearly lateral position.

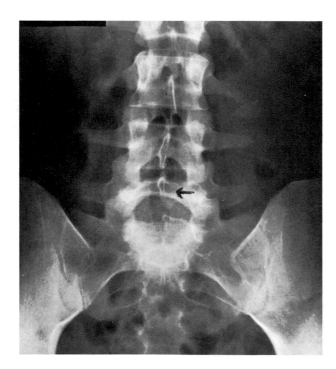

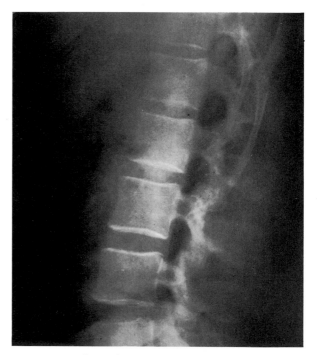

Gas myelograms courtesy Dr. W. Edward Chamberlain.

894

DISKOGRAPHY

Diskography and *nucleography* are terms used to denote the radiologic examination of individual intervertebral disks by means of the injection of a small quantity of one of the water-soluble, iodinated media into the center of the disk through a double-needle entry. This procedure was introduced by Lindblom[1] in 1950, and it has been described in excellent detail by Cloward[2,3] and by Butt.[4]

Diskography is used in the investigation of internal disk lesions that cannot be demonstrated by the myelographic method of examination, such as rupture of the nucleus pulposus. Diskography may be performed separately, or it may be combined with myelography. Cloward[2] states that the diskographic procedure requires no more than thirty minutes, including the processing of the films. He recommends that the patient be given local anesthesia only so that he will be fully conscious and therefore able to inform the physician as to the location of pain when the needles are inserted and the injection is made.

Except for procaine hydrochloride (Novocain), which is added to, and injected with, the contrast solution, and a double-needle rather than a standard spinal-puncture needle, the instrument setup is the same as for spinal puncture (page 874). The double-needle combination consists of an outer, large-bore needle (20-gauge) used to perform the spinal puncture and reach the annulus fibrosus of the disk, and a longer, fine needle (26-gauge), which is then passed through the guide needle and advanced to the center of the nucleus pulposus. The needle lengths are usually 2 and 2½ inches, respectively, for cervical entry, and 3½ and 5 inches for lumbar entry. The position of the needles is determined radiographically before the contrast medium is injected.

[1]Lindblom, Kurt: Technique and results in myelography and disc puncture, Acta Radiol. 34:321-330, 1950.
[2]Cloward, R. B., and Buzaid, L. L.: Discography, Amer. J. Roentgen. 68:552-564, 1952.
[3]Cloward, R. B.: Cervical discography: a contribution to the etiology and mechanism of neck, shoulder, and arm pain, Ann. Surg. 150:1052-1064, 1959.
[4]Butt, W. P.: Discography—some interesting cases, J. Canad. Ass. Radiol. 17:167-175, 1966.

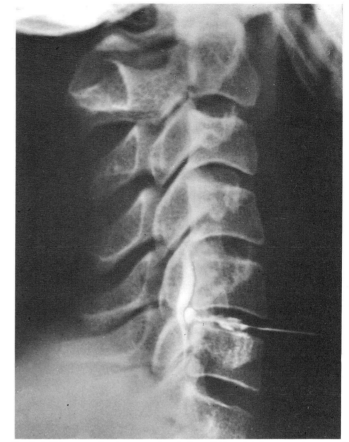

Cervical diskogram showing acute herniation of disk with fragment into spinal canal.

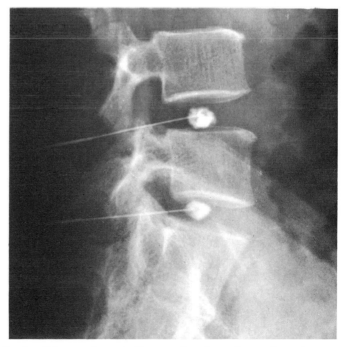

Lumbar diskogram demonstrating normal nucleus pulposus of round contour type.

Radiographs and diagnostic information courtesy Dr. Ralph B. Cloward.

895

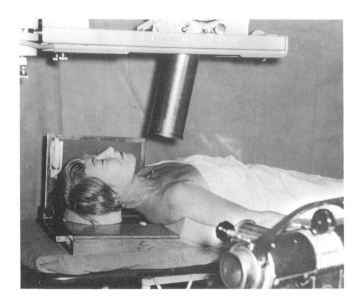

CERVICAL DISKOGRAPHY

In the absence of biplane equipment, cervical diskography requires the use of a cassette tunnel with a slot to hold a vertically placed film and the use of a mobile unit for cross-table lateral projections. The positioning of the patient and the placement of the film and x-ray tube for both frontal and lateral projections are shown in the opposite photograph. The central ray is directed at a cranial angle of 10 degrees for the anteroposterior projection; this angulation is adequate because of the reduction of the lordotic curve, caused by elevating the patient's head.

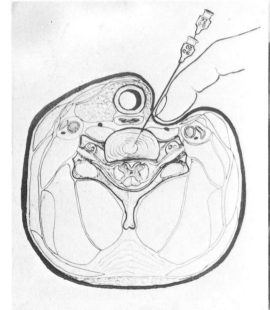
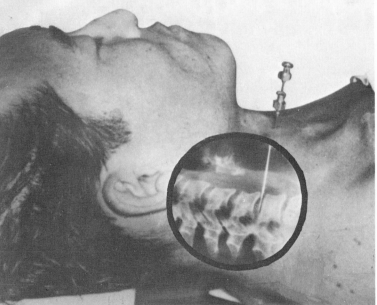

Cervical diskography demonstrated by composite photograph. Drawing shows technique of disk puncture.

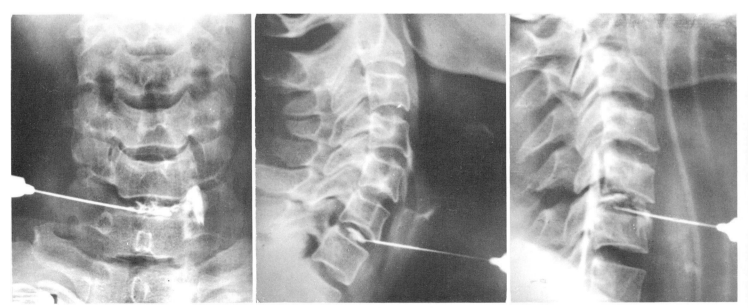

Left lateral disk rupture with Hypaque extending beyond disk space.

Normal disk (nucleus pulposus).

Lacerated disk and fracture dislocation.

Illustrations and diagnostic information courtesy Dr. Ralph B. Cloward.

896

LUMBAR DISKOGRAPHY

For lumbar diskography the patient is placed in the lateral position for the introduction of the needles and the contrast medium and for the first diskogram. A radioparent support is adjusted under the body so that the long axis of the spine is horizontal.

After the injection of the contrast agent, and with the needles in situ, a direct lateral projection is made and inspected. When this study shows that an adequate amount of the medium has been injected, the needles are removed and the puncture site or sites are dressed. The patient is then adjusted in the supine position, with the thighs flexed enough to place the back in contact with the table. For the frontal projection of the last two disk spaces, the thighs are flexed to the lithotomy position, and the central ray is then directed at a cranial angle of 10 to 20 degrees. Lastly, the patient is placed in the erect position for flexion and extension, weight-bearing, lateral studies of the abnormal disk or disks. (The lateral projections are shown on the following page.)

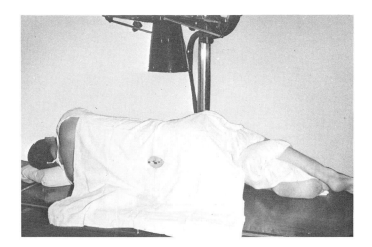

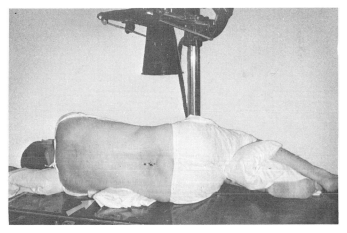

Sterile drape removed to show adjustment of spine.

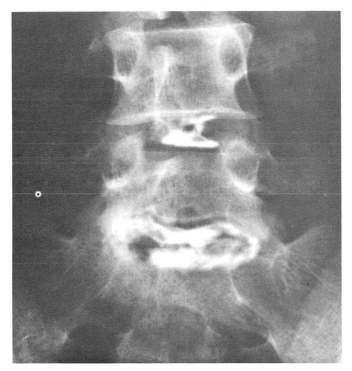

Complete rupture of lumbosacral disk. Contrast solution fills entire interspace, indicating disorganization of entire annulus fibrosus.

Illustrations and diagnostic information courtesy Dr. Ralph B. Cloward.

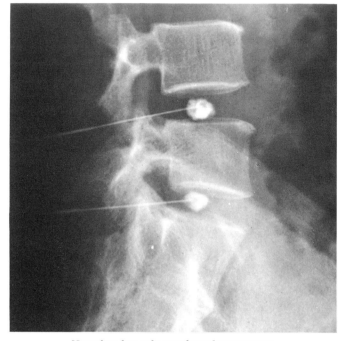

Normal nucleus pulposus of round contour type.

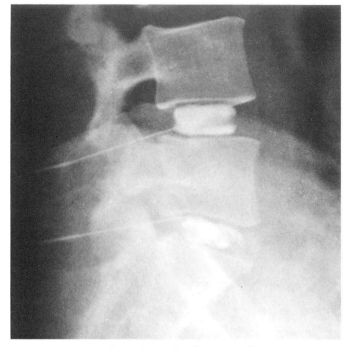

Normal nucleus pulposus of oval or rectangular type.

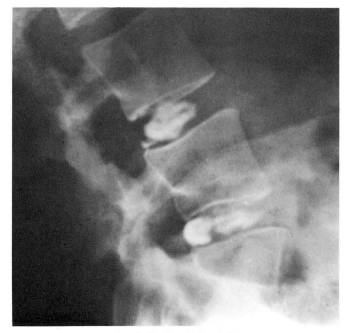

Weight-bearing flexion study.

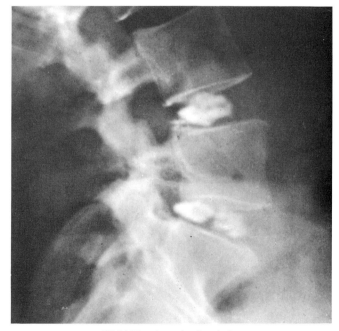

Weight-bearing extension study.

Radiographs and diagnostic information courtesy Dr. Ralph B. Cloward.

Stereotactic surgery

Stereotactic and *stereotrophic surgery* are terms used to denote a highly specialized neurosurgical therapeutic technique. This technique usually requires contrast-filling of the ventricular system, and biplane radiographic or biplane television equipment for the precise three-dimensional guidance of a slender surgical instrument through a burr hole in the cranium to a predetermined point deep within the brain substance.

Stereotactic surgery is used in the treatment of various diseases of the nervous system, some of which cause a loss of control of bodily movement and some of which cause intractable pain. The most frequent use of this surgical technique may be for the treatment of Parkinson's disease. Stereotactic surgery is often the method of choice for the treatment of such conditions because the diseased structure can be reached and surgically destroyed with a slender, specialized instrument (electrode, probe, needle, etc.) guided through a small burr hole in the cranium, thus eliminating the need for open surgery with its attendant risks. The therapeutic lesion can be made by electrical, mechanical, chemical, low temperature, ultrasonic, or radiation techniques.

The tip of the surgical instrument must be placed in the target area with an accuracy greater than 1 mm. deviation from the target point in order to avoid, as far as possible, unintended lesions in adjacent areas. In addition to biplane radiographic equipment or the biplane television equipment found in some large neurologic installations, this precise placement requires a specialized instrument-guidance system known as a stereotactic frame or a stereotactic device. Numerous types of stereotactic devices are in use. Basically, they consist of a frame into which the neurosurgeon immobilizes the patient's head with the attached fixation screws and which incorporates an external reference system and an adjustable instrument-guidance device. The frame also has two frontal and two lateral radiopaque centering devices that the radiologist or the neurosurgeon uses to align the stereotactic frame so that its geometric center coincides with the intersection of the pathways of the frontal and lateral central x-ray beam. The two lateral centering devices on the illustrated (Todd-Wells) stereotactic frame are a removable circle on one side and a cross on the other side, each embedded in a plastic support. Radiographic verification of the frame alignment should show exact superimposition of the two frontal centering devices in the frontal projection, and the center of the cross exactly centered to the center of the circle in the lateral projection. The headrest of the frame is adjustable in vertical and horizontal planes so that the target area can be accurately centered to the external reference system.

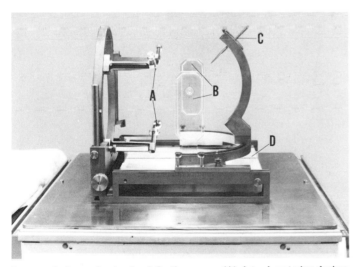

Stereotactic frame showing head fixation screws (**A**), lateral centering devices (**B**), and frontal centering devices (**C** and **D**).

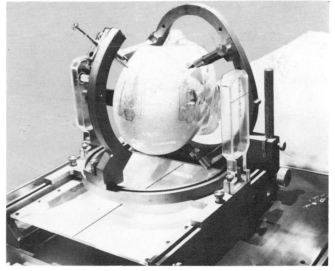

Stereotactic frame with dry skull in place.

Photographs courtesy Dr. Harold L. Stitt.

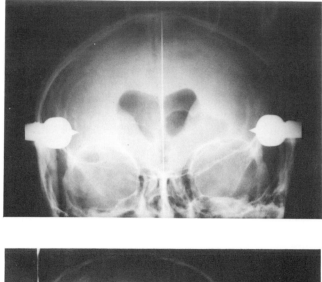

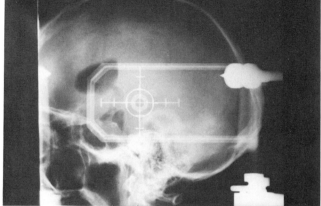

Patient's head fixed in frame. Air has been injected into the ventricles, and the lateral and frontal centering devices aligned.

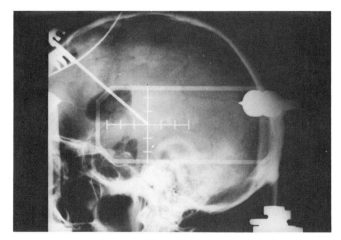

Lateral circular marker was removed, and the head moved to place the lateral cross-hair centering device at a predetermined point on the line between the anterior and posterior commissures (determined by the air and the calcified pineal).

Radiographs and legends courtesy Dr. Harold L. Stitt.

Accurate localization of the radioparent target structure in three dimensions requires internal as well as external reference points. Because of the anatomic variation in the bony structures, internal reference points must be established by introducing a contrast medium (air and/or iodized oil) into the cerebral ventricular system to outline reliable landmarks such as the anterior and posterior commissures and the intraventricular foramen. The pineal body can be used as a reference point when it is calcified. The location of the target structure relative to the reference points is measured, and the reference system coordinates then calculated.

Because the target coordinates must be exactly calculated for accurate localization of the target structure, one of the major problems in stereotaxis is magnified distortion of both the internal and external reference points due to divergence of the x-ray beam at standard focal-film distances. When a large, high-ceilinged room is available, the biplane x-ray tubes are mounted at long focal-film distances (12 feet or more) in order to eliminate image magnification by using only the central, perpendicular band of radiation. When the room size does not permit such an installation, the focal-film distance must be standardized so as to produce radiographic images of constant and known magnification. The measurements of the magnified radiographic images can then, by simple proportion, be transposed to the true measurements on the stereotactic frame for accurate localization of the target structure.

Alignment of the radiopaque centering devices is made in frontal and lateral directions by radioscopy and/or a series of radiographs. After the alignment of the stereotactic frame, the neurosurgeon positions and immobilizes the patient's head in the frame. A nurse assistant is responsible for the surgical supplies and for the care of the patient. Local anesthesia is utilized.

The technologist is responsible for establishing exposure factors that will consistently produce films clearly defining both the ventricular system and the external reference points. He must exactly align the biplane x-ray tubes and fix them in position at the standardized focal-film distance. He must see that the equipment is dust free, and that all radiographic supplies and identification markers are at hand before the patient is brought into the room. Each set of films must be processed as made for immediate interpretation by the radiologist and the neurosurgeon.

A final pair of films is made to verify accurate alignment of the patient's head, as shown by the ventricular outlines, and to show the relationship between the ventricular reference system and the external reference system. The neurosurgeon measures the location of the target structure relative to the ventricular reference points and calculates the reference system coordinates. He then sets the stereotactic instrument-guidance device to the calculated coordinates and guides the surgical instrument toward its target. Interval films are obtained as requested by the neurosurgeon. When the target structure is reached, the position of the instrument is recorded with biplane films, and the surgical lesion is then made.

Cerebral angiography

A CHART OF THE INTRACEREBRAL CIRCULATION[1]

Bert C. Bean, M.D.

Department of Radiology, Buffalo General Hospital, Buffalo, New York

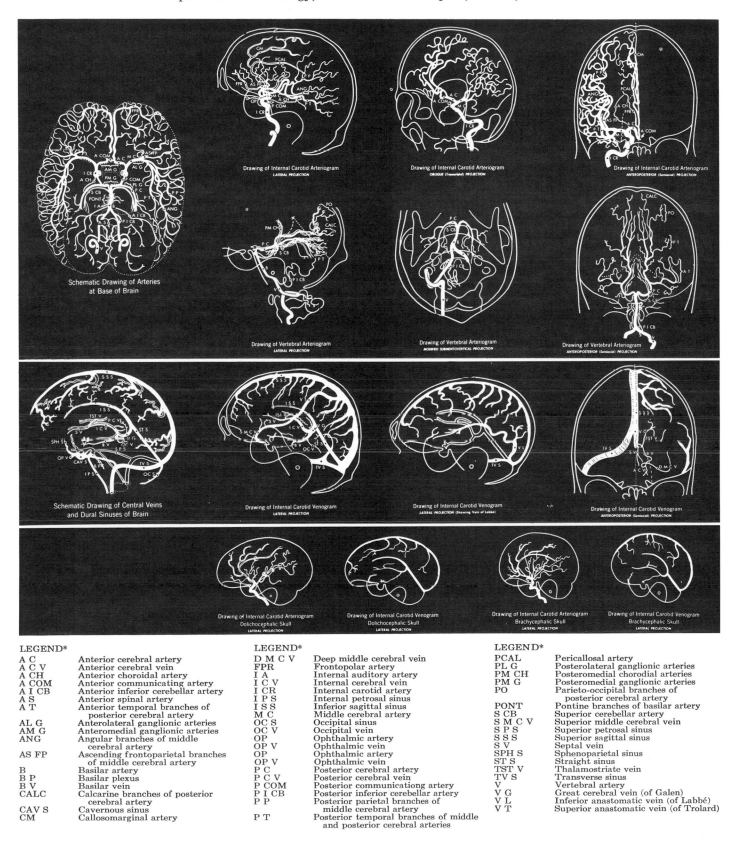

*Anatomic terms used are based on N. A. wherever possible; otherwise terms employed are those commonly referred to in anatomic texts.
[1]Bean, Berten C.: A chart of the intracerebral circulation, ed. 2, Med. Radiogr. Photogr. **34**:25, 1958. Courtesy Dr. Bean and Eastman Kodak Co.

LEGEND*

A C	Anterior cerebral artery
A C V	Anterior cerebral vein
A CH	Anterior choroidal artery
A COM	Anterior communicating artery
A I CB	Anterior inferior cerebellar artery
A S	Anterior spinal artery
A T	Anterior temporal branches of posterior cerebral artery
AL G	Anterolateral ganglionic arteries
AM G	Anteromedial ganglionic arteries
ANG	Angular branches of middle cerebral artery
AS FP	Ascending frontoparietal branches of middle cerebral artery
B	Basilar artery
B P	Basilar plexus
B V	Basilar vein
CALC	Calcarine branches of posterior cerebral artery
CAV S	Cavernous sinus
CM	Callosomarginal artery

LEGEND*

D M C V	Deep middle cerebral vein
FPR	Frontopolar artery
I A	Internal auditory artery
I C V	Internal cerebral vein
I CR	Internal carotid artery
I P S	Internal petrosal sinus
I S S	Inferior sagittal sinus
M C	Middle cerebral artery
OC S	Occipital sinus
OC V	Occipital vein
OP	Ophthalmic artery
OP V	Ophthalmic vein
OP	Ophthalmic artery
OP V	Ophthalmic vein
P C	Posterior cerebral artery
P C V	Posterior cerebral vein
P COM	Posterior communicating artery
P I CB	Posterior inferior cerebellar artery
P P	Posterior parietal branches of middle cerebral artery
P T	Posterior temporal branches of middle and posterior cerebral arteries

LEGEND*

PCAL	Pericallosal artery
PL G	Posterolateral ganglionic arteries
PM CH	Posteromedial chorodial arteries
PM G	Posteromedial ganglionic arteries
PO	Parieto-occipital branches of posterior cerebral artery
PONT	Pontine branches of basilar artery
S CB	Superior cerebellar artery
S M C V	Superior middle cerebral vein
S P S	Superior petrosal sinus
S S S	Superior sagittal sinus
S V	Septal vein
SPH S	Sphenoparietal sinus
ST S	Straight sinus
TST V	Thalamostriate vein
TV S	Transverse sinus
V	Vertebral artery
V G	Great cerebral vein (of Galen)
V L	Inferior anastomatic vein (of Labbé)
V T	Superior anastomatic vein (of Trolard)

CEREBRAL ANGIOGRAPHY—cont'd

Cerebral angiography is the term used to denote radiologic examinations of the blood vessels of the brain by means of injecting them with a radiopaque contrast medium. The procedure was introduced by Egas Moniz[1] in 1927. It is performed in the investigation of intracranial aneurysms or other vascular lesions and to demonstrate tumor masses, which are shown by displacement of the normal cerebrovascular pattern or by the tumor's circulation.

The brain is supplied by four trunk vessels—the right

and left common carotid arteries, which supply the anterior circulation, and the right and left vertebral arteries, which supply the posterior circulation. These paired arteries branch from the arch of the aorta and ascend through the neck, as shown in the accompanying diagram and arteriogram.

It will be noted that the left common carotid artery arises directly from the aortic arch. The right common carotid artery arises with the right subclavian artery about 1½ inches higher at the bifurcation of the innominate artery. The left subclavian artery arises directly from the arch of the aorta. The vertebral arteries arise from the subclavian arteries.

[1]Egas Moniz, A. C.: L'encéphalographie artérielle, son importance dans la localisation des tumeurs cérébrales, Rev. Neurol. 2:72-90, 1927.

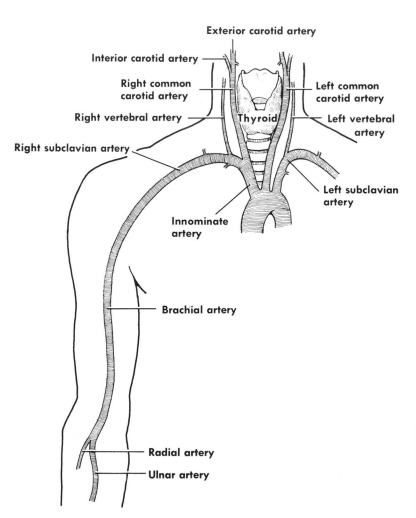

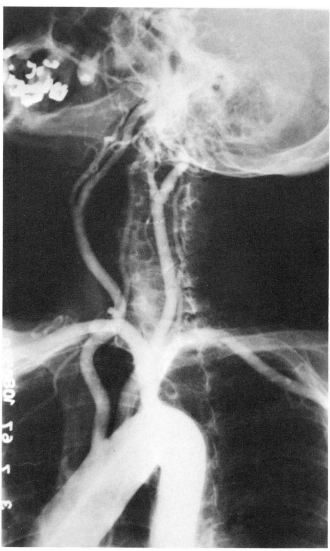

Transfemoral aortic arch arteriogram in right oblique position. Note excellent opacification of brachiocephalic arteries.

Radiograph and legend courtesy Dr. K. Y. Chynn.

Each common carotid artery passes upward and somewhat lateralward along the side of the trachea and larynx to the level of the fourth cervical vertebra, where each divides into internal and external carotid arteries. The latter vessel contributes to the supply of the meninges but not to that of the intracerebral circulation. The internal carotid artery enters the cranium through the carotid foramen and then bifurcates into the anterior and middle cerebral arteries. They, in turn, branch and rebranch to supply the anterior circulation of the respective hemisphere of the brain.

The vertebral arteries ascend through the cervical transverse foramina and then pass medialward to enter the cranium through the foramen magnum. The vertebral arteries unite to form the basilar artery, which, after a short upward course along the posterior surface of the dorsum sellae, bifurcates into the right and left posterior cerebral arteries.

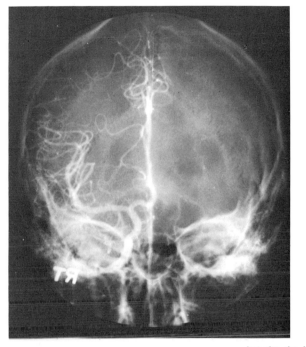
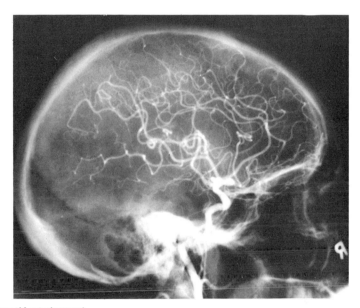

Anterior circulation (carotid arteriograms).

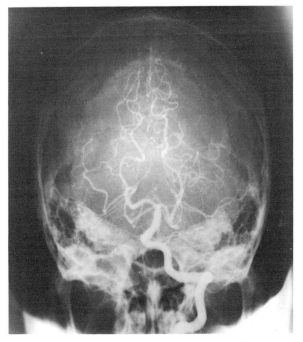
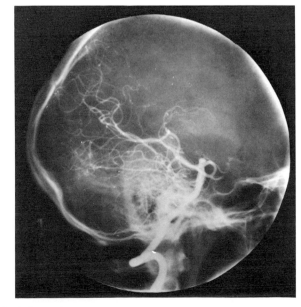

Posterior circulation (vertebral arteriograms).

Radiographs courtesy Dr. John A. Goree.

CEREBRAL ANGIOGRAPHY—cont'd

INJECTION SITES

A radiopaque contrast solution (at present one of the water-soluble, iodinated compounds is used) is injected into the cerebral arteries of the side under investigation. The injection is made by way of the common or internal carotid artery for the demonstration of the anterior circulation, and by way of the vertebral artery for the demonstration of the posterior circulation. While fundamentally the same in that the injection is made into the artery of choice, the surgical techniques differ somewhat. In the *closed*, or *percutaneous*, method, the radiologist inserts the needle into the artery through the skin. In the *open* method, the first part of which may be carried out in the operating room, the neurosurgeon makes an incision and exposes the artery. The patient is then transported to the radiology department, where the needle is introduced into the exposed artery for the injection of the contrast solution.

An injection made into an artery above the point of its origin coincides with the direction of the flow of blood and is referred to as an *anterograde*, or antegrade, injection. Injections made distal to the point of the vessel's origin are made against the direction of blood flow and are called *retrograde* injections. An exception to this is the *retrograde carotid* injection, in which the needle is inserted directly into the vessel but against the direction of blood flow. This injection technique is used when there is a suspected stenosis of the cervical portion of the carotid artery. Note the direction of the needle in the two radiographs below.

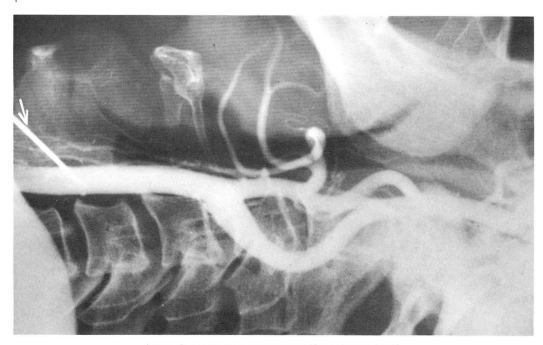

Antegrade percutaneous common carotid arteriogram (neck).

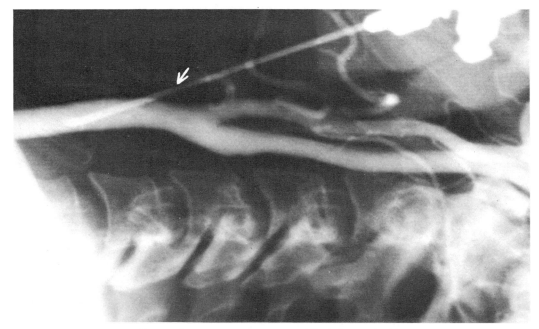

Retrograde percutaneous common carotid arteriogram (neck).

Radiographs courtesy Dr. John A. Goree.

Retrograde injections are employed for the demonstration of the extracranial portions of the arteries supplying the brain, and are used by many radiologists to opacify the intracranial vessels. Retrograde injections may be made by direct puncture of the brachial or subclavian artery, or by catheterization of the subclavian artery or the aortic arch. Catheterization of either vessel may be performed by way of the brachial, axillary, or femoral artery. The catheter is passed, under radioscopic observation, to a point at or near the orifice of the vessel being investigated. In conjunction with an image intensifier, cineradiography and 70 or 90 mm. spot films may be utilized in these examinations. Without special equipment, conventional filming of the extracranial vessels usually consists of two exposures, each requiring a high-pressure injection of a comparatively large volume of the contrast solution in order to obtain retrograde flow. The views taken are a lateral projection of the head and neck and an anteroposterior projection of the neck. For the inclusion of the intracranial vessels on the anteroposterior projection, the head is usually rotated to an oblique or a lateral position. For the inclusion of the aortic arch, the film must project about 2 inches below the level of the sternal angle (see the film on page 902).

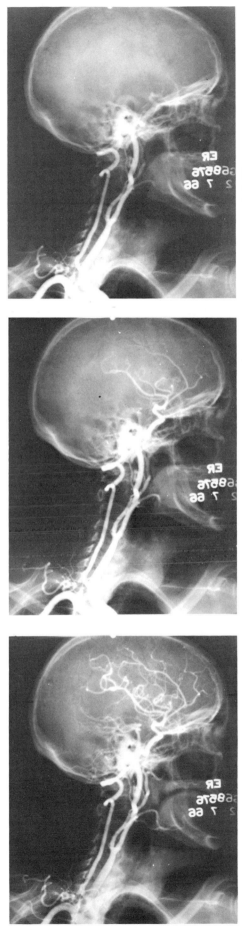

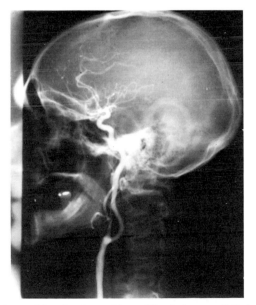

Lateral intracranial and extracranial carotid arteriogram. Catheter in right common carotid artery orifice via femoral artery catheterization.

Courtesy Dr. Irwin Johnsrude.

Three-film sequence of intracranial and extracranial arteries by right brachial retrograde injection.

Radiographs courtesy Dr. John A. Goree.

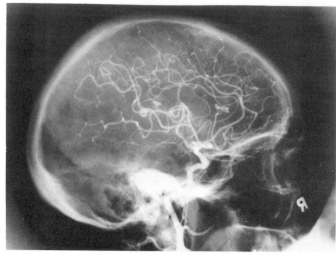

Arterial phase.

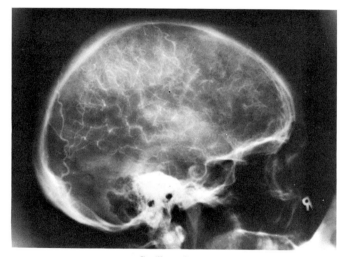

Capillary phase.

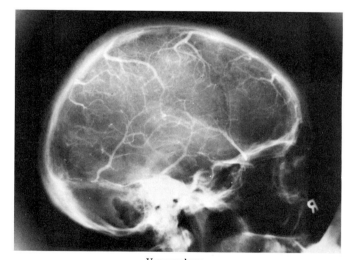

Venous phase.

Serial studies of percutaneous carotid injection courtesy Dr. John A. Goree.

CEREBRAL ANGIOGRAPHY—cont'd

CIRCULATION TIME

According to the estimation of Egas Moniz,[1] only three seconds is the usual time required for the blood to circulate from the internal carotid artery to the jugular vein, the circulation time being slightly prolonged by the injected contrast solution. Greitz,[2] who measured the cerebral circulation time as "the time between the points of maximum concentration [of contrast medium] in the carotid siphon and in the parietal veins," found a normal mean value of 4.13 seconds. Thus it is seen that *time* is a highly important factor in cerebral angiography. The technologist must bear in mind that a delay of even one second can sometimes render the projection valueless. Of course, the time factor is somewhat less critical when serial filming is employed.

The contrast solution is injected as rapidly as possible in order to minimize its dilution with blood. At the radiologist's signal, the first exposure is made either during or immediately after the completion of the injection and is rapidly followed with serial studies of the arterial and venous circulation. The number of films that can be obtained and the time interval between their exposure depend upon the equipment used.

Films made during the arterial phase of circulation delineate the cerebral arteries and are called *arteriograms.* While there is a considerable variation in the circulation time, particularly in pathologic cases, films made from about three to six seconds later capture the venous phase of circulation, demonstrate the cerebral veins, and are called *venograms* or *phlebograms.* Films may be made during the intermediate, or capillary, phase of circulation. It is suggested that they be called *capillariograms.*

[1]Egas Moniz, A. C.: L'angiographie cérébrale, Paris, 1934, Masson & Cie.
[2]Greitz, T.: A radiologic study of the brain circulation by rapid serial angiography of the carotid artery, Acta Radiol., supp. 140, 1956.

EQUIPMENT

Because of the rapidity of the circulation time, an injection of contrast material must be made for each view required unless a roentgenographic unit permitting simultaneous biplane exposures is employed. Where an automatic, high-speed film changer is available, it is possible to make exposures at intervals of one-half second or less. Full information concerning the construction and operation of each of the numerous special units is supplied by the manufacturer.

With standard equipment and the manual method of changing cassettes, it is necessary for one technologist to work from the control room and one from the examining table. Under this circumstance, it is not possible to make more than three exposures on one injection, and usually only two exposures can be made. Perfectly coordinated teamwork between the radiologist and the technologists is essential to a successful result with the manual method. The technologist should discuss the entire procedure with the examining physician and, if necessary, practice it with him until the timing is perfect and the signals clearly understood before participating in an actual examination with him for the first time. Furthermore, regardless of how often the technologists have participated in the manual method, they should rehearse the procedure shortly before the patient is due to arrive, until they achieve perfect timing and coordination.

Tomography of the midline blood vessels may be performed by a single sweep movement of the head.[1] Instead of having the patient nod his head to-and-fro as in pneumographic autotomography, an assitant rotates the head through a small arc in one direction only during a short exposure.

Subtraction techniques (pages 916 to 920) are now widely used in cerebral angiography, and where a small-focal spot tube having high heat capacity is available, serial magnification angiograms can be obtained.

PREPARATION OF PATIENT

Other than the withholding of the preceding meal, preliminary preparation of the patient depends upon his condition and is accordingly determined by the radiologist and the referring physician. Whenever possible, adult patients are examined under local anesthesia in

[1]Smith, J. T., Goree, J. A., Jimenez, J. P., and Harris, C. C.: Cerebral angio-autotomography, Amer. J. Roentgen. 112:315-323, 1971.

conjunction with sedation. Adequate sedation minimizes the intensity of the burning pain felt along the course of the injected vessel and in the areas supplied by it during the rapid injections of the iodinated medium. The sedative has the further advantage of lessening the possibility of a reaction resulting in reflex movement during initial arterial filming at or before the end of each injection.

A sensitivity test is usually performed prior to the examination, and if necessary, the patient is desensitized with an antihistaminic drug.

PREPARATION OF EXAMINING ROOM

It cannot be said too often that radiographic examining rooms and every item in them should be as scrupulously clean as any other room used for medical purposes. The room should be fully prepared, with every item needed or likely to be needed on hand before the patient is admitted. Cleanliness and advance preparation are of vital importance in examinations that must be carried out under aseptic conditions.

The radiographic machine and all working parts of the equipment should be checked, and the controls should be adjusted for the exposure technique to be employed. Identification markers and all accessories, such as cassettes, cassette holder, and grid-front cassettes for horizontal projections, should be conveniently located. Compression and restraining bands should be ready for application. Right-angle projections, exposed singly or simultaneously, are made with the head in the basic position, which obviates the use of a head clamp or a cross-table compression band. Immobilization of the head by suitable strapping must be adapted to the type of equipment employed. Arrangements should be made for immediate processing of the films as the examination proceeds.

The sterile and nonsterile items required for the introduction of the contrast medium vary according to the method of injection. The supplies specified by the radiologist for each procedure should be listed in the angiographic procedure book. Sterile trays or packs, set up to specifications, are usually obtainable from the central sterile-supply room. Otherwise, it is the responsibility of a qualified member of the technologic staff to prepare them. Extra sterile supplies should always be on hand in case of an accident. Preparation of the room includes having full emergency equipment immediately available.

CEREBRAL ANGIOGRAPHY—cont'd

RADIATION PROTECTION

As in all roentgen ray examinations, the patient is protected by a minimum radiation filtration of 2 mm. of aluminum, by sharp restriction of the beam of radiation to the area being examined, and by avoidance of repeat exposures. In angiography each repeated exposure necessitates a repeated injection of the iodinated compound. For this reason, only skilled and specially trained technologists should be assigned to take part in these examinations.

Where a mechanical injection device is not used, the radiologist's hands must be protected by a lead shield. A simply constructed device that is widely used for this purpose consists of a counterweighted sheet of lead rubber, suspended from the ceiling so that it can be easily lowered and raised as required. All parts of this overhead device or other shielding arrangement must be kept strictly free of dust for the protection of the sterile field.

Any assistant required to remain in the examining room during the filming procedure must be supplied with a lead apron and, depending on his proximity to the radiation field, with lead gloves.

POSITION OF PATIENT

All cerebral angiographic injection methods require that the patient be adjusted in the supine position and so kept throughout the examination. Regardless of whether the patient is awake, suitable supports should be placed under points of strain—the small of the back, the knees, and the ankles—and he should be covered according to room temperature. Wrist restraints and compression bands across the body are applied as indicated by the patient's condition.

In preparation for percutaneous puncture of the carotid artery, the head is usually extended to some degree. This is done to elevate and tautly stretch the vessel for the purpose of placing it in a more accessible and stable position for the insertion of the needle. Without a skull unit that can be lowered to place the head in extension over the end of the table, it may be necessary to elevate the shoulders on a pillow or other support. After the needle has been seated in the vessel, great care must be exercised to avoid dislodging it when removing the shoulder support and when positioning and immobilizing the head. The position of the needle can be determined with anteroposterior and cross-table lateral projections of the neck during the injection of a small amount of contrast material. This filming is best done with the use of rapid Polaroid film.

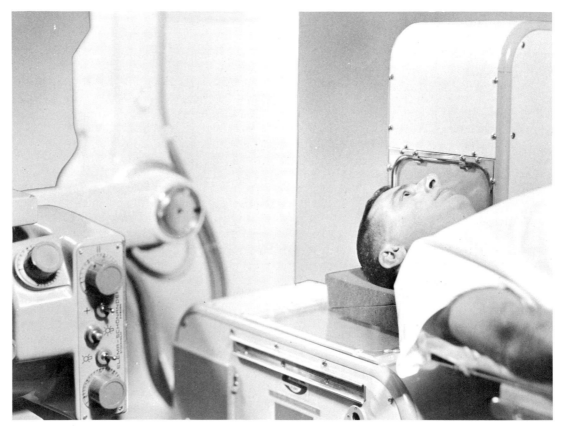

Lateral cerebral angiogram position.

POSITION OF HEAD

The centering and angulation of the central ray required for the demonstration of the anterior circulation differs from that required for the demonstration of the posterior circulation, but the same head position is used for the basic anteroposterior and lateral projections of both regions. For the initial right-angle studies, the head must be elevated on a radioparent support so that it is centered for horizontally projected lateral views. The head is then adjusted to place its median sagittal plane *exactly perpendicular* to the headrest and, consequently, *exactly parallel* with the laterally placed cassette holder. The *infraorbitomeatal line* is used for exact adjustment of the base of the skull. This localization line is used because, due to the danger of displacing the puncture needle, the head can so infrequently be flexed enough to place the orbitomeatal line perpendicular to the horizontal plane. The central ray angulation for caudally inclined antero-posterior and oblique anteroposterior projections may be based from the vertically placed infraorbitomeatal line, or, as advocated by Greitz and Lindgren,[1] the central ray may be adjusted so that it is parallel to the floor of the anterior fossa, as indicated by a line extending from the supraorbital margin to a point 2 cm. cranial to the external auditory meatus.

The literature on cerebral angiography contains numerous projection variations concerning the degree of central ray angulation, the base from which it should be angled or the line that it should parallel, and the degree of part rotation for oblique studies. The most frequently employed views, and reasonably standard specifications for obtaining them, have been selected for inclusion in this text.

The number of views required for satisfactory delineation of a lesion depends upon its nature and location. Oblique projections and/or variations in central ray angulation are taken to separate the shadows of vessels that overlap in the basic views and to evaluate any existing abnormality.

[1]Greitz, T., and Lindgren, E. In Abrams, H. L., editor: Angiography, Boston, 1961, Little, Brown & Co., pp. 41-49.

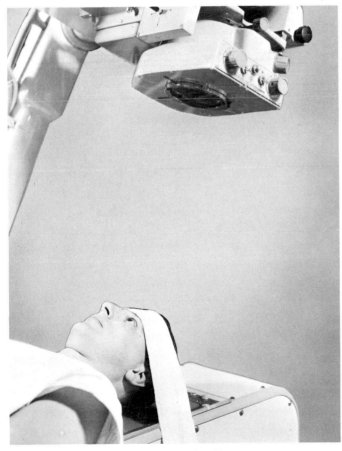

Supraorbital carotid position.

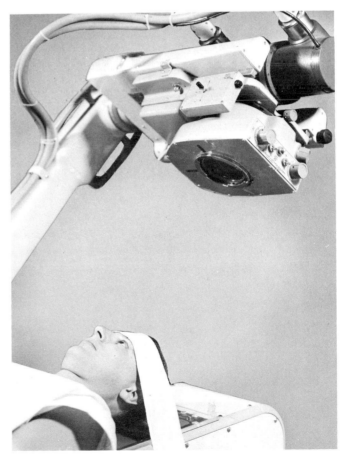

Half-axial vertebral position.

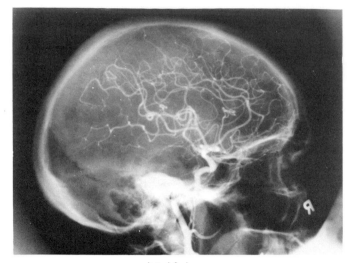

Arterial phase.

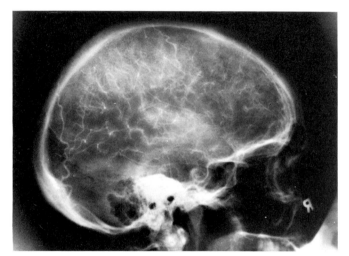

Capillary phase.

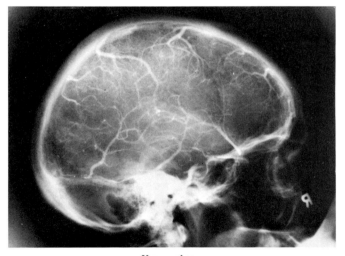

Venous phase.

Serial percutaneous carotid angiograms courtesy Dr. John A. Goree.

CEREBRAL ANGIOGRAPHY—cont'd
Anterior circulation projections
LATERAL PROJECTION

The patient's head is elevated on a suitable support so that it is centered to the vertically placed film. The head is extended enough to place the infraorbitomeatal line perpendicular to the horizontal, and it is then adjusted to place the median sagittal plane *exactly* vertical, and thereby parallel with the plane of the film. Immobilization must be adapted to the type of equipment being employed.

Lateral views of the anterior or carotid circulation are made with the central ray directed horizontally to a point slightly cranial to the auricle and midway between the forehead and the occiput. This centering allows for optimum anatomic variation.

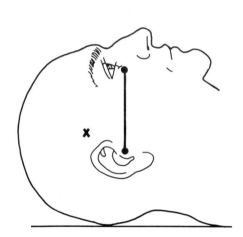

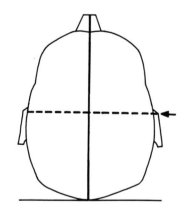

SUPRAORBITAL ANTEROPOSTERIOR PROJECTION

Unless simultaneous biplane projections are being made, the support is removed and the head is rested directly on the table for frontal studies. The head is adjusted so that its median sagittal plane is centered over, and *exactly* perpendicular to, the midline of the grid, and so that it is extended enough to place the infraorbitomeatal line vertical. The head is then immobilized.

The aim in this view is to superimpose the supraorbital margins on the superior margin of the petrous ridges so that the vessels are projected above the floor of the anterior cranial fossa. This result is achieved in a majority of patients by directing the central ray along a line passing 2 cm. cranial to, and parallel with, a line extending from the supraorbital margin to a point 2 cm. cranial to the external auditory meatus; the latter line coincides with the floor of the anterior fossa.

SUPRAORBITAL OBLIQUE PROJECTION

For the demonstration of the region of the anterior communicating artery, the above head position is maintained, except that it is rotated about 30 degrees away from the injected side. The central ray is directed as for the above direct supraorbital projection.

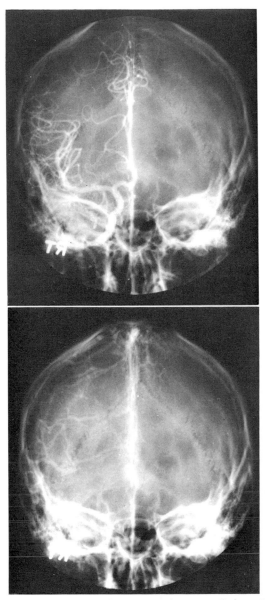

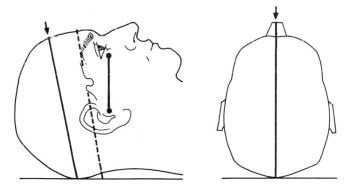

Serial percutaneous carotid angiograms showing, respectively, arterial and venous phases of circulation.

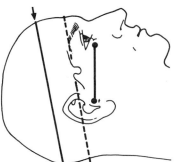

Central ray parallel with Greitz-Lindgren line.

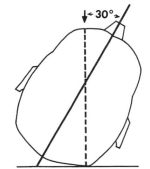

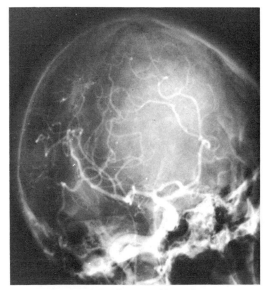

Supraorbital oblique carotid arteriogram.

Radiographs courtesy Dr. John A. Goree.

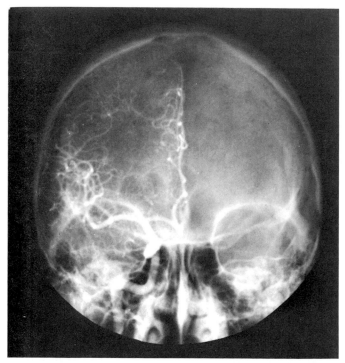

Percutaneous carotid arteriogram. Transorbital anteroposterior projection.

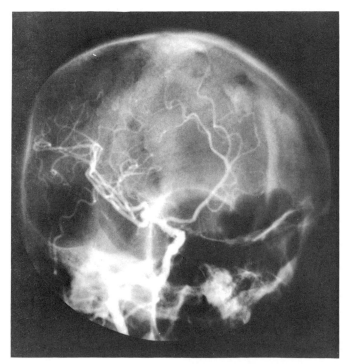

Percutaneous carotid arteriogram. Transorbital oblique projection.

Radiographs courtesy Dr. John A. Goree.

CEREBRAL ANGIOGRAPHY—cont'd
Anterior circulation projections—cont'd

TRANSORBITAL ANTEROPOSTERIOR PROJECTION

This view demonstrates the middle cerebral artery and its main branches within the orbital shadow.

The head is adjusted in the basic anteroposterior position. The central ray is directed through the midorbits at an average angle of 20 degrees toward the head; it should coincide with a line passing through the center of the orbit and a point about 2 cm. cranial to the auricle of the ear.

TRANSORBITAL OBLIQUE PROJECTION

This view demonstrates the internal carotid bifurcation, the anterior communicating, and the middle cerebral arteries within the orbital shadow.

From the basic position, the head is rotated about 30 degrees away from the injected side. The central ray is angled as for the above direct transorbital anteroposterior projection and centered to the midorbit of the uppermost side.

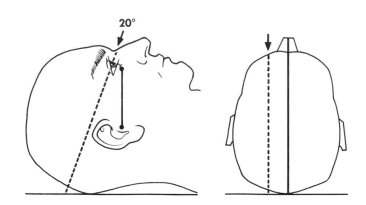

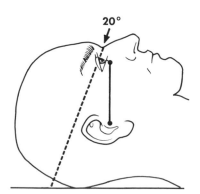

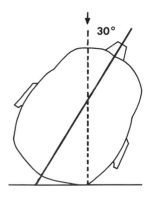

HALF-AXIAL PROJECTIONS

Half-axial anteroposterior and/or oblique projections are used in carotid angiography, when indicated, for further evaluation of vessel displacement or of aneurysms.

1. For a half-axial anteroposterior projection, the head is adjusted in the basic position. The central ray is directed to the region of the hairline at an average angle of 30 degrees toward the feet; it exits at the level of the external auditory meatus.

2. For a half-axial oblique projection, the head is rotated 35 to 45 degrees away from the injected side. The central ray is angled as for the half-axial anteroposterior projection.

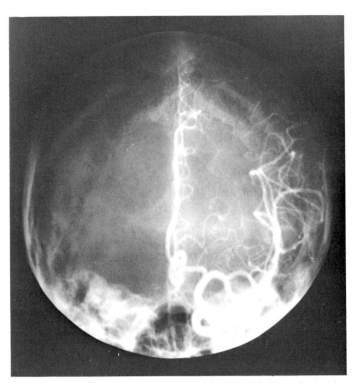

Percutaneous carotid arteriogram, half-axial anteroposterior projection.

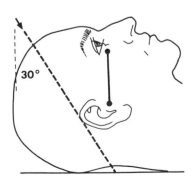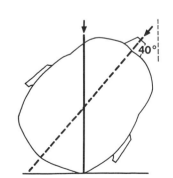

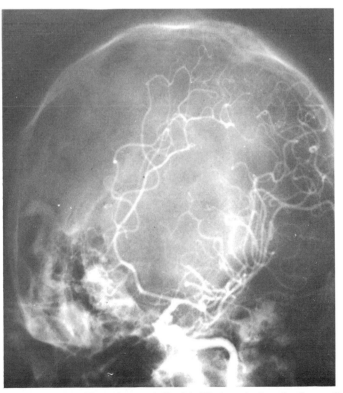

Percutaneous carotid arteriogram, half-axial oblique projection showing small internal carotid artery aneurysm at posterior communicating junction.

Radiographs and diagnostic information courtesy Dr. John A. Goree.

913

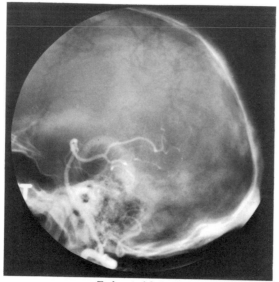

Early arterial phase.

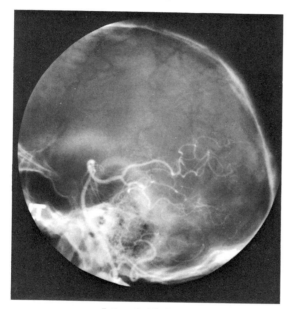

Later arterial phase.

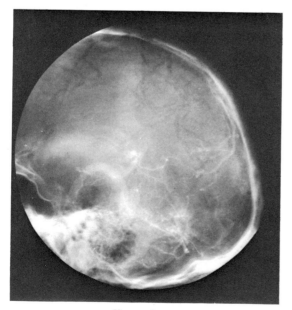

Venous phase.

Contrast medium for above serial angiograms (and for posterior circulation studies shown on page 903) was introduced by percutaneous retrograde injection into left brachial artery.

Radiographs and legend courtesy Dr. John A. Goree.

CEREBRAL ANGIOGRAPHY—cont'd
Posterior circulation projections
LATERAL PROJECTION

The patient's head is elevated on a suitable support, so that it is centered to the vertically placed film. It is extended enough to place the infraorbitomeatal line perpendicular to the horizontal plane and is then adjusted to place the median sagittal plane *exactly* vertical, and thereby parallel with the plane of the film. The head must be rigidly immobilized.

Lateral views of the posterior, or vertebral, circulation are made with the central ray directed horizontally to the mastoid process at a point about 1 cm. cranial to, and 2 cm. posterior to, the external auditory meatus.

The exposure field can be restricted to the middle and posterior fossae for lateral studies of the posterior circulation, the inclusion of the entire skull being neither necessary nor, from the standpoint of optimum technique, desirable.

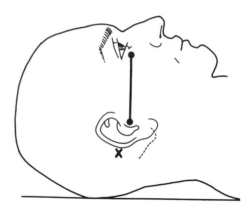

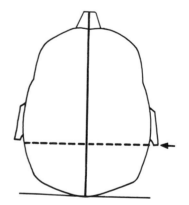

HALF-AXIAL ANTEROPOSTERIOR PROJECTION

Except for simultaneous biplane projections, the support is removed and the head is rested directly on the table for frontal studies. The head is adjusted so that its median sagittal plane is centered over, and is exactly perpendicular, to the midline of the grid, and the head is extended enough so that the infraorbitomeatal line is vertical. It is then immobilized.

The central ray is directed to the region of the hairline at an angle of 30 to 35 degrees toward the feet; it exits at the level of the external auditory meatuses.

SUBMENTOVERTICAL PROJECTION

A modified submentovertical projection is sometimes employed in the investigation of the posterior circulation. It is also used for the anterior circulation when a middle fossa lesion is suspected.

The success of this position depends not only upon the length of the patient's neck (how well the head can be extended) but upon the site of injection. It is usually attempted only in the retrograde procedures.

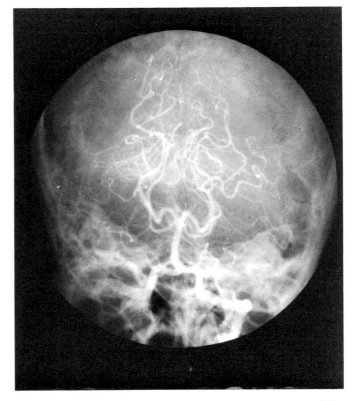

Half-axial anteroposterior projection, arterial phase of posterior circulation.

Courtesy Dr. John A. Goree.

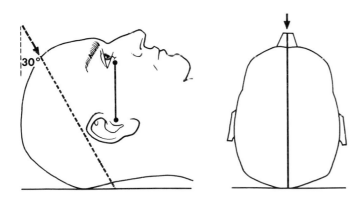

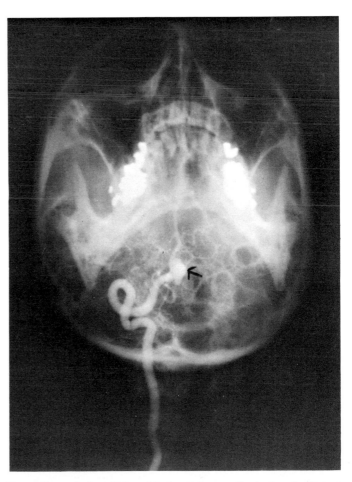

Transaxillary selective right vertebral arteriogram. Basal view showing excellent opacification of right vertebral artery and aneurysm (arrow) at vertebrobasilar junction.

Radiograph and diagnostic information courtesy Dr. K. Y. Chynn.

915

Composite-mask subtraction
White-over-white technique

Contributed by
Roy D. Strand, M.D.

Assistant Professor in Radiology, Harvard Medical School, Boston, Mass.;
Radiologist, The Children's Hospital Medical Center, Boston, Mass.

and

Donald L. Sucher

Special Procedures Illustrator
Department of Radiology, The Children's Hospital
Medical Center, Boston, Mass.

Photographic subtraction, introduced by Ziedses des Plantes,[1] is a technique with which bone structure images are subtracted or canceled out from a film of the bones plus opacified vessels, leaving an unobscured image of the vessels. The technique is applicable in all forms of angiography, wherever the vessels are superimposed by bone structures.

The purpose of subtraction in angiography is to fully define all vessels containing contrast material and at the same time eliminate the confusing overlying bone images. A few terms idiomatic to the subtraction technique must first be defined.

Zero or base film (also called the **control film**) must show the bone structures only, and there must be *no patient motion whatever* between it and the subsequent contrast studies. For these reasons, the zero film is exposed just before contrast medium is injected into the vessels.

Reversal film (also called a **positive mask** or **diapositive**) is a reverse-tone duplicate of the x-ray image, showing black changed to white and white to black. This positive transparency is obtained by exposing a single emulsion film through the traditional x-ray film.

Registration is the matching of one film over another so that the bony landmarks are *precisely* superimposed. So composed, the films are taped together to prevent slippage. Composites herein discussed may involve two or more films.

The simplest method of photographic subtraction consists in obtaining a positive mask, or reversal, of the first film of the angiographic series, the one that does not contain contrast material. When the reversal film is superimposed over a film in the series that contains contrast material, the positive and negative images of the bones tend to cancel each other out, and only the vessels can be seen. The vessels are not canceled out because they were present on only one film. A print is made of this combination of films either by a contact printer or by a device similar to the one herein described and illustrated.

The reversal of the zero film is not usually the exact reversal of the density of the selected angiographic film, so the subtraction result is imperfect. The imperfection can be corrected with what is called *second-order subtraction*. This is done by producing another film, called a *secondary*, or *correction*, *mask*, which compensates for the slight differences. Hanafee and Shinno[2] led the way toward improved subtraction methods. Their method of second-order subtraction consists in superimposing the zero film on its own reversal and making an additional print of the faint image that results from the transmission of light through the two films, which in theory would be the exact opposite of each other. This produces a faint film that does correct for the small "photographic mistake" between the first two. The reversal of the zero film, the correction film, and the film containing contrast material are carefully registered, and this combination is exposed to obtain the final subtraction film.

[1]Ziedses des Plantes, B. G.: Subtraktion: eine roentgenographische Methode zur separaten Abbildung bestimmter Tiele des Objekts, Fortschr. Roentgenstr. **52**:69-79, 1935.

[2]Hanafee, W., and Shinno, J. M.: Second-order subtraction with simultaneous bilateral carotid, internal carotid injections, Radiology **86**:334-341, 1966.

916

MATERIALS

1. The printer consists of lamp, timer, and print box (see photograph opposite).
   a. Kodak Honeycomb Lamp with attached timer. The lamp contains a 6-volt, 50-watt bulb and has a ¾-inch exposure aperture.
   b. The print box is positioned 52 inches below the lamp. It consists of a felt-padded base and a glass plate lid and is large enough to accommodate two films side by side for simultaneous exposure.
2. Films
   a. Kodak commercial film (4127) or Kodak RP/SU subtraction film.
   b. Kodolith Ortho film type 3 (6556).
3. Processing solutions
   a. Kodak liquid x-ray developer and replenisher.
   b. Kodak liquid x-ray fixer and replenisher.
4. A horizontally oriented illuminator. This is used to obtain precise superimposition of the films.

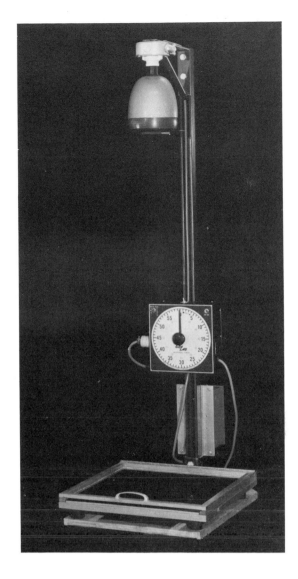

SUBTRACTION PROCEDURE (See figures on this and the facing page)

The objective of the subtraction technique is to obtain a high-contrast film of the vessels only. In the technique described below, a form of second-order subtraction, the correction mask is translucent where the vessels are, so that no grayness is created by the correction film. Thus this method is called the *white-over-white technique*. When correctly applied, this form of second-order subtraction approaches the goal of total elimination of all bony structures, leaving a display of the vessels in high contrast reproduction.

The medium-contrast grade of subtraction film is used in steps 1 and 2, and a high-contrast grade of film for step 3. The light source on the illustrated printer is above, so the subtraction film is placed, emulsion side up, under the film or the film-mask combination to be printed.

Step 1. In order to obtain masks having identical contrast and density, place the following side by side on the print box for simultaneous printing: the zero film (**a**), which produces reversal film (**b**); and the selected film of the angiographic series (**c**), which produces reversal film **d**. Process the mask films. Note that during step 1, two films are exposed side by side, simultaneously.

Step 2. Superimpose reversal film **d** over zero film (**a**), and make secondary reversal film (**e**). Process this film.

Step 3. Superimpose reversal film **b**, secondary reversal (**e**), and the selected film of the contrast series (**c**). Print to produce the final subtraction film (page 920).

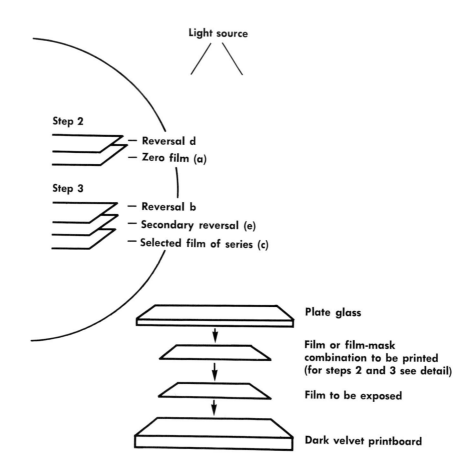

918

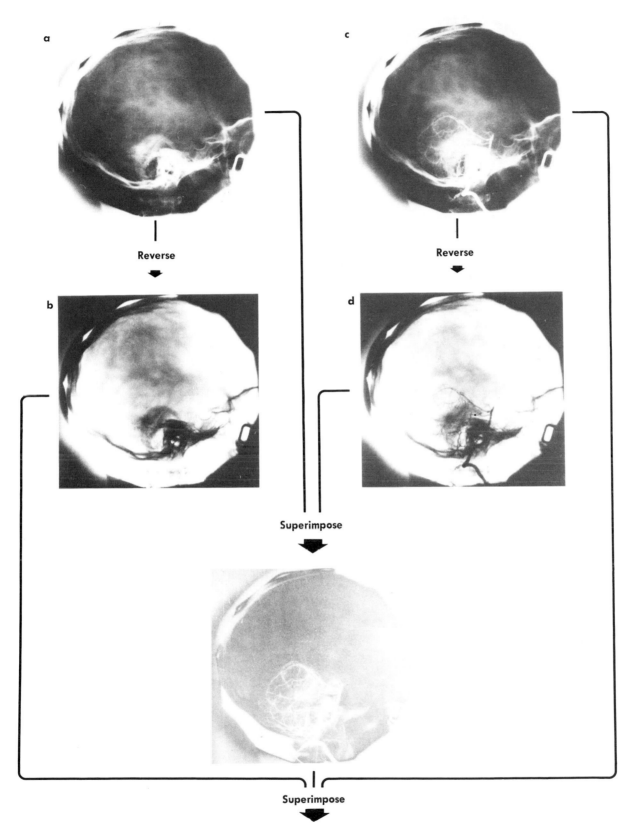

Diagrammatic representation of the steps in composite-mask subtraction. Notations **a** and **c** indicate the zero film and the contrast-containing film of interest in the series. These are simultaneously exposed to light as described in the procedure to obtain their respective reversals, **b** and **d**. The original zero film and the reversal film of interest are superimposed to produce the composite mask, **e**, which will correct for imperfect subtraction when superimposed over **b** and **c** to obtain the final film (see following page).

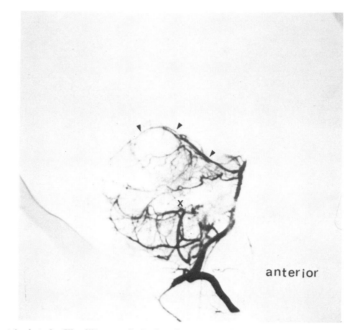

Completed subtraction film of a lateral vertebral study. The filling was limited to the posterior fossa circulation. The superior cerebellar arteries and their branches are the most superior group of vessels (arrows). The choroidal point of the posterior inferior cerebellar artery is readily identifiable (immediately below the x). Directly posterior to the x are inferior vermis branches. The more inferiorly placed curvilinear vessels are hemispheric branches.

DISCUSSION

Inherent advantages of this technique are that considerable latitude is allowed in the choice of film, processing techniques, and equipment. When manual processing is used, Kodak commercial film has been quite satisfactory for the initial and secondary masks (steps 1 and 2). Kodak subtraction film (RP/SU), processed either manually or by an automatic 90-second processor, has given equally good results.

The final film is best printed on a relatively high-contrast grade of film, given long exposure, and then "pulled" after a few seconds of developing. Kodolith Ortho film type 3 has been used as a high-contrast film by us for five years; its use is described by Joyce and Dalrymple.[1] Underdeveloping is of course impossible with automatic processors. However, if manual processing facilities are not available, satisfactory results can be ob-

[1]Joyce, J. W., Dalrymple, G. V., Jungkind, F. F., Scott, P. D., and Davasher, B. G.: Improved contrast in subtraction technique, Radiology 94:157-159, 1970.

tained using Kodak subtraction film with automatic processing.

In the production of the masks for the first two steps, the type of film is not critical, nor is the exposure, as long as both original reversals have the same contrast and density. To accomplish identical contrast and density of the masks, we have found it beneficial to expose them simultaneously in the same print box.

In the superimposing of the combinations of films on the horizontal illuminator, the registration is made easier by eliminating any peripheral light. This is particularly necessary in superimposing the final-step films because of the extreme density of the composite masks.

With the system we use, the exposure times are in the order of three seconds for step 1, one minute for step 2, and three to seven minutes for step 3. Once the subtraction technique is standardized, it can be carried out as a routine darkroom procedure.

Circulatory
system

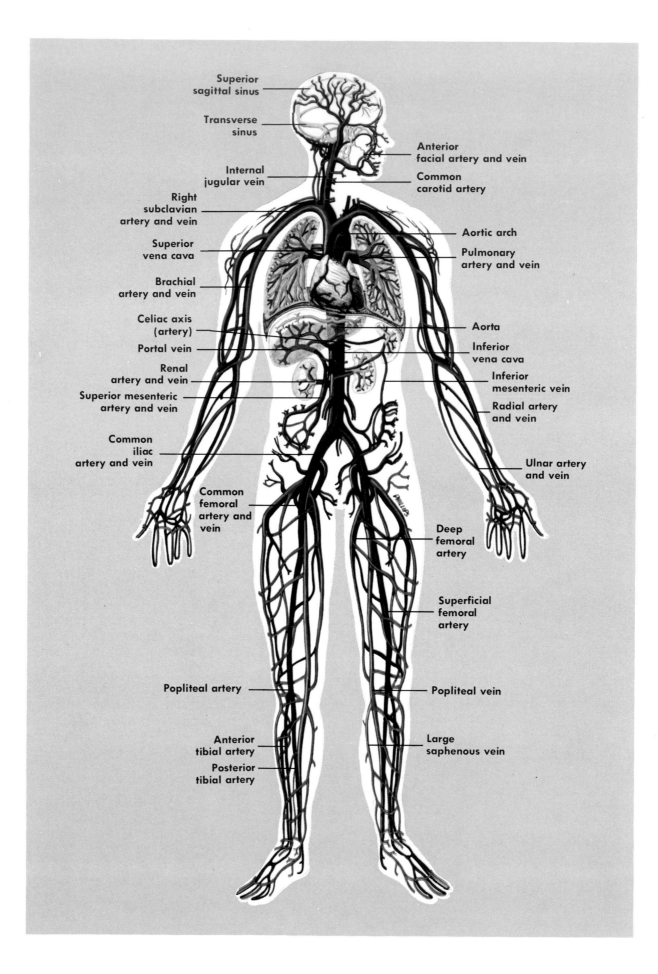

Superior
sagittal sinus

Transverse
sinus

Anterior
facial artery and vein

Internal
jugular vein

Common
carotid artery

Right
subclavian
artery and vein

Aortic arch

Superior
vena cava

Pulmonary
artery and vein

Brachial
artery and vein

Celiac axis
(artery)

Aorta

Portal vein

Inferior
vena cava

Renal
artery and vein

Inferior
mesenteric vein

Superior mesenteric
artery and vein

Radial artery
and vein

Common
iliac
artery and vein

Ulnar artery
and vein

Common
femoral
artery and
vein

Deep
femoral
artery

Superficial
femoral
artery

Popliteal artery

Popliteal vein

Anterior
tibial artery

Large
saphenous vein

Posterior
tibial artery

Circulatory system

The circulatory system comprises two complex systems of intimately associated vessels through which fluid is transported throughout the body in a continuous, unidirectional flow. The circulating fluid performs the dual function of carrying oxygen and nutritive material to the tissues and of collecting and transporting carbon dioxide and other waste products of metabolism from the tissues to the organs of excretion—the skin, the lungs, the liver, and the kidneys. The major portion of the circulatory system transports blood and is called the *blood-vascular system*. The minor portion, called the *lymphatic system*, collects from the tissue spaces the fluid that is filtered out of the blood vessels and conveys it back to the blood-vascular system. The fluid conveyed by the lymphatic system is called *lymph*.

BLOOD-VASCULAR SYSTEM

The blood-vascular system consists of a rhythmically contracting muscular organ called the *heart* and, branching out from and back to the heart, two systems of tubular vessels called *arteries, capillaries,* and *veins*. One of these systems traverses the lungs to discharge carbon dioxide and to take up oxygen for delivery to the remainder of the body tissues; this system of vessels is known as the *pulmonary circulation*. The second system branches throughout the body to the various organs and tissues and is called the *systemic circulation*. The heart serves as a pumping mechanism to keep the blood in constant circulation throughout the vast system of blood vessels. The arteries convey the blood from the heart to the capillaries, from whence the veins convey the blood back to the heart for redistribution.

From the main trunk vessel arising at the heart—the *pulmonary artery* for the pulmonary circulation, and the *aorta* for the systemic circulation—the arteries progressively diminish in size as they divide and subdivide along their course, finally ending in minute branches called *arterioles*. The arterioles divide to form the capillary vessels, and the branching process is then reversed: the capillaries unite to form *venules*, the beginning branches of the veins, which in turn unite and reunite to form larger and larger vessels as they approach the heart. The pulmonary veins end in four trunks opening into the heart, two trunk veins leading from each lung. The systemic veins are arranged in a superficial set, and in a deep set with which the superficial veins communicate; both sets converge toward a common trunk vein. The systemic veins end in two large vessels opening into the heart; the *superior vena cava* leads from the upper portion of the body, and the *inferior vena cava* leads from the lower portion.

The capillaries connect the arterioles and venules to form networks that pervade all organs and all other tissues supplied with blood. The capillary vessels have exceedingly thin walls, and it is through the thin walls of the capillaries that the essential functions of the blood-vascular system take place—the blood constituents are filtered out, and the waste products of cell activity are absorbed. The exchange takes place through the medium of *tissue fluid*, which is derived from the blood plasma and is drained off by the lymphatic system for return to the blood-vascular system. The tissue fluid undergoes modification in the lymphatic system and is then called *lymph*.

The *heart* is the central organ of the blood-vascular system, and it functions solely as a pump to keep the blood in circulation. It is approximately cone-shaped, and measures approximately 4¾ inches in length, 3½ inches in width, and 2¼ inches in depth. It is enclosed in a double-walled, fibrous sac called the *pericardium*, and it is situated obliquely in the middle mediastinum, largely to the left of the median sagittal plane. The base of the heart is directed upward, backward, and to the right.

Its apex rests on the diaphragm and against the anterior chest wall, and is directed downward, forward, and to the left.

The muscular wall of the heart is called the *myocardium*, and because of the force required to drive blood through the extensive systemic vessels, it is about three times as thick on the left side as on the right side. The membrane that lines the heart is called the *endocardium*. The thin, closely adherent membrane that covers the heart is called

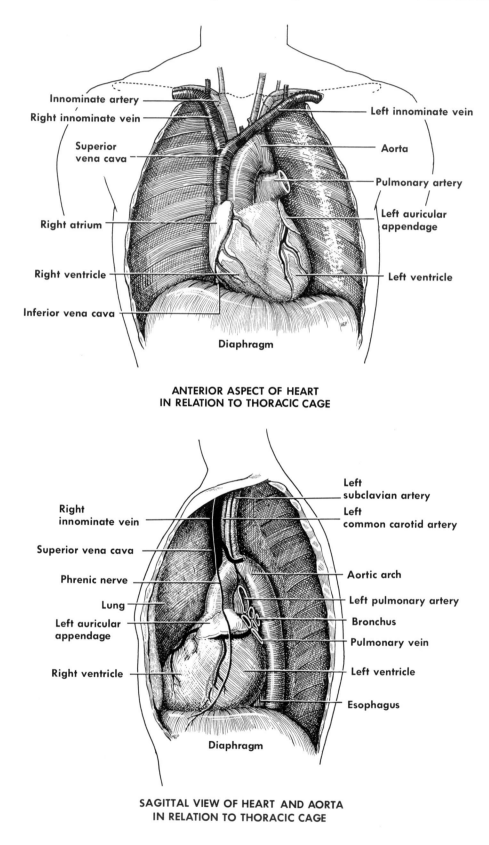

ANTERIOR ASPECT OF HEART
IN RELATION TO THORACIC CAGE

SAGITTAL VIEW OF HEART AND AORTA
IN RELATION TO THORACIC CAGE

924

the *epicardium*, or, because it also serves as the inner wall of the pericardial sac, the *visceral pericardium*. The narrow, fluid-containing space between the two walls of the sac is called the *pericardial cavity*.

The cavity of the heart is divided by septa into right and left halves, and each half is subdivided by a constriction into two cavities, or chambers. The two upper chambers are called *atria*, and each *atrium* consists of a principal cavity and of a lesser one called the *auricula*. The two lower chambers of the heart are called *ventricles*. The opening between the right atrium and the right ventricle is controlled by the *tricuspid valve*, and the opening between the left atrium and the left ventricle is controlled by the *bicuspid*, or *mitral*, *valve*. The atria function as receiving chambers, and the ventricles as distributing chambers. The right side of the heart handles the venous, or deoxygenated, blood, and the left side handles the arterial, or oxygenated, blood. The aorta arises from the left ventricle, and the pulmonary artery from the right ventricle. The pulmonary veins, two right and two left, open into the left atrium. The superior and inferior venae cavae open into the right atrium.

The *aorta* arises from the upper part of the left ventricle and passes upward and to the right for a short distance. It then arches backward and to the left and descends along the left side of the vertebral column to the level of the fourth lumbar vertebra, where it divides into the right and left *common iliac arteries*. The common iliac arteries diverge from each other as they pass to the level of the lumbosacral junction, where each ends by dividing into the *internal iliac*, or *hypogastric, artery* and the *ex-*ternal iliac artery*. The internal iliac artery passes into the pelvis. The external iliac artery passes to a point about midway between the anterior superior iliac spine and the pubic symphysis, and then enters the thigh to become the *femoral artery*.

The arteries are usually named according to their location. The several portions of the aorta are described according to direction, these portions being the *ascending aorta*, the *arch of the aorta*, and the *descending aorta*. The last division, the descending aorta, has thoracic and abdominal portions. The systemic arteries branch out, treelike, from the aorta to all parts of the body except the lungs. Each organ has its own vascular circuit which, arising from the trunk artery, leads back to the trunk vein for return to the heart.

The *pulmonary artery*, the main trunk of the pulmonary circulation, arises from the right ventricle of the heart, passes upward and backward for a distance of about 5 cm., and then divides into two branches, the *right* and *left pulmonary arteries*. These vessels enter the root of the respective lung and, following the course of the bronchi, divide and subdivide to form a dense network of capillaries surrounding the alveoli of the lungs. Through the thin walls of the capillaries the blood discharges carbon dioxide and absorbs oxygen from the air contained in the alveoli. The oxygenated blood passes onward through the pulmonary veins for return to the heart. It will be noted that in the pulmonary circulation, the deoxygenated blood is transported by the arteries, and the oxygenated blood is transported by the veins.

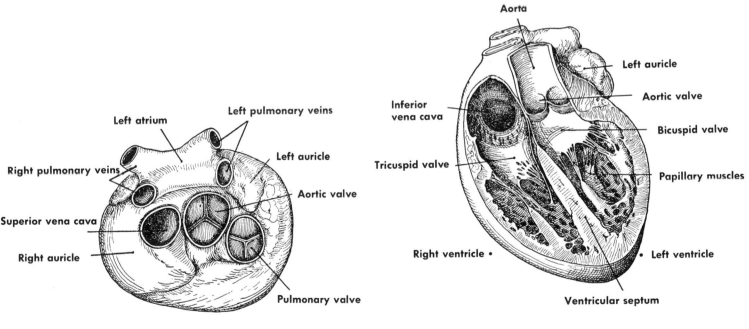

SUPERIOR ASPECT OF HEART

SECTION OF HEART SHOWING VENTRICULAR CHAMBERS, VENTRICULAR SEPTUM, AND PAPILLARY MUSCLES

925

As shown in the diagram below, the oxygenated (arterial) blood leaves the left ventricle by way of the aorta and is carried through the arteries to all parts of the body except the lungs. The deoxygenated (venous) blood is collected by the veins and returned to the right atrium, through the superior vena cava from the upper part of the body and through the inferior vena cava from the lower part of the body. This circuit, from the left ventricle to the right atrium, is called the *systemic circulation*. The venous blood passes from the right atrium into the right ventricle and out through the pulmonary artery and its branches to the lungs. After being arterialized, or oxygenated, in the capillaries of the lungs, the blood is conveyed to the left atrium of the heart through the pulmonary veins. The circuit from the right ventricle to the left atrium is called the *pulmonary circulation*.

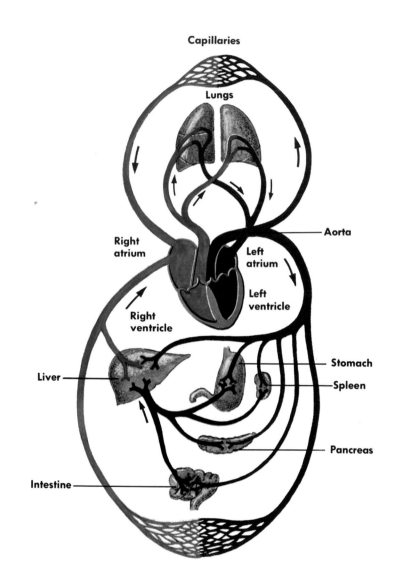

The heart contracts (systole) in pumping blood into the arteries, and relaxes, or dilates (diastole), in receiving blood from the veins. One phase of contraction (referred to as the *heartbeat*) and one phase of dilatation are called a *cardiac cycle*. In the average adult one cycle lasts eight-tenths of a second. However, the *heart rate*, or number of pulsations per minute, varies with size, age, and sex, being faster in small individuals, in young individuals, and in females. The heart rate is also increased with exercise, food, and emotional disturbances.

The velocity of blood circulation varies with the rate and intensity of the heartbeat, and it also varies in the different portions of the system in accordance with their distance from the initial pressure of the intermittent waves of blood issuing from the heart. The speed of flow is thus highest in the large arteries arising at or near the heart, because these vessels receive the full force of each wave of blood pumped out of the heart. The arterial walls expand during the pressure of receiving each wave. They then rhythmically contract, gradually diminishing the pressure of the advancing wave from point to point until the flow of blood is normally reduced to a steady, non-pulsating stream through the capillaries and veins. The *beat*, or contraction and expansion of an artery, which may be felt with the fingers at a number of points, is called the *pulse*.

Greisheimer[1] calculated that a complete circulation of the blood through both the systemic and pulmonary circuits, from a given point and back again, requires about twenty-three seconds and an average of twenty-seven heartbeats. In certain contrast examinations of the cardiovascular system, tests are made on each subject to determine the circulation time from the point of injection of the contrast medium to the site of interest. The circulation time is influenced by body position, that is, whether the patient is erect or recumbent.

[1]Greisheimer, Esther M.: Physiology and anatomy, ed. 4, Philadelphia, 1942, J. B. Lippincott Co., p. 470.

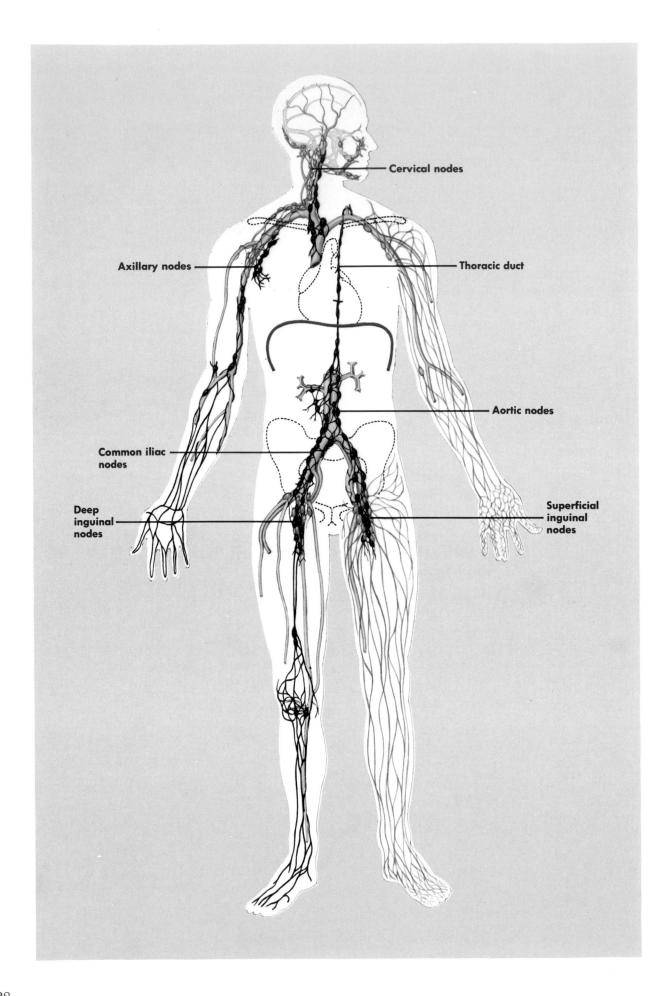

928

LYMPHATIC SYSTEM

The lymphatic system consists of an elaborate arrangement of closed vessels concerned with collecting fluid from the tissue spaces and transporting it to the blood-vascular system. The lymphatic vessels are almost entirely arranged in a superficial set (shown in the facing drawing in green) that lies immediately under the skin and accompanies the superficial veins, and a deep set (shown in black) that accompanies the deep blood vessels and with which the superficial lymphatics communicate. Unlike the blood-vascular system, the lymphatic system has no pumping mechanism. The conducting vessels are richly supplied with valves to prevent backward flow, while the movement of the lymph through the system is believed to be maintained largely by extrinsic pressure from the surrounding organs and muscles.

The lymphatic system begins in complex networks of thin-walled, absorbent capillaries situated in the various organs and tissues. The capillaries unite to form larger vessels, which in turn form networks and unite to form still larger vessels as they approach the terminal collecting trunks. The terminal trunks end at their opening into the large veins at the base of the neck.

The lymphatic vessels are small in caliber and have delicate, transparent walls. Along their course the collecting vessels pass through one or more nodular structures called lymph glands, or nodes. The nodes occur singly but are usually arranged in chains, or in groups, of two to twenty. The nodes are situated so that they form strategically placed centers toward which the conducting vessels converge. The nodes vary from the size of a pinhead to the size of an almond or larger. They may be spherical, oval, or kidney-shaped. Each node has a hilus through which the arteries enter and veins and efferent lymph vessels emerge; the afferent lymph vessels do not enter at the hilus. In addition to the lymphatic capillaries, blood vessels, and supporting structures, each lymph node contains masses, or follicles, of lymphocytes that are arranged around its circumference and from which cords of cells extend through the medullary portion of the node.

A number of conducting channels, here called afferent lymph vessels, enter the node opposite the hilus and break up into wide capillaries that surround the lymph follicles and form a canal known as the peripheral, or marginal, lymph sinus. The network of capillaries continues into the medullary portion of the node, widens out to form medullary sinuses, and then collects into several efferent vessels that leave the node at the hilus. The conducting vessels may pass through several nodes along their course, each time undergoing the process of widening into sinuses. Lymphocytes, a variety of white blood cells formed in the lymph glands, are added to the lymph while it is in the nodes. It is thought that a majority of the lymph is here absorbed by the venous system, and that only a small part is passed on through the conducting vessels.

The absorption and interchange of tissue fluids and of cells takes place through the thin walls of the capillaries. The lymph passes from the beginning capillaries through the conducting vessels, which eventually empty their contents into terminal lymph trunks for conveyance to the blood-vascular system. The main terminal trunk of the lymphatic system, the lower, dilated portion of which is known as the cisterna chyli, is called the thoracic duct. This duct receives the lymphatic drainage from all parts of the body below the diaphragm and from the left half of the body above the diaphragm. The thoracic duct extends from the level of the second lumbar vertebra to the base of the neck, where it ends by opening into the venous system at the junction of the left subclavian and internal jugular veins. Three terminal collecting trunks, called the right jugular, the subclavian, and the bronchomediastinal trunks, receive the lymphatic drainage from the right half of the body above the diaphragm. These vessels open into the right subclavian vein, either separately or, occasionally, after uniting to form a common trunk called the right lymphatic duct.

Visceral and peripheral angiography

Contributed by

Richard G. Lester, M.D.

Professor and Chairman, Department of Radiology
Duke University Medical Center, Durham, N. C.

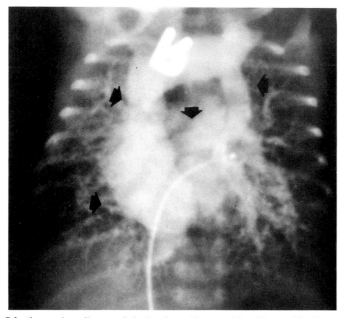

Selective angiocardiogram. Injection into right ventricle of heart. Blue infant with total anomalous pulmonary venous connection. Upper arrows on left point to anomalous vein; upper arrow on right points to dilated superior vena cava; lowest arrow points to right atrium filling through anomalous return.

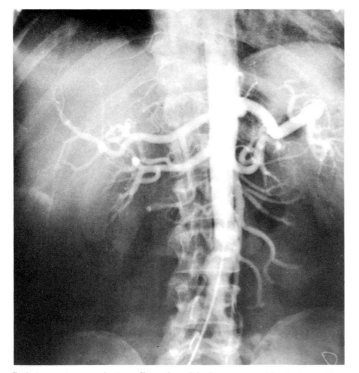

Catheter aortogram. Aorta, celiac axis and its branches, renal arteries, and superior mesenteric arteries shown. Patient has atherosclerosis.

Angiography is a general term used to denote radiologic examinations of vascular structures within the body as they are opacified by an injection of an organic, iodinated contrast solution. A variety of angiographic examinations are performed in the radiology department, and a number of terms are applied to these studies. The terminology used depends upon (1) the vascular structures opacified, and (2) the method of injection.

Arteriography refers to opacification studies of arterial vessels. Frequently, venous structures can also be seen in later stages of such examinations.

Venography is a term denoting opacification studies of peripheral or central veins. *Lymphography*, opacification studies of lymph vessels and lymph nodes, is explained in the next discussion.

Cerebral angiography, opacification studies of the blood vessels of the brain, has been covered in the preceding discussion of the central nervous system.

Angiocardiography is a study to investigate the interior of the heart. The great vessels (e.g., the pulmonary arteries) can also be seen during such examinations.

Aortography refers to opacification studies of either the thoracic aorta (thoracic aortography) or the abdominal aorta (abdominal aortography, lumbar aortography).

Angiographic examinations may also be denoted by the route of injection. Selective angiography is performed through a catheter placed at the site of interest; for example, renal arteriography is performed by passing a catheter into the abdominal aorta and into the mouth of the renal artery to be investigated. Angiography may be performed via needle injection directly into the area of interest (e.g., peripheral arteriography may be performed by injection into the femoral artery), or the injection may be made by the venous route. An example of the latter procedure is "venous aortography," in which a large bolus of contrast material is injected into a peripheral vein, from whence the material passes through the right side of the heart, the lungs, and the left side of the heart; films of the aorta are made at preselected times.

Arteriographic examinations may also be separated into peripheral studies (studies of extremity arteries) and visceral studies (studies of arteries of the chest or abdomen; e.g., renal arteriography).

PURPOSE

Angiographic examinations may have several different diagnostic functions under a variety of circumstances. In most situations, the most crucial purpose of the examination is the precise anatomic delineation of pathologic processes involving vessels themselves.

In other cases, angiographic studies are of dynamic (physiologic) significance. For example, the motion of the pulmonary valve can be studied during selective angiocardiography.

In still other cases, vascular studies are performed for the purpose of organ opacification. Such studies may be particularly valuable in the evaluation of tumors.

The choice of equipment and the method of vascular procedure often depends upon the kind of information desired. Generally speaking, rapid-film units (vide infra) are superior to cine (x-ray motion-picture) devices when anatomic detail is of paramount importance. Conversely, cine devices are superior when dynamic function must be evaluated.

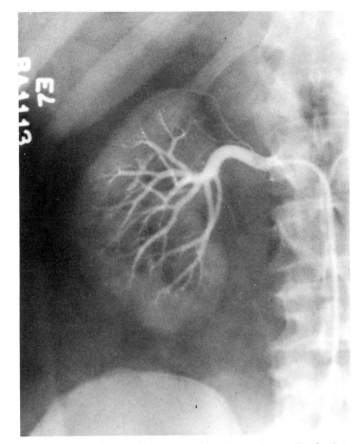

Selective renal arteriogram. Catheter passed from femoral artery. Tip of catheter in renal artery.

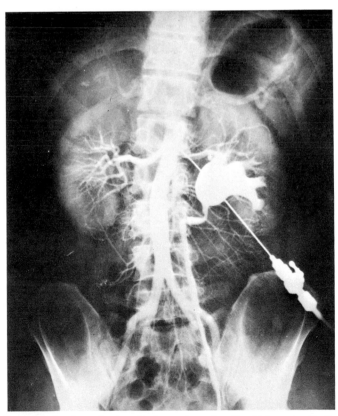

Renal arteries shown by translumbar aortography. Opacified renal collecting system on left (retrograde pyelogram).

Radiograph courtesy Dr. Ned Shnayerson.

931

CONTRAST MEDIA

A wide variety of opaque contrast media are used in angiographic studies. All the materials currently in use are organic iodine solutions. They vary as to chemical nature (e.g., some are sodium salts while others are methylglucamine salts) and in the concentration of the drug per milliliter of solution. The more concentrated media are more opaque; however, they are also more viscous. The choice of contrast media will vary with various angiographic examinations. The choice of such material must be made by the examining radiologist.

In at least one special circumstance, the radiologist may elect to perform the examination by decreasing the density within the heart. In the case of pericardial effusion, radiologists may inject a gas (carbon dioxide) either intravenously or through a catheter into the right atrium of the heart. This examination is simple and safe, but important precautions must be observed. The patient must be placed in the left lateral decubitus position (right side of the thorax up), and the films must be made in the anteroposterior direction by cross-table projection. The carbon dioxide is injected in a carefully measured quantity (usually 50 cc. and not more than 100 cc.). The filming may be performed with a rapid film changer, or films may be changed by hand. Following this examination, it is absolutely essential that the patient maintain the left lateral decubitus position until the carbon dioxide is absorbed by blood passing through the right atrium. In no case should the patient be turned into the supine position until the radiologist specifically instructs the technologist. If this precaution is not observed, an air embolus to a pulmonary artery may result. Even more significant complications may result in patients with pericardial effusion associated with certain congenital heart diseases if this important postexamination routine is not observed.

INJECTION TECHNIQUES

The injection of contrast material may be made by hand with a syringe. More often, a mechanical device is employed to inject a known quantity of the contrast material in a predetermined period of time.

EQUIPMENT

Angiocardiography and selective visceral arteriography require the use of rapid film changers and/or cine devices. Simpler angiographic procedures (e.g., peripheral arteriography, venography) may be performed with conventional Potter-Bucky systems. The decision as to the type of x-ray equipment to be used must obviously be made by the examining radiologist.

A number of rapid film changers are available. All these devices move films and permit exposures at intervals of a fraction of a second. With one device as many as twelve films per second can be made. Others have a maximum speed of six films per second or less. Some devices use cut films, whereas others roll films. In some devices cassettes are moved; in others, screens are apposed to the film by the device during the exposure and moved from this location during the film travel. Rapid film changers may be used either singly or in combination at right angles in order to obtain simultaneous frontal and lateral evaluations of the vascular system under investigation. The latter units are called biplane rapid film changers.

EQUIPMENT—cont'd

Cine apparatus, consisting basically of a camera that photographs the output phosphor of an image intensification system, can achieve sequential exposures up to rates of sixty per second or more, with resultant true motion-picture radiography. These cameras utilize 16 mm. or 35 mm. film rather than the "true" size of film used in rapid film changers. Detail achievable with cine units is not as satisfactory as with the rapid film changers. However, many more events can be photographed with the cine devices, and dynamic function can be evaluated more satisfactorily in this manner.

Many image intensification devices include television circuitry. With such devices, angiographic examinations may be videotaped, or motion-picture photography of the video viewer (Kine) may be utilized.

Rapid film work requires high-power generators. Since high milliampere-second techniques are essential to good contrast, and since short exposures are essential in moving fields, generators must be capable of high current output.

Angiographic rooms frequently contain a great deal of equipment other than specifically radiologic devices. Monitoring systems capable of continuous recording of electrocardiographic data, pressure information from within the heart and great vessels, and, at times, other data may be present. Emergency equipment may include devices for resuscitation, devices for defibrillation of the heart, anesthesia apparatus, etc. The technologist must familiarize himself with the use of each of these pieces of apparatus.

ANGIOGRAPHIC TEAM

While the team of physician and technical specialists in the angiographic room may include such personnel as an anesthetist, a laboratory technician, and a nurse, the basic members of the group are the physician-radiologist and the radiologic technologist. In many cases the technologist will be required to learn and observe sterile techniques, to operate monitoring devices and emergency equipment, and to assist the physician in the performance of the procedure, all in addition to the operation of the radiographic apparatus. Where the technologist is required to operate the nonradiologic apparatus, the physician will ordinarily make certain that the technologist is properly instructed. However, acquiring a knowledge of simple nursing techniques and of sterile procedure is part of the basic preparation of the radiologic technologist.

ANGIOCARDIOGRAPHY

Angiocardiography is the term used to denote opacification studies of the heart and of the great vessels about the heart. Such studies may be performed after the injection of a bolus of contrast material into a peripheral vein of either the upper or the lower extremity; filming of the heart takes place after a suitable interval to permit the opacified blood to reach the thorax. This method is called *forward angiocardiography* or *venous angiocardiography*.

Alternatively, a catheter may be passed from a peripheral vein under radioscopic control through the vena cava and into one of the chambers of the right side of the heart. This more detailed method is called *selective angiocardiography*. In this method, the catheter may be placed in the right atrium, the right ventricle, or the pulmonary artery for detailed study of these areas and of areas beyond the site of injection. By means of a special technique, the catheter may even be passed across the atrial septum into the left atrium and left ventricle.

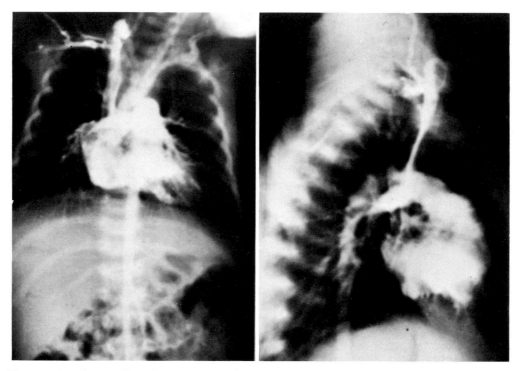

Venous angiocardiogram. This infant is cyanotic, suffering from another type of total anomalous pulmonary venous connection (page 930). Early part of study to show opacification of right side of heart, right-to-left shunt of opacified blood into left atrium, and filling of aorta.

In still another method of evaluating the chambers of the left side of the heart, a catheter is passed from a peripheral artery into the aorta in retrograde fashion, around the arch of the aorta, and across the aortic valve into the left ventricle. This method is sometimes called *left ventriculography* or *retrograde cardioangiography*.

These and other selective techniques permit detailed evaluation of the chambers of the heart, the valves, and the great vessels surrounding the heart. These studies are utilized in studying a wide variety of congenital and acquired heart diseases. Filming may be performed either with rapid film changers or with cine cameras.

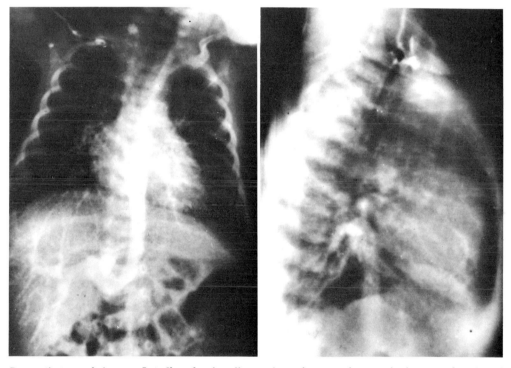

Same patient as on facing page. Late films of angiocardiogram show pulmonary veins emptying into anomalous channel that is directed downward through the diaphragm to connect with the portal vein (normally, pulmonary veins empty into left atrium).

AORTOGRAPHY AND
VISCERAL ARTERIOGRAPHY

Aortography is the study of the thoracic or abdominal aorta and its branch vessels. The simplest method is *venous aortography*, in which a large bolus of contrast material is injected intravenously; sequential filming of the thoracic or abdominal aorta follows after an appropriate interval selected by the physician on the basis of the circulation time. This method depends upon the circulation of the contrast material from the selected vein through the right side of the heart, the pulmonary circulation, and the left side of the heart, and then into the aorta.

Another method of visualizing the abdominal aorta is *translumbar aortography*. With the patient lying prone on the examining table, a long needle is passed percutaneously into the abdominal aorta and contrast material is injected through the needle. This method permits more satisfactory evaluation of the abdominal aorta. It should be noted that the thoracic aorta is not seen when this method is used.

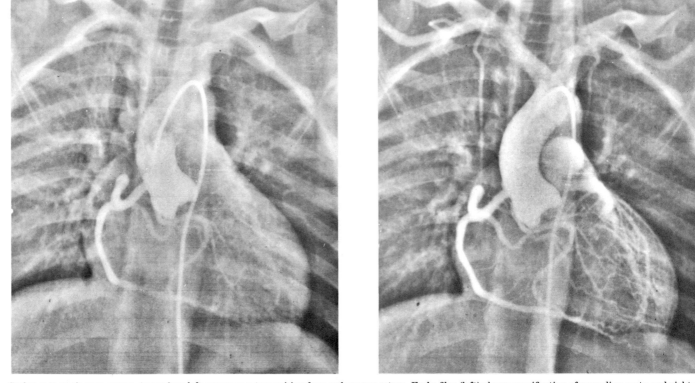

Catheter thoracic aortograms. Anomalous left coronary artery arising from pulmonary artery. Early film (left) shows opacification of ascending aorta and right pulmonary artery. Later film (right) shows opacification of left coronary artery via anastomotic connections from right with subsequent opacification of pulmonary artery.

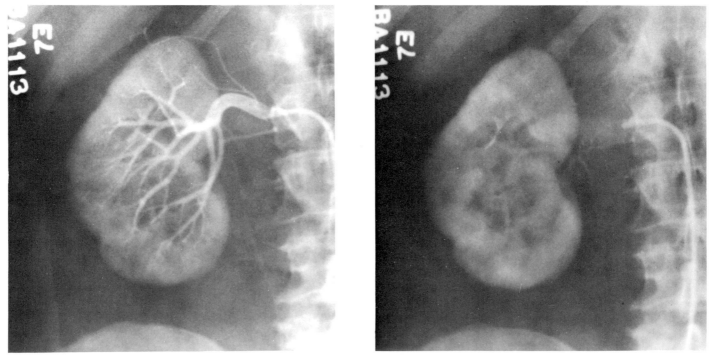

Selective renal arteriograms. Early film (left) shows renal arterial branches. Later film (right) shows nephrogram.

936

The most satisfactory visualization of the aorta is achieved by placing a catheter into the aorta at the desired point. This method of catheter aortography, or selective aortography, is most frequently performed utilizing the Seldinger technique. A specially designed needle is used to puncture the femoral artery. Following satisfactory puncture, a long catheter and a guide wire is passed into the femoral artery. Then the catheter is placed, under radioscopic control, in the desired location in the thoracic or lumbar aorta, contrast material is injected, and films are made at appropriate intervals.

With this catheter technique, branch vessels of the aorta, such as the renal artery, the celiac artery, or the superior mesenteric artery, can be entered selectively and injected for detailed studies of these vessels and their branch vessels. This method is called *selective visceral arteriography*.

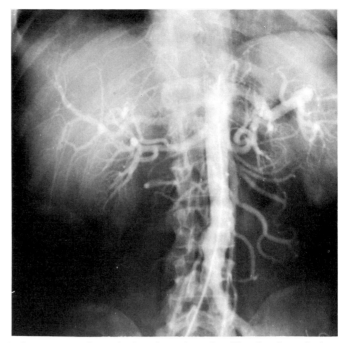

Catheter aortography and visceral arteriography. Tip of catheter in lower dorsal aorta. Celiac axis, renal arteries, superior mesenteric artery, and branches are shown.

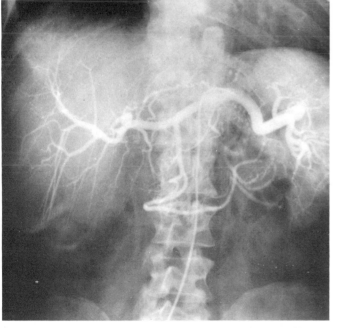

Same patient. Selective celiac arteriogram shows branches of this vessel in much better detail.

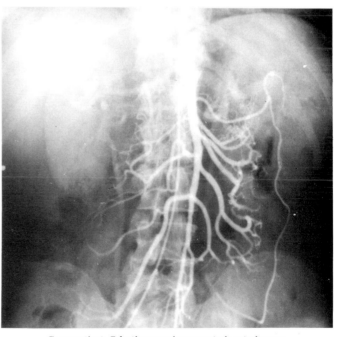

Same patient. Selective superior mesenteric arteriogram.

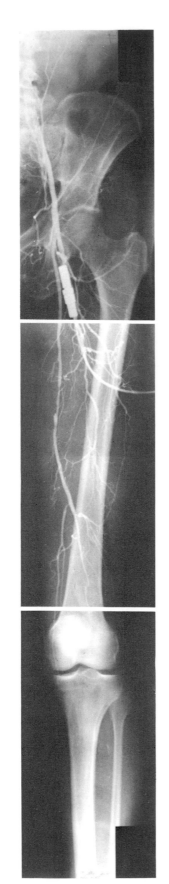

Femoral arteriogram in patient with arteriosclerosis and multiple partial obstructions.

PERIPHERAL ARTERIOGRAPHY AND VENOGRAPHY

All the major arteries of both the upper and the lower extremities may be studied by similar contrast techniques. The veins of the lower extremities, the upper extremities and the venae cavae can be studied by injection studies made at appropriate sites.

In all cases, the precise methods used and the sequence of filming must be determined by the radiologist in charge of the procedures. The exercise of great care in using sterile techniques, in positioning the patient, and in filming the sequence requires careful and informed cooperation between the physician and the radiologic technologist.

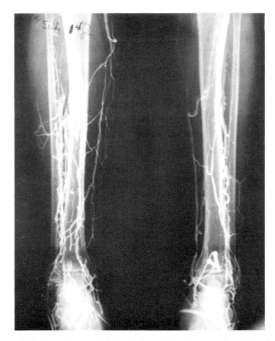

Venogram, Injection of superficial vein in ankle. Shows veins of leg in patient with varicosities and incompetent perforators.

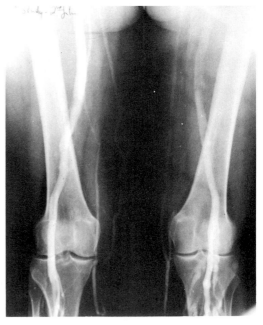

Same patient. Veins of thigh.

Lymphography

Contributed by

David L. Benninghoff, M.D.

Clinical Professor of Radiology, State University of New York,
Downstate Medical Center, Brooklyn, N. Y.
Radiotherapist, Huntington Hospital, Huntington, N. Y.

Lymphography is a general term applied to radiologic examinations of the lymph vessels and nodes after they have been opacified by an injected iodinated contrast medium. The study of the lymph vessels, which may be called *lymphangiography*, is carried out within the first hour following injection of the contrast material. The study of the lymph nodes, which may be called *lymphadenography*, is made twenty-four hours after injection of the contrast medium. The lymph vessels empty the contrast agent within a few hours. The nodes normally retain the contrast substance for no more than three or four weeks. Abnormal nodes may retain the medium for several months, so that delayed lymphadenograms may be made, as indicated, without further injection.

PURPOSE

The primary indication for lymphography is to assess the clinical extent of lymphomas (Hodgkin's disease, lymphosarcoma, reticulum cell sarcoma, and other neoplasms). Lymphography may be indicated in patients in whom there is clinical evidence of obstruction or other impairment of the lymphatic system.

CONTRAST MEDIA

Lymphography is currently performed with the use of an iodinated oil contrast medium and by the direct-injection technique developed by Kinmonth and associates.[1] A water-soluble, iodinated contrast medium may be used to delineate the lymphatic vessels and nodes of the extremities, but these agents are miscible with lymph and undergo dilution, and they diffuse out through the lymphatic walls so rapidly that they cannot be used to study the proximal lymphatics.

The oily contrast medium presently employed is ethiodized oil (Ethiodol). This agent affords opacification of the lymphatic vessels for several hours following the injection. The lymph nodes are outlined on the studies of the vessels, but their internal structure does not become optimally opacified until about twenty-four hours later.

[1]Kinmonth, J. B., Harper, R. A. K., and Taylor, G. W.: Lymphangiography by radiologic methods, J. Fac. Radiologists **6**:217-223, 1955.

Juxta-aortic group

Common iliac group

External chain

External iliac group

Middle chain

Internal chain

Hypogastric group

ILIOPELVIC-AORTIC LYMPHATIC SYSTEM
(After Cuneo and Marcille)
Anterior view

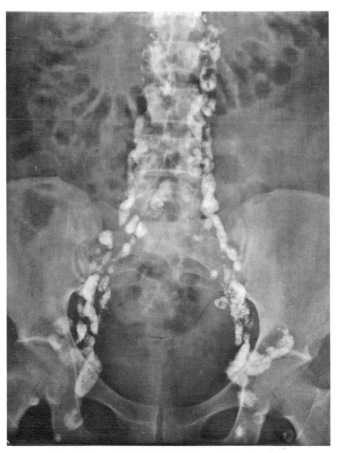

Frontal view of iliopelvic-abdominoaortic lymph nodes.

DYE SUBSTANCE

Ordinarily the peripheral lymphatic vessels cannot be identified easily because of their small size and lack of color. For identification of the lymphatic vessels on the dorsum of the feet and hands, a blue dye that is selectively absorbed by the lymphatics is injected subcutaneously into the first and second interdigital web spaces about fifteen minutes before the examination. The dyes commonly used for this purpose are 11% patent blue violet and 4% sky blue.

Following patent blue violet injection, the patient's urine and skin will be tinted blue. This condition disappears within a few hours.

PRECAUTIONS

As in any procedure involving injection of foreign materials, untoward reactions must be anticipated. The patient must be observed closely, and appropriate medications and resuscitation equipment must be nearby.

INJECTION SITES

Lymphography is limited to easily accessible injection sites—the lymphatics of the feet and of the hands. Most examinations are performed by injection of the lymphatics of the feet. This injection route provides visualization of the lymphatic structures of the lower extremity, the groin, the iliopelvic-abdominoaortic region, and the thoracic duct. Injection of the lymphatics of the hand provides visualization of the upper extremity, and of the axillary, infraclavicular, and supraclavicular regions. Visceral lymphography, that is, visualization of the lymphatic structures of the abdominal and thoracic viscera, is an experimental procedure.

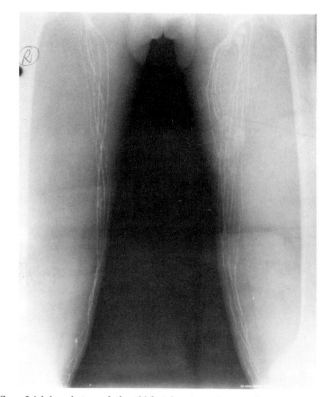

Superficial lymphatics of the thigh taken ten minutes after completion of dorsal pedal lymphatic injection.

INJECTION SUPPLIES

The following items are required for the sterile tray:
1. An insulin or tuberculin syringe for injection of blue dye
2. Three 10 ml. Luer-Lok syringes
3. Two ½-inch, 26-gauge Luer needles
4. Two ¼-inch, 20-gauge Luer needles
5. One No. 3 knife blade holder
6. One No. 10 knife blade
7. One Stevens tenotomy scissors, curved
8. One Knapp Iris scissors, sharp point
9. One Knapp Iris scissors, blunt point
10. Two curved Halsted mosquito clamps
11. Two straight Halsted mosquito clamps
12. One dull, two-pronged retractor (small plastic type)
13. One Thorp forceps
14. One Castroviego suture forceps
15. Four Backhous towel forceps, 3-inch
16. 3-0 black silk sutures
17. 4-0 black silk sutures (atraumatic, with curved cutting-edge needle)
18. One needle holder (Halsey eye)
19. Four surgical towels
20. Two draw sheets
21. Medicine glass
22. Iodine cups (two)
23. Foerstar sponge forceps
24. Polyethylene tubing connected to a 27- or 30-gauge needle for cannulation of the lymph vessel (sterile, disposable lymphography sets supplied by Becton, Dickinson and Co., Rutherford, N. J.)

The following items are required for the service (nonsterile) tray:
1. Skin cleansing agent: 70% alcohol and benzalkonium chloride (Zephiran)
2. Vial of specified sterile blue dye
3. Vial of sterile lidocaine, 1% (Xylocaine)
4. Two vials of sterile contrast medium (Ethiodol)
5. Sponge basin
6. Sterile 2″ × 2″ and 4″ × 4″ gauze squares
7. Adhesive tape

FILMING PROCEDURE

Radiographs are made within the first hour after completion of the injection for the demonstration of the lymph vessels. A second series of radiographs, which may include tomographic studies, is made twenty-four hours later to demonstrate the lymph nodes.

The exposure factors employed for lymphographic studies are the same as those used for bone studies of the respective region.

Tomography and magnification radiography are other techniques sometimes required to obtain better delineation of the opacified lymph nodes.

TECHNIQUE OF LYMPHATIC INJECTION OF FEET

Preceding the examination the feet must be thoroughly washed, and shaved about the sites of injection. The patient is placed in the supine position for the injection procedure and is so kept until the lymphangiographic studies have been completed. The injection need not be made in a radiographic examining room; it may be carried out in an operating room, and the patient may be on a padded stretcher, ready for conveyance to the radiology department.

Both feet are surgically cleansed and draped. The blue dye, 0.1 ml. of 11% patent blue violet or 4% sky blue, is injected subcutaneously into the first and second interdigital web spaces of each foot to stain the lymph for identification of the lymphatic vessels. The dye may be mixed with a local anesthetic to minimize the pain of the injections.

About fifteen minutes after the injection of the blue dye, a local anesthetic (1% lidocaine) is injected subcutaneously in an amount sufficient to distend the tissues overlying the body of the first metatarsal, which is the site of cutdown for exposure and cannulation of the lym-

phatic vessel. A small (2 cm.), longitudinal incision is made over the body of the first metatarsal immediately lateral to the extensor tendon of the great toe. (Some radiologists advocate a transverse incision at this site.) The dye-filled lymphatic is seen as a fine, blue vessel in the subcutaneous tissue. The vessel is dissected free of surrounding tissue and is then cannulated with a 27- or 30-gauge needle connected to polyethylene tubing. The needle is tied securely in the vessel, and the tubing is connected to the syringe containing the contrast medium. An automatic injection device is used. A total of 6 ml. of the contrast medium is slowly injected into each lower extremity over a period of thirty minutes.

That the injection is intralymphatic and not intravenous may, when there is doubt, be determined radiographically with a mobile unit. After completion of the injection, the needle is removed, the overlying skin incision is closed with interrupted silk sutures, and a dressing is applied. The lymphatic vessel is not ligated or disturbed in any way. The patient, still in the supine position, is transported to the radiology department for studies of the lymphatic vessels.

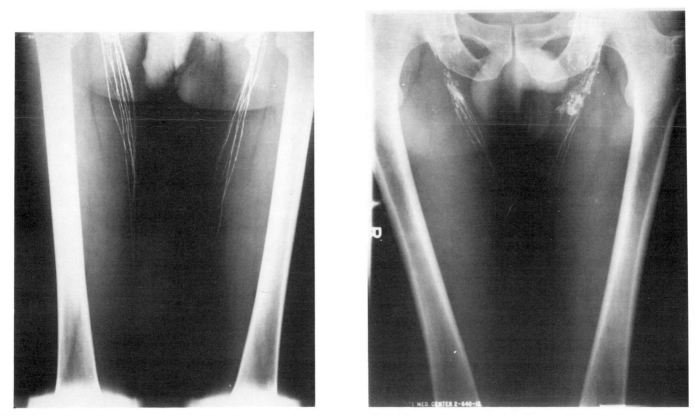

Delayed films of opposite patient. The superficial lymphatic vessels of the thigh are opacified, and the contrast medium is in the superficial inguinal lymph node group.

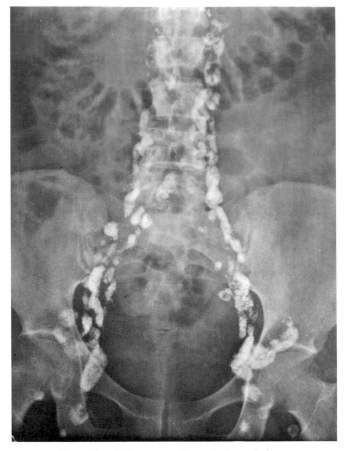

Normal lymphadenogram, anteroposterior projection.

LYMPHOGRAPHY

Iliopelvic-abdominoaortic region

Three radiographs, anteroposterior and 30-degree right and left oblique anteroposterior projections, are taken for each of the two iliopelvic-abdominoaortic studies. The lymphangiograms are taken within the first hour after injection of the contrast medium, and twenty-four hours later, the lymphadenograms are taken.

The exposures are made on $14'' \times 17''$ films that are adjusted to include the lower border of the ischium. The central ray is directed vertically and centered at the level of the iliac crests.

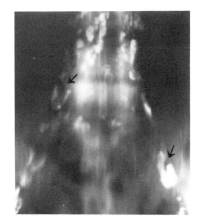

Tomogram demonstrates that the notched areas (arrows) are peripheral defects, most likely fat.

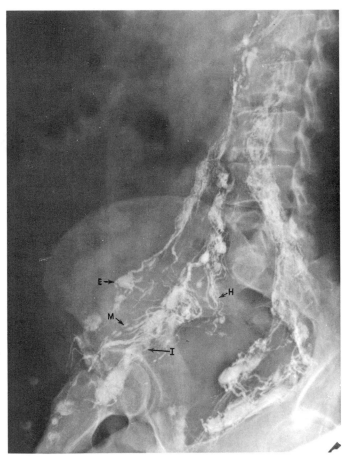

Lymphangiogram of iliopelvic-aortic region. Right anteroposterior oblique projection showing external chain, **E**, middle chain, **M**, and internal chain, **I**, of external and common iliac groups. **H** indicates hypogastric group.

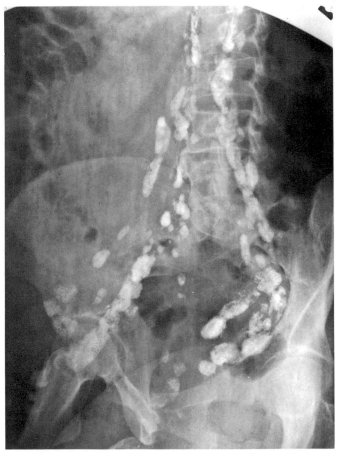

Lymphadenogram (made twenty-four hours later) of same patient.

942

LYMPHOGRAPHY

Thoracic duct

Two radiographs, anteroposterior and left lateral projections, are made for each of two serial studies of the thoracic duct. The contrast medium remains in the thoracic duct for less than an hour after completion of the injection, and the radiologist times these studies accordingly.

The exposures are made on 14″ × 17″ films that are adjusted to place the upper margin of the film 2 inches above the supraclavicular region. The central ray is directed perpendicularly to the midpoint of the film.

Lower extremity

Three anteroposterior projections, centered, respectively, at the level of the midtibias, the level of midfemora, and, for the groins, the level of the symphysis pubis, may be taken for the demonstration of the lymphatic vessels and, twenty-four hours later, for the demonstration of the lymph nodes of the lower extremities.

The exposures are made on 14″ × 17″ films. The central ray is directed vertically.

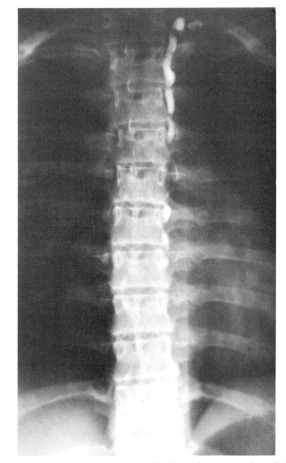

Anteroposterior projection showing opacification of upper portion of thoracic duct. Segmented appearance is caused by valves.

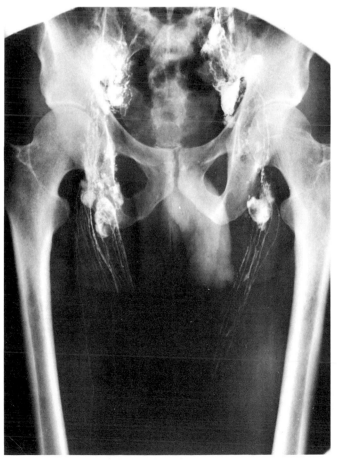

Lymphangiogram of inguinal region and upper thighs.

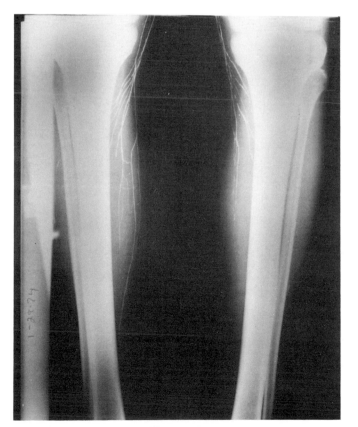

Lymphangiogram of legs ten minutes after injection.

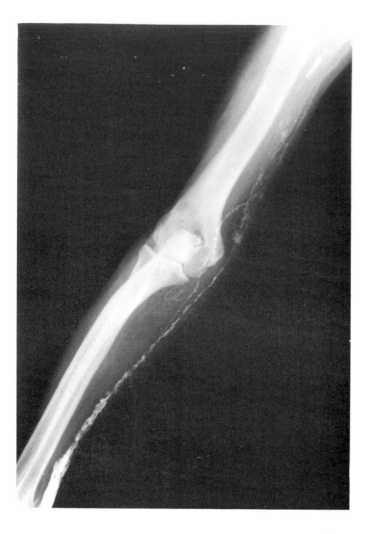

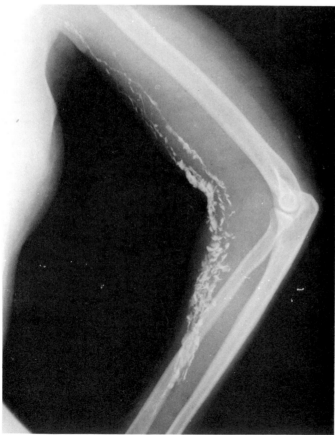

LYMPHOGRAPHY

TECHNIQUE OF LYMPHATIC INJECTION OF HAND

The general procedure is the same as for the feet. Blue dye is injected into the dorsal surface of the first and second interdigital web spaces. A longitudinal skin incision is made on the dorsum of the hand, parallel to, and on the ulnar side of, the tendon of the musculus extensor pollicis longus over the base of the first or second metacarpal. A 30-gauge needle is used for cannulation. Four milliliters of the contrast medium are injected. This quantity is sufficient to visualize the lymphatics of the upper extremity and the lymph nodes of the axilla.

Upper extremity

Anteroposterior and lateral projections are taken on 14″ × 17″ films for both the lymphangiograms and the later lymphadenograms of the arm and forearm. The films are placed diagonally so that they include the entire extremity. The central ray is directed vertically and is centered to the elbow.

Axilla

Anteroposterior and 45-degree, oblique anteroposterior projections are taken for each series of studies of the axilla. These studies may be made on 11″ × 14″ films that are adjusted to include the supraclavicular region. The central ray is directed vertically and is centered to the region of the coracoid process.

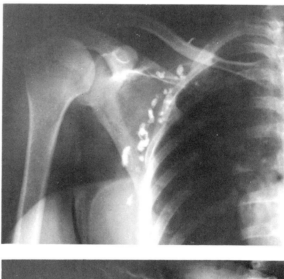

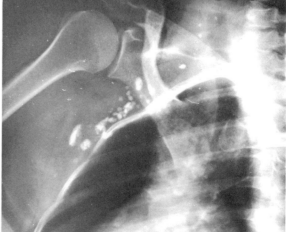

Lymphangiograms of upper extremity, frontal and lateral views. Fluting of vessels and extravasation of contrast medium is shown.

Lymphadenograms of axilla, frontal and oblique views.

944

Pararadiologic imaging modalities

ULTRASONOGRAPHY
AND THERMOGRAPHY

Pararadiologic imaging modalities
Ultrasonography and thermography

Contributed by

Barbara M. Curcio, R.T.

Associate Professor of Radiologic Technology
College of Health and Allied Health Professions
University of Oklahoma Health Sciences Center, Oklahoma City

Ultrasonography and thermography are medical imaging modalities that evolved from technology and instrumentation developed for defense purposes and military use. Each has an interesting history (see bibliography), and its use in medicine is fairly new. These specialties are part of a growing group of nonionizing-radiation imaging methods, which are performed in correlation with radiologic procedures. Many features of the technical aspects of these modalities are related to the importance of positioning and to the cause-and-effect relationship between the production of energy and a resulting film image, and each involves electronic equipment.

There are many nonmedical applications for thermography and ultrasonography, related to industry, ecological studies, and various other sciences, as a review of some of the papers listed in the bibliography will reveal. The discussion here is restricted to the medical uses of these modalities, particularly as they relate to radiologic procedures. A complete training course is beyond the scope of this text, but formal educational programs do exist and the interested technologist is advised to seek information regarding approved schools from the organizations listed below.

American Society of Radiologic Technologists,
    500 N. Michigan Ave., Chicago, Ill. 60611
American Thermographic Society,
    4041 Wilshire Blvd., Los Angeles, Calif. 90010
American Society of Ultrasound Technical Specialists,
    University Hospital, P. O. Box 26901, Oklahoma City,
    Okla. 73190

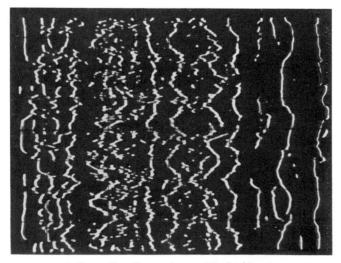

A time-motion ultrasound scan of the fetal heart.

Courtesy Dr. Ross E. Brown.

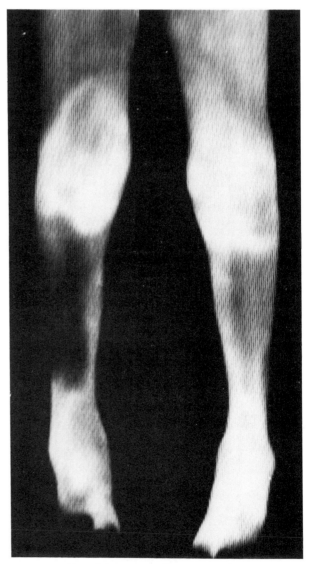

Frontal thermogram of lower extremities.

Courtesy Dr. J. Gershon-Cohen.

ULTRASONOGRAPHY

Ultrasonography is the technical procedure with which the transmitted and reflected properties of an extremely high (*ultra*) sound (*sono*) beam are imaged and recorded (*graph*) after passage through the body. The resultant image is formed by the interaction of the sound beam with the various tissue boundaries or interfaces it encounters during passage through the body. The image may be obtained by various modes, depending on the structure under study. Both stationary and dynamic structures can be evaluated.

Physics of ultrasound

Unlike x rays, which are electromagnetic waves, sound is a matter wave. Sound waves are vibrations in gases, liquids, and solids, and those in the frequency range of from 20 to 20,000 hertz (Hz) are audible. Sound vibrations below 20 Hz are called subsonic, and those above 20,000 Hz are called ultrasonic. Frequencies of 1 to 15 million Hz (or 1 to 15 megahertz [MHz]) are used for medical diagnostic ultrasonography. When ultrasound is transmitted through a medium and strikes a second medium, a part of the energy is reflected at the interface, and the rest of the energy penetrates into the second medium. An interface is a tissue boundary or that point at which the density of the medium is altered. For example, there is an interface between skin and fatty tissue, and another between soft tissue and bone. In ultrasonography diagnostic information is obtained from the sound reflections, or echoes, at tissue boundaries. Because an ultrasound beam travels through tissue at a fixed rate, the distance the beam travels to strike an interface and the distance traveled by the returning echo, when displayed appropriately on the equipment, indicate the proportional distances between the structures traversed.

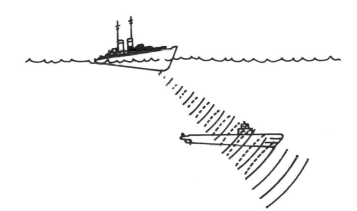

Diagram of principles of sonar in detecting enemy vessels. Medical ultrasound was developed from the principles of sonar utilized in World War II.

Courtesy Dr. Ross E. Brown.

947

Equipment and methodology

Ultrasound equipment produces an adjustable current to stimulate a polarized ceramic (piezoelectric) crystal housed in a device called the transducer. The transducer is used to transmit a pulsed ultrasound beam through the patient. When stimulated electrically (about 500 times per second) the crystal in the transducer converts the energy to ultrasonic impulses. These are then transmitted into the tissues. The strength (sensitivity) of the propagated sound beam must be adjustable to facilitate identification of minute differences in tissue densities (interfaces) of a structure; this could be compared to the effect of kilovoltage in radiography. Since the transducer is stimulated only a portion of the time, it also receives the returning echoes, which are reflected back after contact with tissue interfaces. It does this during the so-called "silent periods" when it is not transmitting. A receiver/amplifier component then processes the minute electrical signal produced from the surface of the crystal by the returning echo, and the reflected echoes are identified on an oscilloscope. The oscilloscope is calibrated by a synchronizer so that the position of the returning echo spikes or echo dots constitutes a direct indication of the distance between the transducer and the tissue borders or interfaces that give rise to the echoes. Finally, the equipment must include a means of making permanent records of the oscilloscope image. Recording is commonly obtained with the use of a Polaroid camera, although other methods of photography may be utilized.

It is also possible to utilize the Doppler effect in a low-energy, high-frequency, continuous ultrasound method. The Doppler effect relates to the alteration in the frequency of sound waves reflected from a moving target, such as a pulsating structure or moving cells within a blood vessel. The frequency of the reflected sound differs from that of the transmitted sound, and the difference in frequency is converted to audible signals. For this method of continuous ultrasound, a transducer having both a transmitting and a receiving crystal is required.

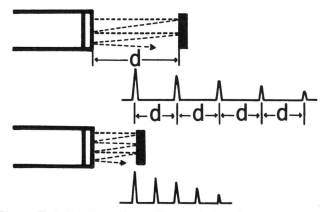

Diagram illustrating the need for amplification of echoes that occur at increasing distance from the transducer. This amplification is performed by the amplifier/receiver mechanism in the equipment.

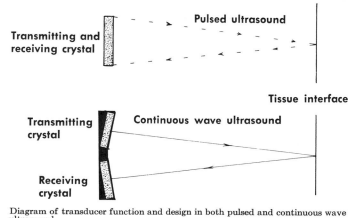

Diagram of transducer function and design in both pulsed and continuous wave ultrasound.

Above diagrams courtesy Dr. Ross E. Brown.

948

Methods of display (imaging)

There are several methods of portraying the echo. In the A-mode method, echoes are recorded as vertical spikes, with the height of the spike proportional to the strength of the echo. The horizontal distance between spikes represents the depth of the reflecting interface. The A-mode method is always performed with the transducer maintained in a fixed position, and it is used to determine the depth of a reflecting interface.

In the B-mode method, the echoes are recorded as dots along a linear trace. The strength of the echoes is recognized by the intensity and size of the dots recorded. The even, horizontal distance between dots is proportional to the depth of the reflecting interface. The B-mode method is used in two ways. First, with the transducer maintained in a fixed position, it is used to evaluate moving structures in the body, and this variation is called the *TM (time-motion)* presentation. The trace moves vertically on the oscilloscope during recording, and the displayed contour of the moving, reflecting interface indicates the amplitude and velocity of the moving structure. The second variation of the B-mode method is one in which the transducer is moved across the patient, and this variation is called *B-mode scan*, or *B-scan*, ultrasonography. In the presentation, a composite image of infinite numbers of B-mode dots produces a two-dimensional, cross-sectional representation of the structures scanned in either a longitudinal or a transverse plane.

A-mode, B-mode and its variations of TM and B-mode scan, and the Doppler method of continuous ultrasound constitute the present methodology in diagnostic ultrasound. The clinical applications of the various methods are summarized in the following list.

A-mode presentation
Echoencephalography
Fetal cephalometry
Ophthalmologic ultrasound
Detection of pericardial effusion
Echoaortography
Determining solid versus cystic tumors

B-mode presentation
TM (time-motion)
Mitral valve motion
Detection of pericardial effusion
Echoaortography
B-mode scan
Hepatic scans
Placental localization
Intrauterine fetal growth, maturity, or death
Determining solid versus cystic tumors
Tumors of the breast

Doppler ultrasound
Detection of intrauterine life
Placental localization
Detection of multiple pregnancy
Assessment of arterial patency
Detection of venous incompetence
Detection of venous occlusion

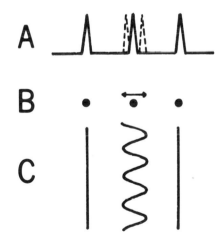

Diagram of characteristics of pulsed ultrasound display modes. **A**, A-mode spike. **B**, B-mode dot. **C**, Vertical trace of B-mode utilized in time-motion (TM), which is influenced by dynamic status of reflected interface.

Courtesy Dr. Ross E. Brown.

949

Selected clinical applications

ECHOENCEPHALOGRAPHY

Echoencephalography is a test to determine the position of the midline structures of the brain. In this examination the A-mode method is used, and the transducer is placed slightly above and anterior to the superior root of the right ear, and the sound beam transmitted across the skull from temple to temple. Echoes are obtained from the near side of the skull, the midline, the far side of the skull, and the skin. These echoes are imaged on the oscilloscope and electronically stored there. The transducer is then placed on the left temporal area, the image is reversed on the oscilloscope screen, and the aforementioned structures are again imaged. The beam echoes received in the right-to-left transmission are portrayed as vertical spikes pointing upward, and those from the opposite transmission as vertical spikes pointing downward. The Polaroid camera is then used to photograph the echoes that have been stored on the oscilloscope. In a normal skull the midline structures are aligned with each other. The accepted normal deviation is 3 mm. If the ultrasound study demonstrates a deviation of more than 3 mm., the physician considers the possibility of the presence of a space-occupying lesion causing the shift in the midline structures.

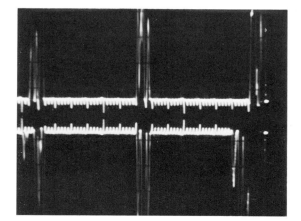

Echoencephalography. Upper spikes represent A-mode echoes of right-to-left transmission of ultrasound beam. Lower spikes represent A-mode echoes of left-to-right transmission of ultrasound beam. A deviation of more than 3 mm. between the two central spikes is considered abnormal and related to a shift of midline structures of the brain. In this scan, the midline structures are normal.

Scan and diagnostic information courtesy Dr. Ross E. Brown.

PLACENTAL LOCALIZATION AND OTHER OBSTETRIC APPLICATIONS

Placental localization

Since B-mode scanning provides a two-dimensional display of the abdomen, it is used for placental localization. Ultrasonography is an effective means of localizing the placenta—determining the site of implantation as anterior, posterior, fundic, or in the lower uterine segment (placenta previa) and its location on either side of the midline.

Before ultrasonic examination of the uterus is performed, the patient's bladder must be full, thus pushing the fetal head up and away from the pubic bones. The patient is placed on the table in the supine position with the abdomen uncovered. The abdomen is divided into four quadrants by two lines intersecting at the umbilicus. Paraffin oil or gel is applied between the transducer and the skin, serving as a coupling agent to prevent air from absorbing the sound waves. The transducer is then gently pressed against the skin and moved in small strokes back and forth across the abdomen. Scans are made in several planes at the discretion of the physician. The various planes provide two-dimensional representations of the outline of the placenta, which appears as small dot-shaped echoes and of the area between the placenta and the fetus; in some cases, the placental site is represented by an echo-free zone. A posterior placental site may be difficult to identify, because of the angulation of the reflecting surface or insufficient penetration of the sound beam due to the patient's size.

The B-mode scan technique is also used to detect fetal death. When death occurs, the amniotic fluid penetrates the epidermis and underlying tissues, forming fluid interspaces, and the resulting two-dimensional scan shows a blurring of the fetal outline. In some cases the scan shows destruction of the normal contours of the head, thereby indicating fetal death.

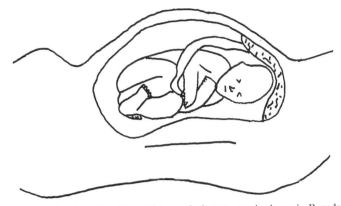

Schematic drawing of location of fetus and placenta previa shown in B-mode scan below.

Drawing by Pamela Seagrove, R.T.

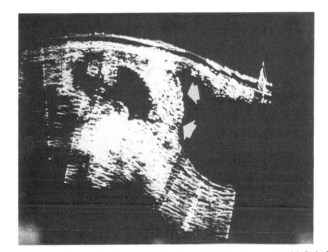

B-mode scan of fetus and placenta previa (arrows). Placenta is massed inferiorly to fetus.

Diagnostic B-mode longitudinal scan courtesy Dr. Ross E. Brown.

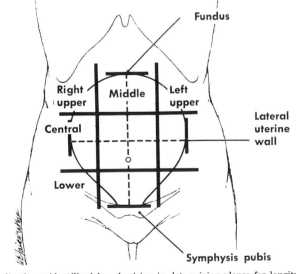

Localization grid utilized by physician in determining planes for longitudinal and transverse B-mode scans of maternal pelvis for placental localization.

Courtesy Dr. Ross E. Brown.

951

Placental localization—cont'd

The Doppler shift phenomenon is another technique used to locate the placenta and monitor the fetus. The Doppler method records sound waves and converts them to audible signals. A Doppler ultrasound unit such as the Doptone[1] or the Ultrasound Monitor[2] is used in this method. The fetal heart sound is detected first, then the placental sounds. The point on the fundus where these sounds are easiest to appreciate is considered to be the center of the placenta. The examining physician ma-

[1]Gould, Inc., Instrument Systems Division, 384 Santa Trinita, Sunnyvale, Calif. 94086.
[2]Hewlett-Packard Co., 175 Wyman St., Waltham, Mass. 02154.

neuvers the ultrasound instrument in several directions at his discretion to identify fetal and placental sounds. The Doppler ultrasound unit can detect several sounds. Maternal vessels have a single "bellowing" sound synchronous with the maternal pulse; the fetal heart has a sharp, rapid "gallop," which can be detected as early as twelve weeks; fetal vessels have a single sound synchronous with the fetal heart; placental sounds are complex, low-pitched "windlike" sounds that are superimposed over the high-pitched sounds of the umbilical cord; fetal movement causes a single "banging" sound. The examining physician is experienced in identifying these sounds. When the ultrasound unit detects no fetal tones or movement, it is concluded that fetal death has occurred.

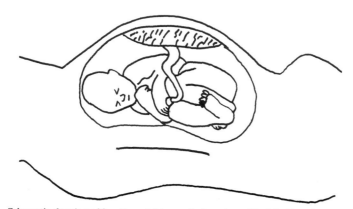

Schematic drawing of location of fetus and placenta outlined in B-mode scan below.

Drawing by Pamela Seagrove, R.T.

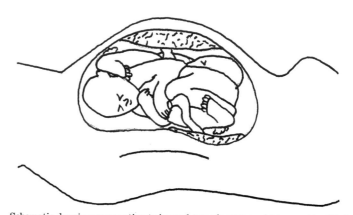

Schematic drawing representing twins and two placentas, which were identified on scan shown below.

Drawing by Pamela Seagrove, R.T.

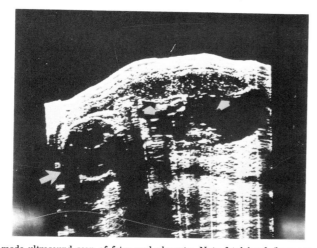

B-mode ultrasound scan of fetus and placenta. Note fetal head (long arrow) and outline of small, dotlike echoes that outline the anteriorly implanted placenta (short arrows).

Diagnostic B-mode longitudinal scan courtesy Dr. Ross E. Brown.

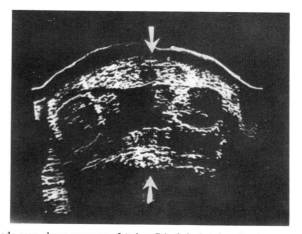

B-mode scan shows presence of twins. Stippled, dot-shaped echoes represent two placental sites, one anterior and the other posterior (arrows).

Diagnostic B-mode longitudinal scan courtesy Dr. Ross E. Brown.

Calculation of fetal heart rate

By the use of more than one ultrasonic display mode, the fetal heart rate can be calculated. The final step utilizes a time-motion mode. After locating the fetus with B-mode scanning, electronic markers are placed along the trace in positions above and below the fetal echoes. The transducer is then placed so that it traverses the fetus and is moved fractionally, using A-mode, until echoes are detected that are undergoing rapid amplitudinal and positional changes at a frequency attributable to fetal heart rate. Without moving the transducer, the display is converted to the time-motion mode, which changes the echo patterns to linear traces that can be interpreted to determine the fetal heart rate.

Fetal cephalometry

Fetal cephalometry, a technique by which the size of the fetal head can be determined and predicted by the use of ultrasound techniques, is another important contribution to non–ionizing-radiation techniques now available for in utero evaluation of the fetus. By a combination of A-mode and B-mode ultrasonography, a demonstration of the biparietal diameter of the fetal head can be obtained, and from this information an estimate of the size and weight of the fetus at term can be predicted.

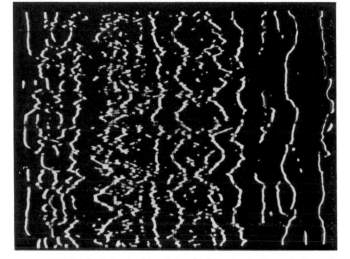

Time-motion scan of the fetal heart. The scan represents the final step in determining fetal heart rate. Since the linear traces of the B-mode time-motion scan take a known rate of time to travel the vertical sweep of the oscilloscope, the heart rate can be determined.

Diagnostic fetal heart scan and legend courtesy Dr. Ross E. Brown.

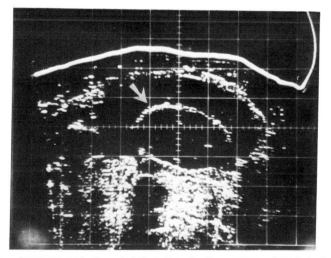

B-mode scan reveals characteristic pattern in the presence of fetal death, destruction of the normal contours of the fetal head (arrow).

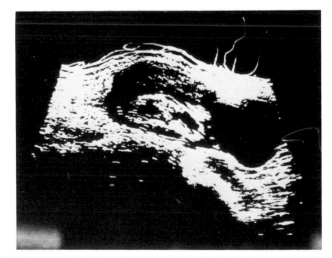

B-mode scan typical of another pattern associated with the presence of fetal death, the presence of amniotic fluid that has penetrated the epidermis and underlying tissues of the fetus. Fluid interspaces have been formed, causing a blurring of the fetal outline.

Above diagnostic B-mode scans courtesy Dr. Ross E. Brown.

953

THERMOGRAPHY

Infrared thermography is the technical procedure by which the body's naturally emitted radiation of heat is collected, measured, and imaged. The resultant thermo *(heat)* graph *(picture)* is a visible, pictorial record of the body's otherwise invisible, spontaneously emitted infrared heat radiation. In thermography, the heat radiation emanating from the skin of the subject is collected and changed electronically into a visible signal, which is then used to make the "thermogram" or thermal display. This display may be recorded on Polaroid film, conventional photographic film, or facsimile paper, or it can be displayed on a cathode tube. Computer tape and digital recording are also utilized. In the three instruments most widely used in medicine,[1-3] the image is produced on a television-like cathode tube and viewed at the "real-time" the subject is examined. After proper adjustments of the equipment have been made to perfect the thermal image, it is recorded permanently by photographic filming of some kind.

Physics of infrared thermography

Infrared radiation is radiant energy having wavelengths that lie just beyond the red end of the visible spectrum

[1]Thermovision: AGA Corp., 550 County Ave., Secaucus, N. J. 07094.
[2]Spectrotherm: Spectrotherm Corp., 3040 Olcott St., Santa Clara, Calif. 95051.
[3]ThermIscope: Texas Instruments, Inc., P. O. Box 1444, Houston, Texas 77001.

and are detected by their thermal (heat) effect. This radiation is a part of the same electromagnetic spectrum of wavelike radiation that includes radio waves, light waves, ultraviolet rays, cosmic rays, and roentgen rays. As just stated, the infrared portion of the electromagnetic spectrum falls just below visible light. All things in nature emit infrared energy, or heat, as a function of their temperature, and all objects in nature seek to remain in thermal equilibrium with their surroundings. Circulation and the internal and surface body mechanisms contribute to the maintenance of human thermal equilibrium. Of utmost importance is the skin. Like other objects in nature, people are constantly emitting infrared radiation. Although heretofore invisible, this spontaneously emitted radiant energy, which is fundamental to all nature, is the physical basis for thermography. The significance of temperature in relation to disease has long been recognized. The birth of contemporary medical thermography occurred in the early 1950s with the declassification of sophisticated, noncontact heat-sensing devices that had been developed for defense and military intelligence projects. A short time after their declassification, these infrared sensing devices were adapted for experimental medical use, and the development of modern medical techniques followed.

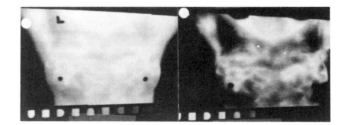

Too little contrast	Too much contrast
Range, 6.5° C.	Range, 4° C.

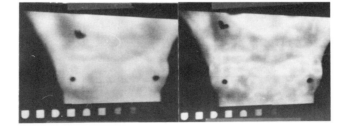

Out of focus	Properly exposed
Range, 5.5° C., near correct	Range, 5° C.

Four thermograms of the breasts on the same patient illustrate the importance of proper focus, contrast, and brightness in obtaining thermal image.

Equipment and methodology

Since the first medical thermograph was built, the science of thermography has grown steadily. Several different types of infrared thermography devices are now available. An excellent historical summary is provided by Gershon-Cohen,[1] and a description and categorization of technical instruments by Curcio and Haberman.[2]

The input of an infrared detector is the radiant energy being spontaneously emitted by the subject. The output is a signal which can be used to make a visible picture that can be interpreted by the examiner. This heat picture or display must be of sufficient optical resolution to reveal details of temperature differences, and must portray the smallest temperature differences considered to have clinical significance.

In a typical thermogram, temperature is represented in shades of gray. The most commonly used method repre-

sents warmer levels of temperature in lighter shades of gray (whiter areas) and cooler levels in darker shades. Some physicians favor and utilize a reversal of this polarity. Most apparatus is designed to provide both types of polarity, and the selection is the option of the user. In thermographic imaging, focus, contrast, and brightness must be considered. Focus is a function of the proper distance of the patient from the sensing device. Contrast may also be termed the sensitivity of the particular thermogram and consists of the gradients of tones between black and saturated white displayed on the thermogram. Contrast is a function of the range of temperatures, and the sensitivity setting of the instrument should depend on the temperature ranges being emitted by the part examined. Brightness relates to the overall lightness or darkness of the thermal image and to optimum appreciation by the human eye. The most satisfactory brightness for a thermogram is reached when the warmest temperature of the subject approaches but does not reach saturated white.

[1]Gershon-Cohen, J.: A short history of medical thermometry, Ann. N. Y. Acad. Sci. **121**:4-11, 1964.

[2]Curcio, B., and Haberman, J.: Infrared thermography: a review of current medical application, instrumentation and technique, Radiol. Techn. **42**:233-247, 1971.

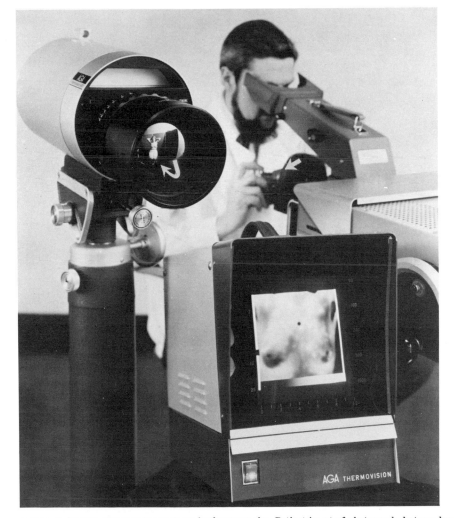

AGA Thermovision unit demonstrating equipment components necessary in thermography. Patient is out of photograph, but can be seen reflected in mirror lens of camera (curved arrow). In foreground is "slave unit" that provides an enlargement of the conventional cathode ray image, which the operator is viewing on the control panel in the background. A camera is attached to the control panel to record real-time image on cathode ray tube. The larger slave unit shown here is not employed in general medical use. This arrangement is for a direct scan.

Courtesy AGA Corp.

Equipment and methodology—cont'd

The emitted radiation must be allowed to flow unhampered and unrestricted to the sensing device. Clothing must be removed, and cross radiation of heat from adjacent body parts eliminated. Since infrared radiation travels in a straight line, the patient may be examined by direct scanning, in which case he or she is directly in front of the instrument, or by the use of an angled mirror that will reflect the radiation into the system when the patient is examined in the recumbent position. A body part whose total surface cannot be evaluated in one position must be arranged in several positions to allow evaluation of the entire surface. In summary, since the patient provides the source of radiation for this imaging modality, he or she must be arranged in such a way as to allow optimum reception of the radiation by the infrared sensing device, and the instrument must be adjusted to receive all the temperature information being emitted by the source. Finally, the recording method must accurately record the thermal image demonstrated at the moment (referred to as the "real-time") of the examination.

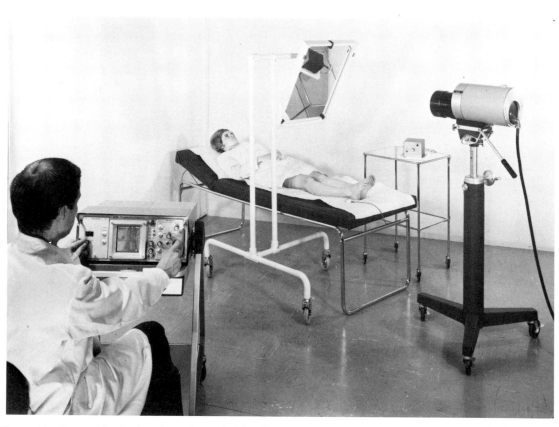

Position of AGA Thermovision for use with reflecting mirror. This method is utilized when patient can be more conveniently examined in the recumbent position. Note thermal "real-time" image on cathode ray tube on control panel.

Courtesy AGA Corp.

Selected clinical applications

Skin temperatures are the result of heat generated by tissue metabolism, the conduction of heat by vascular sources, and the heat of underlying tissues and organs. Skin temperature may also be influenced by external conditions such as the temperature of the immediate surroundings, humidity, and evaporation. Physiologic and pathologic changes affect body tissue temperature and produce surface temperature changes. For all these reasons, the production of a photographic map of body surface temperatures is significant in medical diagnosis.

BREAST DISEASE

One of the most widely used applications of thermography is in the evaluation of breast cancer. The work of Haberman[1] has shown that breast thermograms should be evaluated qualitatively as to the overall thermal pattern as well as quantitatively. Thermograms are considered positive if an abnormal overall pattern is coupled with a significant temperature elevation in one area.

[1]Haberman, J. D.: The present status of mammary thermography, CA **18:**314-321, 1968.

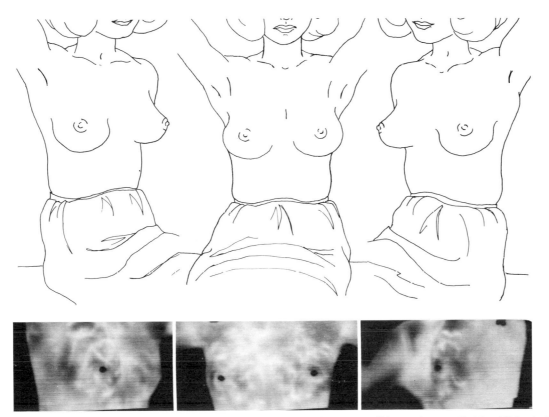

Frontal and oblique positions for routine breast thermography. Frontal position is not sufficient to scan all breast tissue, so that in addition to frontal surface, the lateral surface of each breast must be turned to sensing device and evaluated separately.

Drawings by Carole Peters; thermograms courtesy Dr. J. Gershon-Cohen.

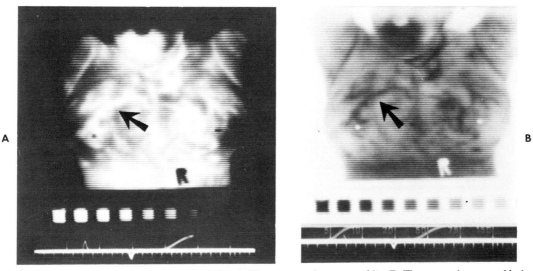

Thermograms made with both types of polarity. **A,** The warmer veins appear white. **B,** The same veins appear black.

957

Nuclear medicine and nuclear medicine technology

Nuclear medicine and nuclear medicine technology

Contributed by

William J. Setlak, N.M.T. (A.R.R.T.), B.S.

Education Director, Nuclear Medicine Technology Training Program
Northwestern Memorial Hospital, Chicago, Ill.

Since this discussion is an introduction to nuclear medicine and nuclear medicine technology, you will encounter a new language. The glossary at the end of the discussion, although limited, will aid you in understanding some new terms.

NUCLEAR MEDICINE

Nuclear medicine originated in a rather unscientific location—under the Stagg Field grandstands at the University of Chicago. Here, in December of 1942, the Nuclear Age began with man's control of the fission of uranium. This event signaled the birth of the reactor and influenced the creation of a new medical science and medical technology.

Nuclear medicine is that science which employs radioactive materials for diagnosing various human diseases. During the past thirty years, this science developed into a recognized medical specialty. The major factors responsible for its dynamic growth are (1) development of new and improved radioactive compounds, (2) advancements in radiation-detecting equipment, and (3) cultivation of new methods for patient test diagnosis. These same factors are also responsible for the growth of nuclear medicine technology. Advancements occurring in any science generate advancements in its technology. For this reason, nuclear medicine and nuclear medicine technology are dependently interrelated, and to describe nuclear medicine technology, it is also necessary to discuss the major aspects of nuclear medicine.

One approach to describing a relatively new science is to compare and contrast it with a familiar science. Nuclear medicine and radiology are comparable because each utilizes radiation; however, the contrast between the two fields involves the source of radiation and the method of its detection.

In nuclear medicine examinations, the radioactive compound administered to the patient concentrates in a particular organ. Sensitive instruments detect the gamma rays emerging from the radioactive compounds and provides diagnostic information. In radiologic examinations, x-radiation generated in a tube passes through the patient and exposes a film. The processed film produces an image of the particular organ system and also provides diagnostic information.

Because of this essential difference, each field specializes in the diagnosis of certain diseases. For example, there is no radiologic method for evaluating thyroid function or for routinely imaging the thyroid gland. Conversely, there is no procedure in nuclear medicine that can visualize a stomach ulcer. Of course, many studies performed in both fields contribute supportive diagnostic information. A patient suspected of having a brain lesion will usually undergo a nuclear medicine brain scan. If this study is abnormal or causes disease to be suspected, a cerebral angiogram may be performed to confirm the initial findings. The information supplied by one test therefore supports the information contributed by the other test. In general, the approach of the two fields to testing with radiation is complementary rather than competitive.

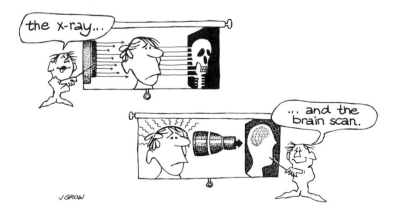

Radioactive compounds

The use of radioactive compounds and radiation detectors is the foundation of the science and technology of nuclear medicine.

The term *radioactive* was introduced by Mme. Curie. Her discovery and isolation of radium, in 1898, completely changed the physical concept of matter. At that time, matter was considered inert unless acted on by external forces. However, Mme. Curie demonstrated that certain elements possess the ability to spontaneously change themselves into different elements. According to her, these elements are not inert but "active." Radioactivity is a nuclear phenomenon exhibited by the atoms of certain elements. The nucleus of an atom (e.g., an atom of radium) contains excess energy and is excited or unstable. As the excited nucleus spontaneously transforms to a more stable state, it emits energy in the form of radiation. The three types of radiation emitted are alpha, beta, and gamma. Experiments conducted by physicists indicated that alpha and beta rays are actually small particles of ejected nuclear mass. Further experiments revealed that the gamma ray is identical, in properties, to Roentgen's x ray. The only difference is that gamma rays originate from the nucleus of unstable elements.

The basic unit of radioactivity is the curie. It is defined as that amount of any radioactive material present to have 37 billion atoms undergoing transformation per second. This amount of radioactivity is too large for diagnostic examinations; instead the subunits millicurie (one-thousandth curie) and microcurie (one-millionth curie) are used.

Radioactive elements exist in nature or are artificially produced in cyclotrons and nuclear reactors. All the radioactive compounds employed in nuclear medicine are artificially produced.

The physicist Ernest Rutherford observed another unique phenomenon of radioactive elements. They display a characteristic that he called *half-life*. Physical half-life is the time period required for one half of any amount of radioactive material to undergo transformation. This time period is a distinct constant for each different radioactive substance and cannot be altered by temperature, pressure, or chemical reactions. For example, the half-life of radium-226 is 1,620 years, and that of technetium-99m is only six hours. Two other half-life characteristics also applicable to radioactive compounds are

biologic and effective. Biologic half-life refers to the time required for the patient to eliminate one half of a substance through the normal process of elimination (urine, feces, exhalation, perspiration). The eliminated material may be either stable or radioactive. Effective half-life is a combination of both the physical and the biologic. It refers to the time required for the patient to eliminate one half of a radioactive compound through the process of physical decay and biologic elimination. The half-life characteristics and the type of radiation emitted indicate the amount of exposure a patient receives from a certain quantity of a particular radioactive compound.

Radioactive compounds, commonly called radionuclides or radiopharmaceuticals, are used as tracers in nuclear medicine examinations of patients. A tracer is any substance that can be identified when introduced into a biologic system. Information regarding structure, function, absorption, secretion, excretion, and volume is obtained by identifying or detecting the tracer. The identifiable characteristic of all radioactive tracers is the emitted radiation.

The two types of tracers utilized in nuclear medicine are radioisotopes and "labeled" compounds.

Isotopes are different atomic forms of the same element. This difference is due to the variation of neutrons in the nucleus. Although isotopes have different neutron numbers, they possess the same proton number and are chemically identical even when one is radioactive. Therefore the chemical reaction of a radioisotope in a biologic system will be the same as that of the stable isotope. For example, the thyroid gland uses iodine for producing hormones. Since the thyroid cannot chemically differentiate between radioactive iodine (^{131}I) and stable iodine (^{127}I), ^{131}I will serve as a tracer for evaluating thyroid function. Thyroid disorders are determined by detecting and measuring the ^{131}I concentrating in the gland or circulating in the blood as hormone. A scanning instrument, which will be discussed later, produces images of the thyroid containing the radioactive tracer. This scan image

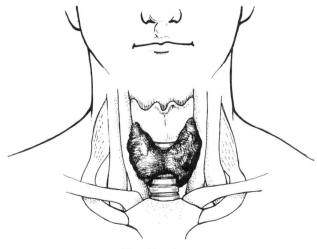

Thyroid anatomy.

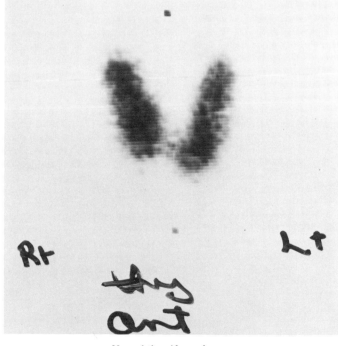

Normal thyroid scan image.

Radioactive compounds—cont'd

reveals thyroid structure and indicates various types of abnormalities. Although any radioisotope of iodine can serve as a thyroid tracer, ^{123}I, ^{125}I, and ^{131}I are commonly used.

The second type of tracer, the labeled compound, is composed of radioactive molecules attached to various chemical and protein complexes. For example, a radioactive technetium-99m molecule is chemically attached to a long-chained phosphate molecule. This reaction forms a technetium-99m–polyphosphate complex, which is used for imaging the skeletal system. Since phosphate is used in the construction of bone cells, this labeled complex will concentrate in the skeletal system. Bone abnormalities are demonstrated on scans as areas of increased tracer concentration.

Most of the radiopharmaceuticals employed in nuclear medicine are labeled compounds. The characteristics of an ideal radiopharmaceutical are (1) short half-life, (2) absence of toxicity, (3) delivery of a low radiation dose, (4) ease of detection, and (5) ready availability. The radionuclide ^{99m}Tc is presently used as a label for many compounds because it has nearly ideal properties. ^{99m}Tc has a short physical half-life and emits only gamma rays, which are easily detected. Because of these properties, ^{99m}Tc compounds generally deliver low radiation exposure to the patient.

Commercial radiopharmaceutical companies produce a large variety of tracer compounds, which are supplied in two forms. The labeled compound is either used as received, or it has to be chemically prepared in the department. In the past this preparation was an intricate procedure accomplished only by a chemist. However, radiopharmaceutical companies have recently developed the "kit" preparation. The kit contains all the materials and chemical ingredients in sterile form to make an "instant radiopharmaceutical." The preparation involves only following a simple recipe and mixing the appropriate radionuclide with the kit ingredients. The technologist can now prepare in his own department many different compound tracers. Advantages of the kit are (1) storage until needed, (2) speed and ease of preparation, and (3) immediate availability. This last feature is extremely important in emergency test procedures. A table of the most commonly used radiopharmaceuticals is included at the end of this discussion.

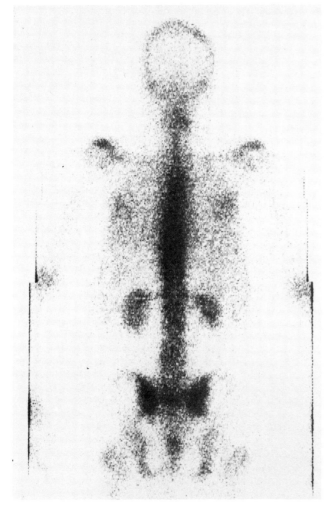

Normal bone scan image.

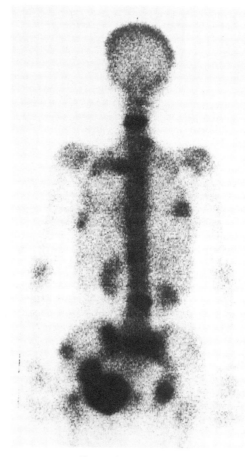

Abnormal bone scan image.

Radiation-detecting equipment

Detection of the radiopharmaceutical with sensitive instruments is essential for performing all nuclear medicine procedures.

Two principal types of instruments for detecting radiation are ionization and scintillation counters.

Instruments that record ionizing events are ion-collecting detectors. A Geiger-Müller counter is an example of this type of detector. It is composed of a gas chamber, high voltage supply, positive and negative electrodes, amplifier, and meter. The radiation that enters the chamber interacts with the gas molecules and produces positive and negative ions. Each ion pair collected by the respective electrode generates a small pulse, which is amplified and recorded by the meter. The number of pulses recorded indicates not only the presence of radiation but also its intensity. Since the gas chamber is rather inefficient for gamma-ray detection, these instruments are seldom used for such test procedures. They are generally used to monitor radiation contamination.

Scintillation instruments detect radiation by recording "light flash" events. These instruments are composed of a scintillation probe, electronic analyzer, and read-out system. The probe, which is the "sensing" portion of the instrument, contains a sodium iodide crystal, photomultiplier tube, and amplifier. When a gamma ray interacts with the molecular composition of the crystal, a light flash, or scintillation, is produced. The photomultiplier tube converts this scintillation into an electric pulse that is proportional in height to the gamma-ray energy. Each pulse is then amplified and directed to the analyzer, which electronically accepts or rejects pulses according to height. Since pulse height represents energy, the analyzer will therefore differentiate between various gamma-ray energies. This is an important feature because each radionuclide emits gamma rays with a characteristic energy. To detect a particular radionuclide, the analyzer is set to accept those pulses corresponding to the gamma-ray energy emitted by that radionuclide. After the pulse has been analyzed and accepted, it is directed to the read-out system. This system contains a sealer or rate meter and, in special detectors, a photodisplay unit. The scaler or rate meter displays the accepted pulses as "counts" per unit of time. The photodisplay unit, which will be described later, produces images on film.

Because the crystal of the scintillation probe is a solid medium, it is highly efficient for detecting gamma rays. Scintillation detectors of various designs are employed in nuclear medicine, and the type of instrument used depends on the study performed.

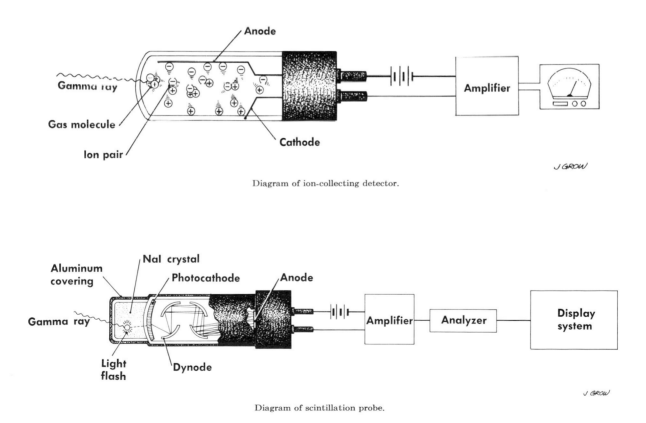

Diagram of ion-collecting detector.

Diagram of scintillation probe.

965

PHOTODISPLAY UNIT FOR ORGAN IMAGING—cont'd

The number and relative densities of the dots form a pattern of the radiopharmaceutical contained within the organ. In some scans, normal areas are demonstrated by an increase in dots, and abnormalities show up as "cold" areas containing no dots. Certain abnormalities of the thyroid, lung, liver, spleen, and pancreas are indicated in this manner. In other scans, normal areas contain no dots, and abnormalities are displayed by an increase in dots. Certain abnormalities of the brain, bone, and thyroid are demonstrated in this manner. Since the scan is a two-dimensional image of a three-dimensional object, several views of the organ are necessary for complete evaluation.

The camera is a stationary detector with a large collimated probe that views an entire organ at one time. Its photodisplay unit, the oscilloscope, is more complex than that of the scanner. Detected gamma rays are momentarily displayed on the oscilloscope screen as small light dots or "blips." A Polaroid, 35 mm. or 70 mm. camera mounted on the oscilloscope photographs the dot display. A composite dot image, called a *scintiphoto* or *photoscan*, is produced by accumulating thousands of dots on the film. This scintiphoto dot pattern (opposite page) supplies the same diagnostic information as the scan. Any organ image produced with the camera can also be obtained with the scanner. The diagnostic information obtained from either instrument is equivalent, but the camera has one major advantage. It can produce rapid, sequential scintiphotos of the organ undergoing evaluation. The 35 mm. or 70 mm. camera mounted to the oscilloscope can be set to make several rapid, short-time exposures of the dot image display. Dynamic movement of the tracer into and out of the organ is sequentially photographed in this manner. Dynamic camera studies provide information concerning blood flow to the heart or to transplanted kidneys. Vascular diseases of the brain and major blood vessels and abnormalities such as aneurysms and deep vein thrombosis are also demonstrated by this technique.

Scanners and cameras both exhibit distinct advantages and limitations in organ imaging; however, it is beyond the scope of this text to discuss them in depth.

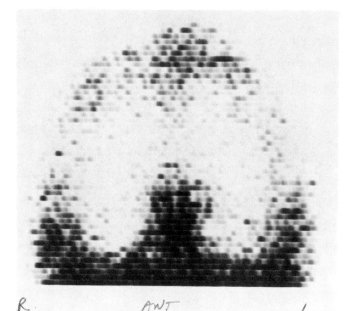

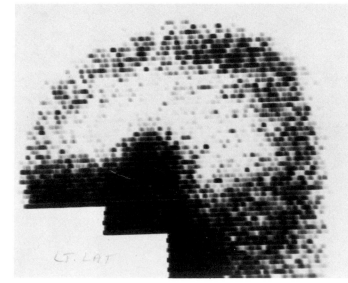

Abnormal brain scan image.

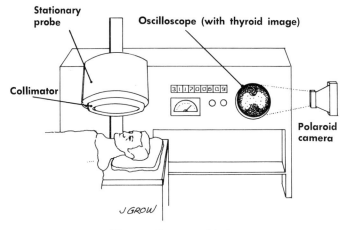

Diagram of a camera detector.

A complex sci
support and se
Just as radiolog
medicine techno

Nuclear medic
using radiophar
obtain diagnosti
nologist has to a
to the clinical te
understanding r
and an awaren
comprehending
pharmacology. I
general knowled
matics. To per
individual has to
methods of clini
not only underst
but is also awar
or alter test rest

Nuclear medic
major areas of
in vivo testing,
departments one
the categories. I
tend to speciali
greater variety o
a large daily pa
vidual will func
than in all areas

RADIOPHARI

Any qualified
technologist; ho
pend on the dep
departments wi
patients will req
individual's day
pharmaceutical
patient doses. /
compounds prep
to each patient

It is the techi
sary radionucli
always be certa
supply of a pai
situation when
partment does
ceutical.

Because this
compounds, he
to minimize exp
is the one most
nation, he or sh
tion procedures

The technolo
ceives the corr
amount. Too n
and too little a

IN VITRO A

The technolo
testing functioi
metric flasks, p

ADVANCES IN ORGAN IMAGING

Advancements in nuclear medicine are particularly evident in the area of imaging. The major influence is the constant improvement of instrument design and function and the development of accessory imaging equipment.

Today, rectilinear scanners are equipped with upper and lower probes, several pulse analyzers, and two to three photodisplay units. These instruments not only produce simultaneous anterior and posterior views, but they can also simultaneously image two organ systems containing two different radionuclides. Also, some instruments have minification devices that display total body images on a $14'' \times 17''$ film.

An accessory presently available for camera imaging is the video tape recorder. This device operates in a manner similar to the "instant video tape replay" used in television broadcasting. All the information from the patient's camera study is recorded and stored on tape. After the completion of the study, the tape is replayed, and static or dynamic scintiphotos are obtained from the oscilloscope replay monitor. These taped examinations can be replayed as often as necessary to obtain optimum diagnostic images. The patient-study can be stored for future reference, or the tapes can be erased and reused. This invaluable accessory adds considerable versatility to imaging techniques, and it is almost a necessity for performing some of the more complex dynamic studies.

Current instrumentation research

Current research in instrumentation includes the development of semiconductor detectors, tomographic imaging, and fluorescent scanning.

The semiconductor crystal, lithium-drifted germanium, is superior to sodium iodide for gamma-ray detection. This improved detecting medium increases the overall quality and detail of organ-imaging studies.

The tomographic instrument is capable of producing multiple in-depth section images. This detector, which is analogous to the radiographic tomography unit, provides more accurate information as to the location of abnormalities within an organ system.

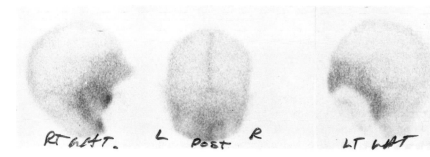

Normal brain scintiphoto.

Radiation protection—cont'd

methods of protection are somewhat easier to achieve in radiography than in nuclear medicine. In radiologic examinations the x rays are directed at the patient and are generated for a short time. The shielded x-ray tube is at a distance, and the technologist usually works behind barriers. In nuclear medicine examinations the technologists are in direct contact with the radiation source while preparing a radiopharmaceutical and injecting the compound into the patient. The patient, after receiving the radiopharmaceutical, is constantly emitting radiation during the entire examination. Since many imaging procedures require one to two hours to complete, the technologist is exposed for a longer period of time. Even though these circumstances are not ideal for protection, the annual radiation exposure in nuclear medicine personnel is generally comparable to that in radiology personnel. One reason is that the total amount of radiation emitted from the radiopharmaceutical is small compared to the amount of x rays generated during radiologic examinations.

In addition to the general methods of protection, the nuclear medicine technologist must be aware of two radiation precautions that are not necessary in radiography. The first precaution involves possible contamination with radioactive materials. Since radiopharmaceuticals are usually in liquid form, there always exists the possibility of a spill. Splashing or spilling radioactive solutions on people and equipment constitutes contamination. It is difficult to avoid, and accidents will happen no matter how carefully the individual works. If contamination occurs, the spill should be confined to a small area and absorbed with paper towels. The contaminated towels are then discarded into a container for radioactive waste. To ensure that contamination has been removed, the area is washed repeatedly with detergents and allowed to dry. A Geiger-Müller counter is used to survey the area. If the area is still contaminated, the washing procedure is repeated.

Hands are the most frequent site of personal contamination; therefore individuals handling radioactivity must always wear disposable gloves. It is much easier to dispose of contaminated gloves than to wash away several layers of contaminated skin.

The second radiation precaution involves the handling of radioactive waste material. Needles, syringes, vials, test tubes, and blood samples containing radioactivity must be given special attention. This waste has to be stored in containers until the radioactivity has decayed to a low radiation level. Waste from short–half-life radionuclides presents no major problem because it takes only a few days for the radioactivity to decay. Conversely, waste from longer–half-life radionuclides will have to be stored for weeks and sometimes months before a low radiation level is attained. When the waste is no longer considered radioactive, it is disposed of as regular garbage.

Table of radiopharmaceuticals

Radionuclide	Symbol	Physical half-life	Chemical form	Diagnostic use
Chromium	^{51}Cr	27.8 days	Sodium chromate	Red blood cell volume; red blood cell survival
Cobalt	^{57}Co	272 days	Cyanocobalamin (vitamin B_{12})	Pernicious anemia
Fluorine	^{18}F	1.8 hours	Sodium fluoride in water	Bone imaging
Gallium	^{67}Ga	77 hours	Gallium citrate	Hodgkin's disease; tumor imaging
Gold	^{198}Au	64 hours	Gold colloid	Liver imaging
Indium	^{111}In	66 hours	Indium chloride	Cerebro spinal fluid imaging
Iodine	^{123}I	13.3 hours	Sodium iodide	Thyroid function and imaging
	^{125}I	60 days	Sodium iodide	Thyroid imaging
			Triiodothyronine	Thyroid hormone assay
			Thyroxine	Thyroid hormone assay
	^{131}I	8.1 days	Sodium iodide	Thyroid function and imaging
			Rose bengal	Liver function and imaging
			Hippuran	Renal function
			Macroaggregated albumin	Lung imaging
			Human serum albumin (^{131}I and ^{125}I)	Plasma volume
Iron	^{59}Fe	45 days	Ferric chloride	Red blood cell production
Mercury	^{197}Hg	65 hours	Chlormerodrin	Brain and renal imaging
	^{203}Hg	48 days	Chlormerodrin	Brain and renal imaging
Selenium	^{75}Se	127 days	Selenomethionine	Pancreas imaging
Strontium	^{85}Sr	64 days	Strontium chloride	Bone imaging
Technetium	^{99m}Tc	6 hours	Sodium pertechnetate	Brain imaging; thyroid imaging
			Sulfur colloid	Liver-spleen imaging
			Human albumin microspheres	Lung imaging
			Human serum albumin	Cardiovascular imaging
			DTPA	Renal imaging
			Polyphosphate	Bone imaging
			Diphosphonate	Bone imaging
			Pyrophosphate	Bone imaging
Xenon	^{133}Xe	5.3 days	Xenon gas	Lung ventilation imaging

Specialization

The science of nuclear medicine is the environment in which the technologist functions. As this environment expands in complexity, it influences the expansion of the technologist's responsibility. In order to adapt, the technologist is required to operate more complicated equipment and perform more complicated tests. The dynamic growth of nuclear medicine is actually creating a new species of technologist—the specialist. Radiopharmacy technology is an example of the current trend in specialization, for this species of technologist already exists in larger institutions. Specialization is also evident in the areas of in vitro testing and organ imaging. Soon, technologists will be trained to excell in performing only radioassay studies. In the near future, imaging technology will consist of two distinct specialists: the scanning procedure experts and the dynamic study experts. And the most important specialists will be the technologists responsible for training these experts—the clinical instructor and the training program director.

The only limiting factor to technology specialization is the growth rate of nuclear medicine. Since the science and technology of nuclear medicine are in an early stage of development, the major advancements and specializations are yet to come.

No matter how specialized the technologist, it is his or her clinical performance that is important to the patient's test diagnosis. Both physician and patient rely on the technologist's skill and ability to perform accurate examinations. Clinical performance is perfected by experience, and it is through experience that the technologist develops judgment. Technical judgment is the ability to decide whether a test has been performed correctly and accurately. To develop this quality the technologist not only has to understand test procedures but also must know the criteria that distinguish normal from abnormal results. A competent technologist is able to judge the validity of his or her clinical performance and the test results. A competent technologist is a master of his art.

GLOSSARY OF SELECTED NUCLEAR MEDICINE TERMS

activity. A shortened form of the word **radioactivity;** used when referring to the amount of radioactivity in a dose, bottle, test tube.

camera. An imaging instrument with large stationary probe; views an entire field at one time.

collimator. A device attached to scintillation probe; made of lead and contains holes; function is to limit field of view and eliminate scatter radiation.

contamination. Radioactivity in places where it should not be—such as on the technologist's hands.

crystal. A radiation-detecting medium, emits light when gamma rays interact; sodium iodide commonly employed; size varies: $3'' \times 2''$ in scanners, $12'' \times \frac{1}{2}''$ in cameras.

decay or **disintegration.** Transformation of a radioactive nucleus, resulting in the emission of radiation.

fission. The "breaking apart" of the uranium-235 nucleus, liberating energy and neutrons; the neutrons are used in producing radioactive isotope in the reactor.

gamma ray. Electromagnetic radiation originating from radioactive nucleus; causes ionization in matter; identical in properties to the x ray.

half-life. The physical characteristic that is specific for each radioactive substance; the time it takes radioactive material to decay to one half of its initial activity; types are biologic and effective.

in vitro. Occurring in the test tube; isolated from the organism.

in vivo. Occurring within the organism.

ionization. Disruption of atoms or molecules by removing orbital electrons; process producing + and − ions.

isotope. Atoms of an element possessing the same proton number but a different neutron number; can be stable or radioactive.

nuclear. Of or pertaining to the nucleus of an atom; used in reference to radioactive atoms.

nuclear symbol notation. $^A_Z X$ X = Chemical symbol
A = Mass number
Z = Atomic number

Examples: $^{131}_{53}I$; $^{51}_{24}Cr$; $^{57}_{27}Co$

pernicious anemia. Defective red blood cells due to the patient's inability to absorb vitamin B_{12}.

probe. Sensing component of scintillation detectors; contains sodium iodide crystal and photomultiplier tube.

radiation. Energy emitted by unstable nuclei; may be particles (e.g., alpha, beta) or electromagnetic (e.g., gamma).

radioactive. Pertaining to atoms of elements that undergo spontaneous transformation, resulting in the emission of radiation.

radionuclide. A general name for a specific radioactive substance; for example ^{99m}Tc, ^{131}I, or ^{51}Cr.

radiopharmaceutical. A chemical compound or protein complex containing radioactive atoms or molecules; used as a tracer in patient testing.

reactor. Cubicle where radioactive isotopes are artificially produced.

scan. Dot image produced on film representing structure of organ containing a radiopharmaceutical; also called scintiscan, scintiphoto, or photoscan.

scanner. Imaging device with moving probe assembly; probe moves in rectilinear motion and maps the radioactivity within an organ.

scintillation. Light flash occurring when gamma rays interact within certain crystals; sodium iodide and cesium iodide are two types of scintillating media.

tracer. Substance possessing characteristics that are identifiable when introduced into a biologic system; it stands out from the surrounding environment.

transformation. Spontaneous, active changing of an unstable nucleus; synonymous with decay or disintegration.

unstable. In an excited, active state; with a nucleus possessing excess energy.

Principles of
radiation therapy

Principles of radiation therapy

Carole A. Sullivan, R.T.

Associate Professor, Department of Radiologic Technology
College of Health and Allied Health Professions
University of Oklahoma Health Sciences Center, Oklahoma City

and

Carl R. Bogardus, Jr., M.D.

Professor and Vice-chairman, Department of Radiologic Sciences
University of Oklahoma College of Medicine, Oklahoma City

The use of ionizing radiation in the treatment of disease has almost as long a history as does the diagnostic applications of the x-ray beam. Emil H. Grubbé, a chemist and roentgen pioneer, administered the first therapeutic application of x rays to a patient who had an advanced carcinoma of the left breast on January 29, 1896, in Chicago, Illinois.[1]

The specialty of radiation therapy technology is no longer considered an adjunct skill to be learned by the diagnostic x-ray technologist. It is a separate specialty requiring an additional period of education and training, and separate certification for this specialty is now required. Information regarding educational programs in radiation therapy technology is available from the organizations listed below.[2,3]

A detailed outline of this complex and sophisticated branch of radiologic technology is not within the scope of this text. However, because it is a closely allied radiation specialty, a brief explanation of the rationale, significance, and technical principles of the therapeutic applications of ionizing radiation is appropriate in a text designed for diagnostic technologists. A glossary of radia-

tion therapy terms is appended to this discussion. A list of references for further study may be found in the bibliography.

Rationale and significance of radiation therapy

The basis of radiation therapy is the selective destruction of diseased tissue by ionizing radiations, for the single purpose of destroying unhealthy tissue while avoiding serious damage to neighboring normal tissue.

The concepts of radiosensitivity and radiocurability have been derived from careful study of the response of normal and malignant tissue to irradiation. No single form of treatment or combination thereof, whether surgery, radiation therapy, or chemotherapy, is ideally suited for every case. Radiation therapy demands more than the skills of beam direction. Total dose planning, treatment planning, care of the patient during and after treatment, and careful follow-up are integral parts of the management of the patient.

The physician practitioner of radiation therapy is called a radiation therapist. Under his or her direction radiation therapy is administered to the patient for the purpose of curing or palliating disease, 99% of which is malignant. For these reasons, a brief review of cancer and the basic physical principles utilized in radiation therapy are appropriate here.

[1]Grigg, E. R. N.: Trail of the invisible light, Springfield, Ill., 1965, Charles C Thomas, Publisher.

[2]Committee on Education in Radiologic Technology, American Medical Association, 307 N. Michigan Ave., Chicago, Ill. 60611.

[3]American Registry of Radiologic Technologists, 2600 Wayzata Blvd., Minneapolis, Minn. 55405.

CANCER

Cancer has been defined in numerous ways, among which are (1) as tissue in which the normal cell-growth controlling mechanism is impared[1]; (2) as a group of diseases of unknown causes; (3) as a genetic disease of somatic cells[1]; or (4) as a spontaneous autoaggressive disease initiated by random gene mutation.[1] Cancer or malignant cells may arise in any body tissue and at any age. Statisticians have estimated that in the year 2000 approximately 400,000 people will die of cancer.[2]

Our knowledge of cancer at this time, however, is extensive and detailed; we know a great deal about the circumstances under which it may occur, some of the predisposing factors, its behavior in the body, its manner of spread, and, fortunately, how to attack it successfully. But the most intimate secret, exactly how and why the cancer cell differs from the normal cell, still eludes us.[3]

Cancer becomes a destructive process when cells cease to live in harmony and begin to invade and destroy neighboring cells. Before this invasion occurs, the malignant cells have already undergone changes in size, shape, and histologic pattern. This transition from normal to malignant appears to be a gradual, continuous process of increasing change. The malignant transformation may start in one area or in multiple areas simultaneously. Malignant cells may invade local tissue by direct extension or disseminate widely by means of the lymphatic system or through the blood system.

[1]Florey, H.: General pathology, Philadelphia, 1970, W. B. Saunders Co.
[1]Burch, R. J.: New approach to cancer, Nature **225**:512, 1970.
[2]Grant, R. N., and Silverberg, E.: Cancer statistics, 1970, New York, 1970, American Cancer Society, Inc.
[3]Walter, J., and Miller, H.: A short textbook of radiotherapy for technicians and students, ed. 3, Boston, 1969, Little, Brown & Co.

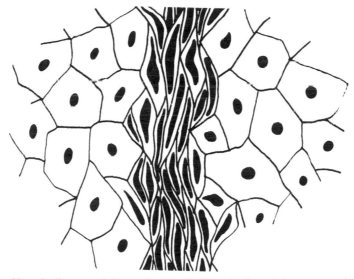

Normal cells surrounded by malignant cells. Normal cells are being compressed and will be ultimately destroyed.

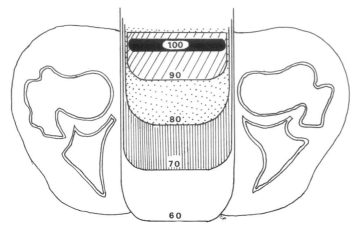

Contour of the pelvis, with an isodose demonstrating the fall-off of dose as the beam passes through the body.

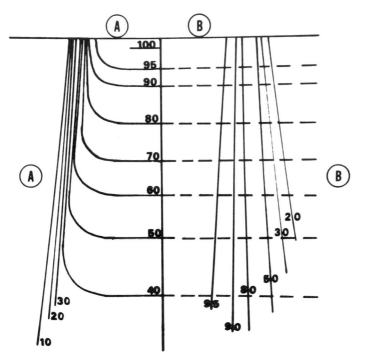

Difference between an isodose curve, *A*, and decrement lines, *B*.

Treatment-planning principles

A malignant tumor may lie close to the surface of the body, deep within the patient and/or in close proximity to critical structures whose function would be impaired or permanently damaged by radiation. Treatment planning consists in applying one or more three-dimensional beams of x-, gamma, or electron radiation to three-dimensional structures of various configuration(s) and composition(s). It is performed manually or with the aid of a computer. When done manually, it may take several hours to produce a dose distribution for the approval of the radiation therapist, and then the distribution may or may not be acceptable. This is particularly true if the distribution is for novel or sophisticated beam arrangements.

Computer technology now adapted for radiation-therapy treatment planning provides the capability of obtaining several treatment plans in a minimal time frame. The use of digital computers in radiotherapy is little more than fifteen years old. The first paper was published by Tsien.[1] At the same time, the radiotherapy community had begun worldwide conversion from orthovoltage x-ray machines to ^{60}Co units and supervoltage units. Although computers have been available for fifteen years or so, they have come into common use in radiation therapy departments within the past five years.

In the first stage of computer history, efforts were made toward the speed-up of dose-distribution calculations. In the second stage, the computer became a practical tool by accumulating a large number of isodose charts. In the third and present stage, computer-aided optimization of a treatment plan is being practiced. The selected treatment plans described on the following page utilize both manual and computer methods of treatment planning.

[1]Tsien, K. D.: The application of automatic computing machines to radiation therapy treatment planning, Brit. J. Radiol. **28**:432-439, 1955.

Selected clinical methods

To give the reader a better understanding of the principles described herein, a brief discussion of common methodology utilized in the treatment of specific malignant diseases is presented.

HODGKIN'S DISEASE

Hodgkin's disease is a systemic cancer of the lymph system. The unquestioned treatment of choice for all but the late stages of Hodgkin's disease is radiation therapy, since the disease process is radiosensitive and locally radiocurable. An overwhelming majority of cases of Hodgkin's disease originate within the lymph node system; consequently radiation-therapy treatment planning requires serious consideration of the systemic nature of the disease. Large mantle fields are utilized for irradiation of the lymph node system above the diaphragm to include the base of the skull, with lead blocks shielding the lungs, humeral heads, and the cervical spine, the latter from the posterior field only. This technique has been described at length.[1]

The periaortic, pelvic, and inguinal lymph nodes are irradiated with large fields in the shape of an inverted Y. This lower field adjoins the mantle field, thus assuring adequate treatment to the entire lymph node system. The total midline dose delivered is about 4,000 rads in 4 to 6 weeks. The dosimetric aspects of this technique are acutely concerned with (1) accurate and reproducible lung shielding and (2) dose uniformity throughout the anatomic areas of varying thickness and contour. The technique is intended to achieve ±5% dose uniformity in the midline of the body.

[1]Kaplan, H. S., and Rosenberg, S. A.: Treatment of Hodgkin's disease, Med. Clin. N. Amer. **50:**1591-1610, 1966.

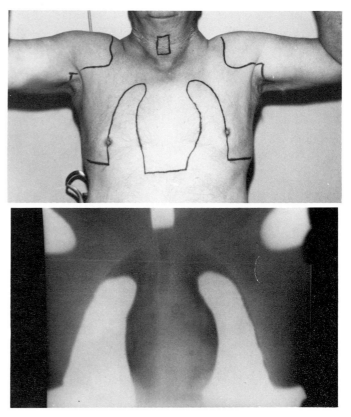

Photograph of patient with a diagnosis of Hodgkin's disease, stage II. Outlined are those areas encompassed by the mantle field and the anatomic areas to be shielded by lead blocks.

Radiograph of same patient demonstrates the lead blocks and the anatomic areas being treated.

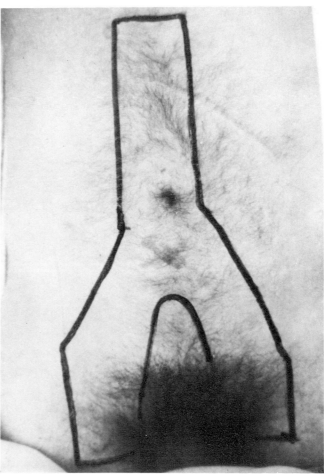

Photograph of patient with a diagnosis of Hodgkin's disease, stage II. Outlined are those areas encompassed by the inverted Y field and the anatomic areas being treated.

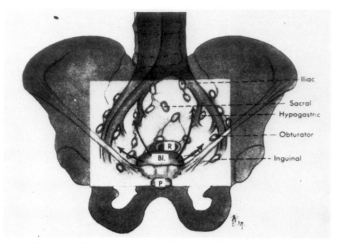

12″ × 12″ beam utilized to encompass the regional lymph nodes in the treatment of carcinoma of the prostate.

Courtesy Dr. W. T. Moss.

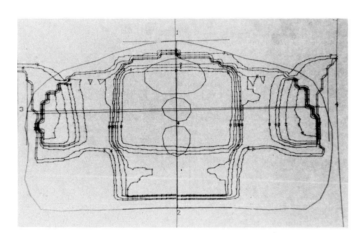

Computer isodose plan demonstrates the dose distribution within the pelvis when treating carcinoma of the prostate. The plan reflects the four-field modality to encompass the prostate gland plus a reasonable margin and regional lymph nodes.

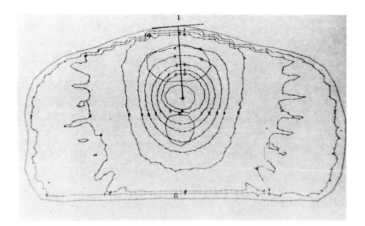

Computer isodose plan demonstrates the dose distribution in the pelvis. The plan reflects a desirable distribution when supplementing dose to the prostate gland or as the desirable dose for treating an early primary cancer of the prostate.

Selected clinical methods—cont'd

CANCER OF THE PROSTATE

Prostatic cancer is the most common cancer in men over 50 years of age and is the leading cause of cancer deaths in men over 75. Carcinomas of the prostate are primarily adenocarcinomas. Early diagnosis of cancer of the prostate can be expected only from routine examination of the prostate gland by rectal palpation in an asymptomatic patient. The most significant laboratory examination is the acid and alkaline phosphotase determinations. Selection of patients for radiation therapy has varied as a result of limited knowledge of the radiocurability of various clinical stages, the palliation provided when cure is not obtained, and the lack of precise data regarding sequelae.[1] Generally, patients with disease in stages I, II, and III are irradiated when not candidates for radical prostatectomy. It should be noted that the probability of cure in the early stages treated with radiation therapy is excellent.

The prostate gland lies between the pubis and the rectum and encircles the bladder neck. The extension of primary disease and the involvement of regional lymph nodes cannot easily be determined. This difficulty, coupled with the fact that only a small portion of these cancers are diagnosed in the early stages, means that a large treatment volume is required.

The volume should encompass regional nodes in the more advanced cancers. As this volume is increased, the incidence of sequelae increases, and tolerated dose is decreased. A single anterior and two oblique beams, or a four-field box technique, are satisfactory for delivering the first 5,000 to 5,500 rads to a volume encompassing pelvic nodes along with the primary cancer. The remaining 1,500 to 2,000 rads are delivered via smaller fields. Rotational therapy and/or adding additional booster doses to the primary disease is utilized in treating smaller volumes.

[1]Ackerman, L. V. and Del Regato, J. A.: Cancer diagnosis, treatment, and prognosis, ed. 4, St. Louis, 1970, The C. V. Mosby Co.

MEDULLOBLASTOMA

Certain tumors have a characteristic by which they may spread to any point in the nervous system. This has led to the development of special radiation-therapy treatment techniques. The best example is medulloblastoma of the cerebellum, common in children and young adults. This tumor has a tendency to metastasize throughout the cerebro-spinal pathway; fortunately, it is also radiosensitive. The optimal radiation therapy technique treats the entire central nervous system in one volume.[1] When multiple small fields are utilized for the spinal treatment, recurrences may appear at the point of portal abutment, and the survival rate is certainly not as high as with the single field treatment.

The optimal method delivers a reasonable distribution of dose throughout a long volume by utilizing a long field to encompass the entire spinal canal and when possible the entire brain. The dose to the brain may be supplemented when the size of the patient prevents an encompassing single field arrangement.

MAXILLARY ANTRUM CARCINOMA

Treatment of maxillary antrum carcinoma varies in different institutions. These tumors are usually squamous cell in origin and vary in degrees of differentiation. The tumor spreads by local infiltration, and the patient is usually asymptomatic until erosion through the bony wall of the sinus occurs. The diagnosis is generally made on the bases of patient's history and clinical examination, with radiography playing an important role in determining the extent of bony erosion.

The aim of radiation therapy is to deliver an adequate uniform dose to the tumor volume while sparing the base of the brain and the contralateral eye.[2] External beam irradiation presents a problem due to the obliquity of the surface of the cheek and the eccentric position of the antrum plus the proximity of the antrum to the lens of the eye and the brain. The technique generally accepted uses a pair of vertically hinged anterior and lateral wedge fields. The geometry presents a zone of homogeneous high dose (arrows on the diagram) in the area of the antrum with sharp fall-off at surrounding structures.

[1]Moss, W. T., Brand, W. N., and Battifora, H.: Radiation oncology: rationale, technique, results, ed. 4, St. Louis, ˇ ˙ The C. V. Mosby Co.
[1]Fletcher, C. H.: Textbook of radiotherapy, ed. 2, Philadelphia, 1973, Lea & Febiger.

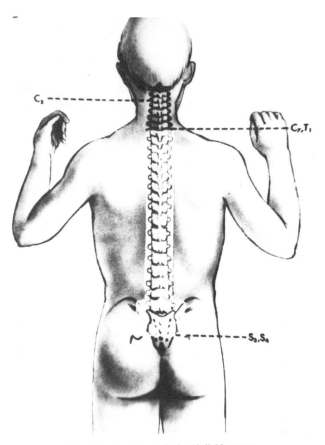

Spinal treatment portal of medulloblastoma.

Courtesy Dr. W. T. Moss.

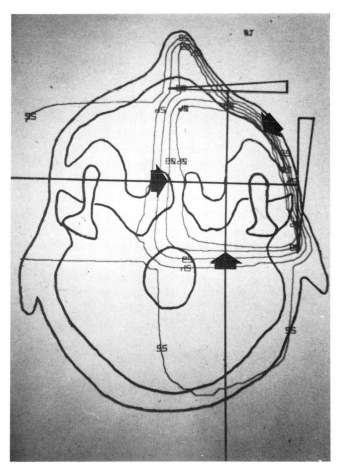

Computer isodose plan demonstrates the dose distribution of two 8 × 8 cm. wedged portals. The wedge filter changes the shape of the isodose line to compensate for irregular surfaces.

GLOSSARY OF SELECTED RADIATION THERAPY TERMS

absorbed dose. The amount of ionizing radiation absorbed per unit mass of irradiated material as it passes through matter.

accelerator (particle). A device that accelerates charged subatomic particles to very great energies. These particles produce x rays and neutrons and may be used for direct medical irradiation and basic physical research. Medical units include linear accelerators, Van de Graaff units, betatrons, and cyclotrons.

air dose. The dose of radiation measured in roentgens in free air, uncorrected for absorption or backscatter.

attenuation. Removal of energy from a beam of ionizing radiation when it traverses matter, by disposition of energy in the matter traversed and/or by deflection of energy out of the beam.

betatron. An electron accelerator that uses magnetic induction to accelerate electrons in a circular path.

bolus. Tissue-equivalent material placed around curved, irregularly shaped anatomic areas to obtain more uniform dosage distribution. Examples include rice, beeswax, Vaseline gauze.

cancer. Term commonly applied to malignant disease.

carcinogen. Any cancer-producing substance or material such as nicotine, radiation, or ingested uranium.

chemical dosimeter. A detector for indirect measurement of radiation by indicating the extent to which the radiation causes a definite chemical change to take place. Example: thermoluminescent dosimeter (TLD).

cobalt-60 (^{60}Co). A radioisotope with a half-life of 5.2 years. Emits two gamma energies, 1.17 and 1.33 mev.

collimator. A diaphragm or system of diaphragms made of a radiation-absorbing material, which define the dimension and direction of a beam.

compensating filter. Filter designed to modify the dose distribution within the patient. Filters may be designed to account for patient shape, size or position.

dose rate. The radiation dose delivered per unit of time, usually roentgens per minute.

dosimeter. A device that measures radiation exposure, such as a film badge, ionization chamber, or Geiger counter.

field size. The geometric area defined by the collimator of a radiotherapy unit at the skin surface.

filter. An attenuator inserted in the beam near the source to modify the beam quality in a desired way. Materials utilized most often are copper, aluminum, and lead.

fractionation. The dividing of a total planned dose into a number of smaller doses to be given over a longer period of time. Consideration must be given to the biologic effectiveness of the smaller doses.

Grenz rays. X rays generated at 20 kvp or less.

half-value layer. The thickness of attenuating material inserted in the beam to reduce the beam intensity to half value.

ionization. The process in which one or more electrons are added to or removed from atoms, thereby creating ions. High temperatures, electrical discharges, or nuclear radiations can cause ionization.

isodose curve. Curve or line drawn to connect points of identical amounts of radiation in a given field.

metastasis. The transmission of cells or groups of cells from a primary tumor to one or more sites elsewhere in the body.

penumbra. Geometric unsharpness around the periphery of a beam of radiation, caused by divergent rays emitted from the periphery of the radiating source (focal spot), the width of the penumbra being proportional to the size of the source.

percent–depth dose. Dose at depth per hundred units at a reference location, usually the skin or maximum ionization depth.

phantom. A volume of material approximating the density and effective atomic number of soft tissue or bone.

rad (radiation *absorbed* *dose*). The basic unit of absorbed dose of ionizing radiation. One rad is the absorption of 100 ergs of radiation energy per gram of absorbing material.

radiation dosimetry. The measurement of the amount of radiation delivered to a specific area.

radiation therapist. A doctor of medicine specializing in the use of ionizing radiation in the treatment of disease.

radiation therapy. A medical specialty in which disease is treated with ionizing radiations.

radiation therapy technologist. A person who has been trained to assist the radiation therapist in the use of ionizing radiation in the treatment of disease and who works under his direction.

radiocurable. Referring to neoplastic cells susceptible to cure (destruction) by ionizing radiation.

radiosensitivity. The responsiveness of cells to radiation.

radium (Ra). A radionuclide (atomic number, 88; atomic weight, 226; half-life, 1,622 years) that is used clinically for radiotherapy. Radium, in conjunction with its subsequent transformations, emits alpha and beta particles and gamma rays. Radium in an encapsulated form is used for various intracavitary radiotherapy applications, as that for cancer of the cervix.

roentgen (r). The unit of exposure dose, based on the extent of ionization in air and defined as 2.58×10^{-4} coulombs per kilogram of dry air. This value is equivalent to 1 electrostatic unit of charge per cubic centimeter, or 0.001293 gram, of dry air; 1.16×10^{12} ion pairs in 1 gram of air; 2.08×10^9 ion pairs per cubic centimeter of air; or the absorption of 87 ergs of energy per gram of air.

scattering. A process in which the trajectory of a particle or photon is changed. Scattering is caused by collisions with atoms, nuclei, and other particles.

sequelae. Reaction or side effects of ionizing radiation on tissue.

skin sparing. In supervoltage beam therapy, the reduced skin injury per roentgen exposure when electron equilibrium is not present at the advance portal but occurs below the skin. Occurs anywhere from 0.5 to 5.0 cm. depending on the energy.

Van de Graaff generator. An electrostatic machine in which electrically charged particles are sprayed on a moving belt and carried by it to build up a high potential on an insulated terminal. Charged particles are then accelerated along a discharge path through a vacuum tube by the potential difference between the insulated terminal and the opposite end of the machine. A Van de Graaff accelerator is often used to inject particles into larger accelerators.

wedge filter. A filter of triangular shape, which decreases in thickness from the base of the triangle to its apex; used to produce inclination of the isodose lines. Use of such filters permits design of customized isodose summations, which deliver very uniform dosage to anatomic areas otherwise difficult to treat properly.

Volume three
Bibliography

PALATE, PHARYNX, AND LARYNX

1896 Macintyre, John: Roentgen rays in laryngeal surgery, J. Laryng. **10**:231, 1896.

Scheier, Max: Ueber die Photographie der Nase und des Kehlkopfes mittels Röntgenstrahlen, Laryng. Gesell. **4**:XII, 1896.

1900 Macintyre, John: The roentgen rays in the diagnosis of the nose and throat, Brit. Laryng. Rhinol. Otolaryng. Ass. II, V, 1900.

1901 Eijkman, P. H.: Der Schlingakt, dargestellt nach Bewegungsphotographien mittels Röntgenstrahlen, Arch. Ges. Physiol. B XCIX, Ref. Fort. B VII, 3, 160, 1901.

1903 Eijkman, P. H.: Radiographie des Kehlkopfes, Fortschr. Roentgenstr. **7**:196-206, 310-318, 1903.

1907 Eijkman, P. H.: Die Bewegung der Halsorgane, Fortschr. Roentgenstr. **11**:130, 196, 280, 1907.

Grumnach: Die Röntgentechnik zur Untersuchung der Mund, Schlund, und Nasenhöhle bei der Phonation, Arch. Laryng. **19**: 1907.

1908 Wasserman, M.: Die Bedeutung des Röntgenverfahrens auf dem Gebiet der Rhinologie und Laryngologie, Fortschr. Roentgenstr. **12**:293, 1908.

1909 Spiess, Gustav: Die Röntgenuntersuchung des oberen Luftwege. In Atlas und Grundriss der Röntgendiagnostik der inneren Medizin, München, 1909, J. F. Lehmann.

1912 Réthi, A.: Die röntgenologische Untersuchung des Kehlkopfes und der Luftröhre, Deutsch. Med. Wschr. **38**:1937, 1912.

1913 Thost, Arthur: Archiv und Atlas des normalen und kranken Kehlkopfes des Lebenden im Röntgenbild, Fortschr. Roentgenstr. **31**:1-50, 1913.

1914 Iglauer, Samuel: Value of roentgenography in the diagnosis of the larynx and the trachea, J.A.M.A. **63**:1827-1831, 1914.

Réthi, A.: Meine neue Methode bei der Röntgendarstellung des Kehlkopfes und der Luftröhre, Laryng. Rhinol. Otol. **6**:28-33, 1914.

Weingaertner, M.: Das Röntgenverfahren in der Laryngologie, Berlin, 1914, Meusser.

1922 Coutard, H.: Note préliminaire sur la radiographie du larynx normale et du larynx cancéreux, J. Belg. Radiol. **13**:287, 1922.

1925 Grandy, C. C.: Roentgenographic demonstration of adenoids, Amer. J. Roentgen. **14**:114, 1925.

1926 Goalwin, Harry A.: Some of the newer methods of the x-ray examination of the paranasal sinuses, the optic canals, the pharynx and larynx, Laryngoscope **36**:235-256, 1926.

1927 Kelemen, G.: Röntgenuntersuchung mit Kontrastmittel bei Kehlkopftuberculose, Arch. Ohr. Nas. Kehlkopfheilk. **117**:225, 1927-1928.

Mosher, H. P., and MacMillan, A. S.: X-ray study of movements of the tongue, epiglottis and hyoid bone in swallowing, Laryngoscope **37**:235-262, 1927.

Sgalitzer, Max: Zur röntgenologischen Darstellung von Pharynxtumoren, Fortschr. Roentgenstr. **36**:1249-1254, 1927.

1928 Brown, Samuel, and Reineke, Harold G.: The roentgenological study of the neck, Amer. J. Roentgen. **20**:208, 212, 1928.

Hickey, Preston M.: Radiography of normal larynx, Radiology **11**:409-411, 1928.

1929 Schüller, Arthur: X-ray examinations of deformities of the nasopharynx, Ann. Otol. **38**:109-129, 1929.

1930 Barclay, A. E.: The normal mechanism of swallowing, Brit. J. Radiol. **3**:534-536, 1930.

Gutzmann, Herman: Röntgenaufnahmen von Zunge und Gaumensegel bei Vocalen und Dauerkonsonanten, Fortschr. Roentgenstr. **41**:392-404, 1930.

Hay, P. D., Jr.: The neck, Ann. Roentgen. **9**:1-99, 1930.

Pancoast, H. K.: Roentgenology of the upper respiratory tract with special reference to the larynx and adjacent structures, J.A.M.A. **95**:1318-1321, 1930.

1932 Oppenheimer, A.: Der Schluckakt. In Becker, R., and Oppenheimer, A.: Normale und pathologische Funktionen der Verdauungsorgane im Röntgenbild, Leipzig, 1932, Georg Thieme.

Sussman, M. L.: The value of roentgenologic examination of the neck, Arch. Otolaryng. **15**:371-381, 1932.

Thost, A.: Die Kehlkopftuberkulose am Lebenden im Röntgenbild, Beitr. Klin. Erforsch. Tuberk. **79**:113-141, 1932.

Wotzilka, G.: Die Bedeutung der Röntgenuntersuchung des Kehlkopfes für die Diagnose und Prognose der Kehlkopftuberkulose, Mschr. Ohrenheilk. **66**:406-408, 1932.

1933 Baldenweck, L., and Gauillard, R.: Récherches sur la radiographie normale et pathologique du larynx, J. Radiol. Electr. **17**:353-362, 1933. Abst.: Amer. J. Roentgen. **32**:573, 1934.

Pancoast, H. K.: Roentgenology of the pharynx and upper esophagus, Amer. J. Cancer **17**:373-395, 1933.

1934 Baldridge, O. E.: The larynx, Xray Techn. **6**:79-81, 1934.

Ducuing, J., Ducuing, L., DeBertrand-Pibrac, and Marquès: La radiographie de l'appareil pharyngolaryngé normale, Bull. Soc. Méd. Paris **22**:415-434, 1934.

Jönsson, G.: Method for roentgen examination of the hypopharynx and upper air passages, Acta Radiol. **15**:144-166, 1934.

Kjellberg, Sven Roland: Einige Studien über das Aussehen des weichen Gaumens an Röntgenbildern, Teils bei normalen, Teils bei einigen pathologischen Zuständen, Acta Radiol. **15**:677-681, 1934.

Taylor, H. K., and Nathanson, Louis: A roentgenological study of tuberculosis of the larynx and neck, Amer. J. Roentgen. **32**:589, 1934.

Worning, Börge: Roentgen examination of laryngeal and hypopharyngeal tumors, Acta Radiol. **15**:12-13, 1934.

Zuppinger, A., and Rüedi, L.: Zur Darstellung des Sinus maxillaris, des Epipharynx und der Trachea mit Kontrastmittel, Fortschr. Roentgenstr. **49**:176-190, 1934.

1936 O'Bannon, R. P.: Radiography of the larynx and pharynx, Xray Techn. **7**:95-98, 134, 1936.

Portmann, G., Mathey-Cornet, R., and Roussett, H.: Contribution à l'étude de la radiographie en phoniatrie, Rev. Laryng. **57**:845-897, 1015-1054, 1936.

Taylor, H. K., and Nathanson, Louis: The roentgenogram in laryngeal tuberculosis, Quart. Bull. Sea View Hosp. **1**:299-313, 1936.

1937 Brown, Samuel, McCarthy, J. E., and Reineke, H. G.: The neck—a roentgenologic study, Radiology **29**:701-714, 1937.

Canuyt, G., and Gunsett, A.: La méthode des coupes radiographiques: tomographie, ou planigraphie appliquée au cancer du larynx, Presse Méd. **45**:1559-1561, 1937.

Canuyt, G., and Gunsett, A.: Tomographies frontales du larynx et des tumeurs laryngées, Bull. Ass. Franc. Cancer **26**:398-413, 1937.

Kerr, H. H., and Bradley, T.: Diverticulum of the larynx, Surgery **2**:598-606, 1937.

1938 Baclesse, F.: Le diagnostic radiographique des tumeurs malignes du pharynx et du larynx; étude anatomotopographique et radiographique, Paris, 1938, Masson & Cie.

Ciurio, L., and Oliveri, A.: Technique and results of roentgenography of the larynx in the anterior position, Radiol. Méd. **25**:834-842, 1938. Abst.: Int. Abstr. Surg. **68**:431, 1939.

Genz, Fritz: Contribution à la technique de l'examen radiographique de larynx, Ann. Otolaryng., pp. 733-740, August, 1938.

Ledoux-Lebard, R., Garcia-Calderon, T., and Djian, A.: La radiographie du larynx de face et sa technique, Bull. Soc. Radiol. Méd. Paris **26**:93, 1938. Abst.: Amer. J. Roentgen. **40**:938, 1938.

Waldapfel, Richard D.: Methodik der Röntgenuntersuchung des Kehlkopfes, Fortschr. Roentgenstr. **53**: 1938.

Young, Barton D.: Soft tissues of air and food passages of the neck, New York, 1938, Thomas Nelson & Sons.

1939 Canuyt, G., and Gunsett, A.: Planigraphies de face du larynx, J. Radiol. **23**:193-202, 1939.

Hartung, Adolph, and Grossman, J. W.: Examination of the larynx and adjacent structures with intrapharyngeal films, Amer. J. Roentgen. **42**:481-489, 1939.

Howes, William E.: Sectional roentgenography of the larynx, Radiology **33**:586-597, 1939.

Lindgren, Erik: Ueber die Röntgenuntersuchung der Larynx, Fortschr. Roentgenstr. **59**:273-285, 1939.

Shannon, E. H., and Veitch, A. H.: Diseases of the hypopharyngeal region producing dysphagia, Amer. J. Roentgen. **42**:173-185, 1939.

Waldenström, Jan, and Kjellberg, Sven Roland: The roentgenological diagnosis of sideropenic dysphagia, Acta Radiol. **20**:623-625, 1939.

1940   Calthrop, G. T.: Radiological demonstration of the adenoids, Lancet **1**:1005, 1940.

Leborgne, F. E.: Tomographic study of cancer of the larynx, Amer. J. Roentgen. **43**:493-499, 1940.

Young, Barton R.: Recent advances in the examination of the air and food passages of the neck, Amer. J. Roentgen. **44**:519-529, 1940.

1941   Caulk, Ralph M.: Tomography of the larynx, Amer. J. Roentgen. **46**:1-10, 1941.

Pendergrass, Eugene P., and Young, Barton R.: The roentgen diagnosis of neoplasm of the air and food passages, with particular reference to the larynx, Radiology **36**:197-211, 1941.

Zachrisson, C. G.: Beitrag zur Röntgenanatomie der Larynx, Acta Radiol. **22**:859-865, 1941.

1942   Caulk, Ralph M.: La tomografía de la laringe, Rev. Radiol. Fis. **9**:1-10, 1942.

Johnstone, A. S.: A radiological study of deglutition, J. Anat. **77**:97-100, 1942.

1943   Belanger, W. J., and Dyke, C. G.: Roentgen diagnosis of malignant nasopharyngeal tumors, Amer. J. Roentgen. **50**:9-18, 1943.

Greisman, B. L.: Mechanism of phonation demonstrated by planigraphy of the larynx, Arch. Otolaryng. **38**:17-26, 1943.

Templeton, F. E., and Kredel, R. A.: The cricopharyngeal sphincter, Laryngoscope **53**:1-12, 1943.

1946   Clerf, Louis H.: Diseases of the upper air passages. In Pillmore, George U., editor: Clinical radiology, Philadelphia, 1946, F. A. Davis Co., vol. 1, pp. 123-153.

Farinas, Pedro L.: Mucosography of the respiratory tract, Radiogr. Clin. Photogr. **22**:38-41, 1946.

Mathey-Cornat, R., and Pellegrino: Sur l'exploration radiologique et le diagnostic des fractures du larynx, J. Radiol. Electr. **27**:419-422, 1946.

Weitz, H. L.: Roentgenography of adenoids, Radiology **47**:66-70, 1946.

1947   Moreau, W. H., and Moreau, George E.: La radiografia simple della laringe, Radiologia **10**:7-16, 1947.

Young, Barton R.: The soft tissues of the air and food passages of the neck. In Golden, Ross, editor: Diagnostic roentgenology, ed. 3, New York, 1947, Thomas Nelson & Sons, vol. 11, pp. 895-912.

1951   Fletcher, G. H., and Matzinger, K. E.: Value of soft tissue technic in the diagnosis and treatment of head and neck tumors, Radiology **57**:305-329, 1951.

1952   MacMillan, A. S., and Kelemen, G.: Radiography of the supraglottic speech organs, Arch. Otolaryng. **55**:671-688, 1952.

1954   O'Bannon, R. P., and Grunow, O. H.: The larynx and pharynx radiographically considered, Southern Med. J. **47**:310-316, 1954.

1955   Brauer, W.: Die Methodik der Larynx-Kontrast-Schichtersuchung, Fortschr. Roentgenstr. **82**:521-525, 1955.

Epstein, B. S.: A roentgenographic aid to the diagnosis of radiopaque foreign bodies in the upper intrathoracic esophagus, Amer. J. Roentgen. **73**:115-117, 1955.

Ramsey, G. H., and others: Cinefluorographic analysis of the mechanism of swallowing, Radiology **64**:498-518, 1955.

1957   Powers, W. E., McGee, H. H., and Seaman, W. B.: Contrast examination of the larynx and pharynx, Radiology **68**:169-177, 1957.

1958   Gay, Brit B., Jr.: A roentgenologic method for evaluation of the larynx and pharynx; technique of examination, Amer. J. Roentgen. **79**:301-305, 1958.

Randall, P., O'Hara, A. E., and Bakes, F. P.: A simple roentgen examination for the study of soft palate function in patients with poor speech, Plast. Reconstr. Surg. **21**:345-356, 1958.

1959   Green, R. I.: Radiological appearances of soft palate with reference to treatment of cleft palate, J. Fac. Radiologists **10**:27-39, 1959.

1960   Ogura, J. H., and others: Laryngograms; their value in the diagnosis and treatment of laryngeal lesions, Laryngoscope **70**:780-809, 1960.

Smith, C. C., and others: Utilization of roentgenology in the study of speech mechanisms, Amer. J. Roentgen. **84**:213-219, 1960.

1961   Green, R. I.: Speech defects; radiology of speech defects, Radiography **27**:331-338, 1961.

Gunson, Edward F.: Radiography of the pharynx and upper esophagus; shoestring method, Xray Techn. **33**:1-8, 1961.

Medina, J., and Seaman, W. B.: Value of laryngography in vocal cord tumors, Radiology **77**:531-542, 1961.

Nylén, B. O.: Cleft palate and speech, Acta Radiol., supp. 203, pp. 1-124, 1961.

Powers, W. E., Holtz, S., Ogura, J., Ellis, B. L., and Mac Gavran, M. H.: Contrast examination of the larynx and pharynx; accuracy and value in diagnosis, Amer. J. Roentgen. **86**:651-660, 1961.

1962   Fabrikant, J. I., and others: Contrast laryngography in the evaluation of laryngeal neoplasms, Amer. J. Roentgen. **87**:822-835, 1962.

Owsley, W. C., Jr.: Palate and pharynx; roentgenographic evaluation in management of cleft palate and related deformities, Amer. J. Roentgen. **87**:811-821, 1962.

1963   O'Hara, A. Edward: Roentgen evaluation of patients with cleft palate, Radiol. Clin. N. Amer. **1**:1-11, 1963.

1964   Klein, R., and Fletcher, G. H.: Evaluation of the clinical usefulness of roentgenologic findings in squamous cell carcinoma of the larynx, Amer. J. Roentgen. **92**:43-54, 1964.

Pastore, P. N., May, M., and Gildersleeve, G. A.: Laryngopharyngogram as a diagnostic aid, Laryngoscopy **74**:723-733, 1964.

Powers, W. E., Holtz, S., and Ogura, J.: Contrast examination of the larynx and pharynx; inspiratory phonation, Amer. J. Roentgen. **92**:40-42, 1964.

Sloan, R. F., and others: Recent cinefluorographic advances in palatopharyngeal roentgenography, Amer. J. Roentgen. **92**:977-985, 1964.

1965   Caplan, L. H., and Naimark, A.: The transtracheal approach to laryngography, Radiology **85**:439-441, 1965.

Jing, Bao-Shan, and McGraw, J. P.: Contrast nasopharyngography in the diagnosis of tumors, Arch. Otolaryng. **81**:365-371, 1965.

Lehmann, Q. H.: Reverse phonation; a new maneuver for examining the larynx, Radiology **84**:215-221, 1965.

1966   Hanson, D. J., and Manor, R. E.: Tomography of the larynx, Med. Radiogr. Photogr. **42**:152-153, 1966.

Maguire, G. H.: The larynx; simplified radiological examination using heavy filtration and high voltage, Radiology **87**:102-109, 1966.

Staple, T. W., and Ogura, J. H.: Cineradiography of the swallowing mechanism following supraglottic subtotal laryngectomy, Radiology **87**:226-230, 1966.

1967   Graf, H., and Fuchs, W. A.: Die Röntgenuntersuchung des Epipharynx mit positivem Kontrastmittel, Fortschr. Roentgenstr. **106**:133-144, 1967.

Johnson, T. H., Green, A. E., and Rice, E. N.: Nasopharyngography; its technic and uses, Radiology **88**:1166-1169, 1967.

Khoo, F. Y., Chia, K. B., and Nalpon, J.: A new technique of contrast examination of the nasopharynx with cinefluorography and roentgenography, Amer. J. Roentgen. **99**:238-248, 1967.

Ryan, James: Pericricoid laryngography, Australas. Radiol. **11**:234-241, 1967.

Thornbury, J. R., and Latourette, H. B.: Comparison study of laryngography techniques; 150 KVP plain roentgenography vs. positive contrast roentgenography, Amer. J. Roentgen. **99**:555-561, 1967.

1968   Bloch, S., and Quantrill, J. R.: The radiology of nasopharyngeal tumors, including positive contrast nasopharyngography, S. Afr. Med. J. **42**:1030-1036, 1968.

Howell, T. R., Gildersleeve, G. A., and King, E. R.: The role of roentgenographic studies in the evaluation and staging of malignancies of the larynx and pharynx, Amer. J. Roentgen. **102**:138-144, 1968.

Johannesson, S.: Roentgenologic investigation of the nasopharyngeal tonsil in children of different ages, Acta Radiol. [Diagn.] **7**:299-304, 1968.

Margolin, F. R., and Steinbach, H. L.: Soft tissue roentgenography of thyroid nodules, Amer. J. Roentgen. **102**:844-852, 1968.

1969 Matoba, N., and Kikuchi, T.: Thyroidolymphography; a new technique for visualization of the thyroid and cervical lymph nodes, Radiology **92**:339-342, 1969.

Skolnick, M. L.: Video velopharnyngography in patients with nasal speech, with emphasis on lateral pharyngeal motion in velopharyngeal closure, Radiology **93**:747-755, 1969.

1970 Johnson, T. H., Jr.: Spray aerosol laryngography, Arch. Otolaryng. **92**:511-513, 1970.

Morgan, J. A., Gyepes, M. T., Jones, M. H., and Disilets, D. T.: Barium-impregnated chocolate fudge for the study of chewing mechanism in children, Radiology **94**:432-433, 1970.

Potter, G. D.: Sclerosis of the base of the skull as a manifestation of nasopharyngeal carcinoma, Radiology **94**:35-38, 1970.

Zamel, N., Austin, J. H. M., Graf, P. D., Dedo, H. H., Jones, M. D., and Nadel, J. A.: Powdered tantalum as a medium for human laryngography, Radiology **94**:547-553, 1970.

1971 Chittinand, S., Patheja, S. S., and Wizenberg, M. J.: Barium nasopharyngography, Radiology **98**:387-390, 1971.

Johnson, T. H., and Feist, J. H.: Laryngography; the procedure of choice for benign laryngeal lesions, Amer. J. Roentgen. **111**:109-114, 1971.

1972 Ma, H. T. G., and Reed, R.: High KV filtration tomograms of the larynx, J. Canad. Ass. Radiol. **23**:119-124, 1972.

1973 Kamdar, K. N., and Ramesh, K. O.: Palatography; a study of velopharyngeal closure, Australas. Radiol. **17**:26-31, 1973.

Olofsson, J., Renouf, J. H. P., and Van Nostrand, A. W. P.: Laryngeal carcinoma; correlation of roentgenography and histopathology, Amer. J. Roentgen. **117**:526-539, 1973.

BODY CAVITIES, ANATOMY

1906 Addison, C.: In Ellis' demonstration of anatomy, ed. 12, New York, 1906, Wm. Wood & Co.

1917 Mills, W. R.: The relation of bodily habitus to visceral form, position, tonus, and motility, Amer. J. Roentgen. **4**:155-169, 1917.

RADIOGRAPHY OF THE THORACIC VISCERA

1936 Fuchs, A. W.: A radiographic view-finder, Radiogr. Clin. Photogr. **12**:2-7, 1936.

TRACHEA, THYROID, AND THYMUS

1899 Blake: The relation of the trachea and bronchi to the thoracic wall as determined by x-ray, Amer. J. Med. Sci. **117**:313, 1899.

1905 Pfeiffer, W.: Die Darstellung der Trachea im Röntgenbild, besonders bei Struma, Bruns' Beiträge, 1905.

1910 Albers-Schönberg, H. E.: Tracheadarstellung. In Röntgentechnik, ed. 3, Berlin, 1910, Gräfe & Sillem, chap. 26.

1921 Pfahler, G. E.: New roentgenographic technic for study of the thyroid, Amer. J. Roentgen. **8**:81-83, 1921.

1928 Eiselberg, A., and Sgalitzer, D. M.: X-ray examination of the trachea and the bronchi, Surg. Gynec. Obstet. **47**:53-68, 1928.

1932 Mitchell, Margaret: Goiter and thymus technic, Xray Techn. **3**:120, 1932.

1941 Clute, Howard M., and Lawrence, K. B.: Intrathoracic goiter, Amer. J. Surg. **54**:151, 1941.

1946 Echternacht, Arthur P.: The thymus gland. In Pillmore, George U., editor: Clinical radiology, Philadelphia, 1946, F. A. Davis Co., vol. 1, pp. 422-424.

Sgalitzer, Max.: Roentgenological examination of the power of resistance of the tracheal wall, Amer. J. Roentgen. **56**:355-360, 1946.

1956 Lentino, W., Marchetto, I., and Poppel, M. H.: A modification of the routine lateral view of the chest to permit visualization of the superior mediastinum, Amer. J. Roentgen. **75**:767-770, 1956.

1960 Segal, R. L., Zucherman, H., and Friedman, E. W.: Soft tissue roentgenography; its use in diagnosis of thyroid carcinoma, J.A.M.A. **173**:1890-1894, 1960.

1964 Hare, W. S. C.: Pneumomediastinography and the thymus, J. Coll. Radiol. Aust. **8**:266-271, 1964.

Heckman, K.: Die frontale Diagonalaufnahme, Röntgenblaetter **17**:551-558, 1964. Abst.: Amer. J. Roentgen. **94**:263, 1965.

1965 Kreel, L., and James, V.: Pneumo-mediastinography by the transternal method; a technique for radiographic visualization of the thymus gland, Radiography **31**:133-137, 1965.

1966 Sumerling, M. D., and Irvine, W. J.: Pneumomediastinography, Amer. J. Roentgen. **98**:451-460, 1966.

1967 Berne, A. S., and others: CO_2–O_2 pneumomediastinography with polytomography for the preoperative evaluation of bronchogenic carcinoma, Radiology **88**:519-525, 1967.

PULMONARY APICES

1908 Groedel, F. M.: Ueber gleichzeitige Aufnahme der beiden Lungenspitzen mit zwei Antikathoden, mittels der Stereoröhre, Fortschr. Roentgenstr. **12**:183, 1908.

Groedel, F. M.: Ueber Lungenspitzenaufnahmen, Verh. Deutsch. Röntgen. **4**:47, 1908.

1912 Kreuzfuchs: Die radiologische Untersuchung der Lungenspitzen, München. Med. Wschr. **59**: 1912.

1919 Sahatschief, A.: Ueber die Röntgenuntersuchung der Lungenspitzen in der antero-posterioren (ventrodorsalen) Lage, Fortschr. Roentgenstr. **26**:197-198, 1919.

1921 Bray, H. A.: A suggestion for improving the visibility of the apical field on the chest radiogram, Amer. J. Roentgen. **8**:602-603, 1921.

1922 Peltssohn, F.: Kompression der Lungenspitzen; ein Hilfsmittel zur Verbesserung der Durchleuchtung und Aufnahmetechnik, Fortschr. Roentgenstr. **30**:283, 1922.

1923 Ziegler, J.: Die Röntgenuntersuchung der Lungenspitzen, Z. Tuberk. **39**:7-20, 1923.

1925 Baum, Felix, and Black, L. T.: The importance of the apical roentgenogram in pulmonary tuberculosis, Amer. Rev. Tuber. **12**:228-230, 1925.

Gassul, R.: Zur Technik der verbesserten Lungenspitzendarstellung, Deutsch. Med. Wschr. **51**:655, 1925.

1926 Appelrath, H.: Eine neue Technik der Lungenspitzenaufnahme, Fortschr. Roentgenstr. **34**:526-528, 1926.

1927 Grynkraut: Sur un procède d'exploration des sommets pulmonaires en oblique, Bull. Mém. Soc. Radiol., May, 1927.

1930 Barsóny, Theodor, and Koppenstein, Ernst: Röntgenuntersuchung der Lungen in vorüber gebeugter Stellung, Röntgenpraxis **2**:409-414, 1930.

Barsóny, Theodor, and Koppenstein, Ernst: Röntgenuntersuchung des Lungenspitzenfeldes in frontaler Strahl-enrichtung, Röntgenpraxis **2**:275-281, 1930.

Barsóny, Theodor, and Koppenstein, Ernst: Röntgenuntersuchung des Lungspitzenfelds mit axialer Strahlenrichtung, Röntgenpraxis **2**:326-330, 1930.

Castellani, Fabio: Una nuova proiezione per l'esame radiologico dell'apice polmonare, Rev. Radiol. Fis. **2**:365-369, 1930.

1931 Barsóny, Theodor, and Koppenstein, Ernst: Begriff der Lungenspitze, zugleich Methoden zur röntgenologischen Darstellung der anatomischen Lungenspitze, Röntgenpraxis **3**:385-394, 1931.

Castellani, Fabio: Ancora su di una modalità personale di tecnica per l'esame radiologico dell'apice, Riv. Radiol. Fis. Med. **6**:793-802, 1931.

1932 Liverani, Ettore: Sulla semeiologia radiologica dell'apice polmonare, Radiol. Med. **19**:493-512, 1932.

1933 Fiorenzi, Oliviero: Contribution technique et anatomo-clinico-radiologique à l'exploration des sommets pulmonaires, Radiol. Med. **20**:460, 1933.

Fiorenzi, Oliviero: Sulla esplorazione radiologica dell' apice polmonare, Radiol. Med. **20**:460-491, 1933.

Zawadowski, Witold: Étude de la statique au niveau des sommets et des parties supérieures des poumons, J. Radiol. Electr. **17**:603-612, 1933.

1935 Zintheo, C. J., Jr.: Technic for roentgenography of the chest apex, Xray Techn. **7**:53-54, 1935.

1937 Twining, E. W.: Lateral view of the lung apices, Brit. J. Radiol. **10**:123-131, 1937.

1938 Salkin, D.: Expiratory roentgenograms for pulmonary apical detail, Amer. J. Roentgen. **39**:363-367, 1938.

Zintheo, C. J., Jr.: Auxiliary techniques in chest roentgenography, Amer. Rev. Tuber. **37**:14-30, 1938.

1939 Mark, F. M., and Taylor, H. K.: A lateral view of the pulmonary apex and upper dorsal spine, Quart. Bull. Sea View Hosp. **4**:189-195, 1939.

1940 Mayer, Herbert: Roentgen aspect of the upper retroesophageal pulmonary borders, Amer. J. Roentgen. **43**:169, 1940.

Remo, L., and Lustok, M.: Angular roentgenography of the pulmonary apex, Amer. Rev. Tuber. **42**:738-746, 1940.

Thomas, A. G.: Positions for demonstrating pulmonary apical lesions, Xray Techn. **12**:50-51, 77, 1940.

1946 Flaxman, A. J.: Apical tuberculosis with roentgen technique, Amer. Rev. Tuber. **54**:1-8, 1946.

1950 Hoffstaedt, E. G.: Radiological demonstration of apical lung lesions, Radiol. Clin. **19**:164-169, 1950.

1951 Cohen, A. G., and Geffen, A.: Roentgenographic methods in pulmonary disease, Amer. J. Med. **10**:375-385, 1951.

1959 Rundle, F. F., de Lambert, R. M., and Epps, R. G.: Cervicothoracic tumors; a technical aid to their roentgenologic localization, Amer. J. Roentgen. **81**:316-321, 1959.

1965 Jakimow, I. L., and Sheehan, F. R.: Kyphotic view, Dis. Chest **47**:636-640, 1965.

1968 Jacobson, G., and Sargent, E. N.: Apical roentgenographic views of the chest, Amer. J. Roentgen. **104**:822-828, 1968.

LUNGS

1897 Williams, Francis: The roentgen rays in thoracic diseases, Amer. J. Med. Sci. **114**:665-687, 1897. Also Yale Med. J. **6**:233-240, 1900.

1901 Cowl: Ueber verschiedene Projektionen des Thorax und über den diagnostischen Wert von Aufnahmepaaren, Fortschr. Roentgenstr. **5**:129, 1901.

1907 Beck, Carl: The roentgen method in the surgery of the chest, Surg. Gynec. Obstet. **6**:683-694, 1907.

Hickey, P. M.: The tubular diaphragm in roentgenography of the chest, Amer. Quart. Roentgen. **1**:14-19, 1907.

1913 Groedel, F. M.: Das Thoraxbild bei zentrischer und exzentrischer Röntgenprojektion, Fortschr. Roentgenstr. **20**:541, 1913.

Sonnenkalb, Victor: Die Darstellung des pneumatischen Systems beim Lebenden, Verh. Deutsch. Otol. Gesell. **32**:367, 1913.

1914 Albert-Weil, E.: La radiographie des adénopathies thoraciques, J. Radiol. Electr. **1**:183-193, 1914.

1916 Hulst, H. M.: Some aspects of special interest bearing on the roentgenological diagnosis of tuberculosis of the lungs, Amer. J. Roentgen. **3**:465-474, 1916.

1919 Miller, W. S.: Stereoroentgenograms of the injected lung as an aid to the study of the lung architecture, Bull. Hopkins Hosp. **30**:34, 1919.

1920 Chaoul, H., and Stierlin, E.: Klinische Röntgendiagnostik der Erkrankungen der Brustorgane. In Chirurgie der Brustorgane, 1920. Abst.: Yearbook of Radiology, p. 243, 1932.

1921 Evans, William A.: The value of lateral and oblique roentgen-ray studies of the chest, Amer. J. Roentgen. **8**:106-112, 1921.

1922 Garcin, J.: Anatomie radiologique des poumons, J. Radiol. Electr. **6**:110-121, 1922.

Gilson, M.: Exploration radiologique des interlobes pulmonaires à l'état pathologique, J. Radiogr. **6**:14-20, 1922.

Thompson, J. C., and Barlow, Nathan: Roentgenray technique for the demonstration of small pneumothorax, Amer. J. Roentgen. **9**:235-240, 1922.

1924 Heuser, Carlo: Roentgenology of pneumonia, Semana Méd. **2**:91, 1924.

LeWald, L. T., and Green, N. W.: The value of the lateral projection in the roentgen ray examination of the chest, Arch. Surg. **8**:265-286, 1924.

Porro, Nicholó: L'esame radiologico del torace dei decubiti laterali ed in quelli supino e prono all'ortoscopio, Radiol. Med. **11**:212-226, 1924.

Sampson, Homer L.: Roentgenographic chest technique, Amer. J. Roentgen. **11**:373-375, 1924.

1925 Fleischner, Felix: Mediastino-interlobar pleuritis; a frequent occurrence in mediastinal gland tuberculosis, Klin. Wschr. **4**:875-877, 1925. Abst.: Amer. J. Roentgen. **15**:263, 1926.

Heuser, Carlo: Roentgenography of hydatid cyst of the lung, Amer. J. Roentgen. **13**:529, 1925.

Pritchard, J. S.: The value of lateral and oblique roentgen light exposure in the diagnosis of thoracic affections, Michigan, 1925. Reprint: Arch. Surg. **10**:557-566, 1925.

1926 Fleischner, Felix: Das Röntgenbild der interlobären Pleuritis und seine Differentialdiagnose, Ergebn. Med. Strahlenforsch. **2**:197-248, 1926. Abst.: Yearbook of Radiology, p. 238, 1932.

Groedel, F. M.: Die anatomische Qualitätsdiagnose der Lungentuberkulose aus dem Röntgenbild, Acta Radiol. **6**:469-472, 1926.

1927 Correra, T.: Contributo allo studio radiologico della pleura; la proiezione cranio-dorso-ventrale del torace, Radiol. Med. **14**:553-564, 1927.

Gerhartz, Heinrich: Röntgenologische Technik bei der Untersuchung der Lungen. In Handbuch der biologischen Arbeitsmethoden, abt. 5⁴, t. II, pp. 1487-1501, 1927.

Pancoast, H. K., Baetjer, F. H., and Dunham, K.: The healthy adult chest; clinical and roentgenological report, Amer. J. Roentgen. **17**:507-527, 1927.

1928 Chapman, John E.: The value of the lateral exposure in the roentgen examination of the chest, Radiology **10**:139-149, 1928.

Eiselberg, A., and Sgalitzer, D. M.: X-ray examination of the trachea and the bronchi, Surg. Gynec. Obstet. **47**:53-68, 1928.

Pottenger, F. M.: Certain factors militating against accurate correlation of physical and roentgen ray examinations of the chest, Amer. J. Med. Sci. **175**:676, 1928.

1929 Holbeach, C. H.: Chest radiology, Brit. J. Radiol. **2**:366-368, 1929.

1930 Bethea, O. W.: The use of lead markers in x-ray examinations of the chest, Radiol. Rev. **52**:243, 1930.

Klemperer, F., and Ahlenstiel, Rolf: Röntgenuntersuchung der Lungen. In Ergebnisse der gesamten Tuberkuloseforschung, v. 1, Leipzig, 1930.

Sante, L. R.: The chest, Ann. Roentgen. **11**:3-53, 1930.

Tartagli, D.: La proiezione di profilo obliquo anteroposteriore per l'esame radiologico laterale di un solo pulmone, Radiol. Med. **17**:1388-1395, 1930.

1931 Baldwin, V. C.: Rapid chest technic, Xray Techn. **3**:62-64, 1931.

de Beaujeu, J. A.: Sur l'examen radiographique de profil pour la localisation des affections intrathoraciques, J. Radiol. **15**:129-140, 1931.

Brown, J. M.: Lung technic, Xray Techn. **3**:60-61, 1931.

Danielius, Gerhard: Röntgenologie der oberen medialen Lungenabschnitte, Fortschr. Roentgenstr. **44**:626-634, 1931.

Jenkinson, E. L.: Pneumothorax, Amer. J. Roentgen. **25**:237-240, 1931.

Malins, Margery M.: Radiography of the chest, Xray Techn. **3**:65-68, 1931.

Rigler, L. G.: Roentgen diagnosis of small pleural effusions, J.A.M.A. **96**:104-108, 1931.

Rigler, L. G.: Roentgenologic observations on the movement of pleural effusions, Amer. J. Roentgen. **25**:220-229, 1931.

Rigler, L. G.: The roentgenography of the pleural effusions, Xray Techn. **3**:56-59, 1931.

Schall, L.: Die Interlobärspalten, Ergebn. Tuberk. **2**:405, 1931.

Sparks, J. V., and Wood, Franklin: Localization of pleural adhesions, Brit. J. Radiol. **4**:592-598, 1931.

Twining, E. W.: Radiology of the chest, Brit. J. Radiol. **4**:658-679, 1931.

1932   Allen, B. M.: X-ray diagnosis of the chest with special reference to fluid, Delaware Med. J. **4**:204-208, 1932.

Liebmann, E.: Pleuraerkrankungen. In Lehrbuch der Röntgendiagnostik, ed. 3, Leipzig, 1932, Georg Thieme, v. 2, pp. 910-931.

Pancoast, H. K., and Pendergrass, Eugene: Localization of foreign bodies in the lung by roentgen examination, Amer. J. Roentgen. **27**:225-233, 1932.

1933   Bridge, Ezra: Definition in chest radiography, Xray Techn. **5**:1-3, 1933.

Daan, Albert: Der Lobus venae azygos im Röntgenbilde, Acta Radiol. **14**:375-389, 1933. Abst.: Amer. J. Roentgen. **32**:574, 1934.

Manges, W. F.: Roentgen diagnosis and localization of opaque foreign bodies in the air passages, Amer. J. Roentgen. **29**:368-383, 1933.

Meyer, Herman: The technician in cases of pneumonia, Xray Techn. **4**:101-104, 1933.

Peltasohn, F., and Neumann, W.: Die Röntgendarstellung der unteren Pleuragrenze, Fortschr. Roentgenstr. **47**:519-529, 1933.

Pigorini, Luigi: Sopra il lobo inferiore, Radiol. Med. **20**:857-877, 1933. Abst.: Amer. J. Roentgen. **32**:573, 1934.

Rigler, L. G., and Erickson, L. G.: Inferior accessory lobe of the lung, Amer. J. Roentgen. **32**:464-486, 1933.

Société de radiologie médicale de France: Séance spéciale consacrée à la technique de la radiographie pulmonaire, Bull. Soc. Radiol. Med. Paris **21**:170-272, 1933.

Wilsey, R. B.: The physical foundations of chest roentgenography, Amer. J. Roentgen. **30**:234-241, 388-400, 523-528, 1933.

1934   Brown, Samuel: Roentgenological examination of the chest in lateral decubitus, Amer. J. Roentgen. **31**:41-43, 1934.

Determann, A.: Ueber die Verwendung von partieller Filterung bei Röntgenaufnahmen, insbesondere Lungenaufnahmen, Fortschr. Roentgenstr. **49**:170, 1934. Abst.: Yearbook of Radiology, p. 278, 1934.

Fray, Walter W.: Radiography of the thorax and its contents, Xray Techn. **5**:118-124, 1934.

Greenberg, Sidney: The superior value of the expiratory roentgenogram in the diagnosis of incomplete pneumothorax, Amer. J. Roentgen. **32**:330, 1934.

Kent, Cynthia McG.: Bucky diaphragm technic in chest radiography, Xray Techn. **5**:124-126, 1934.

Korol, Ephraim, and Scott, H. A.: The use of chest roentgenograms taken with breath held in expiration, Amer. J. Roentgen. **31**:266, 1934.

Levitin, Joseph: The roentgenological position of the potential interlobar spaces, Radiology **23**:629, 1934.

Moulle, Georges: De la méthode dans l'examen radiologique du poumon, Paris, 1934, Masson & Cie.

Wilsey, R. B.: The focal spot in chest radiography, Xray Techn. **6**:68-73, 1934.

Zintheo, Clarence J., Jr.: A diaphragm and plate divider for chest roentgenography, Radiology **23**:594-597, 1934.

1935   Anthony, A., and Schwarz, W.: Beitrag zur röntgenologischen Erkennung des Lungenemphysems, Röntgenpraxis **7**:461-463, 1935. Abst.: Radiology **25**:519, 1935.

Bagnaresi, Giacomo: Influenza del decubito sull'aspetto radiografico e sugli spostamenti del lobo medio nell'in-

filtrazione pneumonica, Radiol. Med. **22**:915-928, 1935. Abst.: Amer. J. Roentgen. **37**:129, 1937.

Ellison, R.: Oblique films for the study of adhesions in artificial pneumothorax, Amer. J. Roentgen. **34**:592-595, 1935.

Gershon-Cohen, J.: Radiographic examination of the chest employing an opaque plastic for equalization of radiographic densities, Radiogr. Clin. Photogr. **11**:10-13, 1935.

Laurell, Hugo: Der Nachweis minimaler, bei gewöhnlicher Lungenuntersuchung oft unsichtbarer Pleuraexsudate, Acta Radiol. **16**:691-704, 1935. Abst.: Amer. J. Roentgen. **37**:132, 1937.

Levitin, Joseph, and Brunn, Harold: A study of the roentgenologic appearance of the lobes of the lung and the interlobar fissures, Radiology **25**:651, 1935.

Mitchell, E. S.: Radiography of the chest, Xray Techn. **7**:14-16, 26, 1935.

Pancoast, H. K., and Pendergrass, E. P.: Roentgen technic with especial reference to examination to diagnose or exclude silicosis, J. Indus. Hyg. **16**:165, 1935.

Peirce, C. B.: Extra-pulmonary tumors of the thorax, Radiology **24**:467-479, 1935.

Rigler, Leo G.: A roentgen study of the mode of development of encapsulated interlobar effusions, J. Thorac. Cardiov. Surg. **5**:295-303, 1935.

Sampson, Homer L.: A double-exposure roentgenological chest technique, Amer. Rev. Tuber. **31**:50-53, 1935.

Stivelman, B. P.: Interlobar pleural effusions, Amer. J. Roentgen. **34**:475-481, 1935.

Weyl, Charles, and Warren, S. R.: Apparatus and technique for roentgenography of the chest, Springfield, Ill., 1935, Charles C Thomas, Publisher.

Wolff, A. O.: Contribution à la topographie des ganglions intrathoraciques surtout à l'égard de la tuberculose des ganglions bronchiques, Acta Radiol. **16**:675-681, 1935. Abst.: Amer. J. Roentgen. **37**:131, 1937.

Zintheo, Clarence J., Jr.: Laboratory notes on chest roentgenography, Xray Techn. **6**:116-120, 147, 1935.

1936   Allison, B. H.: Special technic for chests, Xray Techn. **8**:71-75, 1936.

Fleischner, Felix: Ueber das Wesen der basalen horizontalen Schattenstriefen im Lungenfeld, Wien. Arch. Int. Med. **28**:461, 1936.

Gershon-Cohen, J.: The roentgen examination of the chest, Amer. J. Roentgen. **35**:279, 1936.

Weyl, C., Warren, S. R., Jr., and O'Neill, D. B.: A survey of chest roentgenographic technique, Amer. J. Roentgen. **35**:534-539, 1936.

Weyl, C., Warren, S. R., Jr., and O'Neill, D. B.: The choice of certain technical factors for chest roentgenography, Amer. J. Roentgen. **35**:534-539, 1936.

Wilsey, R. B.: Experiences with the newer technics in chest radiography, Xray Techn. **8**:45-52, 1936.

1937   Delherm, Thoyer, Rozat, P., and Bernhard, J.: Essais de planigraphie; squelette; poumons, Presse Méd. **45**:765-767, 1937.

Eschbach, Heinrich: Zur zweckmässigen Aufnahmetechnik der Lungen bei ausgedehnter massiver Verschattung, Fortschr. Roentgenstr. **56**:486, 1937.

Hirsch, I. S., and Schwarzschild, M.: Directed roentgenography of the thorax, Amer. J. Roentgen. **37**:13-20, 1937.

Inouye, Kazuo: Darstellung von Flüssigkeitsansammlungen und Verdickungen der Pleura im Röntgenbild durch Schrägaufnahme, Fortschr. Roentgenstr. **55**:471-477, 1937.

Peirce, C. B., and Stocking, B. W.: The oblique projection of the thorax, Amer. J. Roentgen. **38**:245-267, 1937.

Pendergrass, E. P., and Hodes, P. J.: The healthy chest, Amer. J. Roentgen. **38**:15, 1937.

Sobolev, V. I.: Ueber röntgenologische Seitenuntersuchung bei Erkrankungen der Lunge, Vestn. Rentgen. Radiol. **18**:102-107, 1937.

Ulrich, K.: Zur splitterlokalisation im Rücken, Röntgenpraxis **9**:770-773, 1937.

1938   Holmes, G. W.: Hemoptysis and the position of the

roentgen examination in its diagnosis, Radiology 31:131-136, 1938.

Maltinsky, M. M.: Special technic of the chest with the high speed Bucky and rotating target tube, Xray Techn. 10:131-133, 143, 1938.

Pesauera, G. S.: The evolution of chest roentgenographic technique, Amer. J. Roentgen. 40:405-409, 1938.

Zintheo, C. J., Jr.: Auxiliary techniques in chest roentgenography, Amer. Rev. Tuber. 37:14-30, 1938.

1939 Byers, D. E.: Technical aspects in the examination of the chest, Xray Techn. 11:96-98, 1939.

Dudley, M. L.: Value of the high speed Bucky in chest x-ray examinations, Xray Techn. 11:95, 124, 1939.

Eller, Virginia H.: The value of anterior-oblique views in chest radiography, Xray Techn. 10:222-224, 247, 1939.

Grandgérard, Roger: La radiotomie thoracique en décubitus latéral, J. Radiol. 23:118, 1939.

Schubert, Brunhilde: Zur Darstellung im Sagittalbild nicht erkennbarer Kavernen, Röntgenpraxis 11:30-31, 1939.

Wilson, H. M.: Exploration of the thorax by body-section roentgenography, Radiology 33:598-604, 1939.

Zintheo, C. J., Jr.: The art of chest radiography, Xray Techn. 10:269-276, 299, 1939.

1940 Cahoon, J. B., Jr.: Lateral chest technic, Xray Techn. 12:55-56, 78, 1940.

Choice (The) of methods of roentgen examination of the chest for diagnostic surveys, Medical series, Bulletin no. III, Pittsburgh, 1940, Air Hygiene Foundation of America, Inc.

Kraft, E., and Herman, Myron: Tomographic diagnosis of pulmonary cavities, Quart. Bull. Sea View Hosp. 5:279, 1940.

Lindblom, Knut: Half-axial projection in accentuated lordosis for roentgen studies of the lungs, Acta Radiol. 21:119-125, 1940.

Petsing, H. G.: The evolution of the chest technic, Xray Techn. 11:125-131, 155, 1940.

Westermark, Nils: On tuberculosis of bronchial lymphglands, Acta Radiol. 21:403-412, 1940.

1941 Frangella, Alfonso: La radiografía de tórax a altos voltajes, Rev. Radiol. Fis. 8:119-128, 1941.

Rabin, C. B.: A technique for the more precise localization of pulmonary abscesses, Amer. J. Roentgen. 46:130-131, 1941.

Rabin, C. B.: Precise localization of pulmonary abscess; the "spot" method, J. Thorac. Cardiov. Surg. 10:662-671, 1941.

Rabin, C. B.: Radiology of the chest. In Golden, Ross, editor: Diagnostic roentgenology, ed. 2, New York, 1941, Thomas Nelson & Sons, vol. 1, pp. 65-195.

Saralegui, J. A., and Valotto, Juan: Control radiográfico del torax superior por la proyección antero-posterior ascendente, Arch. Instituto Municipal Radiol. Fisioter. (Buenos Aires), pp. 149-161, 1941.

1942 Adams, Ralph and Davenport, L. F.: La técnica de la bronquial y un sistema de nomenclatura bronquial, Rev. Radiol. Fis. 9:217-224, 1942.

Fariñas, Pedro L.: Mucosography of the respiratory tract, Radiology 39:84-87, 1942.

Scott, W. G., and Lionberger, John: Studies of the pulmonary vessels by means of body-section radiography, Radiology 39:157-165, 1942.

Tager, Stephen: Use of over-penetrated film technic in the diagnosis of cavities, Radiology 39:389-394, 1942.

Young, B. R.: The value of body section roentgenography (planigraphy) for the demonstration of tumors, non-neoplastic diseases and foreign bodies in the neck and chest, Amer. J. Roentgen. 47:83-88, 1942.

1943 Gordon, Joseph, and Taylor, H. K.: The postthoracoplasty roentgenogram with special reference to posture, Radiology 40:42-48, 1943.

Kerley, Peter: Anatomical and pathological factors in chest radiography, Radiography 9:9-16, 1943.

Young, B. R.: Recent advances in roentgen diagnosis of diseases of the chest including body section roentgenography, New York J. Med. 43:140-143, 1943.

1944 James, J. H.: Radiography of the chest, Radiography 10:65-70, 1944.

Lavner, Gerald, and Copelman, B.: The antero-posterior lordotic projection in the roentgenographic examination of the lungs, Radiology 43:135-141, 1944.

Ponthus, P., and Girgis, A.: Sur une modification de la position lordotique de Fleischner pour l'exploration des scissures, J. Radiol. Electr. 26:67, 1944-1945.

1946 Bishop, Paul A.: Lung abscess. In Pillmore, G. U., editor: Clinical radiology, Philadelphia, 1946, F. A. Davis Co., vol. 1, p. 333.

Cole, Lewis G.: Pneumoconiosis. In Pillmore, G. U., editor: Clinical radiology, Philadelphia, 1946, F. A. Davis Co., vol. 1, pp. 263-269.

Flaxman, A. J.: Apical tuberculosis with roentgen technique, Amer. Rev. Tuber. 54:1-8, 1946.

Richman, S.: The lateral decubitus position in x-ray examinations of the chest, J. Mount Sinai Hosp. N. Y. 13:83-85, 1946.

Salkin, David: Pulmonary tuberculosis. In Pillmore, George U., editor: Clinical radiology, Philadelphia, 1946, F. A. Davis Co., vol. 1, pp. 155-161.

1947 Rabin, Coleman B.: Radiology of the chest. In Golden, Ross, editor: Diagnostic roentgenology, ed. 3, New York, 1947, Thomas Nelson & Sons, vol. 1, pp. 61-68.

Rakofsky, Max, and Satinsky, Victor: Roentgenological aspects of battle injuries of the chest, Amer. J. Roentgen. 57:583-600, 1947.

1948 Nemec, Stanley S.: Differential diagnosis of retrocardiac shadows, Radiology 50:174-182, 1948.

1949 Kjellberg, S. R.: Importance of prone position in the roentgenologic diagnosis of slight mitral disease, Acta Radiol. 31:178-181, 1949.

1951 Atwell, Sherman W.: Standardized oblique roentgenography of the chest, Dis. Chest 19:585-588, 1951.

Cohen, A. G., and Geffen, A.: Roentgenographic methods in pulmonary disease, Amer. J. Med. 10:375-385, 1951.

1955 Kinslow, W. E.: A special lordotic position, Xray Techn. 27:108-109, 1955.

1956 Lentino, W., Marchetto, I., and Poppel, M. H.: A modification of the routine lateral view of the chest to permit visualization of the superior mediastinum, Amer. J. Roentgen. 75:767-770, 1956.

Zinn, B., and Monroe, J.: The lordotic position in fluoroscopy and roentgenography of the chest, Amer. J. Roentgen. 75:682-700, 1956.

1957 Abo, Stanley: Roentgenographic detection of minimal pneumothorax in the lateral decubitus position; costophrenic sign, Amer. J. Roentgen. 77:1066-1070, 1957.

1958 Watson, W.: Gridless radiography at high voltage with airgap technique, Xray Focus (Ilford) 2:12, 1958.

1959 Rundle, F. F., de Lambert, R. M., and Epps, R. G.: Cervicothoracic tumors; a technical aid to their roentgenologic localization, Amer. J. Roentgen. 81:316-321, 1959.

1963 Berlin, H. S., Unger, S. M., Corbin, L. J., Jacobson, H. G., and Poppel, M. H.: Wide angle roentgenography, Amer. J. Roentgen. 90:189-197, 1963.

Tuddenham, W. J.: Problems of perception in chest roentgenology; facts and fallacies, Radiol. Clin. N. Amer. 1:277-289, 1963.

1964 Jackson, F. I.: The air-gap technique; and an improvement by anteroposterior positioning for chest roentgenography, Amer. J. Roentgen. 92:688-691, 1964.

1965 Jakimow, I. L., and Sheehan, F. R.: Kyphotic view, Dis. Chest 47:636-640, 1965.

1966 Ekimsky, B.: Comparative study of lateral decubitus views and those with lateral body inclination in small pleural effusions, Vestn. Rentgen. Radiol. 41:43-49, 1966. (In Russian.) Abst.: Radiology 87:1135, 1966.

Kattan, K.: High kilovoltage oblique roentgenography of the chest; its advantage in differential diagnosis in diseases of the lung and pleura, Dis. Chest 50:605-610, 1966.

Sumerling, M. D., and Irvine, W. J.: Pneumomediastinography, Amer. J. Roentgen. 98:451-460, 1966.

1967 Berne, A. S., Ikins, P. M., and Bugden, W. F.: CO_2-O_2 pneumomediastinography with polytomography for the preoperative evaluation of bronchogenic carcinoma, Radiology **88**:519-525, 1967.

1968 Shopfner, C. E., Jansen, C., and O'Kell, R. T.: Roentgen significance of the transverse thoracic muscle, Amer. J. Roentgen. **103**:140-148, 1968.

Simecek, C.: Diagnostic pneumomediastinography, Dis. Chest **53**:24-29, 1968.

1969 Turner, A. F., and Jacobson, G.: The Valsalva maneuver in the diagnosis of left ventricular aneurysm, Radiology **93**:9-12, 1969.

Westfall, R. E.: Obliteration of segmental pulmonary artery borders; a method of localizing right lower lobe infiltrates, Dis. Chest **56**:305-309, 1969.

1970 Bauer, R. G.: High kilovoltage chest radiography with an air gap, Radiol. Techn. **42**:10-14, 1970.

Jacobson, G., Bohlig, H., and Kiviluoto, R.: Essentials of chest radiography (editorial), Radiology **95**:445-450, 1970.

Miller, R. E.: Simple apparatus for decubitus films with horizontal beam, Radiology **97**:682-683, 1970.

Pfister, R. C., Oh, K. S., and Ferrucci, J. T.: Retrosternal density; a radiological evaluation of the retrosternal-premediastinal space, Radiology **96**:317-324, 1970.

Resnick, D.: The angulated basal view; a new method for evaluation of lower lobe pulmonary disease, Radiology **96**:204-205, 1970.

Sargent, E. N., and Turner, A. F.: Emergency treatment of pneumothorax; a simple catheter technique for use in the radiology department, Amer. J. Roentgen. **109**:531-535, 1970.

Zanca, P.: Roentgenographic measurements of diaphragmatic motion-respiratory compliance, Amer. J. Roentgen. **110**:717-724, 1970.

1973 Kattan, K. R., and Wiot, J. F.: How was this roentgenogram taken, A.P. or P.A.? Amer. J. Roentgen. **117**:843-845, 1973.

Sear, H. S., Friedenberg, M. J., and Bean, J.: Improvement of chest roentgenography by respirator-controlled pulmonary inflation, Radiology **106**:503-505, 1973.

HEART AND MEDIASTINUM

1906 Guilleminot: The exploration of the thorax by orthodiagraphy, Arch. Roentgen Ray **10**:212, 1906.

1908 Groedel, Franz: The examination of the heart by x-ray, Arch. Roentgen Ray **12**:93, 1908.

1909 Claytor, A. Thomas, and Merrill, Walter H.: Orthodiagraphy in the study of the heart and great vessels, Amer. J. Med. Sci. **138**:549, 1909.

1912 Groedel, Franz: Die Röntgendiagnostik der Herz und Gefässerkrankungen, Berlin, 1912, H. Meusser.

1913 Groedel, M.: The picture of the thorax in central (sagittal, frontal and oblique) and eccentric projection [Das Thoraxbild bei zentrischer (sagittaler, frontaler, schräger) und exzentrischer Roentgenprojektion], Fortschr. Roentgenstr. **20**:541-554, 1913. Abst.: Amer. J. Roentgen. **1**:181, 1913-1914.

Thomas, George F.: The roentgen diagnosis of lesions in the region of the mediastinum, Amer. J. Roentgen. **1**:132, 1913-1914.

1914 Josué, O., Delhern, L., and Laquerrière, A.: Note sur l'instrumentation et la technique de la téléradiographie du coeur et de l'aorte, J. Radiol. Electr. **1**:305-311, 1914.

1916 Crane, A. W.: Roentgenology of the heart, Amer. J. Roentgen. **3**:513-524, 1916.

1918 Bardeen, C. R.: Determination of the size of the heart by means of the x-ray, Amer. J. Anat. **23**:423, 1918.

Holmes, George W.: The use of the x-ray in the examination of the heart and the aorta, Boston Med. Surg., p. 478, Oct. 10, 1918.

Vaquez, H., and Bordet, E.: Le coeur et l'aorte, Paris, 1918, Baillière.

1920 Delherm, M. M., and Thoyer-Rozat: L'image radiologique de l'aorte; son trajet—ses rapports—son calibre, J. Radiol. Electr. **4**:97-106, 1920.

Eyster, J. A. E., and Meek, Walter J.: Instantaneous radiographs of the human heart at determined points in the cardiac cycle, Amer. J. Roentgen. **7**:471, 1920.

Martin, Charles: Roentgen-ray study of the great vessels, J.A.M.A. **74**:13, 1920.

Vaquez, H., and Bordet, E.: The heart and the aorta, ed. 2 (trans. from French by James Albert Honey and John Macy), New Haven, Conn., 1920, Yale University Press.

1921 Laubry, C., Mallet, L., and Hirschberg, F.: L'examen radiologique du coeur en position transverse gauche, Arch. Mal. Coeur **14**:394-406, 1921.

Martinez, Gonzales: Some recent advances made in France on the technique of the roentgen diagnosis of diseases of the heart and its vascular pedicle, Amer. J. Roentgen. **8**:491, 1921.

1922 Karschner, G. R., and Kennicott, R. H.: A practical method of roentgen examination of the heart, based upon a study of one hundred consecutive normal and abnormal cases, Amer. J. Roentgen. **9**:305, 1922.

1924 Klason, T.: New methods of radiological investigation of the heart, Acta Med. Scand. **7**(supp.):237, 1924.

1925 Ledbetter, Paul V., Holmes, George W., and White, Paul D.: The value of the x-ray in determining the cause of aortic regurgitation, Amer. Heart J. **1**:196-212, 1925.

1926 Gallino, Martin Marianda: Radiología del corazón, Buenos Aires, 1926, Pedro García.

Knappenberger, George E.: The x-ray in cardiac diagnosis, Radiology **7**:297-305, 1926.

1927 Brown, Samuel, and Weiss, H. B.: Lateral views of the heart and aorta, J.A.M.A. **88**:226-229, 1927.

Gerhartz, Heinrich: Technik der röntgenologischen Untersuchung des Thorax mittelschattens des Herzens und der grossen Gefässe. In Handbuch der biologischen Arbeitsmethoden, abt. 54, t. II, p. 1503, 1927.

1928 Groedel, F. M.: Orthodiagraphy (translated from Schittenhelm der Röntgendiagnostik), New York Acad. Med., Oct., 1928.

Stumpf, P.: Die Gestaltänderung des schlagenden Herzens im Röntgenbild, Fortschr. Roentgenstr. **38**:1055-1067, 1928.

1929 de Beaujeu, Jaubert A.: Sur la radiologie des pleurésies médiastins et costo-médiastinales, Arch. Electr. Méd., no. 551, Nov., 1929.

Rigler, L. G.: Visualized esophagus in diagnosis of diseases of heart and aorta, Amer. J. Roentgen. **21**:563-571, 1929.

Vallebona, A.: La registrazione radiografica dei movimenti del cuore, Radiol. Med. **16**:1004-1015, 1929.

1930 Brown, S., and Reinecke, H. G.: Roentgenological study of superior and posterior mediastinum, Amer. J. Surg. **10**:452-468, 1930.

De Abreu, M.: Études radiologiques sur le poumon et de médiastin, Paris, 1930, Masson & Cie.

Klason, T.: On the horizontal orthoprojection of the heart, Acta Radiol. **11**:57-77, 1930.

O'Kane, George, Andrews, Fred D., and Warren, Stafford L.: A standardization roentgenologic study of the heart and great vessels in the left oblique view, Amer. J. Roentgen. **23**:373-383, 1930.

Paterson, R.: Value of roentgenologic study of esophagus and bronchi in cases of heart disease, especially mitral disease, Amer. J. Roentgen. **23**:396-405, 1930.

1931 Heusel, Charles N.: Problems in cardiac roentgenography, Xray Techn. **2**:114-117, 1931.

1932 Fray, Walter W.: Mensuration of the heart and chest in the left posterior-anterior-oblique position; a comparative study, Amer. J. Roentgen. **27**:729, 1932.

Routier, D., and Heim de Balzac, Raymond R.: Découverte radiologique d'un petit anéorisme aortique, Bull. Soc. Radiol. Méd. Paris **20**:125-129, 1932.

1933 Brown, S.: The roentgenological study of the thoracic aorta, Radiology **20**:343-352, 1933.

Sosman, Merrill C., and Wosika, Paul H.: Calcification in aortic and mitral valves, Amer. J. Roentgen. **30**:328-348, 1933.

Sparks, J. V.: The radiology of heart diseases, Brit. J. Radiol. **6**:723-741, 1933.

Strauss, Arthur E.: Roentgenology of the heart, Xray Techn. **4**:105-108, 1933.

1934 Andrus, Paul M.: A new method of the radiographic exploration of the mediastinum and concealed portions of the pulmonary fields, Radiology 23:97-101, 1934.

Dann, David S.: Further observations on the roentgen examination of the aorta, Radiology 23:208, 1934.

Perona, Pietro: Lo stato attuale e gli odierni orientamenti della radiologia cardiaca, Atti Congresso Ital. Radiol. Med. 11:124-129, 1934.

Roesler, H.: Relation of shape of heart to shape of chest, Amer. J. Roentgen. 32:464-486, 1934.

1935 Schwedel, J. B., and Gutman, E. B.: The esophagus in diseases of the heart and aorta, Amer. J. Roentgen. 34:164, 1935.

Van Buskirk, E. M.: Graphical method for obtaining the area of the heart shadow in the roentgen ray study of heart disease, Radiology 24:433, 1935.

1936 Barsóny, T., and Wald, B.: Das Röntgenbild der oberen-hinteren schwachen Stelle des Mediastinum, Röntgenpraxis 8:88-95, 1936.

LeBorgne, F.: Nueva técnica radiológica per cortes o secciones, An. Ateneo Clin. Quir., pp. 13-15, 1936.

1937 Schwedel, J. B.: Use of barium-filled esophagus in x-ray study of abnormalities of the heart and aorta, Amer. Heart J. 13:723-730, 1937.

1938 Epstein, Bernard S.: The visualization of the aorta by the method of roentgenographic over-penetration, Amer. J. Roentgen. 40:398-400, 1938.

Parkinson, J. B. E., and Thompson, W. A. R.: Cardiac aneurysm, Quart. J. Med. 7:455-468, 1938.

1939 Barclay, A. E., Bancroft, Y., Barron, D. H., and Franklin, K. Y.: A radiographic demonstration of the circulation through the heart in the adult and in the foetus, and the identification of the ductus arteriosus, Brit. J. Radiol. 12:505-517, 1939.

Danelius, G.: Cross-sectional radiography of the heart, Radiology 32:190-194, 1939.

1940 Robinson, Walter W.: Directed roentgenography of the heart and lungs, Xray Techn. 12:1-4, 1940.

Roesler, Hugo: Atlas of cardioroentgenology, Springfield, Ill., 1940, Charles C Thomas, Publisher.

1941 Cole, George C.: The conus arteriosus and the pulmonary artery; improved method of visualization, Amer. J. Roentgen. 45:32-40, 1941.

Levene, George, and Lowman, Robert M.: Roentgen localization of myocardial damage resulting from coronary artery disease, Radiology 36:159-170, 1941.

Roesler, Hugo: Clinical roentgenology of the cardiovascular system. In Golden, Ross, editor: Diagnostic roentgenology, ed. 2, New York, 1941, Thomas Nelson & Sons, vol. 1, p. 197.

1944 Kratcha, Sister Mary R.: Fundamental technical considerations in cardioroentgenology, Xray Techn. 16:1-7, 66-75, 1944.

1946 Echternacht, Arthur P.: Diseases of the mediastinum. In Pillmore, George U., editor: Clinical radiology, Philadelphia, 1946, F. A. Davis Co., vol. 1, pp. 410-412.

Sussman, Marcy L.: Cardiac roentgenography and anatomy. In Pillmore, George U., editor: Clinical radiology, Philadelphia, 1946, F. A. Davis Co., vol. 1, pp. 3-28.

1947 Roesler, Hugo: Clinical roentgenology of the cardiovascular system. In Golden, Ross, editor: Diagnostic roentgenology, ed. 3, New York, 1947, Thomas Nelson & Sons, vol. 1, pp. 197-264.

1949 Kjellberg, S. R.: Importance of prone position in the roentgenologic diagnosis of slight mitral disease, Acta Radiol. 31:178-181, 1949.

1950 Habbe, J. E., and Wright, H. H.: Roentgenographic detection of coronary arteriosclerosis, Amer. J. Roentgen. 63:50-62, 1950.

1954 Gianturco, Cesare: Intrathoracic pressure and position of the patient in the roentgen examination of the mediastinum, Amer. J. Roentgen. 71:870-872, 1954.

1956 Lentino, W., Marchetto, I., and Poppel, M. H.: A modification of the routine lateral view of the chest to permit visualization of the superior mediastinum, Amer. J. Roentgen. 75:767-770, 1956.

BRONCHOGRAPHY

1918 Jackson, C.: The bronchial tree; its study by insufflation of opaque substances in the living, Amer. J. Roentgen. 5:454-455, 1918.

1922 Sicard, J. A., and Forestier, J.: Méthode générale d'exploration radiographique par l'huile iodée, Bull. Mém. 46:463-499, 1922.

1923 Forestier, J., and Leroux, L.: Étude expérimentale radiologique des injections intratrachéales par l'huile iodée, Bull. Mém. 47:299-304, 1923.

1928 Chandler, F. G., and Wood, W. B.: Lipiodol in the diagnosis of thoracic diseases, New York, 1928, Oxford University Press.

1934 Farinas, P. L.: Serial bronchography in the early diagnosis of bronchial carcinoma, Amer. J. Roentgen. 32:747, 1934.

Sante, L. R.: Practical observations on the use of iodized oil in bronchography, Amer. J. Roentgen. 32:32, 763-768, 1934.

1937 Jackson, C. L., and Bonnier, M.: Technique of bronchography, Ann. Otol. 46:771-785, 1937.

1938 Unfug, George: Bronchography, Xray Techn. 9:171-173, 1938.

1939 Wright, Ila: The x-ray technician's part in an examination of the lungs by means of iodized oils, Xray Techn. 11:55-56, 1939.

1942 Adams, Ralph, and Davenport, L. F.: The technic of bronchography and a system of bronchial nomenclature, J.A.M.A. 118:111-116, 1942.

1946 Pappe, J. K.: A simple and practical method of obtaining complete bronchograms, Amer. Rev. Tuber. 54:104-110, 1946.

1947 Okell, E.: Bronchography, Radiography 13:62-65, 1947.

Wisehart, D. E. S.: Bronchography in bronchiectasis in children, Ann. Otol. 56:404-415, 1947.

1948 Blaisdell, I. H.: Bronchography, Laryngoscope 58:288-303, 1948.

Farinas, P. L.: Bronchography by atomization, Radiology 51:491-494, 1948.

Schmidt, H. W.: A method of obtaining good bilateral bronchograms, Proc. Staff Meet. Mayo Clin. 23:71-77, 1948.

1949 Janes, R. G.: A technic for bronchography, Med. Radiogr. Photogr. 25:94-99, 1949.

1951 Nordenstrom, B. E. W., and Norlin, U. A. T.: Bronchography with Metras catheters, Acta Radiol. 35:246-249, 1951.

1952 Meadows, J. A., Jr.: Relatively simple method of bronchography for the radiologist, Southern Med. J. 45:415-420, 1952.

Miller, J. B., and others: New bronchographic technique employing aerosol anesthesia; further experiences in children and adults, Amer. J. Roentgen. 68:229-239, 1952.

1953 Abrams, H. L., and others: The use of delayed films in bronchography, Radiology 61:317-326, 1953.

1954 Crellin, J. A., and others: Bronchographic studies in bronchiectasis before and after pulmonary resection, Amer. Rev. Tuber. 69:657-672, 1954.

Diehl, K. L.: Bronchography; study of its techinques and presentation of improved modification, Arch. Otolaryng. 60:277-290, 1954.

1956 Niknejad, I., Aurelius, J. R., Peterson, D. H., and Rigler, L. G.: The current status of bronchography with water soluble media, Amer. J. Roentgen. 75:701-719, 1956.

Thacker, E. W.: Postural drainage, London, 1956, Lloyd-Luke Co.

1957 Holden, W. S.: The behaviour of contrast medium in the bronchial tree, Brit. J. Radiol. 30:530-536, 1957.

Holden, W. S., and Ardran, G. M.: Observations on the movements of the trachea and the main bronchi in man, J. Fac. Radiologists 8:267-275, 1957.

1958 Beck, R. E., and Hobbs, A. A., Jr.: A technique for bronchography, Amer. J. Roentgen. 79:269-271, 1958.

Rayl, J. E., and Smith, D. E.: Recent advances in bronchography, Dis. Chest 33:235-250, 1958.

1959 Boyan, C. P., and Howland, W. S.: Percutaneous topical

analgesia of larynx and trachea, J.A.M.A. **171**:1822-1825, 1959.

Reams, G. B., and Bosniak, M. A.: Bronchography through puncture of the cricothyroid membrane, J. Thorac. Cardiov. Surg. **40**:117-124, 1959.

Willson, J. K. V.: Cricothyroid bronchography with a polyethylene catheter, Amer. J. Roentgen. **81**:305-311, 1959.

1961 Hemley, S. D., and others: Percutaneous cricothyroid membrane bronchography, Radiology **76**:763-769, 1961.

1962 Waring, W. W., and Killelea, D. E.: Bronchography in infants and children, Pediatrics **30**:378-388, 1962.

1964 Hemley, S. D., and Kanick, V.: Some observations on transcricothyroid bronchography, Amer. J. Roentgen. **92**:578-583, 1964.

Nelson, S. W., Christoforidis, A. J., and Pratt, P. C.: Further experience with barium sulfate as bronchographic contrast medium, Amer. J. Roentgen. **92**:595-614, 1964.

1965 Rossi, P., and others: Transtracheal selective bronchography, Radiology **85**:829-833, 1965.

1966 Cope, C.: Selective bronchial catheterization by a new percutaneous transtracheal technique, Amer. J. Roentgen. **96**:932-935, 1966.

Miller, R. E., Benages, A. G., and McCrea, F. R.: Simplified technic of bronchography, Med. Radiogr. Photogr. **42**:130-144, 1966.

Ryan, Des: Tomobronchography; a study in comparative sectional roentgenology, Australas. Radiol. **10**:347-355, 1966.

1967 Christoforidis, A. J., Nelson, S. W., and Pratt, P. C.: An experimental study of the tissue reaction to the vehicles commonly used in bronchography, Amer. Rev. Resp. Dis. **96**:249-253, 1967.

Grollman, J. H.: A thin-wall double catheter system for transtracheal bronchography, Amer. J. Roentgen. **99**:686-687, 1967.

Lodin, H.: Tomography of the middle and lingular bronchi, Acta Radiol. [Diagn.] **6**:26-32, 1967.

1968 Fennessy, J. J.: Bronchial brushings and transbronchial forceps biopsy in the diagnosis of pulmonary lesions, Dis. Chest **53**:377-389, 1968.

Rinker, C. T., Garrotto, L. J., Lee, K. R., and Templeton, A. W.: Bronchography: diagnostic signs and accuracy in pulmonary carcinoma, Amer. J. Roentgen. **104**:802-807, 1968.

Rybadova, N. I., and Kuznetsov, S. A.: Concerning the method of tomographic examination of the bronchial tree, Vestn. Rentgen. Radiol. **43**:36-43, 1968. (In Russian.) Abst.: Radiology **91**:1249, 1968.

Sargent, E. N., and Turner, A. F.: Percutaneous transcricothyroid membrane selective bronchography; a simple, safe technique for selective catheterization and visualization of segmental and subsegmental bronchi, Amer. J. Roentgen. **104**:792-801, 1968.

1969 Sargent, E. N., and Turner, A. F.: Catheter tip deflector system for selective bronchography, Radiology **93**:936-939, 1969.

1970 Amplatz, K., and Haut, G.: Lateral decubitus bronchography with a single bolus, Radiology **95**:439-440, 1970.

Avery, M. E.: Bronchography: outmoded procedure? Pediatrics **46**:333-334, 1970. Abst.: Radiology **99**:715, 1971.

Beamish, W. E.: Radiologic diagnosis of pulmonary embolism including the application of full-chest tomography, J. Canad. Ass. Radiol. **21**:217-225, 1970.

Dilley, R. B., and Nadel, J. A.: Powdered tantalum: its use as a roentgenographic contrast material, Ann. Otol. **79**:945-952, 1970.

Fennessy, J. J.: Selective catheterization of segmental bronchi with the aid of a flexible fiberoptic bronchoscope, Radiology **95**:689-691, 1970.

Hinchcliffe, W. A., Zamel, N., Fishman, N. H., and others: Roentgenographic study of the human trachea with powdered tantalum, Radiology **97**:327-330, 1970.

Wesolowski, W. E.: A new approach to bronchography: the pleasant ordeal, Radiol. Techn. **41**:291-294, 1970.

1971 Grech, P., and Higginbottom, E.: Inhalation bronchography, Radiography **37**:166-172, 1971.

Willson, J. K., Eskridge, M., and Scott, E. L.: Transbronchial biopsy of benign and malignant peripheral lung lesions, Radiology **100**:541-546, 1971.

1972 Gamsu, G., and Nadel, J. A.: New technique for roentgenographic study of airways and lungs using powdered tantalum, Cancer **30**:1353-1357, 1972.

KYMOGRAPHY

1931 Stumpf, P.: Das röntgenographische Bewegungsbild und seine Anwendung, Fortschr. Roentgenstr. **41**:1-78, 1931.

1932 Delherm, P.: La kymographie, Presse Méd. **40**:515-517, 1932.

1934 Bengt, I.: Roentgenkymography ad modum Stumpf as a method of examining the heart, Acta Radiol. **15**:107-123, 1934.

Hirsch, I. Seth: The recording of cardiac movements and sounds by the roentgen ray, Radiology **22**:403, 720, 1934.

1935 Richter, Hans: Atemtechnik und Zerchfellbewegung im röntgenographischen Bewegungsbild, Fortschr. Roentgenstr. **51**:357-369, 1935.

1936 Scott, W. G., and Moore, Sherwood: Roentgen kymography; its clinical and physiological value in the study of heart diseases, Ann. Int. Med. **10**:306-329, 1936.

Stumpf, P., Weber, H. H., and Weltz, G. A.: Röntgen-kymographische Bewegungslehre innerer Organe, Leipzig, 1936, Georg Thieme.

1937 Scott, Wendell G., and Moore, Sherwood: Roentgen kymography of the respiratory movements of the thorax, diaphragm, lungs, bronchi and mediastinal structures, Amer. J. Roentgen. **37**:721-732, 1937.

Stumpf, Pleikart: Zehn Vorlesungen über Kymographie, Leipzig, 1937, Georg Thieme.

1938 Scott, Wendell G., and Moore, Sherwood: Roentgen kymographic studies of aneurysms and mediastinal tumors, Amer. J. Roentgen. **40**:165-171, 1938.

Stumpf, P.: Roentgen kymography as a diagnostic aid, Radiology **31**:391-397, 1938.

1939 Schmidt, Sister Marie G.: Technic of kymographic examination, Xray Techn. **10**:253-255, 1939.

1940 Schwarzschild, Myron M.: Technical factors in kymography, Xray Techn. **11**:182-184, 205, 1940.

1960 Schmidt, S.: Respiratory kymography in acute abdominal conditions, Acta Radiol. **54**:49-68, 1960.

1963 Respiratory kymography in acute pulmonary disease, Acta Radiol. [Diagn.] **1**:1032-1044, 1963.

1966 Schmidt, S.: Further studies on respiratory kymography in acute abdominal conditions, Radiology **86**:15-26, 1966.

1969 Schmidt, S.: Anatomic and physiologic aspects of respiratory kymography, Acta Radiol. [Diagn.] **8**:409-422, 1969.

ABDOMEN

1900 Williams, Francis H.: X-ray examinations of the abdomen, Boston Med. Surg. J. **23**:1900.

1922 Mallet, Lucien, and Coliez, Robert: Diagnostic radiologique des tumeurs de l'hypocondre gauche, J. Radiol. Electr. **6**:57-67, 1922.

1927 Laurell, Hugo: Acute abdominal cases chiefly from the roentgenological point of view, Acta Chir. Scand. **66**:105-132, 1930. Also Acta Radiol. **8**:109-119, 1927.

1931 Magnusson, W.: On meteorism in pyelography and on the passage of gas through the small intestine, Acta Radiol. **12**:552-561, 1931.

1932 Finsterbusch, R., and Gross, F.: Spontanes Pneumoperitoneum bei Ileus, Röntgenpraxis **4**:585-590, 1932.

Swenson, Paul C., and Hibbard, J. S.: Roentgenographic manifestations of intestinal obstruction, Arch. Surg. **25**:578-600, 1932.

1933 Estiú, Manuel: Nueva posición para el estudio clínico y radiológico del abdomen, Buenos Aires Theses, no. 4721, 1933.

Saito, M.: La radiographie des parois de l'estomac, "pneumo-gastro-pariétographie," Bull. Soc. Chir. Paris **59**:910-912, 1933.

1935 Sante, L. R.: Intestinal obstruction, Amer. J. Roentgen. **34**:744-754, 1935.

1936 Scheibel, Otto: Concerning pitressin in roentgen examination of the abdomen as an agent for reducing shadows caused by intestinal gas, Acta Radiol. **17**:511, 1936.

Stecher, William R.: Roentgenologic aid in the acute abdomen with special reference to intestinal obstruction, Radiology **26**:729-740, 1936.

1937 Hampton, A. O.: A safe method for the roentgen demonstration of bleeding duodenal ulcers, Amer. J. Roentgen. **38**:565-570, 1937.

Kelly, James F., and Dowell, D. H.: The value of the preliminary film without opaque media in the diagnosis of abdominal conditions, Radiology **29**:104-110, 1937.

1938 Golden, Ross: The abdomen. In Golden, Ross, editor: Diagnostic roentgenology, New York, 1938, Thomas Nelson & Sons, pp. 913-935.

1940 Anger, Sister Mary A.: Procedure for various abdominal roentgenographic examinations, Xray Techn. **11**:219-221, 249, 1940.

1941 Rigler, L. G.: Spontaneous pneumoperitoneum, a roentgenologic sign found in the supine position, Radiology **37**:604-607, 1941.

1944 LaFond, John V.: Scout radiographs of acute conditions of the abdomen, Xray Techn. **15**:229, 260, 1944.

1946 Levitin, Joseph: Scout film of the abdomen, Radiology **47**:10-29, 1946.

1947 Baldridge, R. T.: Radiography of the abdomen in suspected ruptured peptic ulcer, Xray Techn. **18**:226-227, 1947.

Golden, Ross: The abdomen. In Golden, Ross, editor: Diagnostic roentgenology, ed. 3, New York, 1947, Thomas Nelson & Sons, vol. 2, pp. 913-935.

Spencer, Jack, and Thaxter, Langdon T.: Acute obstruction of the small bowel, Radiology **49**:611-619, 1947.

1948 Slater, M.: Penetrating wounds of the abdomen, Amer. J. Roentgen. **59**:168-176, 1948.

1951 Frimann-Dahl, J.: Roentgen examination in acute abdominal diseases, Springfield, Ill., 1951, Charles C Thomas, Publisher.

1956 King, J. C.: Trauma to the abdominal and retroperitoneal viscera as it concerns the radiologist, Southern Med. J. **49**:109-119, 1956.

1957 Curry, R. W.: Value of the left lateral decubitus position in the roentgenologic diagnosis of acute abdominal disease, Surg. Gynec. Obstet. **104**:627-632, 1957.

1958 Schultz, E. H., Jr.: An aid to the diagnosis of pneumoperitoneum from supine abdominal films, Radiology **70**:728-731, 1958.

Welsh, H. D., and Fleming, E. G.: Radiographic visualization of subdiaphragmatic air, Med. Radiogr. Photogr. **34**:78-79, 1958.

1960 Samuel, Eric.: The use of contrast media in the investigation of the acute abdomen, Brit. J. Radiol. **33**:82-91, 1960.

1963 Samuel, E., and others: Radiology of the post-operative abdomen, Clin. Radiol. **14**:133-148, 1963.

1965 Buschmann, O., and Kerk, L.: Roentgen diagnosis of renal trauma, Fortschr. Roentgenstr. **103**:683-689, 1965. Abst.: Radiology **87**:192, 1966.

1966 Cornell, W. P., and Ebert, P. A.: Penetrating wounds of the abdominal wall; a new diagnostic technique, Amer. J. Roentgen. **96**:414-417, 1966.

1967 Schorr, S., and Danon, J.: Rupture of the spleen, a new roentgen sign, Amer. J. Roentgen. **99**:616-624, 1967.

1970 Berk, R. N.: Changing concepts in the plain film diagnosis of ruptured spleen, J. Canad. Ass. Radiol. **21**:67-70, 1970.

Bowerman, J. W., and Smithwick, W.: Contrast examination of abdominal stab wounds, Radiology **97**:619-624, 1970.

1971 Lepasoon, J., and Olin, T.: Angiographic diagnosis of splenic lesions following blunt abdominal injury, Acta Radiol. [Diagn.] **11**:257-273, 1971.

Miller, R. E., and Nelson, S. W.: The roentgenologic demonstration of tiny amounts of free intraperitoneal gas: experimental and clinical studies, Amer. J. Roentgen. **112**:574-585, 1971.

1973 Gelfand, D. W.: Positive contrast peritoneography: the abnormal abdomen, Amer. J. Roentgen. **119**:190-197, 1973.

Leigh, P. G. A.: Ruptured spleen: a radiological pitfall and a suggested modification, Brit. J. Radiol. **60**:289-291, 1973.

Miller, R. E.: The technical approach to the acute abdomen, Seminars Roentgen. **8**:267-279, 1973.

Nahum, H., and Levesque, M.: Arteriography in hepatic trauma, Radiology **109**:557-563, 1973.

PERITONEAL PNEUMOGRAPHY

1913 Weber, E.: Ueber die Bedeutung der Einführung von Sauerstoff resp. Luft in die Bauchhöhle für die experimentelle und diagnostische Röntgenologie, Fortschr. Roentgenstr. **20**:453-455, 1913.

1918 Goetze, O.: Die Röntgendiagnostik bei gasgefüllter Bauchhöhle; eine neue Methode, München. Med. Wschr. **65**:1275-1280, 1918.

1919 Stewart, Wm. H., and Stein, A.: Roentgen ray study of the abdominal organs following oxygen inflation of the peritoneal cavity, Amer. J. Roentgen. **6**:533-541, 1919.

1920 Mallet, L., and Band, H.: Le pneumo-péritoine artificiel en radiodiagnostic, J. Radiol. Electr. **4**:23-33, 1920.

1921 Alvarez, W. C.: The use of CO_2 in pneumoperitoneum, Amer. J. Roentgen. **8**:71-72, 1921.

Mallet, Lucien: Le pneumoperitoine en radiodiagnostic, J. Radiol. Electr. **5**:401-409, 1921.

Peterson, R.: The x-ray after the inflation of the pelvic cavity with carbon dioxide gas as an aid to obstetric and gynecologic diagnosis, Surg. Gynec. Obstet. **33**:154-157, 1921.

Sante, L. R.: The detection of retroperitoneal masses by the aid of pneumoperitoneum, Amer. J. Roentgen. **8**:129-134, 1921.

Stein, Arthur, and Stewart, Wm. H.: Pneumoperitoneal roentgen-ray diagnosis, Troy, N. Y., 1921, Southworth Co.

1926 Stein, I. F.: Roentgenographic diagnosis in gynecology; pneumoperitoneum, Surg. Gynec. Obstet. **42**:83-87, 1926.

Stein, I. F., and Arens, R. A.: Iodized oil and pneumoperitoneum combined in gynecologic diagnosis; preliminary report, J.A.M.A. **87**:1299, 1926.

1937 Stein, I. F.: Why pneumoperitoneum? Radiology **28**:391-398, 1937.

1942 Stein, I. F.: Gynecographic aid in diagnosis of ectopic pregnancy, Amer. J. Obstet. Gynec. **43**:400-409, 1942.

1951 Maxfield, J. R., Jr.: Pneumoperitoneum in the study of pelvic structures, J.A.M.A. **146**:920-923, 1951.

1952 Gershon-Cohen, J., and Hermel, M. B.: Pelvic pneumoperitoneum; x-ray appearance of normal female pelvic organs, Amer. J. Obstet. Gynec. **64**:184-187, 1952.

Leucutia, Traian: Pneumoperitoneum and pneumoretroperitoneum (editorial), Amer. J. Roentgen. **68**:655-658, 1952.

1953 Kunstadter, R. H., Guterman, H. S., and Tulsky, A. S.: Transabdominal pneumoperitoneum as an aid in the diagnosis of sex-endocrine disturbances, Amer. J. Dis. Child. **86**:275-283, 1953.

1955 Abrams, B. S., and Hughes, A.: Pneumocography as an aid in the diagnosis of gynecologic disease, Amer. J. Obstet. Gynec. **70**:1115-1125, 1955.

Bétoutières, P., Pélissier, M., Beltrando, L., Paleirac, R., and Candon, J.: Stratigraphie et agrandissement en pneumographie pelvienne chez la femme, J. Radiol. Electr. **36**:94-98, 1955.

Strauss, H. A., and Cohen, M. R.: Gynecography simplified, Amer. J. Obstet. Gynec. **70**:572-581, 1955.

1957 Buice, J. W., and Gould, D. M.: Abdominal and pelvic pneumography, Radiology **69**:704-709, 1957.

Lumsden, K., and Truelove, S. C.: Diagnostic pneumoperitoneum, Brit. J. Radiol. **30**:516-523, 1957.

1958 Gould, D. M., and others: The gynogram, Clin. Obstet. Gynec. **1**:618-628, 1958.
1960 Aparico, C., and King, V.: Pelvic pneumography, Xray Techn. **32**:252-254, 1960.
  Henzl, M., Horský, J., Presl, J., and Valenta, M.: Pneumopelvigraphy of developmental malformations of female internal genitalia, Acta Radiol. **53**:202-208, 1960.
1961 Schulz, E., and Rosen, S. W.: Gynecography; technique and interpretation, Amer. J. Roentgen. **86**:866-878, 1961.
  Šilinková-Málková, E.: Pneumopelvigraphy in diagnosis of gonadal lesions in women, Radiol. Diagn. **2**:59-72, 1961.
1962 Hoffman, M. L.: The importance of pneumoperitoneum, Xray Techn. **33**:381-386, 1962.
1964 Stevens, G. M., and McCort, J. J.: Abdominal pneumoperitoneum, Radiology **83**:480-485, 1964.
1966 Asch, T.: The case for pneumoperitoneum in the diagnosis of inflammatory disease about the diaphragm, Radiology **86**:60-65, 1966.
  Semin, R. N., and others: Combined pneumopelvigraphy and hysterosalpingography in benign gynecological conditions, Radiology **86**:677-681, 1966.
  Stevens, G. M., Weigen, J. F., and Lee, R. S.: Pelvic pneumography, Med. Radiogr. Photogr. **42**:82-127, 1966.
1967 Kendall, B.: Pelvic pneumography, Radiography **33**:3-10, 1967.
  Rådberg, C., and Wickbom, I.: Pelvic angiography and pneumoperitoneum in the diagnosis of gynecologic lesions, Acta Radiol. [Diagn.] **6**:133-144, 1967.
  Richter, K., Mach, S., and Lisewski, G.: Die Pneumopelvigraphie in der gynäkologischen Diagnostik, Fortschr. Roentgenstr. **106**:541-548, 1967.
1968 Lunderquist, A.: Pneumopelvigraphy in the early diagnosis of intersexuality, Amer. J. Roentgen. **103**:202-209, 1968.
1969 Stevens, G. M.: Pelvic pneumography, Seminars Roentgen. **4**:252-266, 1969.
1970 Ghazi, M., Seibel, R. E., and Courey, N. G.: Pelvic pneumography; diagnostic aid in gynecology, Obstet. Gynec. **36**:827-834, 1970.
  Stern, W. Z., and Wilson, L.: Pelvic pneumography with simultaneous hysterosalpingography, Radiology **96**:87-92, 1970.
1973 Meyers, M. A.: Peritoneography; normal and pathologic anatomy, Amer. J. Roentgen. **117**:353-365, 1973.

RETROPERITONEAL PNEUMOGRAPHY

1921 Carelli, H. H., and Sordelli, U.: Un nuevo procedimiento para explorar el riñón, Rev. Asoc. Med. Argent. **34**:424, 1921.
1923 Quinby, W. C.: Perirenal insufflation of oxygen, J. Urol. **9**:13-20, 1923.
1935 Cahill, G. F.: Air injections to demonstrate the adrenals by x-ray, J. Urol. **34**:238-243, 1935.
1941 Menchner, W. H.: Perirenal insufflation, J.A.M.A. **109**:1338-1341, 1941.
1947 Barquin, F. J.: A new technique of perirenal air insufflation, J. Urol. **57**:1-14, 1947.
1948 Ruiz Rivas, M.: Diagnóstico radiológico; el neumorriñón; técnica original, Arch. Esp. Urol. **4**:228-233, 1948.
1950 Alvarez, R., and Mosca, L. G.: El enfisema retroperitoneal, diagnóstico del aneurisma de aorta abdominal y del quiste seroso del riñón, Prensa Med. Argent. **37**:779-781, 1950.
  Ruiz Rivas, M.: Generalized subserous emphysema through a single puncture, Amer. J. Roentgen. **64**:723-734, 1950.
1952 Gershon-Cohen, J., and others: Retroperitoneal pneumography by injection of oxygen into the presacral space, Amer. J. Roentgen. **68**:391-394, 1952.
  Leucutia, Traian: Pneumoperitoneum and pneumoretroperitoneum (editorial), Amer. J. Roentgen. **68**:655-658, 1952.
  Mosca, L. G.: Diagnostic retroperitoneal emphysema, Med. Radiogr. Photogr. **28**:53-61, 1952.

Steinbach, H. L., and others: Extraperitoneal pneumography, Radiology **59**:167-176, 1952.
1953 Lerman, F., and others: Presacral oxygen insufflation, J. Urol. **70**:312-317, 1953.
1954 Joelson, J. J., and others: The radiologic diagnosis of tumors of the adrenal glands, Radiology **62**:488-495, 1954.
1961 Jones, H. E.: The radiology of the adrenal glands, Radiography **27**:68-73, 1961.
1965 McLelland, R., and others: Retroperitoneal pneumography; a safe method using carbon dioxide, Radiol. Clin. N. Amer. **3**:113-128, 1965.
  Robertson, L. H., and others: Retroperitoneal contrast studies; simplified bilateral perirenal carbon dioxide insufflation, J. Urol. **93**:414-416, 1965.
  Schnur, B. M., and Sakson, J. A.: Trans-sacral retroperitoneal pneumography, J. Urol. **94**:701-705, 1965.
1966 Anderson, E. E., and Glenn, J. F.: Translumbar retroperitoneal carbon dioxide insufflation, Amer. J. Roentgen. **98**:212-214, 1966.
1969 Anderson, E. E., and Glenn, J. F.: Carbon dioxide contrast studies in retroperitoneal masses, J. Urol. **101**:530-532, 1969.

SINUS TRACTS AND FISTULAS

1908 Beck, Emil G.: A new method of exploring the boundaries of fistulous tracts and abscess cavities, Arch. Roentgen Ray **13**:11-13, 1908-1909.
1943 Gage, H. C., and Williams, E. R.: The radiological exploration of sinus tracts, fistulae, and infected cavities, Radiology **41**:233-248, 1943. Also Brit. J. Radiol. **16**:8-22, 1943.
1945 Reany, A.: The radiographic demonstration and verification of external abdominal fistulae, Radiography **11**:11-13, 1945.
1947 Pendergrass, R. C., and Ward, W. C.: Roentgenographic demonstration of sinuses and fistulae, Amer. J. Roentgen. **57**:571-577, 1947.
1949 Dell, James M., Jr.: Demonstration of sinus tracts, fistulas, and infected cavities by Lipiodol, Amer. J. Roentgen. **61**:223-231, 1949.
1962 Brekkan, A.: Fistulography with vacuum suction, Acta Radiol. **57**:77-80, 1962.
1965 Stern, W.: New method for demonstrating fistulas of soft tissues, J. Int. Coll. Surg. **44**:688-673, 1965.
1966 Cornell, W. P., and Ebert, P. A.: Penetrating wounds of the abdominal wall: new diagnostic technique, Amer. J. Roentgen. **96**:414-417, 1966.
1969 Miller, W. T., and Sullivan, M. A.: Roentgenologic demonstration of sinus tracts and fistulae, Amer. J. Roentgen. **107**:812-817, 1969.

UPPER ABDOMINAL ORGANS
(DIAPHRAGM, LIVER, SPLEEN, PANCREAS)

1908 Dally-Hals: A contribution to the study of the diaphragm, Arch. Roentgen Ray **13**:21, 1908.
  Lange, Sidney: The relations of the diaphragm as revealed by the roentgen ray, J.A.M.A. **50**:673-676, 1908.
1909 Béclère, H.: Notes sur l'exploration radiologique du foie, Bull. Soc. Radiol. Méd., May, 1909.
1914 Desternes and Baudon: L'exploration radiologique du foie, J. Radiol. Electr. **1**:382-392, 1914-1915.
  Ledoux-Lebard, R.: Quelques exemples de l'utilité de l'examen radiologique du bord inférieur du foie, J. Radiol. Electr. **1**:378-381, 1914-1915.
1920 Ledoux-Lebard, R.: Some examples of the importance of the radiological examination of the inferior surface of the liver, Arch. Radiol. Electr. **24**:163, 1920.
1926 Pfahler, George E.: The measurement of the liver by means of roentgen rays, Amer. J. Roentgen. **16**:558, 1926.
1929 Radt, Paul: Eine Methode zur röntgenologischen Kontrastdarstellung vom Milz und Leber, Klin. Wschr. **8**:2128, 1929.
1930 McNamee, E. P.: Subphrenic abscess, Amer. J. Roentgen. **24**:125-139, 1930.

1931 Brown, Samuel: Roentgenological study of diaphragm, J.A.M.A. **97**:678-681, 1931.

Kadrnka, Silvije: L'hépatosplénographie, J. Radiol. Electr. **15**:291-296, 1931.

1934 Benassi, Enrico: La tecnica radiologica per l'epato-splenografia, Atti Congresso Ital. Radiol. Med., **11**:75, 1934.

Engel, A., and Lisholm, E.: A new roentgenological method of pancreas examination, Acta Radiol. **15**:636-639, 1934.

1938 Kuhlman, Fritz: Die Röntgenuntersuchung des Pankreas, Fortschr. Roentgenstr. **57**:629, 1938.

1943 Borak, J.: Roentgen examination of pancreatic tumors, Radiology **41**:171-180, 1943.

1945 Vickers, Anthony A.: Radiographic investigation of diaphragmatic movements, Brit. J. Radiol. **18**:229-230, 1945.

1946 Poppel, M. H.: Lesions of the pancreas, liver and spleen. In Pillmore, George U., editor: Clinical radiology, Philadelphia, 1946, F. A. Davis Co., vol. 1, pp. 660-697.

1951 Child, C. G., O'Sullivan, W. D., Payne, M. A., and McClure, R. D.: Portal venography, Radiology **57**:691-701, 1951.

Moore, G. E., and Bridenbaugh, R. B.: Roentgen demonstration of the venous circulation in the liver; portal venography, Radiology **57**:685-690, 1951.

1953 Rousselot, L. M., Ruzicka, F. F., and Doehner, G. A.: Portal venography via the portal and percutaneous splenic routes, Surgery **34**:557-569, 1953.

1955 Evans, J. A., and O'Sullivan, W. D.: Percutaneous splenoportal venography, Med. Radiogr. Photogr. **31**:98-107, 1955.

1957 Barton, H. L., and Bennett, H. D.: Hepatography, Amer. J. Roentgen. **78**:710-718, 1957.

1965 Evans, J. A.: Techniques in the detection and diagnosis of malignant lesions of the liver, spleen and pancreas, Radiol. Clin. N. Amer. **3**:567-582, 1965.

Rosch, J.: Roentgenologic possibilities in spleen diagnosis, Amer. J. Roentgen. **94**:453-461, 1965.

1966 Beranbaum, S. L.: Carcinoma of the pancreas; a bi-directional roentgen approach, Amer. J. Roentgen. **96**:447-467, 1966.

1967 Clemett, A. R.: Examination of the pancreas. In Margulis, A. R., and Burhenne, H. J., editors: Alimentary tract roentgenology, St. Louis, 1967, The C. V. Mosby Co.

1973 Ferrucci, J. T., and Eaton, S. B.: Radiology of the pancreas, New Eng. J. Med. **228**:506-510, 1973.

BILIARY TRACT (CHOLEGRAPHY BY ORAL AND INTRAVENOUS METHODS)

1900 Beck, Carl: On the detection of calculi in the liver and gall bladder, Radiographie, no. 38, March, 1900. Abst.: Fortschr. Roentgenstr. **3**:109, 1900; and N. Y. Med. J. **3**:217, 1901.

1909 Beck, Carl: Die Röntgenuntersuchung der Leber und der Gallenblase, München, 1909, J. F. Lehmann.

Béclère, H.: Technique nouvelle de la radiographie des calculs biliares avec présentation de radiograms, Bull. Soc. Méd., May, 1909.

1914 Pfahler, George E.: An improvement in the technique of gall bladder diagnosis, Amer. J. Roentgen. **2**:774-775, 1914-1915.

Pfahler, G. E.: Roentgen rays in diagnosis of gallstones and cholecystitis, J.A.M.A. **62**:1304, 1914.

Stewart, W. H.: Roentgen examination of the gall bladder, Arch, Diagn. **7**:340, 1914.

1915 Cole, Lewis G., and George, A. W.: Roentgen diagnosis of gallstones by improved methods, Boston Med. Surg. J. **172**:326, 1915.

Pfahler, George E.: On improvement in technic of gall bladder diagnosis, Amer. J. Roentgen. **2**:774, 1915.

1919 Aimard: Quelques points de la technique dans le radio-diagnostic de la lithiase biliaire, Bull. Soc. Franc. Électr. Radiol. 1919.

1920 Knox, Robert: The examination of the liver, gall bladder and bile ducts, Arch. Radiol. Electr. **14**:37-54, 119-132, 156-169, 1920.

McLeod, N.: Radiography of the gall bladder, Arch. Radiol. Electr. **15**:141-181, 1920-1921.

1921 Immelman, Max: Die Röntgenuntersuchung des Leber und Gallenblase, Röntgenhilfe, no. 9, 1921.

Knox, Robert: Radiography in the examination of the liver, gall bladder and bile ducts, St. Louis, 1921, The C. V. Mosby Co.

1922 George, Ariel W., and Leonard, Ralph D.: The patho-logical gall bladder. In Annals of roentgenology, New York, 1922, Paul B. Hoeber, Inc., vol. 2.

1923 Thompson-Walker, J., and Knox, Robert: Observations on the lateral position and other methods of exami-nation of the renal and gall bladder areas, Amer. J. Roentgen. **10**:681-696, 1923.

1924 Graham, E. A., Cole, Warren H., and Copher, G. H.: Roentgenological visualization of the gall bladder by the intravenous injection of tetrabromphenolphtha-lein, Ann. Surg. **80**:473-477, 1924.

Haenisch, F.: Die Röntgenuntersuchung der Leber, der Gallenblase und der Gallensteine, Leipzig, 1924, Johann Ambrosius Barth.

Knox, Robert: Radiography of the gall bladder, Acta Radiol. **3**:265-296, 1924.

Marinot, Jean: La radiographie de la vésicule biliare en position debout, Théses de la Faculté de Médecine de Paris, no. 229, Paris, 1924, Louis Arnette.

1925 Anderson, C. C.: The x-ray examination of the gall bladder, New Zeal. Med. J. **14**:201-209, 1925.

Carman, Russel D.: Progress in the roentgenologic ex-amination of the gall bladder, Amer. J. Roentgen. **13**:165-167, 1925.

Clarke, H. T., and Dreger, E. E.: Tetraiodophenol-phthalein sodium salt, Amer. J. Roentgen. **14**:341-342, 1925.

Graham, Evarts A., Cole, Warren H., and Copher, Glover H.: Cholecystography; its development and application, Amer. J. Roentgen. **14**:487-495, 1925.

Graham, Evarts A., Cole, Warren H., and Copher, Glover H.: Cholecystography; the use of sodium tetraiodophenolphthalein, J.A.M.A. **84**:1175-1177, 1925.

Graham, Evarts A., Cole, Warren H., and Copher, Glover H.: The roentgenological visualization of the gall bladder by the use of intravenous injections of sodium tetrabromphenolphthalein, Radiology **4**:83, 1925.

Némours, Auguste: La cholécystographie, J. Radiol. Electr. **9**:449, 1925.

Tandoja, P.: Radiologia delle vie biliari, Atti Congresso Ital. Radiol. Med. **6**:1-76, 1925.

1926 Barcia, P. A., Menendez, C., and Leborgne, F. E.: El estudio radiografico de la vesicula biliar por medio de la tetraiodophenolphtaleina, Ann. Facultad Med. Montevideo **10**:763-782, 1926.

D'Amato, Giuseppe: Cholecystographia, Radiol. Med., Jan., Mar., Sept., 1926.

George, Ariel W.: The practical value of the Graham-Cole method in the diagnosis of the gall bladder dis-ease as compared with the older method, Radiology **6**:292-295, 1926.

Herrnheiser, G., and Hirsch: Die seitliche Aufnahme der Gallenblase, Fortschr. Roentgenstr. **34**:97-99, (Con-gressheft) 1926.

Moller, E., and Ottosen, David: Cholecystography, Acta Radiol. **5**:313-332, 1926.

1927 Barsóny, Theodor, and Breuer, Béla: Neuere Beiträge zur Technik der Cholezystographie, Fortschr. Roent-genstr. **36**:1191-1198, 1927.

Moore, Sherwood: Cholecystography; a summary, Radiology **9**:200-204, 1927.

Vietti, M.: Gallbladder examination in the erect posi-tion, Radiol. Med. **14**:508-523, 1927.

1928 D'Amato, Giuseppe: Cholecystographie, Ergebn. Med. Strahlenforsch. **3**:489-540, 1928.

McCoy, C. C.: Development of the roentgenologic ex-amination of the biliary tract, Radiology **11**:13-26, 1928.

Pillmore, George U.: The technique of gall-bladder

examination, Amer. J. Roentgen. **20**:539-544, 1928.

1929 Bronner, Hans: Die cholezystographische Motilitätsprüfung der Gallenblase und ihre Ergebnisse, Fortschr. Roentgenstr. **39**:23-76, 1929.

Chiray, M., Lomon, A., and Albot, G.: La vesicule biliare, sa topographie radiologique et clinique, son exploration par le palper abdominal, Presse Méd. **37**:1437-1440, 1929.

Coghlan, Harold E.: Estudio radiológico de la vesicula biliar, Santiago de Chile, 1929.

Eller, Virginia H.: Cholecystography and its technic, Xray Techn. **1**:43-46, 1929.

Hummel, J. A.: The technic and management of cholecystography, Xray Techn. **1**:37-38, 1929.

Pracht, Mildred: Gall-bladder technic, Xray Techn. **1**:39-42, 1929.

Sandström, Carl: Ueber die orale Darreichung und die Röntgentechnik, bei Cholezystographien, Acta Radiol. **10**:271-290, 1929.

1930 De Abreu, M.: Radiographie néphro-cholécystique, Paris, 1930.

Held, W. I., and Goldbloom, A. A.: Cholecystography in the left latero-anterior position, Amer. J. Roentgen. **24**:313-316, 1930.

Johannesson, Carl J.: Routine oral cholecystography correlated by gastro-intestinal studies, Radiol. Rev. Chicago Med. Recorder **52**:291-296, 1930.

1931 Desjardins, M. A. U.: L'exploration radiologique dans la cholécystite et la lithiase biliare, J. Radiol. Electr. **15**:65-80, 1931.

Eliasz, E.: Der Wert der gezielten Blendennaufnahemen bie der Cholezystographie, Röntgenpraxis **3**:874-878, 1931.

Kirklin, B. R.: Necessity for accurate technique in oral cholecystography, Amer. J. Roentgen. **25**:595-601, 1931.

Newcomer, N. B., Newcomer, Elizabeth, and Conyers, C. A.: The relations of the antrum and cap to the gall bladder; gastric and duodenal peristalsis as factors in emptying the gall bladder, Radiology **17**:317, 1931.

Vastine, J. H.: A simple technique for intravenous cholecystography, Amer. J. Roentgen. **26**:912-913, 1931.

Walsh, Mabel M.: Routine technic in demonstrating gall bladders after oral administration of the dye, Xray Techn. **2**:118-120, 1931.

1932 Kirklin, B. R.: The role of the radiographer in cholecystography, Xray Techn. **3**:129-133, 1932.

Ridout, Lonnell: Cholecystography revolutionized, Xray Techn. **3**:147-150, 1932.

1933 Akerlund, A.: Beobachtungen bei Cholezystogrammen in aufrechter Körperstellung, Acta Radiol. **14**:74-81, 1933.

Determann, A.: Zur Technik der Gallenblasendarstellung, Röntgenpraxis **5**:611-612, 1933.

Hook, H. H.: Technical considerations in radiography of the gall bladder, Xray Techn. **4**:113-115, 1933.

Kaufmann, W.: Aufnahmetechnisches zur Gallenblasendarstellung, Röntgenpraxis **5**:233-235, 1933.

Ledoux-Lebard, R., and Garcia-Calderon, J.: Technique résultats de l'examen radiographique des voies biliares, Paris Méd. **1**:440-453, 1933.

1934 Bacigalupi, Mario: Sulla utilità della radiografia laterale in colecistografia, Ann. Radiol. Fis. Med. **8**:378-384, 1934.

Béclère, Henri, and Porcher, Pierre: Anatomie radiologique des voies biliares extra-hépatiques et du canal de Wirsung, J. Radiol. Electr. **18**:209, 1934.

Estiu, Manuel, and Nacif, Victorio: El rontgenograma simutanea colecisto duodenal en el diagnóstico de las periduodenitis, Rev. Asoc. Méd. Argent. **48**:1031-1034, 1934.

Feldman, Maurice: Oral cholecystography; a plea for a uniform technique, Amer. J. Roentgen. **31**:227, 1934.

Némours, Auguste: Radiologie de la vésicule biliare, Paris, 1934, Masson & Cie.

Stewart, Wm. H., and Illick, Earl H.: Sources of error in oral cholecystography with methods of correction, Radiology **23**:663-671, 1934.

Ungar, E.: Technische Mängel als Ursache der Nichtdarstellbarkeit der Gallenblase bei der peroralen Cholezystographie, Röntgenpraxis **6**:184, 1934.

1935 Kommerell, Burkhard: Choledochographie, Röntgenpraxis **7**:623-625, 1935.

1936 Collins, E. N., and Root, J. C.: Elimination of confusing gas shadows during cholecystography by the use of pitressin, J.A.M.A. **107**:32, 1936.

Ettinger, Alice: Visualization of minute gallsones, Amer. J. Roentgen. **35**:656-661, 1936.

Seta, Paul R.: De la cholécystographie, Paris theses, 1936.

Whitaker, L. R.: The "double oral" method for cholecystography, Amer. J. Roentgen. **35**:200, 1936.

Zaldin, Samuel: The value of the left anterior oblique position in cholecystography, Radiology **26**:340-341, 1936.

1937 Etzler, Walther: Ein Beitrag zur combinierten Gallenblasenduodenaluntersuchung, Röntgenpraxis **9**:35-36, 1937.

Feldman, Maurice: The roentgenologic importance of the left oblique position in cholecystography, Radiology **29**:89-94, 1937.

Mattson, Segrid E.: Oral cholecystography, Xray Techn. **8**:120-125, 1937.

Prévôt, R.: Zur Röntgendiagnostik der Gallenblase, Röntgenpraxis **9**:689-695, 1937.

1938 Akerlund, A.: Die Verfeinerung der röntgenologischen Gallensteindiagnostik durch Untersuchung der Sedimentierungs und Schichtungsverhaltnissen in der Gallenblase, Acta Radiol. **19**:23, 43, 1938.

Dixon, Frank L.: Oral cholecystography using Pitressin for elimination of intestinal gas, Xray Techn. **9**:145-149, 1938.

Fermin, H. E. A.: Over het Röntgenonderzoek van de Galblaas, Amsterdam, 1938, Scheltema & Holkema.

Gaudentia, Sister Mary: Anatomy and physiology of the biliary tract, Xray Techn. **9**:179-180, 197, 1938.

1939 Dawdy, Edith B.: The technic of making cholecystograms, Xray Techn. **11**:50-52, 65, 1939.

Spillman, Ramsay: The value of radiography of the gall bladder in the upright position, Radiology **33**:77-78, 1939.

1940 Ettinger, Alice: The value of the upright position in gall bladder examinations, Radiology **34**:481-488, 1940.

Newcomer, Nathan B.: The twenty-four hour gall bladder, Radiology **35**:575-583, 1940.

Stenström, B.: Ueber Cholangiographie, Acta Radiol. **21**:549-570, 1940.

1941 Junkmann, K.: Perorale Cholecystographie mit Biliselectan, Klin. Wschr. **20**:125-128, 1941.

Robinson, Walter W.: Oral cholecystography: the basis of standardization of the method, Radiology **36**:131, 1941.

1943 Wachowski, T. J.: Technique for gall-bladder radiography, Xray Techn. **15**:3-5, 1943.

Whelan, Frank J.: Important details in the technique of cholecystography, Xray Techn. **14**:151-153, 1943.

1944 Dannenberg, Max: Cholecystographic studies with Priodax, Amer. J. Roentgen. **51**:328-335, 1944.

Hefke, H. W.: Cholecystography with Priodax; a report on 600 examinations, Radiology **42**:233-236, 1944.

Kent, Thelma: Gall bladder radiography: a table of positions based on two measurements, Xray Techn. **16**:101-107, 1944.

1945 Grandlund, Herbert E.: Technical procedure of the gall bladder examination, Xray Techn. **17**:283-288, 1945.

Henry, Lucas S.: The lateral projection in cholecystography, Radiogr. Clin. Photogr. **21**:9, 24, 1945.

Kirklin, B. R.: Background and beginning of cholecystography, Amer. J. Roentgen. **54**:637-639, 1945.

Whelan, Frank J.: The vertical position in cholecystography, Xray Techn. **17**:289-294, 1945.

1946 Brown, S., and Harper, F.: A new roentgen sign in extrahepatic biliary tract disease, Radiology **47**:239-248, 1946.

Coliez, Robert, and Hickel, Richard: Les calculs biliares "flottant entre deux eaux," J. Radiol. Electr. **27**:238-239, 402-409, 1946.

Donald, Brother: Radiography of the gall bladder, Xray Techn. **18**:5-7, 1946.

Moore, Sherwood: Lesions of the biliary tract. In Pillmore, George U., editor: Clinical radiology, Philadelphia, 1946, F. A. Davis Co., vol. 1, pp. 638-659.

Onstad, Raymond: Tube tilt projection in cholecystography, Xray Techn. **17**:477-478, 1946.

1947 Biancheri, T.: Cholecisti a sinistra, Arch. Ital. Chir. **69**:415-420, 1947.

Brewer, Arthur A.: Cholecystography; a comparative study of the oral and intravenous contrast substances, Radiology **48**:269-273, 1947.

Golden, Ross: The gall bladder. In Golden, Ross, editor: Diagnostic roentgenology, ed. 3, New York, 1947, Thomas Nelson & Sons, vol. 1, pp. 344T-345N.

Howard, Lexie: Radiography in examination of the gall bladder, Xray Techn. **19**:78-79, 1947.

1948 Crowley, Sister Mary de Lellis: The upright position in cholecystography, Xray Techn. **19**:235-237, 280, 1948.

Kirklin, B. R.: A new position for cholecystography, Amer. J. Roentgen. **60**:263-268, 1948.

Whelan, Frank J.: Special cholecystographic technique, Xray Techn. **19**:230-234, 1948.

1949 Lindblom, K.: Axial projection of the gallbladder, Acta Radiol. **32**:189-190, 1949.

1950 Cocchi, U.: Die Nichtgefüllte Gallenblase; ein Beitrag zur Röntgenkontrastdarstellung der Gallenblase nach Wasserstoss oder Karlsbader Salz, Acta Radiol. **33**:115-129, 1950.

1951 Bleich, A. R., and others: Left-upper-quadrant gallbladder, J.A.M.A. **147**:849-851, 1951.

Elsey, E. C., and Jacobs, D. L.: Floating gallbladder stones, Amer. J. Roentgen. **65**:73-76, 1951.

Whelan, Frank J.: Stratification of gallstones in the gallbladder; positions of the gallbladder and of the patient in which stratification can be demonstrated, Xray Techn. **23**:91, 1951.

1952 Maddox, L.: Localization of the gallbladder, Amer. J. Roentgen. **67**:644-645, 1952.

Wilkie, W.: Floating gallstones, S. Afr. Med. J. **26**:357, 1952.

1953 Divilio, L. P.: New roentgen technique for preoperative studies of the biliary tract, Xray Techn. **25**:1-8, 1953.

Etter, Lewis E.: Left-sided gallbladder; necessity for film of the entire abdomen in cholecystography, Amer. J. Roentgen. **70**:987-990, 1953.

Feldman, M., and Meyers, P.: The diagnostic evaluation of erect positioning in cholecystography, Radiology **60**:222-225, 1953.

Friedman, P. S., and Solis-Cohen, L.: Saline concentrations in cholecystography, Amer. J. Roentgen. **70**:437-440, 1953.

Sachs, M. D.: Visualization of the common duct during cholecystography, Amer. J. Roentgen. **69**:745-768, 1953.

Scott, W. G., and Simril, W. A.: Newer radiopaque media for oral cholecystography, Amer. J. Roentgen. **69**:78-87, 1953.

1954 Berk, J. E., Karnofsky, R. E., Shay, H., and Stauffer, H. M.: Intravenous cholecystography and cholangiography, Amer. J. Med. Sci. **227**:361-371, 1954.

Orloff, T. L.: Intravenous choledocholaminography, Amer. J. Roentgen. **72**:804-805, 1954.

Shehadi, W. H.: Oral cholangiography with Telepaque, Amer. J. Roentgen. **72**:436-451, 1954.

Turnbull, A.: Cassette holder for cholecystography in the right lateral decubitus position, Amer. J. Roentgen. **71**:520-521, 1954.

Twiss, J. R., Beranbaum, S. A., Gillette, L., and Poppel, M. H.: Post-cholecystectomy oral cholangiography, Amer. J. Med. Sci. **227**:372-386, 1954.

1955 Stein, G. N., and Finkelstein, A.: Cholangiography, Med. Radiogr. Photogr. **31**:4-18, 1955.

1956 Aldridge, Noel H.: Cholecystography and cholangiography; a review of present methods of examination, Amer. J. Med. Sci. **231**:701-721, 1956.

Cimmino, C. V.: Experiences with upright fluoroscopic spot-film examination of gallbladder, Radiology **67**:74-78, 1956.

Divilio, L. P.: Roentgenographic problems associated with the use of the newer cholecystographic medium, Xray Techn. **28**:227-235, 1956.

Mitchell, David J.: Basic combined cholecystangiography, Brit. J. Radiol. **29**:133-138, 1956.

Phillips, R. I.: Intravenous cholangiography; a consideration of radiographic technique, Xray Techn. **28**:163-168, 1956.

1957 Eliasoph, J., and Marshak, R. H.: Use of prone pressure device in intravenous cholangiography, J. Mount Sinai Hosp. **24**:546-549, 1957.

Esquerra-Gómez, G.: Excretion cholecystocholangiography, Radiology. **69**:94-100, 1957.

Hoffman, C. R.: Phototimed erect compression spot films in cholecystography, Amer. J. Roentgen. **77**:55-60, 1957.

Shehadi, W. H.: Simultaneous intravenous cholangiography and urography, Surg. Gynec. Obstet. **105**:401-406, 1957.

1958 Walker, John H.: Biliary tract roentgenography in the lateral decubitus position, Amer. J. Roentgen. **80**:945-949, 1958.

1959 Chernok, N.: A method for more precise localization of the gallbladder, Xray Techn. **30**:376-379, 1959.

Rabinov, D. I., and Kent, K. H.: Trendelenburg spot roentgenograms in cholecystography, Amer. J. Roentgen. **82**:1020-1023, 1959.

Shapiro, J. H., and others: Oral cholecystography; a review of techniques, Amer. J. Roentgen. **82**:1003-1010, 1959.

1960 Jones, J. A. B., and others: Tomography in intravenous cholangiography, Brit. J. Radiol. **33**:110-118, 1960.

1961 Norman, A., and Saghatoleslami, M.: Oral extrahepatic cholangiography; a simple reliable technic, Radiology **76**:801-804, 1961.

1962 Linsman, J. F.: Pneumatic compression paddle (prone pressure device) in cholecystography and choledochography, Amer. J. Roentgen. **87**:740-744, 1962.

1963 Billimoria, P. E., Judkins, M. P., and Dotter, C. T.: Oral cholecystangiography, Amer. J. Roentgen. **89**:854-858, 1963.

Chesney, D. N.: Radiography of the biliary tract, Radiography **29**:307-323, 1963.

Harper, J. M. E.: Radiography of the biliary tract, Radiography **29**:225-238, 1963.

Shehadi, William H.: Clinical radiology of the biliary tract, New York, 1963, McGraw-Hill Book Co.

Wise, Robert E.: Roentgenology of the liver and biliary tract, Gasteroenterology **45**:644-657, 1963.

1964 Amberg, J. R., and others: The inclined lateral decubitus position for cholecystography, Amer. J. Roentgen. **92**:1128-1130, 1964.

Cliffe, A. E., and Campbell, J. S.: Radiography of the posthepatic bile-collecting system, Med. Radiogr. Photogr. **40**:29-35, 1964.

1966 Darnborough, A., and Geffen, N.: Drip-infusion cholangiography, Brit. J. Radiol. **39**:827-832, 1966.

Feldman, M. I., and Keohane, M.: Slow infusion intravenous cholangiography, Radiology **87**:355-356, 1966.

Shehadi, William H.: Radiologic examination of the biliary tract; plain film of the abdomen; oral cholecystography, Radiol. Clin. N. Amer. **4**:463-482, 1966.

Wax, R. E., and Crummy, A. B.: Drip infusion cholangiography, Radiology **87**:354, 1966.

1967 McDonnell, R. W., and Rice, R. P.: The effect of Neloid on Telepaque cholecystography, Amer. J. Roentgen. **101**:617-618, 1967.

Sargent, E. N., Guth, P. H., and Graffman, M.: Rectal cholecystography, Radiology **88**:997-1001, 1967.

Wangermez, A., and Wangermez, J.: Massive infusion cholangiography, J. Radiol. **48**:827-832, 1967.

1968 Bornhurst, R. A., Heitzman, E. R., and McAfee, J. G.: Double-dose drip-infusion cholangiography; analysis of 107 consecutive cases, J.A.M.A. **206**:1489-1494, 1968.

Cooperman, L. R., Rossiter, S. B., Reimer, G. W., and Ng, E.: Infusion cholangiography, Amer. J. Roentgen. **104**:880-883, 1968.

Foy, R. E., Jr.: Slow-infusion compared with direct-injection cholangiography; application of zonography, Radiology. **90**:576-578, 1968.

Payne, R. F.: Drip infusion cholangiography, Clin. Radiol. **19**:291-295, 1968.

1969 Allen, W. M. C.: Drip infusion cholangiography in cases of failed cholangiography, Brit. J. Radiol. **42:**347-350, 1969.

Cimmino, C. V.: The upside-down view in gallbladder diagnosis, Radiology **92:**645-646, 1969.

Cullinan, J. E., Jr.: Choleroentgenography—history and development of current biliary opacification techniques, Radiol. Techn. **40:**226-235, 1969.

Kotoulas, K., Koureas, P., Salaminios, F., and Michalopoulos, S.: Slow infusion cholecystangiography after the administration of Dolantin (Meperidine or Pethidine), Roentgenblaetter **22:**454-461, 1969. (In German.) Abst.: Radiology **96:**227, 1970.

Nathan, M. H., Newman, A., McFarland, J., and Murray, D. J.: Cholecystokinin cholecystography, Radiology **93:**1-8, 1969.

Rowe, P. W.: Retained needle urography and cholangiography, Radiology **93:**520, 1969.

1970 Dodds, W. J., and Mani, J. R.: The lateral bending maneuver: an aid for cholecystography, Radiology **95:**441-442, 1970.

Gibertini, G., Cortesi, N., Lodi, R., and others: Laparoscopic cholangiography: technique and results, Presse Med. **78:**2471-2474, 1970.

Jensen, R., and Kaude, J.: Oral cholecystography; experimental investigation and clinical comparison of 70 mm film and full-scale radiography, Acta Radiol. [Diagn.] **10:**499-512, 1970.

Lévesque, H. P.: Sabulography, Amer. J. Roentgen. **110:**213-225, 1970.

Nathan, M. H., Newman, A., Murray, D. J., and Camponovo, R.: Cholecystokinin cholecystography; a four year evaluation, Amer. J. Roentgen. **110:**240-251, 1970.

Nolan, D. J., and Gibson, M. J.: Improvements in intravenous cholangiography, Brit. J. Radiol. **43:**652-657, 1970.

Wangermez, A., Wangermez, J., and Debot, P.: Les risques de la cholangiographie-perfusion et les dangers des examens biliaries itératifs, J. Radiol. Electr. **51:**287-290, 1970.

1971 Bilbrey, R. L., and Buonocore, E.: Combined gastrointestinal and gallbladder roentgenograms using fat added to barium meals, Amer. J. Roentgen. **113:**29-33, 1971.

Corcella, A., Bruno, S., Nannelli, U., and Vita, G.: Glucose potentiated perfusion cholangiography, Radiol. Med. **67:**417-428, 1971. (In Italian.) Abst.: Radiology **104:**730, 1972.

Martinez, L. O., Viamonte, M. J., Gassman, P., and Boudet, J.: Present status of intravenous cholangiography, Amer. J. Roentgen. **113:**10-15, 1971.

Ochsner, S. F.: Intramural lesions of the gallbladder, Amer. J. Roentgen. **113:**1-9, 1971.

1973 Moss, A. A., Nelson, J., and Amberg, J.: Intravenous cholangiography, Amer. J. Roentgen. **117:**406-411, 1973.

Rabushka, S. E., Love, L., and Moncada, R.: Infusion tomography of the gallbladder, Radiology **109:**549-552, 1973.

BILIARY DUCTS (CHOLANGIOGRAPHY BY SURGICAL METHODS)

1918 Reich, A. J.: Accidental injection of bile ducts with petrolatum and bismuth paste, J.A.M.A. **71:**1555, 1918.

1922 Tenney, C. F., and Patterson, S. H.: Injection of the bile ducts with bismuth paste and observation on the flow of bile, J.A.M.A. **78:**171-173, 1922.

1927 Piccinino, G., and Pszienza, M.: Iniezione con sostanza opaca di fistola biliare, Arch. Radiol. **3:**939-943, 1927.

1928 Caeiro, J. A.: Las fistulas biliares y su exploración por el lipiodol, Bol. Soc. Cir. B. Air. **12:**855-863, 1928.

1929 Cotte, G.: Sur l'exploration radiologique des voies biliares avec injection de lipiodol après cholécystostomie ou cholédocotomie, Bull. Soc. Nat. Chir. **55:**863-871, 1929.

1930 Gabriel, W. B.: Proof of patency of common bile duct by injection of Lipiodol, Lancet **1:**1014-1015, 1930.

Ginzburg, L., and Benjamin, E. W.: Lipiodol studies of postoperative biliary fistulae, Ann. Surg. **91:**233-241, 1930.

1931 Overholt, R. H.: Biliary tract visualization with radiopaque oils, Surg. Gynec. Obstet. **52:**92-97, 1931.

1932 Mirizzi, P. L.: La colangiografía durante las operaciones de las vias biliares, Bol. Soc. Cir. B. Air. **16:**1133-1161, 1932.

1933 Judd, E. S., and Phillips, J. R.: Patency of biliary ducts, determined by radiopaque oil injection through t-tube previously placed in common bile duct for purpose of prolonged drainage, Surg. Gynec. Obstet. **57:**668-671, 1933.

Mirizzi, P. L.: Cholécystectomie sans drainage, Paris, 1933, Masson & Cie.

1936 Hicken, N. Frederick, Best, R. R., and Hunt, H. B.: Cholangiography; visualization of gallbladder and bile ducts during and after operation, Ann. Surg. **103:**210-229, 1936.

Robins, S. A., and Hermanson, L.: Cholangiography; modified technique for x-ray visualization of bile ducts during operation, Surg. Gynec. Obstet. **62:**684-688, 1936.

1937 Best, R. R., and Hicken, N. F.: Technique of immediate cholangiography, Surg. Gynec. Obstet. **65:**217-219, 1937.

Hufford, C. H.: Postoperative visualization of the biliary tract, Amer. J. Roentgen. **37:**154, 1937.

Hunt, H. B., Hicken, N. F., and Best, R. R.: Exploration of biliary ducts by cholangiography during and following operation, Amer. J. Roentgen. **38:**542-564, 1937.

1938 Best, R. R., and Hicken, N. F.: Cholangiography, Radiogr. Clin. Photogr. **14:**2-6, 1938.

Hulten, O.: Cholangiography during course of operation, Deutsch. Z. Chir. **250:**484-513, 1938.

Mixter, C. G., and Hermanson, L.: A critical evaluation of cholangiography, Amer. J. Surg. **40:**223-231, 1938.

1940 Stenström, B.: Ueber Cholangiographie, Acta Radiol. **21:**549-570, 1940.

1941 Altman, W. S.: Cholangiography; fractional method, Radiology **37:**261-268, 1941.

1945 Lasala, A. J.: Cholangiografía operatoria; la experiencia de 120 casos, Prensa Méd. Argent. **32:**952-967, 1945.

Weinberger, Jacob, and Rosenthal, Abraham: Choledocho-duodenal fistula, Amer. J. Roentgen. **53:**470-473, 1945.

1947 Golden, Ross: Cholangiography. In Golden, Ross, editor: Diagnostic roentgenology, ed. 3, New York, 1947, Thomas Nelson & Sons, vol. 1, pp. 345M-345N.

1949 Hicken, N. F., Stevenson, V. L., Franz, B. J., and Crowder, E.: The technic of operative cholangiography, Amer. J. Surg. **78:**347-355, 1949.

1950 Mirizzi, P. L.: Remarques sur la cholangiographie opératoire associée à quelques procédés accessoires, Mem. Acad. Chir. **76:**592-595, 1950.

1951 Abeatici, S., and Campi, L.: Sur les possibilités de l'angiographie hepatique; la visualization des systèmes portales, Acta Radiol. **36:**383-392, 1951.

Zierold, Arthur: Operating room cholangiograms, Minnesota Med. **34:**439-441, 1951.

1952 Carter, F. R., and Saypol, G. M.: Transabdominal cholangiography, J.A.M.A. **148:**253-255, 1952.

Hight, D., and Lingley, J. R.: The value of cholangiograms during biliary tract surgery, New Eng. J. Med. **246:**761-765, 1952.

Vadheim, J. L., and Rigos, F. J.: Cholangiography as an aid to biliary surgery, Northwest Med. **51:**400-402, 1952.

1953 Murick, A. W., and others: Percutaneous transhepatic cholangiography in diagnosis of obstructive jaundice, J. Surg. **41:**27-31, 1953.

1954 Douglas, T. C., and others: Operating room cholangiography; errors in technique and interpretation, Arch. Surg. **68:**422-429, 1954.

Gius, J. A., Tidrick, R. T., and Hickey, R. C.: Extension of immediate cholangiography in common duct surgery, Surgery **36:**460-467, 1954.

Johnston, E. V., Waugh, J. M., and Good, C. A.: Residual stones in the common bile duct; the question of operative cholangiograms, Ann. Surg. **139**:293-301, 1954.

Young, B. R., and Scanlan, R. L.: New explosion-proof and shock-proof mobile roentgenographic equipment for the operating room, Amer. J. Roentgen. **71**:873-877, 1954.

1955 Stein, G. N., and Finkelstein, A.: Cholangiography, Med. Radiogr. Photogr. **31**:4-18, 1955.

1957 McCabe, E. B., and Heinrich, W. D.: The importance of visualization of the proximal portion of the common duct and hepatic ducts in operative cholangiography, Radiology **69**:240-243, 1957.

McCarty, W. C., and Crickard, G. E.: Operative cholangiography, Radiology **69**:236-239, 1957.

1961 Schulenburg, C. A. R.: Operative cholangiography, S. Afr. Med. J. **35**:202-207, 1961.

1962 Evans, J. A., Glenn, F., Thorbjarnarson, B., and Mujahed, Z.: Percutaneous transphepatic cholangiography, Radiology **78**:362-370, 1962.

Isley, J. K., and Schauble, J. F.: Interpretation of the percutaneous transhepatic cholangiogram, Amer. J. Roentgen. **88**:772-777, 1962.

Stern, W. Z., Schein, C. J., and Jacobson, H. G.: The significance of the lateral view in T-tube cholangiography, Amer. J. Roentgen. **87**:764-771, 1962.

1963 Flemma, R. J., and others: Percutaneous transhepatic cholangiography in the differential diagnosis of jaundice, Surg. Gynec. Obstet. **116**:559-568, 1963.

Shehadi, William H.: Clinical radiology of the biliary tract, New York, 1963, McGraw-Hill Book Co.

1964 Birch, J. R., and others: Transhepatic cholangiography, Canad. Med. Ass. J. **90**:1442-1449, 1964.

Evans, John A.: Specialized roentgen diagnostic technics in the investigation of abdominal disease, Radiology **82**:579-594, 1964.

Ferris, E. J., and others: Percutaneous transhepatic cholangiography, Amer. J. Roentgen. **92**:1131-1138, 1964.

1965 Flemma, R. J., and others: Percutaneous transhepatic cholangiography, Arch. Surg. **90**:5-10, 1965.

Rabinov, K. R., and Simon, M.: Peroral cannulation of the ampulla of Vater for direct cholangiography and pancreatography, Radiology **85**:693-697, 1965.

1966 Berk, J. E.: Visualization of the bile ducts and portal venous system, J.A.M.A. **195**:1020-1024, 1966.

Hermann, R. E.: Operative cholangiography, GP **33**:120-127, 1966.

Hermann, R. E., and Hoerr, S. O.: The value of the routine use of operative cholangiography, Surg. Gynec. Obstet. **121**:1015-1020, 1966.

Mujahed, Z., and Evans, J. A.: Percutaneous transhepatic cholangiography, Radiol. Clin. N. Amer. **4**:535-545, 1966.

Sachs, M. D.: Routine cholangiography, operative and postoperative, Radiol. Clin. N. Amer. **4**:547-569, 1966.

Seldinger, S. I.: Percutaneous transhepatic cholangiography, Acta Radiol., supp. 253, 1966.

1967 Hanafee, W., and Weiner, M.: Transjugular percutaneous cholangiography, Radiology **88**:35-39, 1967.

Kittredge, R. D., and Finby, N.: Percutaneous transhepatic cholangiography, Amer. J. Roentgen. **101**:592-604, 1967.

Thorbjarnarson, B., Mujahed, Z., and Glenn, F.: Percutaneous transhepatic cholangiography, Ann. Surg. **165**:33-40, 1967.

1968 Fogarty, T. J., Krippaehne, W. M., Dennis, D. L., and Fletcher, W. S.: Evaluation of an improved operative technic in common duct surgery, Amer. J. Surg. **116**:177-183, 1968.

Grace, R. H., and Peckar, V. G.: The value of operative cholangiography using an image intensifier and a television monitor, Brit. J. Surg. **55**:933-938, 1968.

Turner, F. W., and Costopoulos, L. B.: Percutaneous transhepatic cholangiography: a study of 115 cases, Canad. Med. Ass. J. **99**:513-521, 1968.

1970 Fazel, I., and Finley, R. K., Jr.: Experience with percutaneous transhepatic cholangiography in a community hospital, Ohio State Med. J. **66**:1193-1200, 1970.

1971 Eaton, S. B., Wirtz, R. D., Eyck, J. R. T., and Richards, J. C.: Iatrogenic liver injury resulting from ductal instrumentation with the Fogerty biliary balloon catheter, Radiology **100**:581-584, 1971.

Herba, M. J., and Kiss, J.: Percutaneous transhepatic cholangiography, J. Canad. Ass. Radiol. **22**:22-29, 1971.

1972 Morettin, L. B., and Dodd, G. D.: Percutaneous transhepatic cholangiography, Amer. J. Dig. Dis. **17**:831-845, 1972.

Peresleny, V., and Cimmino, C.: The oblique view in operating room cholangiography, Radiology **102**:442-443, 1972.

PANCREAS (PANCREATOGRAPHY BY SURGICAL METHODS)

1953 Leger, L.: Surgical contrast visualization of the pancreatic ducts with a study of pancreatic external secretion, Amer. J. Dig. Dis. **20**:8-12, 1953.

1955 Doubilet, H., Poppel, M. H., and Mulholland, J. H.: Pancreatography; techniques, principles, and observations, Radiology **64**:325-339, 1955.

1958 Pollock, A. V.: Pancreatography in the diagnosis of chronic relapsing pancreatitis, Surg. Gynec. Obstet. **107**:765-770, 1958.

1959 Doubilet, H., Poppel, M. H., and Mulholland, J. H.: Pancreatography, Ann. N. Y. Acad. Sci. **78**:829-851, 1959.

Thal, A. P., Goott, B., and Margulis, A. R.: Sites of pancreatic duct obstruction in chronic pancreatitis, Ann. Surg. **150**:49-56, 1959.

1960 Hayes, M. A.: Operative pancreatography, Surg. Gynec. Obstet. **110**:404-408, 1960.

1961 Frimann-Dahl, J.: Radiology in tumors of the pancreas, Clin. Radiol. **12**:73-79, 1961.

1963 Elmslie, R. G., White, T. T., and Magee, D. F.: Pancreatography with particular reference to the activation of pancreatic enzymes, Surg. Gynec. Obstet. **117**:405-410, 1963.

1965 Keddie, N., and Nardi, G. L.: Pancreatography; a safe and effective technic, Amer. J. Surg. **110**:863-865, 1965.

Peskin, G. W., and Johnson, C.: Pancreatic visualization, Amer. J. Med. Sci. **249**:223-229, 1965.

Rabinov, K. R., and Simon, M.: Peroral cannulation of the ampulla of Vater for direct cholangiography and pancreatography, Radiology **85**:693-697, 1965.

1967 Clemett, A. R.: Examination of the pancreas. In Margulis, A. R., and Burhenne, H. J., editors: Alimentary tract roentgenology, St. Louis, 1967, The C. V. Mosby Co.

Trapnell, J. E.: Pancreatography — a reassessment, Brit. J. Surg. **54**:934-939, 1967. Abst.: Radiology **91**:418, 1968; Amer. J. Roentgen. **103**:245, 1968.

1969 Howard, J. M., and Short, W. F.: An evaluation of pancreatography in suspected pancreatic disease, Surg. Gynec. Obstet. **129**:319-324, 1969.

ESOPHAGUS

1896 White: A foreign body in the oesophagus detected and located by the roentgen rays, Univ. Med. Mag. **8**:9, 1896.

1901 Wilms: Die schräge Durchleuchtung des Thorax bei Fremdkörpern im Oesophagus und zur Darstellung der Dorsalwirbelsäule, Fortschr. Roentgenstr. **5**:11-12, 1901-1902.

1905 Bertolotti: Un nuovo metodo di radioscopia esofagea, Riv. Acad. Torino, 1905, nos. 11-12. Abst.: Fortschr. Roentgenstr. **11**:66, 1908.

1906 Holzknecht, G.: Röntgenaufnahmen der Speiseröhre mit Hilfe von Wismutbrei, Gesell. Inn. Med. Kinderheilk. **7**:VI, 1906. Abst.: Fortschr. Roentgenstr. **11**:66, 1908.

1908 Lange, Sidney: The roentgen examination of the esophagus, Arch. Roentgen Ray **13**:231-237, 1908-1909.

1910 Albers-Schönberg, H. E.: Oesophagusdarstellung. In Röntgentechnik, ed. 3, Hamburg, 1910, Gräfe & Sillem, chap. 26.

Williams, H.: X-ray examination of the stricture of the esophagus, Boston Med. Surg. J. **160**:604, 1910.

1911 Jordan, A. C.: The roentgen ray examination of the oesophagus, Arch. Roentgen Ray **15**:348, 1910-1911.

1913 Barclay, Alfred: The stomach and oesophagus; a radiographic study, New York, 1913, The Macmillan Co.

1914 Aubourg and Belot: L'exploration radiologique de l'oesophage, J. Radiol. Electr. **1**:433-443, 1914-1915.

1922 Bowen, Charles F.: Foreign bodies in the bronchus and esophagus, Amer. J. Roentgen. **9**:705, 1922.

1925 Spiess, Gustav: Der Wert der Röntgenuntersuchung für den Nachweiss und klinischen Verlauf bei Fremdkörpern in der Speiseröhre, Fortschr. Roentgenstr. **33**:236, 1925.

Wilon, W. F.: Oesophagoscopie: ein Mittel nichtopake Fremdkörpes durch Röntgenstrahlen nachzuweisen, Brit. Med. J. **1925-I**:656, 1925.

1926 Akerlund, A.: Hernia diaphragmatica hiatus oesophagei vom anatomischen und roentgenologischem Standpunkt, Acta Radiol. **6**:3, 1926.

Manges, Willis F.: Right-oblique-prone posture for study of the esophagus, Amer. J. Roentgen. **16**:374-375, 1926.

1927 Casati, Annibale: Gli spostamenti dell'esofago, Radiol. Med. **14**:593-601, 1927.

Manges, Willis F.: Roentgen diagnosis of foreign bodies in the esophagus, Amer. J. Roentgen. **17**:44, 1927.

1928 Tschendorf, Werner: Die Röntgenuntersuchung der Speiseröhre, Ergebn. Med. Strahlenforsch. **3**:175-288, 1928.

1929 Borquist, A. B.: A technic for radiographing the esophagus, Xray Techn. **1**:18-19, 1929.

1931 Heuser, Carlos: Technical points for the roentgenologist, Radiology **17**:827-828, 1931.

Pulugyay, Joseph: Röntgenuntersuchung und Strahlenbehandlung der Speiseröhre, Handbuch Röntgen. **3**:1931.

1933 Carlsund, Herbert: An aid to the roentgen diagnosis of foreign bodies not visible on ordinary radiography in the hypopharynx and oesophagus, Acta Radiol. **14**:391-398, 1933. Abst.: Amer. J. Roentgen. **32**:572, 1934.

1934 Wright, H. E., and Freeman, E. B.: New method for visualization of the unobstructed esophagus, Radiology **22**:160-162, 1934.

1935 Barsóny, Theodor, and Koppenstein, E.: Zur Röntgenologie der Pars abdominalis der Speiseröhre und der Incisura cardica, Röntgenpraxis **7**:439-446, 1935.

1937 Oppenheimer, Albert: Esophageal varices, Amer. J. Roentgen. **38**:403-414, 1937.

Scott, Wendell G.: Un método de roentgendiagnóstico de cuerpos extraños no opacos situados en el esófago, Rev. Radiol. Fis. **4**:1-4, 1937.

1938 Vickers, F. P.: Radiography of the esophagus and suspected cases of diaphragmatic hernia of the stomach, Radiography **4**:149-151, 1938.

1942 Ledoux-Lebard, R., and Lonlas, A.: Le radiodiagnostic des corps étrangers de l'oesophage (données pratiques), J. Radiol. Electr. **25**:161-163, 1942-1943.

1944 Akerlund, A., and Welin, S.: Roentgen diagnosis of malignant tumors with the boundary region between the pharynx and esophagus, Acta Radiol. **25**:883-911, 1944.

Skarby, Hans-Gösta: Ueber die klinische und röntgenologische Diagnose von Fremdkörpen, speziell Fischgräten im Hypopharynx und Oesophagus unter Angabe einer geeigneten röntgenologischen Methodik, Acta Radiol. **25**:796-823, 1944.

1946 Holinger, Paul H.: Lesions of the esophagus. In Pillmore, George U., editor: Clinical radiology, Philadelphia, 1946, F. A. Davis Co., vol. 1, pp. 463-485.

1947 Amann, Rose: Visualization of non-opaque foreign bodies in the esophagus, Xray Techn. **18**:289-290, 1947.

Golden, Ross: The esophagus. In Golden, Ross, editor: Diagnostic roentgenology, ed. 3, New York, 1947, Thomas Nelson & Sons, vol. 1, pp. 269-289.

Johnstone, H. S.: Foreign bodies in the esophagus, Brit. J. Radiol. **20**:41-42, 1947.

1951 Donaldson, L.: Roentgenologic examination of the esophagus, Surg. Clin. N. Amer. **31**:21-38, 1951.

1955 Epstein, B. S.: A roentgenographic aid to the diagnosis of radiopaque foreign bodies in the upper intrathoracic esophagus, Amer. J. Roentgen. **73**:115-117, 1955.

1956 Freidenfelt, H.: A double contrast method for the roentgen examination of esophageal strictures, Acta Radiol. **46**:499-506, 1956.

1957 Nelson, S. W.: The roentgenologic diagnosis of esophageal varices, Amer. J. Roentgen. **77**:599-611, 1957.

1961 Gunson, Edward F.: Radiography of the pharynx and upper esophagus; shoestring method, Xray Techn. **33**:1-8, 1961.

1963 Swart, B.: Die Technik der Varicendarstellung am Oesophagus, Radiologe **3**:65-75, 1963. Abst.: Radiology **81**:1054, 1963.

1966 Donner, M. W., Silbiger, M. L., Hookman, P., and Hendrix, T. R.: Acid-barium swallows in the radiographic evaluation of clinical esophagitis, Radiology **87**:220-225, 1966.

1968 Mortensson, W., and Sandmark, S.: Roentgen examination of stricture of the lower esophagus, Acta Radiol. [Diagn.] **7**:355-360, 1968.

1969 Feist, J. H., and Riley, R. R.: Diagnosis of esophageal varices, Radiology **93**:861-866, 1969.

1972 Ghahremani, G. G., Port, R. B., Winans, C. S., and Williams, J. R.: Esophageal varices: enhanced radiologic visualization by anticholinergic drugs, Amer. J. Dig. Dis. **17**:703-712, 1972.

ALIMENTARY TRACT
General

1904 Rieder, H.: Beiträge zur Topographie des Magendarmkanals beim lebenden Menschen nebst Untersuchungen über den zeitlichen Ablauf der Verdauung, Fortschr. Roentgenstr. **8**:142, 1904-1905.

Rieder, H.: Radiologische Untersuchungen des Magens und Darmes beim lebenden Menschen, München. Med. Wschr. **51**:1548, 1904.

1906 Hulst, Henry: Roentgenography in diseases of the stomach and intestines, Trans. Amer. Roentgen Ray Soc., 1906.

1907 Hildebrand: Ueber die Methode, durch Einbringen von schattengebenden flüssigkeiten Hohlorgane des Körpers im Röntgenogram sichtbar zu machen, Fortschr. Roentgenstr. **11**:96, 1907.

Groedel, F. M.: Examination of the stomach and intestines by means of roentgen rays, Arch. Roentgen Ray **12**:122-130, 1907-1908; **15**:156-158, 1910-1911.

1910 Albers-Schönberg, H. E.: Röntgentechnik, Magen- und Darmuntersuchungen, Berlin, 1910, Gräfe & Sillem, chap. 28.

Cole, L. G., and Einhorn, Max: Radiograms of the digestive tract by inflation with air, New York Med. J., 1910.

1913 Leonard, Charles Lester: The radiography of the stomach and intestines, Amer. J. Roentgen. **1**:5-38, 1913.

1915 Tousey, Sinclair: Gastro-intestinal radiography in the prone position with the pelvis elevated, Int. Med. J. **22**:1039-1040, 1915.

1916 Jones, Llewelyn L.: Routine technic of barium diagnosis, Amer. J. Roentgen. **3**:477-481, 1916.

1918 Spangler, Davis: Opaque roentgen ray meals and enemas, Amer. J. Roentgen. **5**:175-180, 1918.

1923 Moody, R. O., Van Nuys, R. G., and Chamberlain, W. E.: Position of the stomach, liver, and colon, J.A.M.A. **81**:1924-1931, 1923.

1925 McMally, William D.: Two deaths from the administration of barium salts, J.A.M.A. **84**:1805, 1925.

1926 Moody, R. O., Van Nuys, R. G., and Chamberlain, W.: Visceral anatomy of healthy adults, Amer. J. Anat. **37**:273, 1926.

1928 Taylor, Henry K.: Potter-Bucky table adapted for multiple exposures, Radiology **10**:506-509, 1928.

1929 Artos, Sister Mary: Gastro-intestinal surveys, Xray Techn. **1**:33-36, 1929.

1930 Berg, H. H.: Röntgenuntersuchungen am Innenrelief des Verdauungskanals, Leipzig, 1930, Georg Thieme.

1932 Rose, J. S.: Serial plating in gastro-intestinal work, Xray Techn. **3**:107-113, 1932.

1936 Barclay, Alfred: The digestive tract; a radiological study of its anatomy, physiology and pathology, Cambridge, England, 1936, University Press.

Carty, John R., and Merrill, Vinita: Some essential considerations of the technic of gastrointestinal radiography, Radiology 26:531-534, 1936.

1937 Adkins, Mary E.: The value of laterals in gastro-intestinal series, Xray Techn. 8:153-154, 1937.

Lane, Lulu: Radiography of the gastro-intestinal tract, Xray Techn. 8:150-152, 1937.

1938 Bermond, M.: Contributo alla localizzazione radiologica dei corpi estranei delle vie respiratorie e digestive, Arch. Radiol. 16:5-15, 1938.

Eller, Virginia H.: Spot radiography of the gastrointestinal tract with a fluoro-graphic unit, Xray Techn. 9:225-228, 1938.

Hershenson, Morris A.: Compression blocks in gastric intestinal roentgenography, Amer. J. Roentgen. 40:451-453, 1938.

1939 Frimann-Dahl, J.: Roentgenologic examination of acute abdominal lesions, Acta Radiol. 20:441-442, 1939.

1941 Lofstrom, J. E.: Further observations on elimination of intestinal gas shadows in roentgenography, Radiology 36:34-41, 1941.

1942 Piotrowski, Brother Dominic: Technique for gastrointestinal radiography, Xray Techn. 14:121-123, 133, 1942.

1947 Golden, Ross: The roentgen-ray examination of the digestive tract. In Golden, Ross, editor: Diagnostic roentgenology, ed. 3, New York, 1947, Thomas Nelson & Sons, vol. 1, pp. 265-350.

1956 Davis, L. A., Huang, K. C., and Pirkey, E. L.: Water-soluble nonabsorbable radiopaque mediums in gastrointestinal examinations, J.A.M.A. 160:373-375, 1956.

1957 Henry, G. W.: Detection of gastrointestinal bleeding with a barium-hydrogen peroxide mixture, Amer. J. Roentgen. 78:698-704, 1957.

1959 Templeton, F. E.: Gastrointestinal radiology, Amer. J. Dig. Dis. 4:661-681, 1959.

1960 Shehadi, W. H.: Orally administered water soluble iodinated contrast media, Amer. J. Roentgen. 83:933-941, 1960.

1965 Rosen, R. S., and Jacobson, G.: Visible urinary tract excretion following oral administration of water-soluble contrast media, Radiology 84:1031-1032, 1965.

1966 Dietrich, D. E.: Bowel preparation for outpatient radiography, Radiology 86:488-492, 1966.

Stomach and duodenum; pancreas

1896 Hemmeter, John: Photography of the human stomach by the roentgen method, Boston Med. Surg. J. 25:136, 1896.

1899 Abrams: Eructations and skiagraphy, Philadelphia Med. J. 4:315, 1899.

1906 Einhorn, Max, and Cole, Lewis G.: Roentgenography of the stomach, Med. Record 70:572, 1906.

1913 Beaujeu, M. A.: La radiographie de l'estomac normal, Lyon Méd. 120:832-837, 1913.

Beaujeu, M. A.: Quelques radiographies d'estomacs pathologiques dans le décubitus lateral droit, Lyon Méd. 120:1094-1099, 1913.

1915 American priority in use of bismuth for examination of human stomach (editorial), Amer. J. Roentgen. 2:692, 1915.

1917 Mills, Walter R.: The relation of bodily habitus to visceral form, position, tonus, and motility, Amer. J. Roentgen. 4:155-169, 1917.

1918 Goetze, C.: Die Röntgendiagnostik bei gasgefüllter Bacuhhöhle; eine neue Methode, München. Med. Wschr. 44:1435, 1918.

1921 Guénaux and Vasselle: Technique de l'examen radioscopique du duodenum, J. Radiol. Electr. 5:443-447, 1921.

1922 Lebon and Colombier: L'estomac normal, J. Radiol. Electr. 6:301-320, 1922.

1923 Dufougeré, William, and Dufougeré, A.: De l'emploi des rayons X en stomatologie, Paris, 1923, A. Maloine & Fils.

1926 Vespignani, Arcangelo: La posizione tricliniare destra nell esame radiologico dello stomaco e del duodeno, Radiol. Med. 13:272-281, 1926.

1929 Pendergrass, Robert C.: Roentgenographic examination of the duodenum, Amer. J. Roentgen. 22:355-359, 1929.

1932 Geyman, Milton J.: Evaluation of compression technique in the roentgen examination of duodenal lesions, Amer. J. Roentgen. 28:211-221, 1932.

Grier, G. W.: The advantages of roentgenoscopic control in roentgenography of the stomach, Amer. J. Roentgen. 28:204-210, 1932.

1933 Saito, Makoto: La radiographie des parois de l'estomac, "pneumo-gastro-parietographie," Bull. Chir. Paris 59:910-912, 1933.

1934 Engel, A., and Lysholm, E.: New roentgenological method of pancreas examination and its practical results, Acta Radiol. 15:635-651, 1934.

1936 Kirklin, B. R.: A technic for roentgenoscopic examination of the stomach and duodenum, Radiology 26:521-531, 1936.

1937 Hampton, A. O.: A safe method for the roentgen demonstration of bleeding duodenal ulcers, Amer. J. Roentgen. 38:565-570, 1937.

Schons, Edward: The right oblique horizontal (supine) position in demonstration of the duodenal ulcer crater, Amer. J. Roentgen. 38:42-47, 1937.

1938 Dufour, Pierre: Renseignements fournis par l'étude radiologique de l'estomac en décubitus dorsal, Bull. Soc. Radiol. Méd. Paris 26:116-118, 1938.

Kuhlman, F.: Die Röntgenuntersuchung des Pankreas, Fortschr. Roentgenstr. 57:629-639, 1938.

Schons, E.: La posición horizontal (supina) oblicua derecha para la demonstración del crater de la úlcera duodenal, Rev. Radiol. Fis. 5:69-74, 1938.

1940 Vik, Frances L.: Positioning patients for radiography of the stomach according to body habitus, Xray Techn. 12:85-89, 1940.

1941 Brown, S., McCarthy, J. E., and Fine, A.: Pancreatic tumors, Radiology 36:596-603, 1941.

1944 Templeton, Frederic E.: X-ray examination of the stomach, Chicago, 1944, University of Chicago Press, pp. 507-516.

1945 Thomas, Sydney F.: The value of gastric pneumography in roentgen diagnosis, Radiology 45:128-137, 1945.

1946 Brown, S., and Harper, F. G.: A new roentgen sign in extra-hepatic biliary tract diseases, Radiology 47:239-248, 1946.

Oppenheimer, Albert: The supine projection in the diagnosis of lesions of the corpus and posterior wall of the stomach, Amer. J. Roentgen. 55:454-463, 1946.

1949 Poppel, M. H., Scheinmel, A., and Mednick, E.: The procurement and critical appraisal of the width diameter of the midline retrogastric soft tissues, Amer. J. Roentgen. 61:56-60, 1949.

1951 Clay, R. C., and Hanlon, C. R.: Pneumoperitoneum in differential diagnosis of diaphragmatic hernia, J. Thorac. Cardiov. Surg. 21:57-70, 1951.

Johnstone, A. S.: Diagnosis of early gastric herniation at the esophageal hiatus, J. Fac. Radiologists 3:52-65, 1951.

Lawler, N. A., and McCreath, N. D.: Gastro-esophageal regurgitation, Lancet 2A:369-374, 1951.

Poppel, M. H.: Roentgen manifestations of pancreatic disease, Springfield, Ill., 1951, Charles C Thomas, Publisher.

1952 Evans, John A.: Sliding hiatus hernia, Amer. J. Roentgen. 68:754-763, 1952.

1953 Klami, P.: On the visualization of ulcerative processes using hydrogen peroxide in contrast medium; preliminary report, Acta Radiol. 39:98-104, 1953.

1954 Lockwood, I. H., Smith, A. B., and Shook, L. D.: Lesions in and about the second portion of the duodenum, Amer. J. Roentgen. 71:573-579, 1954.

1955 Liotta, D.: Pour le diagnostic des tumeurs du pancréas: la duodénographie hypotonique, Lyon Chir. 50:455-460, 1955.

1956 Boyd, J. W., Harris, J. R., Butler, E. B., and Donaldson, S. W.: Evaluation of the various methods of demonstrating a hiatus hernia, Amer. J. Roentgen. 75:262-268, 1956.

Wolf, B. S., and Guglielmo, J.: Method for the roentgen demonstration of minimal hiatal herniation, J. Mount Sinai Hosp. 23:738-741, 1956.

1957 Gordon, Sewell S.: The angled posteroanterior projection of the stomach; an attempt at better visualization of the high transverse stomach, Radiology **69**:393-397, 1957.

Hafter, E.: Röntgenologische und klinische Aspekte der Hiatushernie, Radiol. Clin. **26**:382-396, 1957. Abst.: Radiology **71**:458, 1958.

Wolf, B. S., and Guglielmo, J.: The roentgen demonstration of minimal hiatus hernia, Med. Radiogr. Photogr. **33**:90-92, 1957.

1958 Amplatz, K.: A new and simple approach to air-contrast studies of the stomach and duodenum, Radiology **70**:392-394, 1958.

Beranbaum, S. L., and Jacobson, H. G.: Right angle roentgenography of the gastrointestinal tract, Amer. J. Roentgen. **80**:933-944, 1958.

Foegelle, E. F.: Stomach radiography; special emphasis on hiatal hernia, Xray Techn. **30**:167-171, 1958.

Heilbrun, N.: Radiologic study of the cardioesophageal area, New York J. Med. **58**:3280-3283, 1958.

Marshak, R. H., and Gerson, A.: Use of prone pressure device for visualizing hiatus hernia, Amer. J. Dig. Dis. **3**:857-860, 1958.

Schatzki, R., and Gary, J. E.: Face-on demonstration of ulcers in upper stomach in dependent position, Amer. J. Roentgen. **79**:772-780, 1958.

1959 Carmichael, J. H. E.: An evaluation of the toe-touch position in the diagnosis of hiatus hernia, Brit. J. Radiol. **32**:479-482, 1959.

1960 Stein, G. N., and Finkelstein, A.: Hiatal hernia: roentgen incidence and diagnosis, Amer. J. Dig. Dis. **5**:77-87, 1960.

1961 Frimann-Dahl, J.: Radiology in tumors of the pancreas, Clin. Radiol. **12**:73-79, 1961.

Gugliantini, P.: Utilità delle incidenze oblique caudocraniali nello studio radiologico della stenosi congenita ipertrofica del piloro, Ann. Radiol. Diagn. **34**:56-69, 1961. Abst.: Amer. J. Roentgen. **87**:623, 1962.

Sommer, A. W., and Stevenson, C. L.: Hiatal hernia; an evaluation of diagnostic procedures, Amer. J. Dig. Dis. **6**:412-422, 1961.

1962 Frimann-Dahl, J., and Troetteberg, K.: Parietography of the stomach, Brit. J. Radiol. **35**:249-254, 1962.

1963 Martin, J. A.: Esophageal hiatus hernia of the stomach, Amer. J. Roentgen. **90**:799-804, 1963.

1964 Kissler, B., and others: A new method for the roentgenologic opacification of the pancreas, Radiology **83**:611, 1964.

Moldenhauer, W., and Rienck, H.: Die Parietographie, eine Zusatzuntersuchung des Magens [Parietography, an additional study of the stomach], Fortschr. Roentgenstr. **100**:569-578, 1964. Abst.: Amer. J. Roentgen. **92**:1213, 1964.

Pattinson, J. N.: Iodine compounds in the alimentary tract, Radiography **30**:103-109, 1964.

Sim, G. P. G.: An evaluation of tests for hiatus hernia, Brit. J. Radiol. **37**:781-787, 1964.

Stein, G. N., and others: Evaluation of conventional roentgenographic techniques for demonstration of duodenal ulcer craters, Amer. J. Roentgen. **91**:801-807, 1964.

1965 Kissler, B., and others: The roentgenologic diagnosis of pancreatic disease, Radiology **85**:59-64, 1965.

Köhler, Rolf: Parietography of the stomach, Acta Radiol. [Diagn.] **3**:393-406, 1965.

1966 Beranbaum, S. L.: Carcinoma of the pancreas; a bidirectional roentgen approach, Amer. J. Roentgen. **96**:447-467, 1966.

Kalokerinos, J.: Olympus GFT camera gastroscope and Olympus GT5 standard gastrocamera: realm of radiologist, Australas. Radiol. **10**:39-44, 1966.

Porta, E., and Verrengia, F.: Gastric parietography in the preoperative evaluation of surgical therapy of neoplasms of the stomach, Ann. Radiol. Diagn. **39**:492-524, 1966. (In Italian.) Abst.: Radiology **89**:1130, 1967; Amer. J. Roentgen. **103**:241, 1968.

Raia, S., and Kreel, L.: Gas-distention double-contrast duodenography using the Scott-Harden gastroduodenal tube, Gut **7**:420-424, 1966.

Shirakabe, H.: Atlas of x-ray diagnosis of early gastric cancer, Philadelphia, 1966, J. B. Lippincott Co.

Taylor, D. A., and others: A new method for visualizing the gastric wall, Radiology **86**:711-717, 1966.

1967 Bilbao, M. K., Frische, L. H., Dotter, C. T., and Rosch, J.: Hypotonic duodenography, Radiology **89**:438-443, 1967.

Blendis, L., Beilby, J., Wilson, J., and others: Carcinoma of the stomach: evaluation of individual and combined diagnostic accuracy of radiology, cytology and gastrophotography, Brit. Med. J. **1**:656-659, 1967.

Blendis, L., Cameron, A., and Hadley, G.: Analysis of 400 examinations using the gastrocamera, Gut **8**:83-87, 1967.

Gianturco, C.: Rapid fluoroscopic duodenal intubation, Radiology **88**:1165-1166, 1967.

Hanafee, W. N., and Weiner, M.: External guided passage of an intestinal intubation tube, Radiology **89**:1100-1102, 1967.

Kreel, L.: The pancreas: newer radiological methods of investigation, Postgrad. Med. J. **43**:14-23, 1967.

Morrissey, J., Tanaka, Y., and Thorsen, W.: Gastroscopy: review of English and Japanese literature, Gastroenterology **53**:456-476, 1967.

1968 Bilbao, M. K., Rosch, J., Frische, L. H., and Dotter, C. T.: Hypotonic duodenography in the diagnosis of pancreatic disease, Seminars Roentgen. **3**:280-287, 1968.

Brunner, S., Rahbek, J., and Mosbech, J.: Roentgenologic and gastrocamera examinations in the differential diagnosis of gastric ulcer, Amer. J. Roentgen. **104**:598-602, 1968.

Hajdu, N.: The role of translateral films in the barium meal, Clin. Radiol. **19**:33-46, 1968. Abst.: Amer. J. Roentgen. **103**:484, 1968.

Kreissmann, A.: Hypotonic duodenography, Fortschr. Roentgenstr. **108**:464-474, 1968. (In German.) Abst.: Radiology **92**:661, 1969.

Lieber, A., Schaefer, J. W., and Belin, R. P.: Hypotonic duodenography; diagnosis of annular pancreas in an adult, J.A.M.A. **203**:425-427, 1968.

Mallet-Guy, P., Jacquemet, P., Murat, J., and Ejazi, M.: Experience with modern radiologic techniques in pancreatic diseases, Ann. Radiol. **11**:857-863, 1968. (In French.) Abst.: Radiology **93**:1397, 1969.

Schottman, G. W.: Fluoroscopy supply cart, Radiology **90**:1207, 1968.

Sim, G. P. G.: The diagnosis of craters in the duodenal cap, Brit. J. Radiol. **41**:792-794, 1968.

Solomon, A.: Hypotonic duodenography, S. Afr. Med. J. **42**:1039-1040, 1968.

1969 Gelfand, D. W., and Hachiya, J.: The double-contrast examination of the stomach using gas-producing granules and tablets, Radiology **93**:1381-1382, 1969.

Goldstein, H. M., and Zboralske, F. F.: Tubeless hypotonic duodenography, J.A.M.A. **210**:2086-2088, 1969.

Kisseler, B., Buysch, K. H., Paschke, K. G., and Suchan, M.: Simple method for demonstrating the gastric wall, Fortschr. Roentgenstr. **110**:630-639, 1969. (In German.) Abst.: Radiology **94**:729, 1969.

Lawson, T. L., and Margulis, A. R.: A simplified tube control method of hypotonic duodenography, Radiology **92**:1119-1120, 1969.

Meyerhofer, H.: "Conventional" roentgen diagnosis of pancreatic diseases (with special consideration of hypotonic duodenography and percutaneous transhepatic cholangiography), Roentgenblätter **22**:24-34, 1969. (In German.) Abst.: Radiology **93**:1398, 1969.

Sargent, E. N., and Meyers, H. I.: Wire guide and technique for Cantor tube insertion; rapid small bowel intubation, Amer. J. Roentgen. **107**:150-155, 1969.

Solanke, T. F., Kumakura, K., Maruyama, M., and Someya, N.: Double-contrast method for the evaluation of gastric lesions, Gut **10**:436-442, 1969.

Sparberg, M.: Gastroscopy without assistance: description of technique, Gastroint. Endosc. **15**:114-116, 1969.

Stage, P., and Banke, L.: Hypotonic duodenography, Gut **10**:428-432, 1969.

Stordy, S. N., Greig, J. H., and Bogoch, A.: The steak and barium meal; a method for evaluating gastric emptying after partial gastrectomy, Amer. J. Dig. Dis. **14**:463-469, 1969.

Tréheux, A., Fays, J., and Velut, A.: The use of hypotonic duodenography in the diagnosis of post-bulbar ulcers, Ann. Radiol. **12**:451-465, 1969. (In French.) Abst.: Radiology **95**:474, 1970.

1970 Amberg, J. R., and Unger, J. D.: Contamination of barium sulfate suspension, Radiology **97**:182-183, 1970.

Ferrucci, J. T., Benedict, K. T., Page, D. L., and others: Radiologic features of the normal hypotonic duodenogram, Radiology **96**:401-408, 1970.

Gelfand, D. W., and Moskowitz, M.: Massive gastric dilatation complicating hypotonic duodenography; a report of three cases, Radiology **97**:637-639, 1970.

Herrera, C. A.: Normal and pathologic radiology of the esophago-cardio-tuberosity area, Rev. Argent. Radiol. **33**:247-262, 1970. (In Spanish.) Abst.: Amer. J. Roentgen. **112**:862, 1971.

Kadell, B. M., Weiner, M., Johnson, J. N., and Pops, M.: The gastrocamera—a method in vivo: roentgenologic-pathologic correlation, Amer. J. Roentgen. **110**:315-321, 1970.

Poole, G. J.: A new roentgenographic method of measuring the retrogastric and retroduodenal spaces: statisitcal evaluation of reliability and diagnostic utility, Radiology **97**:71-81, 1970.

1971 Calenoff, L., and Sparberg, M.: Gastric pseudolesions: roentgenographic-gastrophotographic correlation, Amer. J. Roentgen. **113**:139-146, 1971.

Hanelin, J.: Some technical aspects in the demonstration of gastric lesions, Seminars Roentgen. **6**:235-253, 1971.

Hines, W. B., Kerr, R. M., Meschan, I., and Martin, J. F.: Roentgenologic and gastrocamera correlation in lesions of the stomach, Amer. J. Roentgen. **113**:129-138, 1971.

1972 Mettler, F. A., and Ghahremani, G. G.: The fuzzy fluid level sign, Radiology **105**:509-511, 1972.

Obata, W. G.: A double-contrast technique for examination of the stomach using barium sulfate with simethicone, Amer. J. Roentgen. **115**:275-280, 1972.

Sear, H. S., and Friedenberg, M. J.: Simplified technique for tubeless hypotonic duodenography, Radiology **103**:210, 1972.

1973 Maurer, H. J., Odegaard, H. I., Mair, I. W. S., and Natvig, K.: Radiological findings in the globus syndrome; conventional radiographic examination of the esophagus and stomach with the additional use of acid barium, Fortschr. Roentgenstr. **118**:446-450, 1973. (In German.) Abst.: Radiology **110**:245, 1974.

Miller, R. E., Chermish, S. M., Rosenak, B. D., and Rodda, B. E.: Hypotonic duodenography with Glucagon, Radiology **108**:35-42, 1973.

Pochaczevsky, R.: "Bubbly barium": a carbonated cocktail for double-contrast examination of the stomach, Radiology **107**:465-466, 1973.

Wendth, A. J.: Hypotonic duodenography; a modified technique using a selective catheter system, Radiology **108**:274, 1973.

Small intestine

1912 Cole, Lewis G.: Radiography of the intestinal tract, Arch. Roentgen Ray, 1912.

Cole, Lewis G.: The value of serial radiography in gastro-intestinal diagnosis, J.A.M.A. **65**:1947, 1912.

1928 Case, James T.: Roentgenological aid in the diagnosis of ileus, Amer. J. Roentgen. **19**:413-425, 1928.

1929 Pesquera, G. S.: Method for direct visualization of lesions in the small intestines, Amer. J. Roentgen. **22**:254-257, 1929.

1938 Ghelew, B., and Mengis, O.: Mise en évidence de l'intestin grêle par une nouvelle technique radiologique, Presse Méd. **46**:444-445, 1938.

1939 Gershon-Cohen, J., and Shay, H.: Barium enteroclysis; method for direct immediate examination of the small intestine by single and double contrast techniques, Amer. J. Roentgen. **42**:456-458, 1939.

Wangensteen, O. H., and Rea, C. E.: Distention factor in simple intestinal obstruction, Surgery **5**:327-339, 1939.

1943 Schatzki, Richard: Small intestinal enema, Amer. J. Roentgen. **50**:743-751, 1943.

1946 Beilin, David S.: Lesions of the duodenum, jejunum and ileum. In Pillmore, George U., editor: Clinical radiology, Philadelphia, 1946, F. A. Davis Co., vol. 1, pp. 543-544.

1947 Frimann-Dahl, J.: Roentgenological examination of ileus, Acta Radiol. **28**:331-351, 1947.

1948 Wyatt, G. M.: Barium sulfate in saline suspension, Radiology **51**:326-330, 1948.

1949 Weintraub, S., and Williams, R. G.: A rapid method of roentgenologic examination of the small intestine, Amer. J. Roentgen. **61**:45-55, 1949.

1959 Golden, Ross: Radiological examination of the small intestine, ed. 2, 1959, Springfield, Ill., Charles C Thomas, Publisher.

Golden, Ross: Technical factors in the roentgen examination of the small intestine, Amer. J. Roentgen. **82**:965-972, 1959.

1960 Greenspon, E. A., and Lentino, W.: Retrograde enterography; a new method for the roentgenologic study of the small bowel, Amer. J. Roentgen. **83**:909-918, 1960.

Martel, W., Whitehouse, W. M., and Hodges, F. J.: Small bowel tumors, Radiology **75**:368-379, 1960.

1961 Morton, J. L.: Notes on small bowel examination, Amer. J. Roentgen. **86**:76-85, 1961.

1962 Friedenberg, M. J.: Roentgen study of the small bowel in adults and children with neostigmine, Amer. J. Roentgen, **88**:693-701, 1962.

Pygott, F.: The small bowel; its radiographic investigation, Radiography **28**:191-203, 1962.

1965 Miller, R. E.: Complete reflux small bowel examination, Radiology **84**:457-463, 1965.

1969 Howarth, F. H., Cockel, R., Roper, B. W., and Hawkins, C. F.: The effect of Metoclopramide upon gastric motility and its value in barium progress meals, Clin. Radiol. **20**:294-300, 1969.

1971 Goldstein, H. M., Poole, G. J., Rosenquist, C. J., and others: Comparison of methods for acceleration of small intestinal radiographic examination, Radiology **98**:519-523, 1971.

1972 Miller, R. E., and Lehman, G.: Localization of small bowel hemorrhage; complete reflux small bowel examination, Amer. J. Dig. Dis. **17**:1019-1023, 1972.

Large intestine

1914 Jangeas and Friedel: L'examen du rectum et de l'anse sigmoïde par les rayons X, J. Radiol. Electr. **1**:257-261, 1914.

1922 Montanari, Arrigo: La posizione laterale sinistra nello studio radiologico del colon destro, Atti Congresso Ital. Radiol. Med. **4**:83-111, 1922.

1923 Fischer, A. W.: Ueber eine neue röntenologische Untersuchungsmethode des Dickdarms: Kombination von Kontrasteinlauf und Luftaufblähung, Klin. Wschr. **2**:1595-1598, 1923.

1925 Fischer, A. W.: Ueber die Röntgenuntersuchung des Dickdarms mit Hilfe einer Kombination von Lufteinblasung und Kontrasteinlauf, Arch. Klin. Chir. **134**:209-269, 1925.

1928 Ottonello, P.: La proiezione laterale sinistrodestra della regione cecale, Atti Congresso Ital. Radiol. Med. **8**:347-348, 1928.

Podesta, V.: La proiezione assiale del colon e del bacino, Atti Congresso Ital. Radiol. Med. **8**:346, 1928.

1929 Ottonello, P.: La proiezione laterale sinistradestra del tratto ileo-ceco-colico, Radiol. Med. **26**:74-90, 1929.

1930 Eisler, F.: Zur Technik der Dickdarmuntersuchung, Röntgenpraxis **2**:741-742, 1930.

Wolf, A.: Das Rektum und das untere Sigmoid, Fortschr. Roentgenstr. **42**:358-363, 1930.

1931 Bertel, G.: Sui metodi d'indagine radiologica per una più esatta interpretazione di alcuni sintomi di affezioni del grosso intestino, Arch. Radiol. **7**:297-334, 1931.

Weber, Harry M.: The roentgenologic demonstration of

polypoid lesions and polyposis of the large intestine, Amer. J. Roentgen. **25**:577-587, 1931.

Wolf, A.: Study of the pathological rectum, Fortschr. Roentgenstr. **44**:342-347, 1931.

1932 Gerson-Cohen, J., and Shay, H.: The colon as studied by the double contrast enema, Amer. J. Roentgen. **27**:838, 1932.

Stewart, W. H., and Stewart, H. E.: A method of more clearly visualizing lesions of sigmoid, Amer. J. Roentgen. **28**:379-384, 1932.

1933 Fricke, O.: A new method of roentgenological presentation of the rectum, Röntgenpraxis **5**:365-368, 1933.

1934 Walther, Hans E.: Die Darstellung der untersten Partien des Dickdarmes im Röntgenbild, Acta Radiol. **15**:487-490, 1934.

1935 Levy, Florence: Visualization of the colon by the combined method, Xray Techn. **7**:76-77, 1935.

1937 Case, James T.: Comparison of methods of roentgen examinations of the colon, J.A.M.A. **108**:2028-2034, 1937.

Pansdorf, Hans: Die Darstellung tiefsitzender Krankheitsprozesse am Sigma im Röntgenbild, Röntgenpraxis **9**:764-769, 1937.

1938 Robins, Samuel A., and Altman, William S.: The significance of the lateral view of the rectum, Amer. J. Roentgen. **40**:598-605, 1938.

1939 Oppenheimer, A., and Saleeby, G. W.: Proctography; roentgenologic studies of the rectum and sigmoid, Surg. Gynec. Obstet. **69**:83-93, 1939.

Wangensteen, O. H., and Rea, C. E.: Distention factor in simple intestinal obstruction, Surgery **5**:327-339, 1939.

1940 Stewart, Wm. H., Huber, Frank, and Ghiselin, F. H.: An improved routine for the roentgen examination of the rectum and sigmoid, Amer. J. Dig. Dis. **7**:244-247, 1940.

1944 Billing, Lars: Zur Technik der Kontrastuntersuchung des Colon sigmoideum, Acta Radiol. **25**:418-422, 1944.

Henderson, N. P.: The value of the opaque enema and its modifications, Brit. J. Radiol. **17**:140-149, 1944.

Oppenheimer, Albert: Roentgen diagnosis of incipient cancer of the rectum, Amer. J. Roentgen. **52**:637-646, 1944.

Pendergrass, R. C., and Cooper, F. W., Jr.: Simple method for study of the colon in the presence of a colostomy, Amer. J. Roentgen. **52**:563, 1944.

Poppel, M. H.: The roentgen demonstration of Meckel's diverticulum, Amer. J. Roentgen. **51**:205-206, 1944.

1946 Brust, John C. M., and Childs, Donald S.: Lesions of the colon, rectum, anus and appendix. In Pillmore, George U., editor: Clinical radiology, Philadelphia, 1946, F. A. Davis Co., vol. 1, pp. 594-597.

Robin, P. A.: A method for barium enema examination of the patient with a colostomy, Amer. J. Roentgen. **55**:782-783, 1946.

1947 Davis, Carl, Jr.: Enema tube perforation of colon, Ann. Surg. **126**:377-379, 1947.

1948 Fletcher, G. H.: An improved method of visualization of the sigmoid, Amer. J. Roentgen. **59**:750-752, 1948.

1950 Gianturco, C.: High-voltage technic in diagnosis of polypoid growths of the colon, Radiology **55**:27-29, 1950.

Loehr, W. M.: A method for improving roentgenograms of the colon after colostomy, Amer. J. Roentgen. **64**:835-836, 1950.

Root, J. C., and Rayle, A. A.: A device for roentgen examination of the colon following colostomy, Radiology **54**:732-734, 1950.

Scheidt, R.: Darmperforation nach Kontrastdarstellung bei stenosierendem Sigma-carcinom, Chirug **21**:602-603, 1950.

Yates, C. W., Moreton, R. D., and Cooper, E. M.: Double-contrast studies of the colon with special reference to preparation and fictitious polyps, Radiology **55**:539-544, 1950.

1951 Cross, F. S.: A new method for obtaining barium enemas in colostomy patients, Surgery **30**:460-464, 1951.

Moreton, R. D., and others: One-stage method of double-contrast study of the colon, Radiology **56**:214-221, 1951.

Raap, Gerard: A position of value in studying the pelvis and its contents, Southern Med. J. **44**:95-99, 1951.

Templeton, F. E., and Addington, E. A.: Roentgenologic examination of the colon using drainage and negative pressure, with special reference to early diagnosis of neoplasms, J.A.M.A. **145**:702-704, 1951.

1952 Greene, E. I., and Greene, J. M.: Traumatic perforation of the colon in a patient with a colostomy, J.A.M.A. **148**:49-50, 1952.

Kleinsasser, L. J., and Warshaw, H.: Perforation of the sigmoid colon during barium enema; report of a case with review of the literature, and experimental study of the effect of barium sulfate injected intraperitoneally, Ann. Surg. **135**:560-565, 1952.

Roman, P. W., and others: Massive fatal embolism during barium enema study, Radiology **59**:190-192, 1952.

Stevenson, C. A.: Technic of double contrast examination of the colon, Surg. Clin. N. Amer. **32**:1531-1537, 1952.

Zheutlin, N., Lasser, E. C., and Rigler, L. G.: Clinical studies on the effect of barium in the peritoneal cavity following rupture of the colon, Surgery **32**:967-979, 1952.

1953 Gianturco, C., and Miller, G. A.: Routine search for colonic polyps by high-voltage radiography, Radiology **60**:496-499, 1953.

Hodges, P. C.: Roentgen examination of the colon, J.A.M.A. **153**:1417-1421, 1953.

Kaufman, P. A., and Swerdlow, H.: Bowel perforation following enema through a permanent colostomy, Arch. Surg. **67**:612-615, 1953.

Klein, R. R., and Scarborough, R. A.: Traumatic perforations of the rectum and distal colon, Amer. J. Surg. **86**:515-522, 1953.

Potter, R. M.: Dilute contrast media in the diagnosis of lesions of the colon, Radiology **60**:500-509, 1953.

1954 Cimmino, C. V.: Radiography of the sigmoid flexure with the Chassard-Lapiné projection, Med. Radiogr. Photogr. **30**:44-45, 1954.

Ettinger, A., and Elkin, M.: Study of the sigmoid by special roentgenographic views, Amer. J. Roentgen. **72**:199-208, 1954.

Govoni, A., Brailsford, J. F., and Mucklow, E. H.: The use of hydrogen peroxide for the elimination of gas from the intestine during roentgenography of the abdominal viscera, Amer. J. Roentgen. **71**:235-238, 1954.

Hill, L. F.: Enemas can be fatal (editor's column), J. Pediat. **45**:751-753, 1954.

Stevenson, C. A.: The development of the colon examination, Amer. J. Roentgen. **71**:385-397, 1954.

1955 Lusted, L. B., and Miller, E. R.: A pneumocolon bottle, Radiology **64**:424-425, 1955.

Welin, S.: Demonstration of polyps in the colon with double contrast method, Fortschr. Roentgenstr. **82**:341-344, 1955.

1956 Osborne, G., Pattinson, G. N., and Ward, M. W. P.: The value of the lateral view of the rectosigmoid, J. Fac. Radiologists **7**:286-290, 1956.

Sánchez, L. A.: The use of hydrogen peroxide to eliminate intestinal gas, Radiología **7**:17-18, 1956. (In Spanish.) Abst.: Radiology **69**:625-626, 1957.

Shapiro, J. H., and Rifkin, H.: Perforation of the colon during a barium enema study, Amer. J. Dig. Dis. **1**:430-436, 1956.

Westing, S. W.: Note on barium enema examination of incontinent patients, Radiology **66**:582-584, 1956.

1957 Hartman, A. W., and Hills, W. J.: Rupture of colon in infants during barium enema; report of two cases, Ann. Surg. **145**:712-717, 1957.

Levene, G.: Rates of venous absorption of carbon dioxide and air used in double contrast examination of the colon, Radiology **69**:571-575, 1957.

Levene, G., and Kaufman, S. A.: An improved technic for double contrast examination of the colon by the use of compressed carbon dioxide, Radiology **68**:83-85, 1957.

Robinson, J. M.: Polyps of the colon: how to find them, Amer. J. Roentgen. **77**:700-725, 1957.

1958 Chuker, G. N., and Gilmer, W. P.: Preparation of the

colon prior to barium enema, Radiology **71**:570-572, 1958.

Grillo, H. C., and Nardi, G. L.: Perforation of the colon during enema into the colonic stoma, Surg. Gynec. Obstet. **107**:659-662, 1958.

Welin, S.: Modern trends in diagnostic roentgenology of the colon, Brit. J. Radiol. **31**:453-464, 1958.

1959   Gillespie, J. B., Miller, G. A., and Schlereth, J.: Water intoxication following enemas for roentgenographic preparation, Amer. J. Roentgen. **82**:1067-1069, 1959.

Grodsky, L.: Perforation of the colon and rectum during administration of barium enema, Dis. Colon Rectum **2**:216-225, 1959.

Lörinc, P., and Brahame, F.: Perforation of the colon during examination by the double contrast method, Gastroenterology **37**:770-773, 1959.

Rosenberg, L. S., and Fine, A.: Fatal venous intravasation of barium during a barium enema, Radiology **73**:771-773, 1959.

Santulli, T. V.: Perforation of the rectum or colon in infancy due to enema, Pediatrics **23**:972-976, 1959.

1960   Forrester, H. C., and Soule, A. B.: The value of routine lateral rectal projection in barium enema study, Acta Radiol. **53**:113-119, 1960.

Furste, W., and Knoernschild, H.: Perforation of the distal large intestine produced by intraluminal traumas, Amer. J. Surg. **99**:665-675, 1960.

Lame, E. L.: A new design for barium rectal tube, Radiology **75**:289-291, 1960.

Margulis, A. R., and Jovanovich, A.: Roentgen diagnosis of submucous lipomas of the colon, Amer. J. Roentgen. **84**:1114-1120, 1960.

Meyers, P. H.: Contamination of barium enema apparatus during its use, J.A.M.A. **173**:1589-1590, 1960.

Nathan, M. H., and Kohen, R.: The Bardex tube in performing barium enemas; evaluation of its use and safety, Amer. J. Roentgen. **84**:1121-1124, 1960.

Porter, E. C.: The risk of barium enema, J. Maine Med. Ass. **51**:422-423, 1960.

Steinbach, H. L., Rousseau, R., McCormack, K. R., and Jawetz, E.: Transmission of enteric pathogens by barium enema, J.A.M.A. **174**:1207-1208, 1960.

1961   Dreyfuss, J. R., Robbins, L. L., and Murphy, J. T.: Disposable plastic unit for barium enema examination, Radiology **77**:834-835, 1961.

Keynes, W. M.: Implantation from bowel lumen in cancer of the large intestine, Ann. Surg. **153**:357-364, 1961.

Levene, G.: Low temperature barium-water suspensions for roentgenologic examination of the colon, Radiology **77**:117-118, 1961.

Pochaczevsky, R., Sherman, R. S., and Meyers, P. H.: Disposable kit for barium enemas, Radiology **77**:831-833, 1961.

1962   Cook, G. B., and Margulis, A. R.: The use of silicone foam for examining the human sigmoid colon, Amer. J. Roentgen. **87**:633-643, 1962.

Pagan-Carlo, J., and others: Hypaque enema as diagnostic aid in evaluation of intestinal obstruction in newborn infant, Amer. J. Roentgen. **88**:571-574, 1962.

Steinbach, H. L., and Burhenne, H. J.: Performing the barium enema; equipment, preparation, and contrast medium, Amer. J. Roentgen. **87**:644-654, 1962.

1963   Hemley, S. D., and Kanick, V.: Perforation of the rectum; a complication of barium enema following rectal biopsy, report of two cases, Amer. J. Dig. Dis. **8**:882-884, 1963.

Pochaczevsky, R., and Sherman, R. S.: A new technique for the roentgenologic examination of the colon, Amer. J. Roentgen. **89**:787-796, 1963.

Riordan, A. F., and others: Bowel preparation for radiologic examination; comparison of techniques, J. Canad. Ass. Radiol. **14**:26-28, 1963.

Shehadi, William H.: Studies of the colon and small intestines with water-soluble iodinated contrast media, Amer. J. Roentgen. **89**:740-751, 1963.

1964   Meyers, P. H., Nice, C. M., Mouton, R., and Stern, H. S.: Controlled standardization in examination of the colon, Southern Med. J. **57**:1429-1431, 1964.

Meyers, P. H., and Richards, M.: Transmission of polio

virus vaccine by contaminated barium enema with resultant antibody rise, Amer. J. Roentgen. **91**:864-865, 1964.

Noveroske, R. J.: Intracolonic pressures during barium enema examinations, Amer. J. Roentgen. **91**:852-863, 1964.

1965   Almen, T.: Simple device for technical improvement of bowel examination of patients with a colostomy, Brit. J. Radiol. **38**:75-76, 1965.

Brown, B. St. J.: Defecography or anorectal studies in children including cinefluorographic observations, J. Canad. Ass. Radiol. **16**:66-76, 1965.

Dahl, L. E.: Colon examinations in patients with colostomies, Acta Radiol. [Diagn.] **3**:30-32, 1965.

Green, W. W., and Blank, W. A.: Colostomy perforations by the irrigating tip, Dis. Colon Rectum **8**:59-61, 1965.

Seaman, W. B., and Wells, J.: Complications of the barium enema, Gastroenterology **48**:728-737, 1965.

1966   Anderson, J. J. F.: Device for colon examination in patients with colostomia, Radiologe **6**:380, 1966.

Dysart, D. N., and Stewart, H. R.: Special angled roentgenography for lesions of the rectosigmoid, Amer. J. Roentgen. **96**:285-291, 1966.

Miller, R. E.: Enema control for difficult patients, Radiology **87**:756-758, 1966.

Noveroske, R. J.: Perforation of the rectosigmoid by a Bardex balloon catheter; report of three cases, Amer. J. Roentgen. **96**:326-331, 1966.

Shea, F. P.: The problem of tannic acid in colon examinations (editorial), Amer. J. Roentgen. **96**:520-522, 1966.

Spiro, R. H., and Hertz, R. E.: Colostomy perforation, Surgery **60**:590-597, 1966.

Stevens, G. M.: The use of a water enema in the verification of lipoma of the colon, Amer. J. Roentgen. **96**:292-297, 1966.

Virtama, P.: Rectal parietography in ulcerative colitis, Acta Radiol. [Diagn.] **4**:344-348, 1966.

1967   Becker, M. H., Genieser, N. B., and Clark, H.: Perforation of the colon during barium enema, New York State J. Med. **67**:278-282, 1967.

Miller, R. E.: The clarity of good technic, Amer. J. Dig. Dis. **12**:418-420, 1967.

Pantone, A. M., and Berlin, L.: Air-contrast examination of the colon: an entity of the past, Amer. J. Dig. Dis. **12**:110-112, 1967.

Welin, S.: Results of the Malmo technique of colon examination, J.A.M.A. **199**:369-371, 1967.

1968   Brekkan, A., and Axen, O.: Roentgen examination of enterostomy openings with use of vacuum suction, Radiology **91**:385-386, 1968.

1969   Laird, D. R.: Colostomy safety tip, Dis. Colon Rectum **12**:59-60, 1969.

Miller, R. E.: A new enema tip, Radiology **92**:1492, 1969.

Nigro, N. D.: A special catheter for colostomy irrigation, Dis. Colon Rectum **12**:61-62, 1969.

1970   Amberg, J. R., and Unger, J. D.: Contamination of barium sulfate suspension, Radiology **97**:182-183, 1970.

Apsimon, H. T.: The single phase double-contrast enema; a technique suitable for the average department, Clin. Radiol. **21**:188-194, 1970.

Brown, R. C., and Cohen, W. N.: A new projection for demonstrating the sigmoid colon, J. Canad. Ass. Radiol. **21**:27-30, 1970.

Burhenne, H. J.: Technique of colostomy examination, Radiology **97**:183-185, 1970.

Mattsson, O.: A safer enema nozzle, Acta Radiol. [Diagn.] **10**:557-560, 1970.

Miller, R. E.: Simple apparatus for decubitus films with horizontal beam, Radiology **97**:682-683, 1970.

Pearl, T., and Goldman, W.: Unravelling the tangled sigmoid: routine angulation of the tube in the detection of occult lesions, Amer. J. Roentgen. **110**:399-405, 1970.

Wener, L.: The angled prone projection: its value in diagnosis of low-lying lesions, Amer. J. Roentgen. **110**:393-398, 1970.

1971 Land, R. E.: Colostomy enema; description of a catheter-nipple device, Radiology **100**:36, 1971.

Pochaczevsky, R., and Meyers, P. H.: A safe, self-retaining, disposable rectal catheter for barium enemas with sealed insufflation bulb and movable external retention cushion, Amer. J. Roentgen. **113**:359-361, 1971.

Waldron, R. L., and Seaman, W. B.: Roentgenographic examination of patients with colostomies, enterostomies, and large fistulous and sinus tracts, Amer. J. Roentgen. **113**:297-300, 1971.

1972 Ferrucci, J. T., Jr.: Hypotonic barium enema examination, Amer. J. Roentgen. **116**:304-308, 1972.

Pochaczevsky, R., and Meyers, P. H.: A new, disposable catheter for selective guided barium enemas; contrast examinations in patients with colostomies, rectal lesions and fistulas and for pediatric colon studies, Amer. J. Roentgen. **115**:392-395, 1972.

1973 Hamelin, L., and Hurtubise, M.: Remote control technique in double-contrast study of the colon, Amer. J. Roentgen. **119**:382-392, 1973.

1974 Miller, R. E.: The barium enema as a cancer detection procedure: its use and abuse. In Radiologic and other biophysical methods in tumor diagnosis. Chicago, 1974, Year Book Medical Publishers, Inc.

URINARY TRACT AND ADRENAL GLANDS

1896 Macintyre, J.: Roentgen rays—photography of renal calculus; description of adjustable modification in focus tube, Lancet **2**:118, 1896.

1900 Albers-Schönberg, H. E.: Zur Technik der Nierensteinaufnahmen, Fortschr. Roentgenstr. **3**:210, 1900.

1904 Close, B.: Radiographie eines durch das Kystoskop diagnostizierten Falles von kompletter Ureterenverdopplung, Deutsch. Z. Chir. **72**:613, 1904.

1906 Voelker, F., and von Lichtenberg, A.: Pyleographie des Nierenbeckens nach Kollargolfüllung, München. Med. Wschr. **53**:105-107, 1906.

1907 Sträter, A.: Die Röntgenographie der Nieren, Verk. Deutsch. Röntgen. **3**:90, 1907.

1910 Lomon, Andre: Die Radiographie der Uretergegend, Bull. Soc. Radiol. Méd. Paris **14**:1910. Abst.: Fortschr. Roentgenstr. **15**:315, 1910.

Pasteau and Bélot: Die radiographische Darstellung der Niere, Paris Chir., Feb.-Mar., 1910. Abst.: Fortschr. Roentgenstr. **14**:448, 1910.

Uhle, A. A., Pfahler, G. E., Mackimey, W. H., and Miller A. G.: Combined cystoscopic and roentgenographic examination of the kidneys and ureter, Ann. Surg. **51**:546, 1910.

1911 Holland, Charles T.: Recent development in pyelography, Arch. Roentgen Ray **16**:134, 1911.

1916 Garratt, John M.: Roentgenographic examination of the urinary bladder, Amer. J. Roentgen. **3**:399-402, 1916.

1918 Kretschmer, Herman L.: A new procedure for the localization of ureteral stone, Surg. Gynec. Obstet. **27**:472-474, 1918.

1919 Pfahler, George E.: Injection of air for the roentgen diagnosis of tumors of the bladder, Amer. J. Roentgen. **6**:371, 1919.

1920 Braash, W. F.: Roentgen examination of the urinary tract made opaque, Amer. J. Roentgen. **7**:584, 1920.

1921 Carelli, H. H., and Sordelli, E.: Un nuevo procedimiento para explorar el riñon, Rev. Ass. Med. Argent. **34**:424, 1921.

Lawrence, W. S.: Remarks on the technique of the roentgen examination of the kidneys, Amer. J. Roentgen. **8**:115-119, 1921.

Sgalitzer, M., and Hryntschak, T.: Roentgen investigation of the bladder in the lateral position, Z. Urol. **15**:10, 1921.

1923 Béclère, Henri: Radiographies rénales de profil, Bull. Soc. Radiol. Méd. Paris **11**:36, 1923.

Nichols, Bernhard H.: Important points in the technique of roentgenological examinations of the urinary tract, Amer. J. Roentgen. **10**:19-27, 1923.

Rowntree, L. G., Sutherland, C. G., Osborne, E. D., and Scholl, A. J., Jr.: Roentgenography of the urinary tract during excretion of sodium iodide, J.A.M.A. **80**:368, 1923.

Thompson-Walker, J., and Knox, R.: Observations on the lateral position and other methods of examination of the renal and gall bladder areas, Amer. J. Roentgen. **10**:681-696, 1923.

1924 Hickey, Preston M.: Roentgen-ray examination of the urinary tract. In Cabot, Hugh, editor: Modern urology, Philadelphia, 1924, Lea & Febiger, vol. 1, pp. 119-137.

1926 Gottlieb, J., and Strokoff, F.: Röntgendiagnostik der Divertikel der Harnblase, Fortschr. Roentgenstr. **35**:574-578, 1926-1927.

1927 Giongo, Franco: Considerazioni sulla pielografia, Radiol. Med. **14**:387-424, 1927.

1929 Mulvey, Marie: The technique for roentgen ray examination of the kidney, Xray Techn. **1**:20, 1929.

Roseno, A., and Jepkins, H.: Intravenous pyelography, Fortschr. Roentgenstr. **39**:859-863, 1929. (In German.) Abst.: Amer. J. Roentgen. **22**:685-686, 1929.

Swick, M.: Darstellung der Niere und Harnwege im Röntgenbild durch intravenöse Einbringung eines neuen Kontraststoffes des Uroselectans, Klin. Wschr. **8**:2087-2089, 1929. Abst.: Amer. J. Roentgen. **23**:686-687, 1930.

Von Lichtenberg, A., and Swick, M.: Klinische Prüfung des Uroselectans, Klin. Wschr. **8**:2089, 1929.

1930 Hirsch, I. Seth: Urography by uroselectan, Radiology **15**:480, 1930.

Maxentia, Sister M.: Kidney technic, Xray Techn. **2**:20-22, 1930.

Swick, M.: Intravenous urography by means of sodium salt of 5-iodo-2 pyridon-N-acetic acid, J.A.M.A. **95**:1403, 1930.

1931 Magnusson, W.: On meteorism in pyelography and on passage of gas through the small intestine, Acta Radiol. **12**:552-561, 1931.

Mertz, H. O.: The lateral pyelogram, J. Indiana Med. Ass. **24**:537-541, 1931.

Ochsner, H. C., and Wishard, W. N., Jr.: Urinary tract roentgenography by means of skiodon, Amer. J. Roentgen. **25**:314-319, 1931.

Young, Hugh H., and Waters, Charles A.: Urological roentgenology. In Case, James T., editor: Annals of roentgenology, vol. 1, New York, 1931, Paul B. Hoeber, Inc.

1932 Barsóny, Theodor, and Koppenstein, Ernst: Verbesserte röntgenologische Darstellung des Harnblasenbodens, Röntgenpraxis **4**:778-781, 1932.

Wesson, M. B., and Fulmer, C. C.: Influence of ureteral stones on intravenous urograms, Amer. J. Roentgen. **28**:27-33, 1932.

1933 Barsóny, Theodor, and Pollack, E.: Intravenous urocystography, Röntgenpraxis, Nov. 15, 1953. Abst.: Yearbook of Radiology, pp. 357-358, 1933.

Swick, M.: Excretion urography with particular reference to newly developed compound; sodium ortho-iodohippurate, J.A.M.A. **101**:1853, 1933.

1934 Mertz, H. O., and Hamer, H. G.: Lateral pyelogram; investigation of its value in urologic diagnosis, J. Urol. **31**:23-55, 1934.

Stewart, Wm. H., Illick, H. Earl, and Kenyon, H. R.: Special device for ureteral compression in intravenous urography, Amer. J. Roentgen. **32**:254-255, 1934.

1935 Sokow, Theodore: Radiographic technic in excretory urography, Xray Techn. **6**:111-113, 1935.

1936 Hilgenfeldt, O.: Das Veratmungspylogram [The respiration pyelogram], Deutsch. Z. Chir. **247**:441-460, 1936.

McKenzie, J. W.: Urography, Xray Techn. **7**:102-103, 1936.

Wesson, M. B., and Ruggles, H. E.: Urological roentgenology, Philadelphia, 1936, Lea & Febiger.

Wugmeister, I.: Die röntgenographische Darstellung divertikulärer Gebilde der hinteren Harnröhre, Röntgenpraxis **8**:313-316, 1936.

1937 Baker, W. E.: Urografia, Rev. Radiol. Fis. **4**:320-322, 1937.

Berger, R. A.: Increasing the value of intravenous urography by improvements in technique, Amer. J. Roentgen. **38**:156-161, 1937.

Boeminghaus: Technik der Röntgenuntersuchung der Harnorgane, Röntgenpraxis **9**:727-749, 1937.

Eller, Virginia H.: Intravenous pyelography, Xray Techn. **8**:112-114, 1937.

Gillies, C. L.: El radiodiagnóstico de las lesiones de los órganos inferiores del aparato urinario, Rev. Radiol. Fis. **4**:243-248, 1937.

Hutchinson, Robert: Compression technique in urography, Brit. J. Radiol. **10**:882-890, 1937.

Kennedy, W. T.: Incontinence of urine in the female; some functional observations of the urethra illustrated by roentgenograms, Amer. J. Obstet. Gynec. **33**:19-29, 1937.

Stevens, W. E., and Smith, S. P.: Roentgenological examination of the female urethra, J. Urol. **37**:194-201, 1937.

1938 Jaches, Leopold, and Sussman, M. L.: Roentgenologic diagnosis of diseases of the urinary tract. In Golden, Ross, editor: Diagnostic roentgenology, New York, 1938, Thomas Nelson & Sons, vol. 2, pp. 583-714.

Menville, J. G.: The lateral pyelogram as a diagnostic aid in perinephritic abscess, J.A.M.A. **111**:231-233, 1938.

Price, R. J.: Pyelo-ureterography in inclined planes, Amer. J. Roentgen. **40**:730-736, 1938.

1939 Beetz, Ruth C.: Technical aspects of intravenous pyelography, Xray Techn. **11**:53-54, 74, 1939.

Hunt, Howard B., Papma, Alfred M., and Anderson, Gladys O.: Excretory urography by intramuscular injection of diodrast, Xray Techn. **10**:201-203, 1939.

1940 Bacon, Ralph O.: Respiration pyelography, Amer. J. Roentgen. **44**:71-82, 1940.

Barnes, A. C.: A method for evaluating the stress of urinary incontinence, Amer. J. Obstet. Gynec. **40**:381-390, 1940.

Shiflett, E. L., and Keith, D. Y.: Lateral pyelography, Amer. J. Roentgen. **43**:664-672, 1940.

1943 Cole, Hazel: Duties of an x-ray technician in urography, Xray Techn. **14**:166-168, 1943.

Pendergrass, E. P.: Excretory urography as a test of urinary tract function; Carmen lecture, Radiology **40**:223-246, 1943.

1944 Walldén, L.: On roentgen diagnosis of space-restricting processes in the small pelvis, Acta Radiol. **25**:856-873, 1944.

1945 Baim, Albert: Intravenous pyelography, Xray Techn. **16**:199, 217, 1945.

Bell, J. C., Heublein, G. W., and Hammer, H. J.: The roentgen examination of the urinary tract, Amer. J. Roentgen. **53**:527-562, 1945.

Edling, Nils: Urethrocystography in the male with special regard to micturition, Acta Radiol., supp. 58, pp. 1-144, 1945.

Pritchard, Walter: Intravenous urograms, J. Urol. **53**:387-392,1945.

1946 Dell, J. M., and Barnwell, C. H.: The normal lateral retrograde pyelogram, Radiology **47**:163-165, 1946.

Hellmer, H.: Tactics and technique for urography, Brit. J. Radiol. **19**:169-172, 1946.

Kennedy, W. T.: The muscle of micturition; its role in the sphincter mechanism with reference to incontinence in the female, Amer. J. Obstet. Gynec. **52**:206-211, 1946.

Lindblom, K.: Percutaneous puncture of renal cysts and tumors, Acta Radiol. **27**:66-72, 1946.

Nichols, Bernard H.: Genito-urinary lesions in male and female. In Pillmore, George U., editor: Clinical radiology, Philadelphia, 1946, F. A. Davis Co., vol. 1, pp. 701-707, 728, 747.

Pereira, Athayde: Roentgen diagnosis of diseases of the neck of the bladder, Amer. J. Roentgen. **56**:489-499, 1946.

Prehn, D. T.: A pyelographic sign in the diagnosis of perinephric abscess, J. Urol. **55**:8-17, 1946.

Wesson, Miley B.: Urologic roentgenology, ed. 2, Philadelphia, 1946, Lea & Febiger.

1947 Coliez, Robert: Les signes radiologiques de stase et de suppression urétero-rénale au cours de l'urographie intra-veineuse, J. Radiol. Electr. **28**:311-342, 1947.

Jaches, Leopold, and Sussman, Marcy: Roentgenologic diagnosis of diseases of the urinary tract. In Golden, Ross, editor: Diagnostic roentgenology, ed. 3, New York, 1947, Thomas Nelson & Sons, vol. 2, pp. 583-715.

Nesbit, Reed M., and Valk, William L.: The oblique projection in urography, Amer. J. Roentgen. **58**:510-513, 1947.

Weens, H. S., and Florence, T. J.: Nephrography, Amer. J. Roentgen. **57**:338-341, 1947.

1948 Ruiz Rivas, M.: Diagnóstico radiológico; el neumorriñón; técnica original, Arch. Espan. Urol. **4**:222-233, 1948.

Zatskin, H. R.: Effective compression in excretory pyelography, Radiology **50**:639-644, 1948.

1950 Ruiz Rivas, M.: Generalized subserous emphysema through a single puncture, Amer. J. Roentgen. **64**:723-734, 1950.

Vesey, J., Dotter, C. T., and Steinberg, I.: Nephrography; simplified technic, Radiology **55**:827-833, 1950.

1951 Braasch, W. F., and Emmett, J. L.: Clinical urology, Philadelphia, 1951, W. B. Saunders Co.

Frei, A.: Zur Röntgenkontrastdarstellung und Beurteilung von Blasendivertikeln, Fortschr. Roentgenstr. **75**:83-88, 1951.

Hunt, L. H.: Urographic technique, Xray Techn. **23**:84-90, 1951.

Wall, B., and Rose, D. K.: Clinical intravenous nephrogram, J. Urol. **66**:305-314, 1951.

Weens, H. S., Olnick, H. M., James, D. F., and Warren, J. V.: Intravenous nephrography; a method of roentgen visualization of the kidney, Amer. J. Roentgen. **65**:411-414, 1951.

1952 Clarke, B. G.: Cystourethrograms in the diagnosis of diseases of the urethra, prostate and bladder neck, J. Maine Med. Ass. **43**:372-376, 1952.

Lindblom, K.: Diagnostic kidney puncture in cysts and tumors, Amer. J. Roentgen. **68**:209-215, 1952.

1953 Boyce, W. H., and others: The dorsal cystogram or "squat shot"; a technique for roentgenography of posterior bladder and pelvic ureters, J. Urol. **70**:969-974, 1953.

Grossman, J. W., and Nalle, B. C.: Abdominal compression; the all-important factor in excretory urography, Amer. J. Roentgen. **69**:851-852, 1953.

Hodgkinson, C. P., and Doub, H. P.: Roentgen study of urethrovesical relationships in female urinary stress incontinence, Radiology **61**:335-345, 1953.

1954 Bailey, K. V.: A clinical investigation into uterine prolapse with stress incontinence treatment by modified Manchester celporrhaphy, J. Obstet. Gynaec. Brit. Emp. **61**:291-301, 1954.

Ettinger, A., and Elkin, M.: The value of plain film in renal mass lesions (tumor and cysts), Radiology **62**:372-382, 1954.

Evans, J. A., Dubilier, W. J., and Monteith, J. C.: Nephrotomography, Amer. J. Roentgen. **71**:213-233, 1954.

Joelson, J. J., and others: The radiologic diagnosis of tumors of the adrenal gland, Radiology **62**:488-495, 1954.

Keats, P. G.: Physical, physiological and hormonal aspects of hydronephrosis, J. Fac. Radiologists **6**:123-133, 1954.

Weens, H. S., and Florence, T. J.: The diagnosis of hydronephrosis by percutaneous renal puncture, J. Urol. **72**:589-595, 1954.

Wickbom, Ingmar: Pyelography after direct puncture of the renal pelvis, Acta Radiol. **41**:505-512, 1954.

1955 Casey, W. C., and Goodwin, W. E.: Percutaneous antegrade pyelography and hydronephrosis; direct intrapelvic injection of urographic contrast material to secure a pyeloureterogram after percutaneous needle puncture and aspiration of hydronephrosis, J. Urol. **74**:164-173, 1955.

Clarke, B. G., Phillips, R. I., Goade, W. J., and Ettinger,

A.: Recent advances in radiography of the urogenital organs, Xray Techn. **27**:175-183, 1955.

Dean, A. L., Jr., Lattimer, J. K., and McCoy, C. B.: The standardized Columbia University cystogram, J. Urol. **78**:662-668, 1955.

Evans, J. A., Monteith, J. C., and Dubilier, W. J.: Nephrotomography, Radiology **64**:655-663, 1955.

Goodwin, W. E., and others: Roentgenographic visualization of the adrenal glands; use of aortography and/or retroperitoneal pneumography to visualize the adrenal glands; combined "adrenalography," J. Urol. **74**:231-242, 1955.

Hope, J. W., and Campoy, F.: The use of carbonated beverages in pediatric excretory urography, Radiology **64**:66-71, 1955.

Rollins, M., and others: Clinical evaluation of a new compound for intravenous urography, Amer. J. Roentgen. **73**:771-773, 1955.

Root, J. C., and Strittmatter, W. C.: Hypaque, a new urographic contrast medium, Amer. J. Roentgen. **73**:768-770, 1955.

Stewart, C. M.: Delayed cystography and voiding cysto-urethrography, J. Urol. **74**:749-759, 1955.

1956 Bailey, K. V.: A clinical investigation into uterine prolapse with stress incontinence, J. Obstet. Gynaec. Brit. Emp. **63**:663-676, 1956.

Davis, H. J., and Cian, L. G.: Positive pressure urethrography; new diagnostic method, J. Urol. **75**:753-757, 1956.

Harrow, B. R.: Experiences in intravenous urography using Hypaque, Amer. J. Roentgen. **75**:870-876, 1956.

Kaufman, J. J., and Russell, M.: Cystourethrography; clinical experience with the newer contrast media, Amer. J. Roentgen. **75**:884-892, 1956.

Lattimer, J. K., and others: The triple voiding technique in children with dilated urinary tracts, J. Urol. **76**:656-660, 1956.

1957 Evans, John A.: Nephrotomography in the investigation of renal masses, Radiology **69**:684-689, 1957.

Rolleston, G. L., and Reay, E. R.: The pelvi-ureteric junction, Brit. J. Radiol. **30**:617-625, 1957.

Steinbach, H. L., and others: The diagnosis of adrenal neoplasms by contrast media, Radiology **69**:664-671, 1957.

1958 Garfinkel, B., and Furst, N. J.: Simultaneous roentgen examination of the urinary and biliary tracts with Duografin, Radiology **70**:243-245, 1958.

Gudbjerg, C. E., and others: Micturition cysto-urethrography; automatic serial technique, Acta Radiol. **50**:310-316, 1958.

Handel, J., and Schwartz, S.: Value of the prone position for filling the obstructed ureter in the presence of hydronephrosis, Radiology **71**:102-103, 1958.

Hodgkinson, C. P., Doub, H. P., and Kelly, W. T.: Urethrocystograms; metallic bead chain technique, Clin. Obstet. Gynec. **1**:668-677, 1958.

Van Velzer, D. A., and Lanier, R. R.: A simplified technic for nephrotomography, Radiology **70**:77-81, 1958.

1959 Jones, D. R.: Nephrotomography, Xray Techn. **30**:487-490, 1959.

Post, H. W. A., and Southworth, W. F. W.: The technique and interpretation of nephrotomograms, Brit. J. Radiol. **32**:734-738, 1959.

1960 Bartley, O., and Helander, C. G.: Double-contrast cystography in tumors of the urinary bladder, Acta Radiol. **54**:161-169, 1960.

Chynn, K. Y., and Evans, J. A.: Nephrotomography in differentiation of renal cyst from neoplasm, J. Urol. **83**:21-24, 1960.

Dunbar, J. S., McEwan, D. W., and Herbert, F.: The value of dehydration in intravenous pyelography; an experimental study, Amer. J. Roentgen. **84**:813-836, 1960.

Hope, J. W., Jameson, P. J., and Michie, A. J.: Voiding urethrography; an integral part of intravenous urography, J. Pediat. **36**:768-773, 1960.

1961 Doyle, F. H.: Cystography in bladder tumors; technique using "steripaque" and carbon dioxide, Brit. J. Radiol. **34**:205-215, 1961.

Dunbar, J. S., Goldbloom, R. B., Pollock, V., and Rad-

ford, R.: An automatic device for voiding urethrography in infants and small children, Radiology **76**:467-471, 1961.

Elkin, Milton: The prone position in intravenous urography for study of the upper urinary tract, Radiology **76**:961-967, 1961.

Jones, H. E.: The radiology of the adrenal glands, Radiography **27**:68-73, 1961.

Smullen, W. C., and others: Equipment aids in intravenous pyelography, Radiology **76**:475-477, 1961.

1962 Amplatz, K.: Two radiographic tests for assessment of renovascular hypertension; a preliminary report, Radiology **79**:807-815, 1962.

Calatroni, C. J., Poliaka, A., and Kohana, A.: A roentgenologic study of stress incontinence in women, Amer. J. Obstet. Gynec. **83**:649-656, 1962.

Elkin, Milton: Supine and prone positions in intravenous urography for diagnosis of bladder lesions, Radiology **78**:904-913, 1962.

Green, T. H., Jr.: Development of a plan for the diagnosis and treatment of urinary stress incontinence, Amer. J. Obstet. Gynec. **83**:632-648, 1962.

1963 Anderson, M. L., and Zatz, L. M.: Voiding cystourethrography in children, Radiol. Techn. **35**:171-175, 1963.

McGowan, R. C.: The voiding cystogram with cineradiography, Xray Techn. **34**:275-280, 1963.

1964 Amplatz, Kurt: Assessment of curable renovascular hypertension by radiographic techniques, Radiology **83**:816-829, 1964.

Freidenberg, M. J., and Carlin, M. R.: The routine use of higher volumes of contrast material to improve intravenous urography, Radiology **83**:405-413, 1964.

Harris, J. H., and Harris, J. H., Jr.: Infusion pyelography, Amer. J. Roentgen. **92**:1391-1396, 1964.

Pochaczevsky, R., and Grabstald, H.: Double contrast barium cystography utilizing carbon dioxide, Amer. J. Roentgen. **92**:365-374, 1964.

Poszvek, H., and Seyss, R.: Zur Tecknik der Pyelographie, Roentgenblaetter **17**:493-499, 1964. Abst.: Amer. J. Roentgen. **93**:776, 1965.

Schencker, B.: Drip infusion pyelography; indications and applications in urologic roentgen diagnosis, Radiology **83**:12-21, 1964.

Smith, M. K.: Bead chain urethrocystography, Radiol. Techn. **35**:385-390, 1964.

Steinberg, I., and Evans, J. A.: Note on intravenous pyelography with 66.8 percent sodium iothalamate; conray-400, iodine content 40 percent, Amer. J. Roentgen. **92**:267-269, 1964.

1965 Benness, G. T.: Double dose urography, J. Coll. Radiol. Aust. **9**:78-82, 1965.

Brodeur, A. E., and others: A potential hazard of barium cystography, Radiology **85**:1080-1084, 1965.

Jacobson, B., and Sundin, T.: Automatic exposure device for voiding cystography, Acta Radiol. [Diagn.] **3**:189-192, 1965.

Lowman, R. M.: Retroperitoneal tumors; a survey and assessment of roentgen techniques, Radiol. Clin. N. Amer. **3**:543-566, 1965.

McElwain, J. T.: Polycystography in evaluating bladder tumors, Radiol. Techn. **37**:127-131, 1965.

Neal, M. P., Jr., and others: Contrast infusion nephrotomography, J.A.M.A. **193**:101-104, 1965.

Sendel, A.: Infusion pyelography, Fortschr. Roentgenstr. **103**:725-729, 1965. (In German.)

Servadio, C.: A modified technique for intravenous pyelography, Brit. J. Urol. **37**:385-389, 1965.

Schencker, B., Marcure, R. W., and Moody, D. L.: Simplified nephrotomography; drip infusion technique, Amer. J. Roentgen. **95**:283-290, 1965.

Shawdon, H. H., and others: Double contrast cystography applied to the diagnosis of tumors in bladder diverticula, Brit. J. Urol. **37**:536-544, 1965.

Shopfner, C. E.: Cystourethrography; an evaluation of method, Amer. J. Roentgen. **95**:468-474, 1965.

Thornbury, J. R., and Immergut, M. A.: Polyview voiding cystourethrography in children, Amer. J. Roentgen. **95**:475-478, 1965.

Wendth, A. J., Jr.: Drip infusion pyelography, Amer. J. Roentgen. **95**:269-282, 1965.

1966 Anderson, K., Karle, H., and Werner, H.: Renovascular hypertension and washout urography, Acta Radiol. [Diagn.] 4:145-154, 1966.

Bartness, J.: Intravenous pyelography without compression, Radiology 87:359, 1966.

Becker, Joshua A.: Drip infusion pyelography; its evaluation as a routine examination, Amer. J. Roentgen. 98:97-101, 1966.

Geraghty, J. A.: An approach to the problem of intestinal gas in diagnostic radiology, Brit. J. Radiol. 39:42-46, 1966.

Gould, H. R., and Peterson, C. G., Jr.: Voiding cystourethrography in children; the use of a rapid film changer, Amer. J. Roentgen. 98:192-199, 1966.

Hartley, W.: Infusion urography, Clin. Radiol. 17:237-241, 1966.

Hoffmann, J., and Ulrich, G.: Cystourethrography and female urinary stress incontinence, Acta Radiol. [Diagn.] 4:1-13, 1966.

Kittredge, R. D., and others: Urethral diverticula in women, Amer. J. Roentgen. 98:200-207, 1966.

Lang, E. K., and others: The diagnosis of suprarenal mass lesions by retroperitoneal gas studies and arteriography, Amer. J. Roentgen. 98:215-221, 1966.

Schencker, B.: Further experience with drip infusion pyelography, Radiology 87:304-308, 1966.

Schreiber, M. H., and others: The normal pyelogram urea washout test, Amer. J. Roentgen. 98:88-95, 1966.

Thornbury, J., Immergut, M. A., Culp, D. A., and Flocks, R. H.: Polyview voiding cystourethrography, J. Urol. 95:264-265, 1966.

1967 Ashley, A. J.: The McCallum suction cannula technique for urethrography, Radiography 33:195-200, 1967.

Becker, J. A.: The nonvisualized kidney: the value of nephrotomography, Radiology 89:676-681, 1967.

Hodge, K. E.: Combined synchronous voiding cinecystourethrography and cystometry in the investigation of vesicourethral reflux in children, J. Canad. Ass. Radiol. 19:342-348, 1967.

Laubenberger, T., and Jahnecke, J.: The percutaneous renal biopsy under radiological control, German Med. Monthly 12:206-208, 1967. (In German.) Abst.: Amer. J. Roentgen. 102:240, 1968.

Lillard, R. L., and others: Four phase nephrotomography in the diagnosis of renal cysts and tumors, Amer. J. Roentgen. 99:593-599, 1967.

Taylor, D. A., Macken, K. L., and Fiore, A. S.: Mannitol pyelography: a simplification of the drip infusion technique, Radiology 88:1117-1120, 1967.

1968 Bandtlow, K.: Urethrozystographie, Röntgenblaetter 21:434-443, 1968. (In German.) Abst.: Amer. J. Roentgen. 105:243, 1969.

Berdon, W. E., Baker, D. H., and Leonidas, J.: Prone radiography in intravenous pyelography in infants and children, Amer. J. Roentgen. 103:444-455, 1968.

Dilella, D.: Radiographic localization of the kidney for renal biopsy, Radiol. Techn. 40:1-9, 1968.

Feldman, M. I., Goade, W. J., Jr., Bouras, L., and Bargoot, F. J.: Total urography by rapid intravenous infusion, J. Urol. 99:220-222, 1968.

Hutch, J. A., and Schopfner, C. E.: The lateral cystogram as an aid to urologic diagnosis, J. Urol. 99:292-296, 1968.

Klawon, Sister M. M.: Urethrocystography and urinary stress incontinence in woman, Radiol. Techn. 39:353-358, 1968.

Lalli, A. F.: Percutaneous translumbar pyelography, Radiology 90:331-333, 1968.

Marchi, B., and Ceci, G. P.: Sphinctero-urethrography, Radiol. Med. 54:904-913, 1968. (In Italian.) Abst.: Radiology 94:486, 1968.

Nogrady, M. B., and Dunbar, J. S.: On the use of the pneumatic compression paddle for improved visualization of the upper urinary tract in pediatric patients, Amer. J. Roentgen. 103:218-222, 1968.

Reisner, K., and van de Weyer, K. H.: Nephrotomography: technic, indications and limitations, Roentgenblaetter 21:9-15, 1968. (In German.) Abst.: Radiology 91:860, 1968.

Scott, W. C.: Infusion pyelography in perspective, Clin. Radiol. 19:83-89, 1968.

Theander, G., and Wehlin, L.: The radiology of pelvic endometriosis, Clin. Radiol. 19:19-32, 1968.

1969 Frodl, F. K. O.: The importance of intravenous urography in the prone position, Fortschr. Roentgenstr. 110:474-479, 1969. (In German.) Abst.: Radiology 95:480, 1970.

Kaude, J. V., Lorenz, E., and Reed, J. M.: Gonad dose to children in voiding urethrocystography performed with 70 mm image-intensifier fluorography, Radiology 92:771-774, 1969.

Kaude, J. V., and Reed, J. M.: Voiding urethrocystography by means of 70 mm image-intensifier fluorography, Radiology 92:768-770, 1969.

Lang, E. K.: Double-contrast gas-barium cystography in the assessment of diverticula of the bladder, Amer. J. Roentgen. 107:769-775, 1969.

Lopez, F. A., Stern, W. Z., Siegelman, S. S., and Jacobson, H. G.: The nephrogram: a valuable indicator of renal abnormalities, Amer. J. Roentgen. 106:614-622, 1969.

Marx, F., and Gunther, H.: Concerning dehydration prior to urography, Fortschr. Roentgenstr. 110:826-830, 1969. (In German.) Abst.: Radiology 95:229, 1970.

Remmers, A. R., Schreiber, M. H., Smith, G. H., and others: The pyelogram urea washout test in the evaluation of renovascular hypertension, Amer. J. Roentgen. 107:750-755, 1969.

Rowe, P. W.: Retained needle urography and cholangiography, Radiology 93:520, 1969.

1970 Dure-Smith, P.: The dose of contrast medium in intravenous urography: a physiologic assessment, Amer. J. Roentgen. 108:691-697, 1970.

Jensen, J. T.: Double-contrast cystography; a new contrast medium and a simplified technique, Acta Radiol. [Diagn.] 10:337-344, 1970.

Lepasoon, J.: Indications for infusion pyelography: a comparison, Radiologe 10:93-99, 1970. (In German.) Abst.: Radiology 97:731, 1970.

Riggs, W., Hagood, J. H., and Andrews, A. E.: Anatomic changes in the normal urinary tract between supine and prone urograms, Radiology 94:107-113, 1970.

Shopfner, C. E.: Pyelo-cystourethrography: methodology, Pediatrics 46:553-565, 1970.

1971 Bates, C. P., and Corney, C. E.: Synchronous cine/pressure/flow cystography: a method of routine urodynamic investigation, Brit. J. Radiol. 44:44-50, 1971.

Cook, I. K., Keats, T. E., and Seale, D. L.: Determination of the normal position of the upper urinary tract on the lateral abdominal urogram, Radiology 99:499-502, 1971.

Lentzen, W., Frik, W., and Schiffer, A.: Is infusion urography superior to conventional urography? Fortschr. Roentgenstr. 114:393-406, 1971. (In German.) Abst.: Amer. J. Roentgen. 113:206, 1971.

McClennan, B. L., and Becker, J. A.: Excretory urography; choice of contrast material, Radiology 100:591-595, 1971.

Navarrete, R. V.: Repeat direct pyelography via needle nephrostomy, Acta Radiol. [Diagn.] 11:33-37, 1971.

1972 Jeans, W. D., and Penry, J. B.: Renal puncture, Clin. Radiol. 23:298-311, 1972.

Sherwood, T., and Stevenson, J. J.: Antegrade pyelography: a further look at an old technique, Brit. J. Radiol. 45:812-820, 1972.

Stolz, J. L., and Fogel, E. J.: The chain cystourethrogram, Radiology 103:204-206, 1972.

1973 Liebeskind, A. L., Elkin, M., and Goldman, S. H.: Herniation of the bladder, Radiology 106:257-262, 1973.

MALE GENITAL TRACT

1913 Belfield, W. T.: Skiagraphy of seminal ducts, J.A.M.A. 60:800-801, 1913.

Belfield, W. T.: Vasostomy and radiography of the seminal ducts, Surg. Gynec. Obstet. 16:569, 1913.

Belfield, W. T.: Vasostomy; radiography of seminal duct, J.A.M.A. 61:1867-1869, 1913.

1914 Thomas, B. A., and Pancoast, H. K.: Observations on the pathology, diagnosis and treatment of seminal vesiculitis, Ann. Surg. 60:313-318, 1914.

1917 Evans, William A.: Roentgenography of the prostate, Amer. J. Roentgen. 4:196, 1917.

1920 Scaduto, G.: La radiografia della prostata, Atti Congresso Ital. Radiol. Med. 3-4:148, 1920-1922.

Young, H. H., and Waters, C. A.: X-ray studies of the seminal vesicles and vasa deferentia after urethroscopic injection of the ejaculatory ducts with thorium; a new diagnostic method, Bull. Hopkins Hosp. 31:12, 1920.

1926 Belfield, W. T., and Rolnick, H. C.: Roentgenography and therapy with iodized oils, J.A.M.A. 86:1831-1833, 1926.

Rolnick, H. C.: Catheterization of the ejaculatory ducts, Surg. Gynec. Obstet. 42:667-670, 1926.

1929 Sargent, J. C.: Interpretation of the seminal vesiculogram, Radiology 12:472-483, 1929.

Smyrniotis, P. C.: Calcification bilharzique des vésicules séminales, J. Egypt Med. Ass. 10:231-235, 1929.

1931 Kidd, F.: Seminal vesiculogram, Brit. J. Urol. 3:177-178, 1931.

1935 Yanagihara, H., and Miyata, T.: Radiography of the vas deferens (ampulla) and seminal vesicles, J. Orient. Med. 23:85-94, 1935.

1938 Peterson, A. P.: Retrograde catheterization in the diagnosis of seminal vesiculitis, J. Urol. 39:662-667, 1938.

1939 Wilhelm, S. F.: Vaso-seminal vesiculography, J. Urol. 41:751-757, 1939.

1943 Gonzales-Iman, F.: Retrograde seminal vesiculography, J. Urol. 49:618-627, 1943.

1945 Bertelsen, A., and Wandall, H. H.: Vasoseminal vesiculography and its clinal application, Acta Radiol. 26:36-45, 1945.

1948 Gee, E. M.: Primary carcinoma of the seminal vesicle; report of two cases, Brit. J. Urol. 20:72-76, 1948.

Heller, M.: Sur une méthode permettant l'étude radiologique de la vésicule séminale, J. Radiol. Electr. 29:151-152, 1948.

Staehler, W.: Die Diagnose der inneren männlichen Genitaltuberkulose im Röntgenbild, Helv. Chir. Acta 15:475-486, 1948.

1949 Pohjola, R., and Tuovinen, P. I.: Vesiculography in vesiculoprostatitis, Ann. Chir. Gynaec. Fenn. 38:221-237, 1949.

1951 Boreau, J., Elbim, A., Hermann, P., Vasselle, B., and Fua, R.: L'epididymographie, Presse Méd. 59:1406-1407, 1951.

Boreau, J., Vasselle, B., and Jagailloux, S.: Étude radiologique des voies génitales normales et pathologiques de l'homme, Presse Méd. 61:1-4, 1951.

1952 Edling, N. P. G.: Roentgen diagnosis of diseases of the prostate, J. Urol. 62:197-207, 1952.

1953 Boreau, Jacques: L'étude radiologique des voies séminales normales et pathologiques, Paris, 1953, Masson & Cie.

Boreau, J., Jagailloux, S., Vasselle, B., and Hermann, P.: Epididymography, Med. Radiogr. Photogr. 29:63-66, 1953.

Comarr, A. E., and Dodenhoff, L.: Safe, simple method of performing urethrograms, J. Urol. 70:980-981, 1953.

Pereira, A.: Roentgen interpretation of vesiculograms, Amer. J. Roentgen. 69:361-379, 1953.

Vasselle, B.: Étude radiologique des voies séminales, These de Paris, 1953.

1954 Puigvert, A., and Romero-Aguirre, C.: La vesiculografía para el diagnóstico de las afecciones de la próstata y vejiga, Acta Iber. Radiol. Cancer. 3:1-31, 1954.

Tucker, A. S., Yanagihara, H., and Pryde, A. W.: A method of roentgenography of the male genital tract, Amer. J. Roentgen. 71:490-500, 1954.

1955 Comarr, A. E., and Bors, E.: Spermatocystography in patients with spinal cord injuries, J. Urol. 73:172-178, 1955.

1956 Bauer, Karl M.: Seltene Erkrankungen der Samenblasen, Z. Urol. 49:287-295, 1956.

Comarr, A. E.: Position of the patient for roentgenologic interpretation of prostatogram, Amer. J. Roentgen. 75:893-895, 1956.

1957 Gambetta, G., and Borini, L.: La stratigraphie des vésicules séminales normales et pathologiques, Acta Urol. Belg. 25:11-34, 1957.

Golji, H.: Clinical value of epididymo-vesiculography, J. Urol. 78:445-455, 1957.

Vanwelkenhuyzen, P.: Les modifications radiologiques des voies séminales par les lésions de la prostate, Acta Urol. Belg. 25:34-52, 1957.

1958 Vanwelkenhuyzen, P.: Remarques sur l'interprétation des vésiculographies en cas de lésions de la prostate, Acta Urol. Belg. 26:38-47, 1958.

1959 D'Alessandro, A.: Contributo allo studio del cancro primitivo delle vesicole siminali, Minerva Urol. 11:71-80, 1959.

1960 Martinelli, V., Micieli, G., and Saracca, L.: Quadri deferentovesiculografici nella ipertrofia prostatica, Ann. Ital. Chir. 37:34-49, 1960.

Osadchuk, V. I.: Experience in the roentgenologic study of the seminal vesicles, Urologiia 25:35-40, 1960.

1961 Marshall, D. F., Leary, G. C., O'Donnell, E. E., and Geer, G. I.: Seminal vesicle carcinoma, J. Maine Med. Ass. 52:145-147, 1961.

Nylander, G., Ryrberg, C. H., and Wilbrand, H.: Comments on the clinical value of seminal vesiculography, Urol. Int. 12:289-306, 1961.

1962 Fetter, T. R., and others: Seminal vesiculography; diagnostic aid in prostatic carcinoma, J. Urol. 87:718-725, 1962.

Ney, C., and Friedenberg, R. M.: Seminal vesiculography, Jew. Mem. Hosp. Bull. (N. Y.) 7:212-216, 1962.

1963 Heller, E., and Whitesel, J. A.: Seminal vesicle cysts, J. Urol. 90:305-307, 1963.

Nisenbaum, L. I.: Cystic adenoma of the seminal vesicle with teratoid nature, Urologiia 28:56-78, 1963.

1964 Elliott, J. P., Jr., and others: Vasoseminal vesiculography as a diagnostic aid in prostatic and seminal vesicle disease, J. Urol. 92:513-516, 1964.

Gil Vernet, S.: La tuberculose génitale masculine, Urol. Int. 18:25-42, 1964.

Mazurek, L. J.: Examen radiologique des voies séminales en incidence dorso-sacrale, Ann. Radiol. 7:69-72, 1964. Abst.: Radiology 83:753, 1964.

1965 Lawson, L. J., and MacDougall, J. A.: Multilocular cyst of the seminal vesicle, Brit. J. Urol. 37:440-442, 1965.

Liliequist, B., and Rais, O.: Roentgenologic procedures in vesiculography, Acta Radiol. [Diagn.] 3:321-334, 1965.

1969 Sugiura, H., and Hasegawa, S.: Transrectal prostatography: its use in prostatic hypertrophy, Amer. J. Roentgen. 107:796-802, 1969.

1971 Sugiura, H., and Hasegawa, S.: Clinical evaluation of transrectal prostatography, Amer. J. Roentgen. 111:157-164, 1971.

1974 Boreau, Jacques: Images of the seminal tracts, New York, 1974, S. Karger.

BREAST

1913 Salomon, A.: Beiträge zur Pathologie und Klinik der Mammakarzinome, Arch. Klin. Chir. 101:573-668, 1913.

1920 Bobrie, Y., and Colombier, R.: Technique spéciale pour la radiographie des parties molles, Bull. Soc. Radiol. Méd. Paris 8:64-66, 1920.

1930 Warren, Stafford L.: A roentgenological study of the breast, Amer. J. Roentgen. 24:113-124, 1930.

1931 Goyanes, J., and others: Sobre la radiografía de la glandula mamaria y su valor diagnóstico, Arch. Esp. Oncol. 11:111-142, 1931.

Romagnoli, M.: La radiologia delle mammelle, Rev. Radiol. Fis. Med. 6:689-728, 1931.

1932 Fray, W. W., and Warren, S. L.: Stereoscopic roentgenography of the breast, Ann. Surg. 95:425-432, 1932.

Lockwood, I. H.: Roentgen-ray study of the mammary gland, Southern Med. J. 25:903, 1932.

Vogel, W.: Die Röntgendarstellung von Mammatumoren, Arch. Klin. Chir. 171: 618-626, 1932.

1933 Seabold, Paul S.: Procedure in the roentgen study of the breast, Amer. J. Roentgen. 29:850-851, 1933.

1935 Bianchini, Alessandro: Lo studio radiologico della mammella muliebre, Radiol. Med. 22:167-172, 1935.

Ledoux-Lebard, R., Garcia-Calderon, J., and Espaillat,

A.: L'examen radiographique du sein, Paris Méd. 1:92-99, 1935.

1937 Gershon-Cohen, J.: Cradle for the roentgen x-ray of the female breast, Radiology 28:234-236, 1937.

Hicken, N. Frederick: Mammography; the roentgenographic diagnosis of breast tumors by means of contrast media, Surg. Gynec. Obstet. 64:593, 1937.

Hicken, N. Frederick: Radiographic demonstration of breast lesions, Radiogr. Clin. Photogr. 13:2-9, 1937.

1938 Friedman, J. L., and Slater, C.: Mammography; soft tissue technique, Amer. J. Surg. 41:310-314, 1938.

Gershon-Cohen, J., and Strickler, Albert: Roentgenologic examination of the normal breast, Amer. J. Roentgen. 40:189-201, 1938.

1939 Hunt, H. B., and Hicken, N. F.: Evaluation of various diagnostic procedures used in the study of the breast with particular reference to roentgenographic examination, Radiology 63:712-723, 1939.

1940 Hoing, Margaret: A workable technic for mastography, Xray Techn. 11:136-137, 1940.

1941 Ehrlich, David E.: Pendant mastography, Radiology 36:488-490, 1941.

1944 Leborgne, Raúl: Diagnóstico de los procesos pathológicos de la mama por la radiografía con la inyección de madios de contraste, Obstet. Gynec. Latino-Amer. 2:551-561, 1944.

1947 Lame, L. Edwin, and Pendergrass, Eugene P.: An addition to the technic of simple breast roentgenography, Radiology 48:266-268, 1947.

Leborgne, Raúl: Estudio radiológico de la glandula mamaria, Arch. Urug. Med. Cir. Especialid. 30:52-63, 1947.

1951 Leborgne, Raúl: Diagnosis of tumors of the breast by simple roentgenography, Amer. J. Roentgen. 65:1-11, 1951.

1952 Gershon-Cohen, J., and Ingleby, H.: Roentgenography of cancer of the breast, Amer. J. Roentgen. 68:1-7, 1952.

Gros, C. M., and Sigrist, R.: La radiographie de la glande mammaire, J. Belg. Radiol. 35:226-268, 1952.

1953 Eubank, M. C.: Technical aspects of breast roentgenography with emphasis on mammography, Xray Techn. 24:309-320, 1953.

Gershon-Cohen, J., and Ingleby, H.: Carcinoma of the breast; roentgenographic technic and diagnostic criteria, Radiology 60:68-76, 1953.

1955 Sprecher, C. C.: X-ray examination of the female breast, Xray Techn. 26:341-342, 1955.

1957 Gros, C. M.: La radiographie des cancers du sein, Sem. Hôp. Paris 33:4275-4280, 1957.

1958 Kremens, V.: Roentgenography of the breast, Amer. J. Roentgen. 80:1005-1013, 1958.

Werner, K., Buttenberg, D., and Zeitz, H.: Zur Röntgenuntersuchung der Mamma, Fortschr. Roentgenstr. 88:690-697, 1958.

1959 Sklaroff, D. M., and others: X-ray examination of the breast, J. Canad. Ass. Radiol. 10:13-16, 1959.

1960 Egan, R. L.: Experience with mammography in a tumor institution; evaluation of 1,000 studies, Radiology 75:894-900, 1960.

Gershon-Cohen, J.: Technical improvements in breast roentgenography, Amer. J. Roentgen. 84:224-226, 1960.

Gould, H. P., Ruzicka, F. F., Sanchez-Ubeda, R., and Perez, J.: Xeroradiography of the breast, Amer. J. Roentgen. 84:220-223, 1960.

1961 Gershon-Cohen, J.: Breast roentgenology, Amer. J. Roentgen. 86:879-883, 1961.

1962 Bražnikov, N. N.: Zur Methodik der Röntgenuntersuchung der Mamma, Radiol. Diagn. 3:547-555, 1962.

Forman, M.: Roentgenography of the male breast, Amer. J. Roentgen. 88:1126-1134, 1962.

Tellem, M., Prive, L., and Meranze, D. R.: Four-quadrant study of breasts removed for carcinoma, Cancer 15:10-17, 1962.

1963 Asch, T.: Mammography; a study of 500 patients, Amer. J. Roentgen. 90:366-372, 1963.

Gershon-Cohen, J., and Berger, S. M.: Mastography, Radiol. Clin. N. Amer. 1:115-143, 1963.

Keats, T. E., Koenig, G. F., Rall, K. L., and Wood, D. D.: Soft tissue roentgenography of the breast, Amer. J. Roentgen. 90:359-365, 1963.

Leborgne, R., Leborgne, F., Jr., and Leborgne, J. H.: Soft tissue radiography of the axilla in cancer of the breast, Brit. J. Radiol. 36:494-496, 1963.

Stanton, L., Lightfoot, D. A., Boyle, J. J., and Cullinan, J. E.: Physical aspects of breast radiography, Radiology 81:1-16, 1963.

1964 Binzer-Pfertzel, C. C.: Mammography and its relation to disease, Radiography 30: 159-162, 1964.

Donovan, R. J.: A new contour cassette for mammographic roentgenography, Amer. J. Roentgen. 91:917-918, 1964.

Egan, R. L.: Mammography, Springfield, Ill., 1964, Charles C Thomas, Publisher.

Funderburk, W. W., Syphax, B., and Ruguero, W.: The value of contrast medium injection in locating lesions of the breast causing discharge, with particular reference to duct papillomas, J. Nat. Med. Ass. 56:127-132, 1964.

Funderburk, W. W., Syphax, B., and Smith, C. W.: Contrast mammography in breast discharge, Surg. Gynec. Obstet. 119:276-280, 1964.

Holohan, F.: Technical considerations in breast radiography, Radiol. Techn. 35:247-251, 1964.

Sherman, R. S.: Areas of concern in mammographic techniques (editorial), Amer. J. Roentgen. 91:1173-1174, 1964.

Siler, W. M., Snyder, R. E., Garrett, R., McLaughlin, J. S., and Sherman, R. S.: The development and use of mammographic technique, Amer. J. Roentgen. 91:910-918, 1964.

1965 Bjørn-Hansen, R.: Contrast mammography, Brit. J. Radiol. 38:947-951, 1965.

Gershon-Cohen, J.: Mammography; some remarks on techniques, Radiol. Clin. N. Amer. 3:389-401, 1965.

Turner, A. E.: A review of technique development; mammography, xeromammoradiography, and thermomammography, Radiol. Techn. 36:325-334, 1965.

1966 Berger, S. M., Curcio, B. M., Gershon-Cohen, J., and Isard, H. J.: Mammographic localization of unsuspected breast cancer, Amer. J. Roentgen. 96:1046-1052, 1966.

Curcio, Barbara M.: Mammography and the radiologic technologist, Radiol. Techn. 38:143-151, 1966.

Egan, R. L.: The technical aspects of mammography, Med. Radiogr. Photogr. 42:2-5, 1966.

Lotz, K., Reichel, W. S., and Tautz, M.: Grundlagen der Mammographie, Fortschr. Roentgenstr. 105:229-239, 1966.

1967 Gershon-Cohen, J., Ingleby, H., Berger, S., and others: Mammographic screening for breast cancer: results of a ten-year survey, Radiology 88:663-667, 1967.

Gros, C. M.: Methodologie, J. Radiol. Electr. 48:638-655, 1967.

Lotz, K., and Tautz, M.: Das Problem der Planparallelität bei der Mammographie, Fortschr. Roentgenstr. 106:276-282, 1967.

Metzenthin, B., Rehm, A., and Fischedick, O.: Das Röntgenbild der männlichen Mamma, Fortschr. Roentgenstr. 106:567-573, 1967.

O'Mara, R. E., Ruzicka, F. F., Osborne, A., and Connell, J.: Xeromammography and film mammography: completion of a comparative study, Radiology 88:1121-1126, 1967.

Scott, W. G.: Mammography and the training program of the American College of Radiology, Amer. J. Roentgen. 99:1002-1008, 1967.

1968 Ap Simon, H. T., Stewart, H. J., and Williams, W. J.: Recording the gross outlines of breast tumors; a pathological assessment of the accuracy of radiographs of breast cancer, Brit. J. Cancer 22:40-46, 1968.

Egan, Robert L.: Technologist's guide to mammography, Baltimore, 1968, The Williams & Wilkins Co.

Egan, R. L., and Fenn, J. O.: Phantoms for evaluating mammography techniques and roentgenographic detail, Amer. J. Roentgen. 102:936-940, 1968.

Lasky, H. J.: A new mammographic technic, Radiology 91:381-382, 1968.

Minagi, H., Tennant, J. C., and Youker, J. E.: Coning

and breast compression; an aid in mammographic diagnosis, Radiology **91**:379-381, 1968.

O'Donnell, E.: Radiographic objectives of mammography, Radiol. Techn. **39**:273-282, 1968.

Strax, P., and Oppenheim, A.: New apparatus for mass screening in mammography, Amer. J. Roentgen. **102**:941-945, 1968.

Wolfe, J. N.: Xerography of the breast, Radiology **91**:231-240, 1968.

1969 Gershon-Cohen, J., and Hermel, M. B.: Modalities in breast cancer detection: xeroradiography, mammography, thermography, and mammometry, Cancer **24**:1226-1230, 1969.

Hermel, M. B., Gershon-Cohen, J., and Byrne, R. N.: Mammographic technique: need for routine spot roentgenograms, Amer. J. Roentgen. **105**:880-884, 1969.

Isard, H. J., Ostrum, B. J., and Shilo, R.: Thermography in breast carcinoma, Surg. Gynec. Obstet. **128**:1289-1293, 1969.

Howland, W. J., Johnson, T. H., and Reagan, T. A.: Laminagraphy of the breast, Radiology **92**:609-612, 1969.

Stevens, G. M.: Variations and supplementary techniques in mammography, Oncology **23**:120-125, 1969.

Wallace, T.: Radiographic identification of calcifications in breast specimens, Radiol. Techn. **40**:211-215, 1969.

Zippin, C.: The epidemiology of breast cancer, Oncology **23**:93-98, 1969.

1970 Curcio, B.: Technique for radiographic localization of non-palpable breast tumors, Radiol. Techn. **42**:155-160, 1970.

Gershon-Cohen, J. G.: Atlas of mammography, New York, 1970, Springer Verlag.

Gershon-Cohen, J., Hermel, M. B., and Birsner, J. W.: Advances in mammographic technique, Amer. J. Roentgen. **108**:424-427, 1970.

Gilbertson, J. D., Randall, M. G., and Fingerhut, A. G.: Evaluation of roentgen exposure in mammography. Part I. Six views, Radiology **95**:383-394, 1970.

Gilbertson, J. D., Randall, M. G., and Fingerhut, A. G.: Evaluation of roentgen exposure in mammography. Part II. Four views, Radiology **97**:641-648, 1970.

Jabczenski, M. A.: Pendent mammography: a new approach to an old technique, J. Canad. Ass. Radiol. **21**:43-45, 1970.

Palmer, R. C., Egan, R. L., and Barrett, B. J.: Preliminary evaluation of absorbed dose in mammography, Radiology **95**:395-397, 1970.

Price, J. L., and Butler, P. D.: The reduction of radiation and exposure time in mammography, Brit. J. Radiol. **43**:251-255, 1970.

1971 Dowdy, A. H., Barker, W., Lagasse, L. D., and others: Mammography as a screening method for the examination of large populations, Cancer **28**:1558-1562, 1971.

Palmer, R. C., Egan, R. L., and others: Absorbed dose in mammography using three tungsten and three molybdenum target tubes, Radiology **101**:697-699, 1971.

Quimet-Oliva, D.: Air axillography, Amer. J. Roentgen. **111**:153-156, 1971.

Shapiro, S., Strax, P., and Venet, L.: Periodic breast cancer screening in reducing mortality from breast cancer, J.A.M.A. **215**:1771-1785, 1971.

Snyder, R. E., and Rosen, P.: Radiography of breast specimens, Cancer **28**:1608-1611, 1971.

Wolfe, J. N., Dooley, R. P., and Harkins, L. E.: Xeroradiography of the breast: a comparative study with conventional film mammography, Cancer **28**:1569-1574, 1971.

1972 Nunnerley, H. B., and Field, S.: Mammary duct injection in patients with nipple discharge, Brit. J. Radiol. **45**:717-725, 1972.

Gurley, L., and Harwood, S.: A practical technique for baseline mammography, Radiol. Techn. **44**:138-145, 1972.

Simon, N., Lesnick, G. J., Lerer, W. N., and Bachman, A. L.: Roentgenographic localization of small lesions of the breast by the spot method, Surg. Gynec. Obstet. **134**:572-574, 1972.

1973 Martin, J. E.: Xeromammography—an improved diagnostic method, Amer. J. Roentgen. **117**:90-96, 1973.

Ostrum, B. J., Becker, W., and Isard, H. J.: Low-dose mammography, Radiology **109**:323-326, 1973.

Rini, J. M., Horowitz, A., Balter, S., and Watson, R.: A comparison of tungsten and molybdenum as target material for mammographic x-ray tubes, Radiology **106**:657-661, 1973.

Strax, P., Venet, L., and Shapiro, S.: Value of mammography in reduction of mortality from breast cancer in mass screening, Amer. J. Roentgen. **117**:686-689, 1973.

Threatt, B., and Appelman, H. D. Mammary duct injection, Radiology **108**:71-76, 1973.

FEMALE REPRODUCTIVE SYSTEM
Hysterosalpingography

1927 Heuser, C.: La uterosalpingoradiografia, Semana Med. **2**:905-906, 1927.

1928 Kolbow, H.: Uterus und Vagina im seitlichen Röntgenbild, Zbl. Gynaek. **52**:2788, 1928.

1930 Robins, S. A.: Hysterosalpingography, Amer. J. Roentgen. **23**:573-575, 1930.

Witwer, E. R., and others: The present status of hysterosalpingography with a review of the literature and a report of 512 personal cases, Amer. J. Roentgen. **23**:125-159, 1930.

1931 Jarchow, J. M.: Gynecological roentgenology, Ann. Roentgen. **13**:1931.

1937 Runstrom, Gösta: Hysterosalpingography by examination in different positions with horizontally directed rays, Acta Radiol. **18**:119-140, 1937.

1942 Kjellberg, S. R.: Hysterosalpinopelvigraphie, Acta Radiol., supp. 43, pp. 40-44, 1942.

Martin, C. L.: Fallopian tube visualization as a treatment for sterility, Amer. J. Roentgen. **47**:894-901, 1942.

1945 Tooker, Dorothy: Uterosalpingography, Xray Techn. **16**:168-171, 1945.

1946 Mandeville, Frederick F.: Roentgenography in gynecology. In Pillmore, George U., editor: Clinical radiology, Philadelphia, 1946, F. A. Davis Co., vol. 1., pp. 758-785.

1947 Robins, Samuel A., and Shapira, Albert A.: Uterotubography. In Golden, Ross, editor: Diagnostic roentgenology, ed. 3, New York, 1947, Thomas Nelson & Sons, vol. 2, pp. 715-721.

1948 Sharman, A.: A new contrast medium (Rayopake) for hysterosalpingography, J. Obstet. Gynaec. Brit. Comm. **55**:770-773, 1948.

1957 Lehfeldt, H., and others: Cineradiography of the female pelvic organs; a preliminary report on a new method, Amer. J. Obstet. Gynec. **74**:413-418, 1957.

1958 Williams, G. A.: Hysterosalpingography, Clin. Obstet. Gynec. **1**:629-644, 1958.

1960 Henry, G. W., and Hunter, R. G.: Hysterosalpingography with water soluble medium (Salpix), Amer. J. Roentgen. **84**:924-928, 1960.

1962 Chérigié, E., and others: Progrès récents en hystérosalpingographie, Ann. Radiol. **5**:515-522, 1962.

1969 Aaro, L. A., and Stewart, J. R.: Hysterosalpingography with image-intensified fluoroscopy, Amer. J. Obstet. Gynec. **105**:1124-1128, 1969.

Fullenlove, T. M.: Experience with over 2000 uterosalpingographies, Amer. J. Roentgen. **106**:463-471, 1969.

Greenbaum, E. I., Podolak, G., and O'Loughlin, B. J.: The use of hysterography in the detection of hydatidiform mole, Amer. J. Roentgen. **105**:885-889, 1969.

Griffiths, H. J. L.: A clinical and radiological evaluation comparing the use of two contrast media in hysterosalpingography—Salpix and Urografin, Brit. J. Radiol. **42**:835-837, 1969.

Norman, O.: Hysterography in cancer of the uterus, Seminars Roentgen. **4**:244-251, 1969.

Senties, L., Perdomo, A., and Luna, R.: Diagnosis of

hydatidiform mole by hysterography through trans-abdominal injection, Obstet. Gynec. **33**:352-357, 1969.

Weiner, M.: Hysterosalpingography in benign pelvic conditions, Seminars Roentgen. **4**:235-243, 1969.

Vaginography

1954 Katzner, P., and Trachtman, B.: Diagnosis of vaginal ectopic ureter by vaginogram, J. Urol. **72**:808-811, 1954.

1963 Coe, Fred O.: Vaginography, Amer. J. Roentgen. **90**:721-722, 1963.

Lambie, R. W., Rubin, S., and Dann, D. S.: Demonstration of fistulas by vaginography, Amer. J. Roentgen. **90**:717-720, 1963.

1964 Wolfson, J. J.: Vaginography for demonstration of ureterovaginal, vesicovaginal, and rectovaginal fistulas, Radiology **83**:438-441, 1964.

1969 Rubin, S., Lambie, R. W., Davidson, K. C., and Herman, E. M.: Barium vaginography, Seminars Roentgen. **4**:212-217, 1969.

Pelvic pneumography

1961 Schulz, E., and Rosen, S. W.: Gynecography; technique and interpretation, Amer. J. Roentgen. **86**:866-878, 1961.

1966 Stevens, G. M., Weigen, J. F., and Lee, R. S.: Pelvic pneumography, Med. Radiogr. Photogr. **42**:82-127, 1966.

1967 Rådberg, C., and Wickbom, I.: Pelvic angiography and pneumoperitoneum in the diagnosis of gynecologic lesions, Acta Radiol. [Diagn.] **6**:133-144, 1967.

1970 Stern, W. Z., and Wilson, L.: Pelvic pneomography with simultaneous hysterosalpingography, Radiology **96**:87-92, 1970.

Fetography and placentography

1900 Fabre and Trillat: Die Radiographie des lebenden Fötus, Arch. Electr. Méd., no. 300, 25, XII, 1900. Abst.: Fortschr. Röntgenstr. **16**:404, 1900.

1923 Candy, T. J.: Radiography of the foetus in utero, Arch. Radiol. Electr. **28**:146-153, 1923.

1930 Baumann: Röntgendiagnostik in der Schwangerschaft und wahrend der Geburt, München. Med. Wschr. **77**:1148-1151, 1930.

Grier, G. W.: The value of a lateral view in the diagnosis of pregnancy, Radiology **14**:571-575, 1930.

1934 Snow, W., and Powell, C. B.: Roentgen visualization of the placenta, Amer. J. Roentgen. **31**:34-40, 1934.

Ude, W. H., Weum, T. W., and Urner, J. A.: Roentgenologic diagnosis of placenta previa, Amer. J. Roentgen. **31**:230-233, 1934.

1935 Burke, F. J.: Amniography, J. Obstet. Gynaec. Brit. Comm. **42**:1096-1106, 1935.

Ude, W. H., and Urner, J. A.: Roentgenologic diagnosis of placenta previa, Amer. J. Obstet. Gynec. **29**:667-669, 1935.

1938 Elward, J. F., and Belair, J. F.: Roentgen diagnosis of pregnancy, Radiology **31**:678-686, 1938.

Ude, W. H., Urner, J. A., and Robbins, O. F.: Roentgenologic diagnosis of placenta previa, Amer. J. Roentgen. **40**:37-42, 1938.

1939 Hubeny, M. J., and Delano, P. J.: A plea for the more frequent use of the lateral roentgenogram in the diagnosis of pregnancy, Radiology **32**:546-549, 1939.

Snow, W.: Late extrauterine pregnancy diagnosed by soft tissue roentgenography, Amer. J. Roentgen. **41**:537-540, 1939.

Snow, W., and Rosensohn, M.: Roentgenologic visualization of the soft tissues in pregnancy, Amer. J. Roentgen. **42**:709-717, 1939.

1940 Dippel, A. L., and Brown, W. H.: Direct visualization of the placenta by soft tissue roentgenography, New Eng. J. Med. **223**:316-323, 1940.

Dippel, A. L., and Brown, W. H.: Roentgen visualization of the placenta by soft tissue technique, Amer. J. Obstet. Gynec. **40**:986-994, 1940.

1941 Ball, Robert P., and Golden, Ross: Roentgenologic sign for detection of placenta previa, Amer. J. Obstet. Gynec. **42**:530-533, 1941.

Cameron, M. F.: Visualization of the placenta by soft tissue radiographs, Ontario Radiographer **2**:12-14, 1941.

1942 Cahoon, John B.: Uses of opaque plastic filters in radiography of the lateral lumbar spine, lateral cervicodorsal spine, and cases of suspected placenta previa, Xray Techn. **13**:242-243, 246, 1942.

Snow, William: Clinical roentgenology of pregnancy, Springfield, Ill., 1942, Charles C Thomas, Publisher, chap. 6.

Vaughan, C. E., Weaver, R. T., and Adamson, D. L.: Roentgenographic visualization of the placenta, utilizing the plastic filter, Canad. Med. Ass. J. **46**:314-321, 1942.

Wigby, P. E.: The diagnosis of placenta previa by means of the lateral soft tissue film of the abdomen, Texas J. Med. **38**:390-394, 1942.

1943 Baylin, G. J., and Lambeth, S. S.: Roentgen diagnosis of placenta previa, Radiology **40**:497-500, 1943.

Cameron, Mary F.: Placentagrams, Xray Techn. **14**:227-230, 1943.

Smith, R. M.: Roentgenologic localization of the placenta without contrast media, Amer. J. Roentgen. **49**:750-755, 1943.

1944 McCort, J. J., Davidson, C. N., and Walton, H. J.: Determination of the placental site in bleeding during the last trimester of pregnancy, Amer. J. Roentgen. **52**:128-135, 1944.

Moir, C.: Fallaceis in soft tissue placentography, Amer. J. Obstet. Gynec. **47**:198-211, 1944.

1945 Bishop, P. A.: The roentgenological visualization of the placenta, Surg. Clin. N. Amer. **25**:1394-1407, 1945.

1946 Alexander, O. M.: A survey of radiographic techniques employed in obstetrical and gynecological practice, Radiography **12**:97-103, 1946.

1947 Robinson, David, and Boyd, William S.: Roentgenographic visualization of the placenta, Amer. J. Roentgen. **58**:730-732, 1947.

1948 Cahoon, John B.: Barium plastic filters in roentgen diagnosis of placenta previa, Xray Techn. **19**:185-188, 1948.

1949 Cameron, M. F.: Placentography, Canad. X-ray News Letter, **5**:2-4, 1949.

Herrman, W. G.: Lateral visulization of the pregnant uterus, Med. Radiogr. Photogr. **25**:83, 1949.

Reid, F.: An aluminum filter for use in localization of the placenta site, Brit. J. Radiol. **22**:81-83, 1949.

Stevenson, C. S.: X-ray visualization of the placenta; experiences with soft tissue and cystographic techniques in the diagnosis of placenta previa, Amer. J. Obstet. Gynec. **58**:15-29, 1949.

1950 McEnerney, P. E.: Technical aspects of arterial visualization of the placenta, Xray Techn. **21**:189-195, 1950.

1951 McGann, M. J.: An aluminum filter for placenta visualization, Xray Techn. **22**:304-305, 1951.

1952 Quist, Carl F.: Soft tissue radiography of the placenta, Acta Radiol. **37**:510-518, 1952.

Reeves, R. J., and Cahoon, J. B.: Lateral radiography of the pregnant uterus; a technical review, Med. Radiogr. Photogr. **28**:2-10, 1952.

1953 Alcántara-Carhajal, R. R.: Iodine wedge filter for roentgenographic use, Radiology **61**:243-245, 1953.

1957 Hodge, K. E.: Gravitational placentography, Radiology **68**:637-647, 1957.

Watson, H. B., and others: Placentography in management of placenta praevia, Brit. Med. J. **2**:490-494, 1957.

1958 Whitehouse, W. M., and others: Reduction of radiation hazard in obstetric roentgenography, Amer. J. Roentgen. **80**:690-695, 1958.

1959 Geffen, A.: Placentography with duo- and tri-speed intensifying screens, Amer. J. Roentgen. **82**:897-901, 1959.

1960 Rossi, P., Rizzi, J., and De Santis, V.: Simultaneous lateral placentography, Radiology **74**:298-299, 1960.

1964 Verco, P. W.: Placental localization; a survey of 275 patients, J. Coll. Radiol. Aust. **8**:205-213, 1964.

1965 Cahoon, J. B.: Formulating x-ray techniques, ed. 6, Durham, N. C., 1965, Duke University Press.

Vickers, A. A.: Placentography simplified, Clin. Radiol. 16:351-362, 1965.

Vickers, A. A.: Restriction of obstetric radiology, Lancet 1:1318-1322, 1965.

1966 Prevatte, P., and Izenstark, J. L.: Roentgenographic and radioisotopic placental localization, Radiol. Techn. 38:1-6, 1966.

1968 Schreiber, M. H., and Morettin, L. B.: The lateral compression roentgenogram of the abdomen in pregnancy, Amer. J. Roentgen. 102:768-772, 1968.

Schwartz, G. S.: Radiation hazards to the human fetus in present-day society: Should a pregnant woman be subjected to a diagnostic x-ray procedure? Bull. N. Y. Acad. Med. 44:388-399, 1968. Abst.: Amer. J. Roentgen. 103:962, 1968.

Tessaro, A. N., and Chasler, C. N.: Amniography as an aid in intrauterine transfusion, Amer. J. Roentgen. 103:195-201, 1968.

1969 Kohorn, E. I., Morrison, J., Ashford, C., and Blackwell, R. J.: Ultrasonic scanning in obstetrics and gynecology, Obstet. Gynec. 34:515-522, 1969.

Spindola-Franco, H., Ceballos-Jabat, J., and Cisneros, H. A.: Value of amniography in determining fetal viability, Acta Radiol. [Diagn.] 8:17-28, 1969.

Weill, F., Colette, C., Zurlinden, B., and others: Radiology without x-rays: placenta localization by thermography and tomoechography, Ann. Radiol. 12:797-810, 1969. (In French.) Abst.: Radiology 96:235, 1970.

1970 Aguero, O., and Zighelboim, I.: Fetography and molegraphy, Surg. Gynec. Obstet. 130:649-654, 1970.

Casselden, P. A.: Soft tissue placentography and the uterine compressor, Radiography 36:125-131, 1970.

1972 Brown, A. A., and Young, G. B.: A study of four methods of placental localization, Amer. J. Obstet. Gynec. 114:24-28, 1972.

Pelvimetry

1898 Pinard, and Varnier: Beckenmessung, Zbl. Gynaek. 22:1145, 1897. Abst.: Fortschr. Roentgenstr. 1:113, 1898.

1900 Wormser: Ueber die Verwertung der R in der Geburtschilfe, Beiträge Geb. Gyn., no. 3, 1900. Abst.: Fortschr. Roentgenstr. 4:139, 1900.

1907 Pfahler, George E.: Radiographic measurement of the diameters of the female pelvis and new technique in radiographing vesical calculi, Amer. Quart. Roentgen. 1:23-27, 1907.

1909 Bouchacourt: Die Radiopelvimetrie, Bull. Soc. Radiol. Paris 1:234-241, 1909. Abst.: Fortschr. Roentgenstr. 15:62, 1909.

1910 Albers-Schönberg, H. E.: Schwangerschaftdiagnose. In Die Röntgentechnik, Hamburg, 1910, Gräfe & Sillem, p. 415.

Manges, Willis F.: Pelvimetry, Amer. Roentgen Ray Soc., 1910. Abst.: Fortschr. Roentgenstr. 17:404, 1910.

1914 Perussia, Felice: Tecnica della radiografia del feto nell'utero materno, Radiol. Med. 1:203-210, 1914.

1916 Van Allen, Harvey: Easy and accurate pelvimetry by the roentgen ray, Amer. J. Roentgen. 3:367-368, 1916.

1921 Chamberlain, W. Edward, and Newell, R. R.: Pelvimetry by means of the roentgen ray, Amer. J. Roentgen. 8:272-276, 1921.

Klason, T.: Radiologische Methoden zur Bestimmung der Conjugata vera, Acta Radiol. 1:308-318, 1921-1922.

Thoms, Herbert: Lateral roentgenograms of the pelvis and the mensuration of the conjugata vera, New Eng. J. Med. 200:829, 1921.

1923 Chassard and Lapiné: Étude radiographique de l'arcade pubienne chez la femme enceinte, J. Radiol. Electr. 7:113-124, 1923.

1924 Portes, L., and Blanche: Études critique des procédés radiopelvimetriques, Gynec. Obstét. 10:416-447, 1924.

1925 Thoms, Herbert: Pelvimetry of superior strait by means of roentgen ray, J.A.M.A. 85:253-256, 1925.

1926 Béclère, H., and Ameline: Radiographie latérale du bassin osseux et des oranges pelviens, J. Radiol. Electr. 10:317, 1926.

Thoms, Herbert: The clinical significance of x-ray pelvimetry, Amer. J. Obstet. Gynec. 12:543-550, 1926.

Heublein, A. C., Robert, D. J., and Ogden, R. T.: Roentgen pelvimetry after Thoms' method with simplification of technique, Amer. J. Roentgen. 20:64-66, 1926.

1927 Johnson, C. R.: Mersuration and localization by means of the roentgen ray, Radiology 8:518-521, 1927.

Thoms, Herbert: X-ray pelvimetry; simplified technique, Surg. Gynec. Obstet. 45:827-828, 1927.

1929 Samuel, Max: Ueber Ausbau und Bedeutung einer röntgenologischen Darstellung der Beckengelenke, Röntgenpraxis 1:944-947, 1929.

Thoms, Herbert: A new method of roentgen pelvimetry, J.A.M.A. 92:1515-1516, 1929.

1930 Barbacci, Gino: Metodo radiografico semplice e preciso di pelvimetria interna, Rev. Radiol. Fis. Med. 2:358-364, 1930.

Thoms, Herbert: Fetal cephalometry in utero, J.A.M.A. 95:21-24, 1930.

1931 Ehrenberg, Claude: Obstetrics from an x-ray standpoint, Xray Techn. 3:49-52, 1931.

Grunspan-de Brancas, Matilda: La radiologie en obstétrique, J. Radiol. Electr. 15:273-290, 1931.

Rowen, L. A.: A simple and accurate method of radiographic pelvimetry, Brit. J. Radiol. 4:432-439, 1931.

Walton, Henry J.: Intrauterine roentgen cephalometry and pelvimetry, Amer. J. Roentgen. 25:758-760, 1931.

1932 Hodges, P. C., and Ledoux, A. C.: Roentgen ray pelvimetry; simplified stereoroentgenographic method, Amer. J. Roentgen. 27:83-95, 1932.

Rowden, L. A.: Radiographic pelvimetry, Brit. J. Radiol. 5:657, 1932.

Thoms, Herbert: Occipito-posterior position and the transversely contracted pelvis, Amer. J. Obstet. Gynec. 24:50, 1932.

1933 Ewer, J. N., and Bowen, C. B.: Roentgen pelvimetry, Amer. J. Roentgen. 29:462-468, 1933.

Orley, A.: The evolution of x-ray pelvimetry, Brit. J. Radiol. 6:345-359, 1933.

Schumacher, P. H.: Die Röntgendiagnostik in der Geburtshilfe, Ergebn. Med. Strahlenforsch. 6:235-321, 1933.

Thoms, Herbert: Roentgen pelvimetry; a description of the grid method and a modification, Radiology 21:125-130, 1933.

1935 Ball, Robert P.: Roentgen pelvimetry and fetal cephalometry, Radiogr. Clin. Photogr. 11:11-17, 1935.

Ball, Robert P., and Marchbanks, S. S.: Roentgen pelvimetry and fetal cephalography, Radiology 24:77-84, 1935.

Weitzner, S. F.: A simple roentgenographic method for accurately determining the true conjugate diameter of the pelvis, Amer. J. Obstet. Gynec. 30:126, 1935.

1936 Cizek, J.: Zur Methodik der röntgenologischen Messung der Conjugata vera, Röntgenpraxis 8:306-312, 1936.

Clark, Erminda R.: The Thoms' method of pelvimetry, Xray Techn. 7:144-146, 1936.

Moses, C. D., and Bodenbender, A. N.: Pelvimetry by the Thoms' method, Radiogr. Clin. Photogr. 12:2-6, 1936.

Pettit, A. V., Garland, H. L., and Dunn, R. D.: Correlation between shape of the female pelvis and clinical course of labor, Western J. Surg. 44:1-20, 1936. Abst.: Yearbook of Radiology, p. 306, 1936.

1937 Hodges, Paul C.: Roentgen pelvimetry and fetometry, Amer. J. Roentgen. 37:644-662, 1937.

Pickham: Zur Technik der Röntgenuntersuchung der Schwangerschaft, Röntgenpraxis 9:835-836, 1937.

Thoms, Herbert, and Wilson, Hugh M.: Lateral roentgenometry of the pelvis; a newly modified technic, Yale J. Biol. Med. 9:305, 1937.

1938 Garland, H. L.: The shape of the female pelvis and its clinical significance, Amer. J. Roentgen. 40:359-370, 1938.

Moloy, Howard C., and Swenson, Paul C.: The use of the roentgen ray in obstetrics. In Golden, Ross, editor: Diagnostic roentgenology, New York, 1938, Thomas Nelson & Sons, vol. 2, p. 755.

Thoms, Herbert, and Wilson, Hugh M.: Roentgen methods for routine obstetrical pelvimetry, Yale J. Biol. Med. **10**:437-444, 1938.

Torpin, R., Holmes, L. P., and Hamilton, W. P.: Roentgen pelvimetry simplifying Thoms' method, Radiology **31**:584, 1938.

1939   Caldwell, W. E., Moloy, H. C., and Swenson, P. C.: The use of roentgen ray in obstetrics; roentgen pelvimetry and cephalometry; technique of pelvioradiography, Amer. J. Roentgen. **41**:305-316, 1939.

Christensen, H.: Eine einfache Methode für die stereometriche Messung, Acta Radiol. **20**:137-147, 1939.

Reuter, E. G., and Reeves, R. J.: Roentgen pelvimetry (simplified method), Amer. J. Roentgen. **42**:847-856, 1939.

1940   Frei, Sister Mary C.: Radiographic technic involved in pelvimetry, Xray Techn. **11**:222-223, 1940.

Hodges, P. C., and Dippel, A. L.: Use of x-rays in obstetrical diagnosis, with particular reference to pelvimetry and fetometry, Surg. Gynec. Obstet. **70**:421-446, 1940.

Snow, William, and Lewis, F.: Simple technique and new instrument for rapid roentgen pelvimetry, Amer. J. Roentgen. **43**:132, 1940.

Thoms, Herbert: A discussion of roentgen pelvimetry and the description of a roentgen pelvimeter, Amer. J. Roentgen. **44**:9-16, 1940.

Thoms, Herbert: The estimation of pelvic capacity, Amer. J. Surg. **47**:691-741, 1940.

Warren, Cora: Radiographic technic involved in pelvimetry, Xray Techn. **12**:52-54, 1940.

1941   Ball, R. P., and Golden, R.: Roentgenologic sign for detection of placenta previa, Amer. J. Obstet. Gynec. **42**:530-533, 1941.

Mulica, Bessie: Technical aspects of roentgen pelvimetry by the Thoms' method, Xray Techn. **13**:6-7, 51, 1941.

Perlberg, Harry J.: Measurement of the true conjugate with the aid of a new lightweight rule, Amer. J. Roentgen. **45**:935-936, 1941.

Taylor, Robert: Pelvic mensuration, Xray Techn. **12**:132-134, 1941.

Thoms, H., and Wilson, H. M.: The roentgenological survey of the pelvis, Yale J. Biol. Med. **13**:831-839, 1941.

1942   Henderson, S. G.: Pelvimetry by perforated plate method, Amer. J. Roentgen. **47**:427-436, 1942.

Steele, K. B., and Javert, C. T.: Roentgenography of obstetric pelvis; combined isometric and stereoscopic technique, Amer. J. Obstet. Gynec. **43**:600-610, 1942.

1943   Ball, Robert P., and Golden, Ross: Roentgenographic obstetrical pelvicephalometry in the erect posture, Amer. J. Roentgen. **49**:731-741, 1943.

Javert, C. T.: Combined isometric and stereoscopic technique for radiographic examination of obstetrical patient, N. Carolina Med. J. **4**:465-473, 1943.

Rita, Sister Helen: A review of the literature on the technical aspects of roentgenography in obstetrics, Xray Techn. **15**:65-73, 96-101, 1943.

1944   Colcher, A. E., and Sussman, Walter: A practical technique for roentgen pelvimetry with a new positioning, Amer. J. Roentgen. **51**:207-214, 1944.

1946   Good, Allen C.: Roentgenography in obstetrics. In Pillmore, George U., editor: Clinical radiology, Philadelphia, 1946, F. A. Davis Co., vol. 1, pp. 786-820.

1947   Allen, E. P.: Standardized radiological pelvimetry, Brit. J. Radiol. **20**:45-54; 108-118; 164-169, 1947.

Moloy, Howard C., and Swenson, Paul C.: The use of the roentgen ray in obstetrics. In Golden, Ross, editor: Diagnostic roentgenology, ed. 3, New York, 1947, Thomas Nelson & Sons, vol. 2, pp. 755-826.

1948   Kendig, T. A.: A simple pelvimeter to be used with triangulation method of pelvimetry, Radiology **50**:395-399, 1948.

Wilson, A. K.: Simplified method of roentgen pelvicephalometry, Amer. J. Roentgen. **59**:688-698, 1948.

1949   Colcher, A. E., and Sussman, W.: Changing concepts of x-ray pelvimetry, Amer. J. Obstet. Gynec. **57**:510-517, 1949.

1950   Isaacs, I.: Roentgen pelvimetry by differential divergent distortion, Amer. J. Roentgen. **63**:669-676, 1950.

March, H. C.: Accurate isometric roentgen pelvimetry

in erect posture, Amer. J. Roentgen. **63**:677-680, 1950.

Van Herick, M., and Good, C. A.: Comparative accuracy of the Chassard-Lapiné and recumbent positions in roentgen measurement of the pelvic outlet, Radiology **54**:392-396, 1950.

1952   Coe, Fred O.: Roentgenographic cephalopelvimetry, Amer. J. Roentgen. **67**:449-457, 1952.

1955   Moir, J. Chassar: The uses and value of radiology in obstetrics. In Browne, F. J., and Browne, J. C. M.: Antenatal and postnatal care, ed. 8, London, 1955, J. & A. Churchill, pp. 614-641.

Schwarz, G. S.: Orthometric pelvimetry; its use in obstetrical roentgenometry, Bull. Sloan Hosp. Women **1**:69-75, 1955.

1956   Schwarz, G. S.: An orthometric radiograph for obstetrical roentgenometry, Radiology **66**:753-761, 1956.

Wakeman, A. C. R.: A simple method of pelvimetry, Brit. J. Radiol. **29**:459-460, 1956.

1957   Grotins, E., and Schwarz, G. S.: The technique of orthometric pelvimetry, Xray Techn. **28**:328-336, 1957.

1958   Bruser, M.: A simple and accurate method of x-ray pelvimetry, Radiology **71**:565-569, 1958.

Davis, G. D., and Hunt, A. P.: Roentgen evaluation of pelvic dystocia, Clin. Obstet. Gynec. **1**:645-657, 1958.

Whitehouse, W. M., and others: Reduction of radiation hazard in obstetric roentgenography, Amer. J. Roentgen. **80**:690-695, 1958.

1960   Alexander, O. M.: Exact lateral pelvimetry; a radiographic technique utilizing a base line, Radiography **26**:170-175, 1960.

Borell, U., and Fernström, I.: Radiologic pelvimetry, Acta Radiol., supp. 191, pp. 70-76, 1960.

Moir, J. Chassar: The uses and value of radiology in obstetrics. In Browne, F. J., and Browne, J. C. M.: Antenatal and postnatal care, ed. 9, London, 1960, J. & A. Churchill, pp. 389-409.

1962   McGowen, M.: Radiographic pelvimetry, Xray Techn. **33**:341-344, 1962.

1964   Borell, U., and Rådberg, C.: Orthodiagraphic pelvimetry with special reference to capacity of distal part of pelvis and pelvic outlet, Acta Radiol. [Diagn.] **2**:273-282, 1964.

1965   Hannah, W. J.: X-ray pelvimetry; a critical appraisal, Amer. J. Obstet. Gynec. **91**:333-341, 1965.

Templeton, A. W.: High kilovoltage pelvimetry, Amer. J. Roentgen. **93**:943-947, 1965.

Vickers, A. A.: Restriction of obstetric radiology, Lancet **1**:1318-1322, 1965.

1966   Diehl, J., and Fernström, I.: Radiologic pelvimetry with special reference to widest transverse diameter of pelvic inlet, Acta Radiol. [Diagn.] **4**:557-568, 1966.

Milne, E. N. C.: Orthodiagraphic shift pelvimetry, J. Canad. Ass. Radiol. **17**:29-37, 1966.

1968   Schwarz, G. S.: Radiation hazards to the human fetus in present-day society: Should a pregnant woman be subjected to a diagnostic x-ray procedure? Bull. N. Y. Acad. Med. **44**:388-399, 1968. Abst.: Amer. J. Roentgen. **103**:962, 1968.

1969   Johnson, T. H., and Reagan, T. A.: A roentgenologic rule and pelvimetry technique, Amer. J. Roentgen. **105**:890-893, 1969.

Percy-Lancaster, R.: Pelvic arthropathy, S. Afr. Med. J. **43**:551-557, 1969.

1970   de Villiers, P. D.: Radiation dose with the orthometric view in x-ray pelvimetry, S. Afr. Med. J. **44**:820-822, 1970.

1971   Murray, J. P.: Semi-orthometric pelvimetry: an appraisal, Brit. J. Radiol. **44**:524-530, 1971.

1972   Brown, R. C.: A modification of the Colcher-Sussman technique of x-ray pelvimetry, Amer. J. Roentgen. **115**:623-629, 1972.

Cockshott, W. P., and Lawson, J.: Radiology of advanced abdominal pregnancy, Radiology **103**:21-29, 1972.

BRAIN AND SPINAL CORD
Cerebral pneumography

1918   Dandy, Walter E.: Ventriculography following the injection of air into the cerebral ventricles, Ann. Surg. **68**:5-11, 1918.

1919   Dandy, Walter E.: Roentgenography of the brain after

the injection of air into the spinal canal, Ann. Surg. **70**:397-403, 1919.

1921 Bingel, Adolf: Enzephalographie, Fortschr. Röntgenstr. **28**:205-217, 1921-1922.

1926 Jüngling, Otto: Ventrikulographie bzw. Enzephalographie im Dienste der Diagnostik von Erkrangkungen des Gehirns, Ergebn. Med. Strahlenforsch. **2**:3-105, 1926.

1927 Grant, F. C.: Ventriculography, Amer. J. Roentgen. **18**:264-269, 1927.

Pendergrass, E. P.: A new arrangement of the Bucky diaphragm for encephalography, Amer. J. Roentgen. **17**:358-359, 1927.

1929 Pancoast, H. K., and Fay, T.: Encephalography: roentgenological and clinical considerations for its use, Amer. J. Roentgen. **21**:421-447, 1929.

1930 Bruya, Carlton D.: Ventriculography, Xray Techn. **2**:47-49, 1930.

1931 Anger, Sister Mary A.: Ventriculography, Xray Techn. **3**:76-78, 1931.

Waggoner, R. W., and Clark, D. M.: A new position used in encephalography, Amer. J. Roentgen. **25**:533-535, 1931.

1932 Dandy, Walter E.: The brain. In Practice of surgery, v. XII. Hagerstown, Md., 1932, W. F. Prior Co., Inc.

1933 Green, Madge: Ventriculography, Xray Techn. **5**:68-72, 1933.

1934 Bruya, Carlton D.: Ventriculography, Xray Techn. **5**:158-161, 1934.

Howard, Campbell: Observations on encephalography, Amer. J. Roentgen. **32**:301-310, 1934.

Kornblum, Karl, and Grant, F. C.: Encephalography, Amer. J. Roentgen. **32**:311-316, 1934.

1937 Davidoff, L. M., and Dyke, C. G.: The normal encephalogram, Philadelphia, 1937, Lea & Febiger.

Lysholm, Erik: Das Ventriculogram, Acta Radiol., supp. 24, 25, 26, 1937 and 1938.

1938 Baker, W. E.: Ventriculography without specialized apparatus, Radiography **4**:163-172, 1938.

Clarke, E. R.: Encephalography, Xray Techn. **9**:142-144, 149, 1938.

1939 Twining, E. W.: Radiography of the third and fourth ventricles, Brit. J. Radiol. **12**:385-418, 1939.

1940 Pancoast, H. K., and Pendergrass, E. P.: Cerebral pneumography. In The head and neck in roentgen diagnosis, Springfield, Ill., 1940, Charles C Thomas, Publisher.

1946 Davidoff, L. M., and Dyke, C. G.: The normal encephalogram, ed. 2, Philadelphia, 1946, Lea & Febiger.

German, William J., and Wilson, Hugh M.: Anatomy and roentgenography of the cranium. In Pillmore, George U., editor: Clinical radiology, Philadelphia, 1946, F. A. Davis Co., pp. 3-18; p. 19; pp. 39-53.

1948 Kubanka, Edward: Encephalography, Roentgenography, pp. 12, 23, 1948.

1950 Ziedses des Plantes, B. G.: Examen du troisième et du quatrième ventricule au moyen de petites quantités d'air, Acta Radiol. **34**:399-407, 1950.

1954 Shapiro, R., and Robinson, F.: Controlled pneumoencephalography; consideration of head position and gas-fluid replacement, J. Neurosurg. **11**:122-127, 1954.

1957 Lindgren, Erik: Radiologic examination of the brain and spinal cord, Acta Radiol., supp. 151, 1957.

Manfredi, R. A., and Kruse, F. J.: Laminography with cerebral pneumography, J. Neurosurg. **14**:374-381, 1957.

Robertson, E. G.: Pneumoencephalography, Springfield, Ill., 1957, Charles C Thomas, Publisher.

1958 Etter, L. E., and Youngue, E. L.: Small pneumoencephalograms as a screening procedure in the study of convulsive disorders, Radiology **70**:23-32, 1958.

Plante, W. H.: Ventriculography and pneumoencephalography, Xray Techn. **29**:305-308, 1958.

1959 Dyken, M.: Pneumoencephalography with direct injection and positional directing of air, J. Neurosurg. **16**:99-106, 1959.

Ralston, B. L., and others: Pantopaque ventriculography in the localization of surgical lesions of the posterior fossa, Amer. J. Roentgen. **81**:972-983, 1959.

Schvarcz, J.: Autotomography of the fourth ventricle and floor of the third ventricle, Acta Radiol. **52**:465-469, 1959.

1960 Kruyff, Evert: Some remarks on encephalography, Amer. J. Roentgen. **84**:38-47, 1960.

Schecter, M. M., and Jing, B. S.: Improved visualization of ventricular system with technic of autotomography, Radiology **74**:593-600, 1960.

1962 Burrows, E. H.: An autotomographic appliance, Amer. J. Roentgen. **87**:366-370, 1962.

New, P. F. J.: Head-holder for pneumoencephalography, Radiology **78**:628-629, 1962.

Scott, M.: A technique for air encephalography using a stretcher with a detachable support for sitting position, Amer. J. Roentgen. **88**:21-23, 1962.

Smith, G. V.: Autotomography of the cerebral ventricular system, Xray Techn. **34**:5-7, 1962.

1963 Amplatz, K.: An improved chair for pneumoencephalography and autotomography, Amer. J. Roentgen. **90**:184-188, 1953.

Gass, H.: Pantopaque anterior basal cisternography of the posterior fossa, Amer. J. Roentgen. **90**:1197-1204, 1963.

Johnston, J. D. H., Alexander, G. H., and Rosomoff, H. L.: A simplified method for the pneumoencephalographic demonstration of the fourth ventricle and aqueduct of Sylvius, J. Neurosurg. **20**:81-83, 1963.

1964 Alker, L. M.: Radiography of the cerebral ventricles, Radiol. Techn. **35**:259-266, 1964.

Diaz, A., and Parera, C. E.: Radiography of the skull and brain, Wilmington, Del., 1964, E. I. du Pont de Nemours & Co.

Gianturco, C., and Miller, G. A.: Tilt-table encephalography, Radiology **83**:46-47, 1964.

Paris, A.: Intra-cranial investigation with the use of contrast media, Radiography **30**:192-203, 1964.

Potts, D. G., and Tavaras, J. M.: A new somersaulting chair for cerebral pneumography, Amer. J. Roentgen. **91**:1144-1149, 1964.

1965 New, P. F. J., and Webster, E. W.: Physical and anatomical considerations in autotomography, Acta Radiol. [Diagn.] **3**:370-384, 1965.

Potts, D. G.: A new universal head unit, Amer. J. Roentgen. **95**:957-961, 1965.

1968 Fredzell, G., Greitz, A., Grepe, A., and Holmstrom, L.: Mimer III and rotating chair, Acta Radiol. [Diagn.] **7**:543-552, 1968.

Kieffer, S. A., Amplatz, K., and Peterson, H. O.: Single-sweep rotation tomography in coronal and lateral planes: its value in pneumoencephalographic diagnosis, Radiology **91**:372-376, 1968.

Siqueira, E. B., Bucy, P. C., and Cannon, A. H.: Positive contrast ventriculography, cisternography and myelography, Amer. J. Roentgen. **104**:132-138, 1968.

Stitt, H. L., Dunbar, H. S., Schick, R. W., and Dunn, A. A.: Pontocerebellar cisternography, Radiology **90**:942-945, 1968.

1969 Alberti, J., Andrews, J., and Wilson, G.: Posterior fossa tomography during encephalography, Acta Radiol. [Diagn.] **9**:128-131, 1969.

Campbell, C. B.: The value of autotomography in the demonstration of the midline ventricular system of the brain, Radiol. Techn. **41**:65-73, 1969.

Gvozdanović, V.: The somersault technique in encephalography and ventriculography, Acta Radiol. [Diagn.] **9**:160-166, 1969.

Wilkinson, H. A.: Selective third ventricular catheterization for Pantopaque ventriculography, Amer. J. Roentgen. **105**:348-351, 1969.

1970 Geilfuss, C. J., and Hargest, T. S.: A modification of the Amplatz pneumographic chair for better head stabilization, Radiology **97**:685-686, 1970.

Baker, H. L.: Pneumoencephalography: a challenge in technique, Seminars Roentgen. **5**:126-137, 1970.

Lang, E. K., and Russell, J. R.: Pantopaque ventriculography: demonstration and assessment of the third ventricle and posterior fossa, J. Neurosurg. **32**:5-15, 1970.

Picaza, J. A., Hunter, S. E., and Cannon, B. W.: Axial

ventriculography, J. Neurosurg. **33**:297-303, 1970.

Pribram, H. F. W.: X-ray equipment, Seminars Roentgen. **5**:122-125, 1970.

1973   Morris, L., and Wylie, I. G.: Tomography in cerebral pneumoencephalography, Clin. Radiol. **24**:221-230, 1973.

White, Y. S., Bell, D. S., and Mellick, R.: Sequelae to pneumoencephalography, J. Neurol. Neurosurg. Psychiat. **36**:146-151, 1973.

Myelography

1919   Dandy, Walter E.: Roentgenography of the brain after the injection of air into the spinal canal, Ann. Surg. **70**:397-403, 1919.

1922   Sicard, J. A., and Forestier, J.: Méthode générale d'exploration radiologique par l'huile iodée (lipiodol), Bull. Soc. Méd. Hôp. Paris **46**:463-469, 1922.

1925   Dandy, Walter E.: The diagnosis and localization of spinal cord tumors, Ann. Surg. **81**:223-254, 1925.

1929   Schmorl, G.: Ueber Knorpelknöten an der Hinterfläche der Wirbelbandscheiben, Fortschr. Roentgenstr. **40**:629-634, 1929.

1934   Mixter, W. J., and Barr, J. S.: Rupture of the intervertebral disc with involvement of the spinal canal, New Eng. J. Med. **211**:210-215, 1934.

1938   Young, B. R., and Scott, M.: Air myelography: substitution of air for Lipiodol in roentgen visualization of tumors and other structures in the spinal canal, Amer. J. Roentgen. **39**:187-192, 1938.

1939   Chamberlain, W. Edward, and Young, B. R.: Air myelography in the diagnosis of intraspinal lesions producing low back and sciatic pain, Radiology **33**:695-700, 1939.

Lindgren, Erik: Diagnosis of tumors of the spinal cord by air or gas myelography, Acta Chir. Scand. **82**:303-318, 1939.

Lindgren, Erik: Myelography with air, Acta Psychiat. Neurol. **14**:385-388, 1939.

Smith, Wayne: Technical problems involved in the study of the spinal canal with Lipiodol, Xray Techn. **10**:164-165, 197, 1939.

1940   Melter, T. B.: Pneumomyelographic radiography, Xray Techn. **12**:47-49, 1940.

1941   Sandford, H., and Doub, H. P.: Epidurography; a method of roentgenologic visualization of protruded intervertebral disks, Radiology **36**:712-716, 1941.

1942   Coombs, W. H. J.: Myelography, Radiology **8**:90-93, 1942.

1943   Nosik, William: Intraspinal Thorotrast, Amer. J. Roentgen. **49**:214-218, 1943.

1944   Lindblom, K.: Protrusion of disks and nerve compression in the lumbar region, Acta Radiol. **25**:195-212, 1944.

Ramsey, George H. S., and Strain, William H.: Pantopaque; a new contrast medium for myelography, Radiogr. Clin. Photogr. **20**:25-33, 1944.

1945   Arbuckle, R. K., Shelden, H. C., and Pudenz, R. H.: Pantopaque myelography; correlation of roentgenologic and neurologic findings, Radiology **45**:356-369, 1945.

Schnitker, Max T., and Booth, George T.: Pantopaque myelography for protruded discs of the lumbar spine, Radiology **45**:370-376, 1945.

1946   Ramsey, George H. S., French, Douglas J., and Strain, William H.: Lesions of the intervertebral discs and spinal cord. In Pillmore, George U., editor: Clinical radiology, Philadelphia, 1946, F. A. Davis Co., vol. 2, pp. 109, 115-124.

Rouse, Opal: Myelography, Xray Techn. **18**:69-70, 1946.

1947   Judd, George: Myelography, Radiography **13**:18-20, 1947.

1948   Bartelink, D. L.: Myelography in intervertebral disc protrusion (horizontal beam examination with the patient prone), Radiology **50**:202-206, 1948.

1950   Bell, A. L. L., and others: An erect method of myelography, Amer. J. Surg. **79**:259-263, 1950.

Camp, J. D.: Contrast myelography past and present; Carmen lecture, Radiology **54**:477-506, 1950.

Lindblom, K.: Technique and results in myelography and disc puncture, Acta Radiol. **34**:321-330, 1950.

1952   Wood, E. H.: Myelography with Pantopaque, Med. Radiogr. Photogr. **28**:47-52, 1952.

1955   Murlagh, F., Chamberlain, W. E., Scott, M., and Wycis, H. T.: Cervical air myelography, Amer. J. Roentgen. **74**:1-21, 1955.

1956   Borrelli, F. J., and Maglione, A. A.: The importance of myelography in spinal pathology, Amer. J. Roentgen. **76**:273-289, 1956.

1957   Lindgren, Erik: Radiologic examination of the brain and spinal cord, Acta Radiol., supp. 151, 1957.

1959   Kvernland, B. N., and others: Upright large volume dynamic myelography, Radiology **72**:562-568, 1959.

1962   Bull, J. W. D., McKissock, W., Bloom, W., Chynn, K. Y., and Potts, D. G.: Atlas of myelography, New York, 1962, Grune & Stratton, Inc.

1963   Amundsen, P., and others: Evaluation of lumbar radiculography (myelography) with water soluble contrast media, Acta Radiol. [Diagn.] **1**:659-665, 1963.

Baker, H. L., Jr.: Myelographic examination of posterior fossa with positive contrast medium, Radiology **81**:791-801, 1963.

Bonte, G., and Delfosse, C.: Diagnostic des myélopathies cervicales d'origine discale par la myélotomographie gaseuse par voie lombaire, Acta Radiol. [Diagn.] **1**:666-674, 1963.

Gass, H.: Pantopaque anterior basal cisternography of the posterior fossa, Amer. J. Roentgen. **90**:1197-1204, 1963.

Roth, M.: Gas myelography by the lumbar route, Acta Radiol. [Diagn.] **1**:53-65, 1963.

Solé-Llenas, J.: Mielografía gaseosa, An. Med. **4**:58-67, 1963.

1964   Crandall, P. H., and Hanafee, W. N.: Cervical spondylotic myelopathy studied by air myelography, Amer. J. Roentgen. **92**:1260-1269, 1964.

Di Chiro, G., and Fischer, R. L.: Contrast radiography of the spinal cord, Arch. Neurol. **11**:125-143, 1964.

1966   Epstein, B. S., and Epstein, J. A.: Myelography utilizing image intensification fluoroscopy, cineradiography, and siphonage to remove the radiopaque, Med. Radiogr. Photogr. **42**:9-11, 1966.

Jacobson, L. H.: A simple way to lower the shoulders in cervical myelography, Radiology **86**:745, 1966.

Liliequist, B.: Gas myelography in the cervical region, Acta Radiol. [Diagn.] **4**:79-92, 1966.

Lodin, H.: Two-needle oxygen myelography, Acta Radiol. [Diagn.] **4**:62-64, 1966.

Rezende, T.: Double-contrast myelography, Acta Radiol. [Diagn.] **5**:1104-1106, 1966.

Westberg, G.: Gas myelography and percutaneous puncture in the diagnosis of spinal cord cysts, Acta Radiol., supp. 252, 1966.

Wilson, G., and others: Comparison of gas and positive contrast in evaluation of cervical spondylosis, Amer. J. Roentgen **97**:648-654, 1966.

1968   Ewart, J.: Epidural myelography, Radiography **34**:93-97, 1968.

Shapiro, R.: Myelography, ed. 2, Chicago, 1968, Year Book Medical Publishers, Inc.

Wende, S., and Beer, K.: The diagnostic value of gas myelography, Amer. J. Roentgen. **104**:213-218, 1968.

1969   Gilland, O., Chin, F., Anderson, W. B., and Nelson, J. R.: A cinemyelographic study of cerebrospinal fluid dynamics, Amer. J. Roentgen. **106**:369-375, 1969.

Jirout, J.: Pneumomyelography, Springfield, 1969, Charles C Thomas, Publisher.

Pribram, H. F. W., Kitchen, R. E., and Neal, M. P., Jr.: A simple biplane myelographic table, Amer. J. Roentgen. **105**:411-412, 1969.

Southworth, L. E., Jimenez, J. P., and Goree, J. A.: A practical approach to cervical air myelography, Amer. J. Roentgen. **107**:486-490, 1969.

Wendth, A. J., and Moriarty, D. J.: A simplified method for the rapid removal of myelographic contrast agent, Radiology **93**:1092, 1969.

1970   Chin, F. K., and Anderson, W. B.: Improvement of

root-sleeve filling in lumbar myelography with oil-soluble media, Radiology **96**:668-669, 1970.

Kieffer, S. A., Peterson, H. O., Gold, L. H. A., and Binet, E. F.: Evaluation of dilute Pantopaque for large-volume myelography, Radiology **96**:69-74, 1970.

1971   Bradac, G. B., and Simon, R. S.: Cervical air myelography—an improved technique, Fortschr. Roentgenstr. **115**:73-78, 1971. (In German.) Abst.: Radiology **102**:489, 1972.

1972   Adams, F. G., and Ward, P.: Value of lateral decubitus screening in myelography, Clin. Radiol. **23**:427-433, 1972.

George, A. E., and Kricheff, I. I.: A catheter technique for myelography, Radiology **104**:435-436, 1972.

Haverling, M.: Transsacral puncture of the arachnoidal sac. An alternative procedure to lumbar puncture, Acta Radiol. [Diagn.] **12**:1-6, 1972.

Heinz, E. R., and Goldman, R. L.: The role of gas myelography in neuroradiologic diagnosis, Radiology **102**:629-634, 1972.

1973   Chynn, K. Y.: Painless myelography: introduction of a new aspiration cannula and review of 541 consecutive studies, Radiology **109**:361-367, 1973.

Hayt, D. B.: Remotely controlled myelography, Amer. J. Roentgen. **118**:677-681, 1973.

Diskography

1950   Lindblom, Kurt: Technique and results in myelography and disc puncture, Acta Radiol. **34**:321-330, 1950.

1952   Cloward, R. B.: Anterior herniation of ruptured intervertebral disc with comments on diagnostic value of discogram, Arch. Surg. **64**:457-463, 1952.

Cloward, R. B., and Buzaid, L. L.: Discography, Amer. J. Roentgen. **68**:552-564, 1952.

1956   Peacher, W. G., and Storrs, R. P.: The roentgen diagnosis of herniated disk with particular reference to diskography (nucleography), Amer. J. Roentgen. **76**:290-302, 1956.

Swanson, F. V.: Discogram, Xray Techn. **28**:178-180, 1956.

1958   Cloward, R. B.: Cervical diskography; technique, indications, and use in diagnosis of ruptured cervical disks, Amer. J. Roentgen. **79**:563-574, 1958.

1959   Cloward, Ralph B.: Cervical diskography; a contribution to the etiology and mechanism of neck, shoulder and arm pain, Ann. Surg. **150**:1052-1064, 1959.

1961   Stuck, R. M.: Cervical diskography, Amer. J. Roentgen. **86**:975-982, 1961.

1962   Collis, J. S., and Gardner, W. J.: Lumbar discography, J. Neurosurg. **19**:452-461, 1962.

1963   Butt, W. P.: Lumbar discography, J. Canad. Ass. Radiol. **14**:172-181, 1963.

Cloward, R. B.: Cervical discography, Acta Radiol. [Diagn.] **1**:675-687, 1963.

Hernández-Ros, A.: Discografía; exploracíon discográfica de la columna lumbar, An. Med. **4**:67-93, 1963.

Meyer, R. R.: Cervical diskography, Amer. J. Roentgen. **90**:1208-1215, 1963.

1964   Feinberg, S. B.: The place of diskography in radiology as based on 2,320 cases, Amer. J. Roentgen. **92**:1275-1281, 1964.

Schaerer, J. P.: Cervical discography, J. Int. Surg. **42**:287-296, 1964.

1966   Butt, W. P.: Discography—some interesting cases, J. Canad. Ass. Radiol. **17**:167-175, 1966.

1967   Edholm, P., Fernström, I., and Lindblom, K.: Extradural lumbar disk puncture, Acta Radiol. [Diagn.] **6**:322-328, 1967.

Grote, W., and Wappenschmidt, J.: Ueber Technik und Indikation zur zervikalen Diskographie, Fortschr. Roentgenstr. **106**:721-727, 1967.

1969   Jirout, J.: Pneumographic examination of lumbar disc lesions; a new method, Acta Radiol. [Diagn.] **9**:727-732, 1969.

1971   Raynor, R. B.: Discography and myelography in acute injuries of the cervical spine, J. Neurosurg. **35**:529-535, 1971.

Stereotactic surgery

1947   Spiegel, E. A.: Stereotaxic apparatus for operations on the human brain, Science **106**:349-350, 1947.

1959   Perl, T., and Ecker, A.: Roentgenographically controlled placement of the needle in the trigeminal root for the treatment of tic douloureux, Amer. J. Roentgen. **82**:830-839, 1959.

1963   Perl, T., and Ecker, A.: Radiographically controlled injections through the foramen ovale for the relief of tic douloureux and of Parkinsonism, Acta Radiol. [Diagn.] **1**:901-912, 1963.

1965   Cobble, S. P., and Brackett, C. E.: Changes in the ventricular size during stereotaxic surgery, Amer. J. Roentgen. **95**:890-898, 1965.

1967   Dobben, G. D., Mullan, S., and Moseley, R. D.: A new biplane neuroradiologic localizing instrument, Radiology **89**:329-331, 1967.

1968   Fox, J. L., and Green, R. C.: Stereotaxic brain surgery. Part I. A geometric consideration of polar coordinates and polar range finding, Acta Neurochir. **18**:57-67, 1968.

Fox, J. L., and Green, R. C.: Stereotaxic brain surgery. Part II. Description of a method using biplane television guidance, Acta Neurochir. **18**:171-185, 1968.

1969   Ecker, A., and Perl, T.: Selective Gasserian injection for tic douloureux; technical advances and results, Acta Radiol. [Diagn.] **9**:38-48, 1969.

Fox, J. L., and Green, R. C.: A new method of stereotaxis, Radiology **92**:259-264, 1969.

Grabow, J. D.: Value of roentgenology in electrode placement techniques in electroencephalography, Acta Radiol. [Diagn.] **9**:54-57, 1969.

Hodges, P. C., and Garcia-Bengochea, F.: Precise alignment of x-ray beams for stereotactic surgery, Amer. J. Roentgen. **105**:260-269, 1969.

Rand, R. W., Heuser, G., Dashe, A., and others: Stereotaxic transsphenoidal biopsy and cryosurgery of pituitary tumors, Amer. J. Roentgen. **105**:273-286, 1969.

Todd, E. M., and Crue, B. L.: An image enlargement scale for stereotactic surgery, Amer. J. Roentgen. **105**:270-272, 1969.

1970   Fox, J. L.: The central x-ray beam in stereotaxis, Amer. J. Roentgen. **110**:166-169, 1970.

1971   Dawson, B. H., Dervin, E., and Heywood, O. B.: Some radiographic problems encountered in stereotactic surgery, Radiography **37**:131-139, 1971.

1972   Leksell, L.: Stereotaxis and radiosurgery, Springfield, Ill., 1972, Charles C Thomas, Publisher.

Cerebral angiography

1927   Egas Moniz, Antonio C.: A prova da encefalografia arterial, Lisboa Med. **4**:301-345, 1927.

Egas Moniz, Antonio C.: L'encéphalographie artérielle, son importance dans la localisation des tumeurs cérébrales, Rev. Neurol. **2**:72-90, 1927.

1928   Egas Moniz, Antonio C.: Nouvelle technique de l'encéphalographie artérielle; quelques cas de localisation de tumeurs cérébrales, Presse Méd. **36**:689-693, 1928.

1934   Egas Moniz, Antonio C.: L'angiographie cérébrale, Paris, 1934, Masson & Cie.

1939   Turnbull, Frank: Cerebral angiography by direct injection of the common carotid artery, Amer. J. Roentgen. **41**:166-167, 1939.

1941   Allen, E., and Camp, J. D.: Angiography in diagnostic roentgenology, New York, 1941, Thomas Nelson & Sons.

Gross, Sidney W.: Cerebral arteriography with diodrast, fifty per cent, Radiology **37**:487, 1941.

Sanchez-Perez, J. M.: Cerebral angiography, Surgery **10**:535-552, 1941.

1943   Sanchez-Perez, J. M.: Cranial seriograph and its utility in neurologic radiology for cerebral angiography, Surgery **13**:661-666, 1943.

1944   Engeset, Arne: Cerebral angiography with perabrodil. (Carotis angiography), Acta Radiol., supp. 55-57, pp. 1-38, 1944.

Stoltz, Sister Mary F.: The technique of angiography, Xray Techn. **15**:219-222, 1944.

1945 List, Carl F., Burge, Curtis H., and Hodges, Fred J.: Intercranial angiography, Radiology **45**:1-14, 1945.

1946 German, William J., and Wilson, Hugh M.: Anatomy and roentgenography of the cranium; cerebral angiography. In Pillmore, George U., editor: Clinical radiology, Philadelphia, 1946, F. A. Davis Co., vol. 2, pp. 53-56.
List, Carl, and Hodges, Fred J.: Angiographic diagnoses of expanding intracranial lesions by vascular displacement, Radiology **47**:319-333, 1946.

1947 Camp, John D., and Allen, Edgar V.: Angiography. In Golden, Ross, editor: Diagnostic roentgenology, ed. 3, New York, 1947, Thomas Nelson & Sons, vol. 2, pp. 1143-1168.
Hodes, Philip J., Perryman, Charles R., and Chamberlain, Richard H.: Cerebral angiography, Amer. J. Roentgen. **58**:543-583, 1947.

1948 Engeset, Arne: About the angiographic visualization of the posterior cerebral artery, especially by intracarotid injection of contrast, Acta Radiol. **30**:152-162, 1948.
Engeset, Arne, and Kvadsheim, Hans: Technical improvements in cerebral angiography, Acta Radiol. **29**:83-86, 1948.
Green, J. R., and Arana, R.: Cerebral angiography, Amer. J. Roentgen. **59**:617-650, 1948.

1949 Bull, J. W. D.: A review of cerebral angiography, Proc. Roy. Soc. Med. **42**:880-890, 1949.
Fineman, S.: A practical serialograph for intracranial angiography, Amer. J. Roentgen. **61**:324-334, 1949.
Sanchez-Perez, J. M., and Carter, R. A.: The time factor in cerebral angiography and an automatic seriograph, Amer. J. Roentgen. **62**:509-518, 1949.
Sugar, O., and others: Vertebral angiography, Amer. J. Roentgen. **61**:166-182, 1949.

1950 Lindgren, E.: Percutaneous angiography of the vertebral artery, Acta Radiol. **33**:389-404, 1950.
Löfstedt, Stig: Intracranial arterial aneurysms, Acta Radiol. **34**:339-349, 1950.
Wise, R. E., and others: Cerebral arteriography, Amer. J. Roentgen. **64**:239-254, 1950.

1951 Curtis, J. D.: Cerebral angiography, Brit. J. Surg. **38**:295-331, 1951.

1952 Kinley, G. J., and Leighninger, D. S.: Aneurysm of anomalous ophthalmic artery presenting in the sphenoid sinus and simulating an aneurysm of the internal carotid artery on routine arteriography, J. Neurosurg. **9**:544-547, 1952.
Krayenbuhl, H.: Diagnostic value of orbital angiography, Brit. J. Ophthal. **42**:180-190, 1952.

1953 Seldinger, S. I.: Catheter replacement of the needle in percutaneous arteriography; a new technique, Acta Radiol. **39**:368-376, 1953.

1954 French, L. A., and Watson, J. C.: Angiography versus pneumoencephalography, Xray Techn. **25**:251-255, 1954.
Lindgren, Erik: Röntgenologie einschliesslich Kontrastmethoden, Olivercroma Tonnis Handb. Neurochir. **2**:189-197, 1954.

1955 Gould, P. L., and others: Vertebral angiography by retrograde injection of the brachial artery, J. Neurosurg. **12**:369-374, 1955.
Hunter, C. R., and Mayfield, F. H.: The oblique view in cerebral angiography, J. Neurosurg. **12**:78-80, 1955.
Plaut, H. F.: Vertebral arteriography of the brain; detailed diagram of the arterial branches in the fronto-occipital roentgen view, Amer. J. Roentgen. **74**:226-231, 1955.

1956 Greitz, T.: A radiologic study of the brain circulation by rapid serial angiography of the carotid artery, Acta Radiol., supp. 140, 1956.

1957 Lindgren, Erik: Radiologic examination of the brain and spinal cord, Acta Radiol., supp. 151, 1957.

1958 Ghirardi, L., Garello, L., and Lertora, M.: Experienze angiografiche cerebrali in proiezione sottomentobregmatica, Ann. Radiol. Diagn. **31**:102-118, 1958.

1959 Boyd-Wilson, J. S.: Oblique views; their place in arteriographic diagnosis of intracranial aneurysms, J. Neurosurg. **16**:297-310, 1959.
Smith, L.: Improvements in cerebral angiographic technique, Xray Techn. **31**:23-27, 1959.
Steinberg, I., and others: Safe and practical intravenous method for abdominal aortography, peripheral arteriography, and cerebral angiography, Amer. J. Roentgen. **82**:758-772, 1959.

1960 Gensini, G. G., and Ecker, A.: Percutaneous aortocerebral angiography, Radiology **75**:885-893, 1960.
Kuhn, R. A.: The normal branchial cerebral angiogram, Amer. J. Roentgen. **84**:78-87, 1960.

1961 Greitz, T., and Lindgren, E.: In Abrams, H. L., editor: Angiography, Boston, 1961, Little, Brown & Co., pp. 41-49.
Kuhn, R. A.: Successful radiographic demonstration of the human circle of Willis, J.A.M.A. **175**:769-772, 1961.
Schramel, R., and others: Visualization of the extracranial cerebral circulation by cardio-angiography, J.A.M.A. **175**:304-305, 1961.
Steinberg, I., and Evans, J. A.: Technique of intravenous carotid and vertebral arteriography, Amer. J. Roentgen. **85**:1138-1145, 1961.

1962 Alexander, D. M., and Simon, G.: Cerebral angiography, Radiography **28**:115-118, 1962.
Krayenbuhl, H.: The value of orbital angiography for the diagnosis of unilateral exophthalmos, J. Neurosurg. **19**:289-301, 1962.
Tatelman, M., and Sheehan, S.: Total vertebral-basilar arteriography via transbrachial catheterization, Radiology **78**:919-929, 1962.
Wolf, B. S., and others: The posterior inferior cerebellar artery on vertebral angiography, Amer. J. Roentgen. **87**:322-337, 1962.

1963 Hanafee, W.: Axillary artery approach to carotid, vertebral, abdominal aorta, and coronary angiography, Radiology **81**:559-567, 1963.
Newton, T. H.: Axillary artery approach to arteriography of the aorta and its branches, Amer. J. Roentgen. **89**:275-283, 1963.
Westcott, J. L., and others: Percutaneous transfemoral selective arteriography of branchiocephalic vessels, Amer. J. Roentgen. **90**:554-563, 1963.

1964 Diaz, A., and Parera, C. E.: Radiography of the skull and brain, Wilmington, Del., 1964, E. I. du Pont de Nemours & Co.
Goree, J. A., and others: Percutaneous retrograde brachial angiography in the diagnosis of acoustic neuroma, Amer. J. Roentgen. **92**:829-835, 1964.
Paris, A.: Intracranial investigation with the use of contrast media, Radiography **30**:192-203, 1964.
Shenkin, H. A., and others: Value of routine urography during cerebral angiography, J.A.M.A. **187**:207-211, 1964.

1965 Baird, R. M., and others: Percutaneous retrograde brachial arteriography, Amer. J. Roentgen. **94**:19-29, 1965.
Du Boulay, G. H., and Jackson, D. C.: Cranial angiotomography, Clin. Radiol. **16**:148-153, 1965.
Hanafee, W., and others: Venography of the cavernous sinus, orbital veins, and basal venous plexus, Radiology **84**:751-753, 1965.
Liliequist, B., and Hellström, L.: Technique of aortocervical angiography, Acta Radiol. [Diagn.] **3**:17-29, 1965.
Marshall, T. R., and Ling, J. T.: Carotid-vertebral and cerebral arteriography, J. Kentucky Med. Ass. **63**:265-269, 1965.

1966 Morris, Leon: Angiographic demonstration of the circle of Willis, Acta Radiol. [Diagn.] **5**:424-427, 1966.
Weibel, J., and Fields, W. S.: Angiography of the posterior cervicocranial circulation, Amer. J. Roentgen. **98**:660-671, 1966.

1967 Koch, R. L., Bieber, W. P., and Hill, M. C.: The hanging head position for detection of site of internal carotid artery occlusion, Amer. J. Roentgen. **101**:111-115, 1967.

Liliequist, B.: Capillary phase in cerebral angiography, Acta Radiol. [Diagn.] **6**:113-125, 1967.

Rabinov, K., and Lavender, P.: The coronal tangential view for the demonstration of extracerebral hematomas, Amer. J. Roentgen. **101**:107-110, 1967.

1968 Leeds, N. E., Isard, H. J., Goldberg, H., and Cullinan, J. E.: Serial magnification cerebral angiography, Radiology **90**:1171-1175, 1968.

1969 Lee, K. F.: A new head positioning device for cerebral angiography and pneumoencephalography, Amer. J. Roentgen. **106**:440-441, 1969.

1970 Morris, L.: A lateral oblique view in cerebral angiography, Radiology **96**:61-65, 1970.

Sones, P. J., Hoffman, J., and Brylski, J. R.: Epidural subtemporal hematoma: angiographic changes involving the meningeal artery, Amer. J. Roentgen. **108**:756-761, 1970.

1971 Baker, H. L.: The clinical usefulness of magnification cerebral angiography, Radiology **98**:587-594, 1971.

Glickman, M. G., Gletne, J. S., and Mainzer, F.: The basal projection in cerebral angiography, Radiology **98**:611-618, 1971.

Goldman, R. L., and Heinz, E. R.: Technique of cerebral angiography, Seminars Roentgen. **6**:7-13, 1971.

Lee, K. F., and Lin, S. R.: An improved technique in orbital venography with the use of Innovar and compression devices, Amer. J. Roentgen. **112**:339-341, 1971.

Pochaczevsky, R., and Levine, S.: Skull immobilizer and positioner, Amer. J. Roentgen. **112**:408-410, 1971.

Smith, J. T., Goree, J. A., Jimenez, J. P., and Harris, C. C.: Cerebral angioautotomography, Amer. J. Roentgen. **112**:315-323, 1971.

Wende, S., Schindler, K., and Moritz, G.: The diagnostic value of the angiographic magnification technique with small focal spot tubes in two planes, Radiologe **11**:471-475, 1971.

1972 Deck, M. D. F., Grossman, C. B., Moody, D. M., and Potts, D. G.: Clinical experience with circular angiotomography, Radiology **105**:591-595, 1972.

1973 Glickman, M. G., McNamara, T. O., and Margolis, M. T.: Arteriographic diagnosis of subtemporal subdural hematoma, Radiology **109**:607-615, 1973.

Gold, L. H. A., Krause, D., and Amplatz, K.: Routine biplane magnification cerebral angiography, Radiology **106**:321-324, 1973.

Skelly, G. A., and Mansour, G.: A simple method of stereoscopic angiography with particular reference to the posterior fossa, Amer. J. Roentgen. **118**:690-694, 1973.

1974 Newton, T. H., and Potts, D. G., editors: Radiology of the skull and brain. Vol. 2, Angiography, St. Louis, 1974, The C. V. Mosby Co.

Composite mask subtraction technique

1935 Ziedses des Plantes, B. G.: Subtraktion: eine roentgenographische Methode zur separaten Abbildung bestimmter Teile des Objekts, Fortschr. Roentgenstr. **52**:69-79, 1935.

1961 Ziedses des Plantes, B. G.: Subtraktion, Stuttgart, 1961, Georg Thieme.

1962 Hanafee, W., and Stout, P.: Subtraction technique, Radiology **79**:658-661, 1962.

Levick, R. K., and Mitchell, J.: A simplified method of subtraction and its application to renal arteriography, Brit. J. Radiol. **35**:843-846, 1962.

1964 Horenstein, R., Lundh, A., and Sjögren, S. E.: A subtraction method, Acta Radiol. [Diagn.] **2**:264-272, 1964.

1965 Chynn, K. Y.: Simplified subtraction technique, Amer. J. Roentgen. **95**:970-975, 1965.

Oldendorf, W. H.: A modified subtraction technique for extreme enhancement of angiographic detail, Neurology **15**:366-370, 1965.

1966 Hanafee, W., and Shinno, J. M.: Second-order subtraction with simultaneous bilateral carotid, internal carotid injections, Radiology **86**:334-341, 1966.

Oldendorf, W. H.: Auto-subtraction; a photographic technique for enhancement of detail in radiographic reproduction, Acta Radiol. [Diagn.] **4**:97-104, 1966.

Wallman, H., and Wickbom, I.: Electronic subtraction, Acta Radiol. [Diagn.] **5**:562-569, 1966.

Wise, R. E., and Ganson, J.: Subtraction technic: video and color methods, Radiology **86**:814-821, 1966.

1967 Dalrymple, G. V., Gaston, S. L., Scott, P. D., and others: A rapid method for producing subtraction technic roentgenograms, Radiology **89**:934-935, 1967.

Kimber, P. M.: Routine photographic subtraction, Radiography **33**:255-258, 1967.

Ruggiero, G., and Mazzacurati, M.: Subtraction technique in encephalography, Invest. Radiol. **2**:326-331, 1967.

Tucker, A. K.: Subtraction in radiology, Radiography **33**:125-129, 1967.

1968 Winkler, N. T.: Roentgenographic subtraction technique, Radiol. Techn. **39**:339-346, 1968.

1969 Benness, G. T.: Television subtraction, Australas. Radiol. **13**:314-318, 1969.

Liliequist, B., and Welander, U.: Colour in subtraction angiography, Acta Radiol. [Diagn.] **8**:1-4, 1969.

1970 Jenkin, C., Pribram, H., and Eisenman, J. I.: Light intensity variation; a novel approach to subtraction technique, Radiology **97**:684-685, 1970.

Joyce, J. W., Dalrymple, G. V., Jungkind, F. F., and others: Improved contrast in subtraction technique, Radiology **94**:157-159, 1970.

Miller, E. R., McCurry, E. M., and Hruska, B. B.: Anisotrophic subtraction and edge-enhancement of roentgenographic images, Radiology **97**:27-32, 1970.

Thiel, A. J.: Photographic subtraction and color addition to enhance cut film, 35 mm slides and 16 mm cine studies of vascular systems, Radiol. Techn. **42**:1-7, 1970.

1971 Hehman, K. N.: Subtraction in cerebral angiography, Seminars Roentgen. **6**:14-16, 1971.

1972 Fiebach, O., and Dorr, K.: A simplified method for photographic subtraction using a 90 second processor, Fortschr. Roentgenstr. **117**:476-478, 1972. (In German.)

Hoffman, R. B., and Rein, B.: The routine use of subtraction in aortic arch studies, Radiology **102**:575-578, 1972.

1973 Athanasoulis, C. A., and others: Angionephrotomography and subtraction; relative value in renal mass lesions, Amer. J. Roentgen. **117**:108-111, 1973.

Lee, I., and Hunter, T. B.: Modified subtraction technique for neuroradiology, Radiology **108**:442-443, 1973.

Miller, E. R.: Photographic anisotrophic subtraction and edge enhancement, Radiology **106**:222-223, 1973.

Rothman, S. L. G., Kier, E. L., Allen, W. E., and Barauskas, L.: A simple technique for photographic image enhancement of subtraction films, Radiology **107**:461-463, 1973.

CIRCULATORY SYSTEM
Anatomy

1942 Greisheimer, E. M.: Physiology and anatomy, ed. 4, Philadelphia, 1942, J. B. Lippincott Co., p. 470.

Visceral and peripheral angiography

1899 Tait, Dudley: Radiography of arteries in the living subject, Amer. Xray J. **4**:1899.

1923 Beberich, J., and Hirsch, S.: Die röntgenographische Darstellung der Arterien und Venen am lebenden Menschen, Klin. Wschr. **2**:2226-2228, 1923.

1924 Brooks, B.: Intra-arterial injection of sodium iodide, J.A.M.A. **82**:1016-1019, 1924.

1929 Dos Santos, R., and others: Arteriographie des membres de l'aorte et de ses branches abdominales, J. Radiol. Electr. **55**:587-601, 1929.

Weiss, S., Robb, G. P., and Blumgart, H. L.: Velocity of blood flow in health and disease as measured by the effect of histamine on the minute vessels, Amer. Heart J. **4**:664-691, 1929.

1931 Dos Santos, R., Lemas, A. C., and Caldas, J. P.: Arteriographie des membres et de l'aorte abdominale, Paris, 1931, Masson & Cie.

Dos Santos, R., Lemas, A. C., and Caldas, J. P.: Les recents progrès dans la technique de l'arteriographie de l'aorte abdominale, Presse Méd. 39:574-577, 1931.

Egas Moniz, A. C., de Carvalho, Lopo, and Lima, A.: Angiopneumographie, Presse Méd. 39:996-999, 1931.

Forssmann, W.: Ueber Kontrastdarstellung der Höhlen des lebenden rechten Herzens und der Lungenschlagader, München. Med. Wschr. 78:489-492, 1931.

1932 Saito, M., and Kamikawa, K.: New modification for the injection method of arteriography (injection in refluence), Amer. J. Surg. 17:16-19, 1932.

Wohlleben, Theo.: Venographie, Klin. Wschr., Oct. 22, 1932. Abst.: Yearbook of Radiology, p. 341, 1933.

1934 Ravina, A.: L'exploration radiologique des vaisseaux pulmonaires par l'injection de substances de contraste, Progrès. Méd., pp. 1701-1705, Nov. 3, 1934.

Veal, Ross J., and McFetridge, Elizabeth: Technical considerations in arteriography of the extremities, Amer. J. Roentgen. 32:64-71, 1934.

1935 Dos Santos, R.: Phlebography of inferior vena cava, J. Urol. 35:586, 1935.

1936 Barker, N. W., and Camp, J. D.: Direct venography in obstructive lesions of the veins, Amer. J. Roentgen. 35:485-489, 1936.

1937 Castellanos, A., Pereiras, R., and Garcia, A.: L'angiocardiografía radio-opaca, Arch. Soc. Clin. Habana 31:9-10, 1937.

Farinas, P. L.: Differential diagnosis of bone tumors of the extremities by arteriography, Radiology 29:29-32, 1937.

1938 Castellanos, A., Pereiras, R. and Vazques Paussa, A.: La angiocardiografía, Rev. Cien. Méd. 1:1-10, 1938.

Castellanos, A., Pereiras, R., and Vazques Paussa, A.: On special automatic device for angiocardiography, Bol. Soc. Cubana Pediat. 10:209-215, 1938.

Dos Santos, J. C.: Direct venography: conception, technique, first results, J. Int. Chir. 3:625, 1938.

Pereiras, R.: Aspecto arteriográfico en dos casos de tumores malignos del sistema oseo, Bol. Soc. Cubana Pediat. 10:377-386, 1938.

Robb, George P., and Steinberg, Israel: Practical method of visualization of the chambers of the heart, the pulmonary circulation, and the great blood vessels in man, J. Clin. Invest. 17:507, 1938.

Zehnder, M.: Zur Technik der Arteriographie, Zbl. Neurochir. 2:281, 1938.

1939 Castellanos, A., and Pereiras, R.: Counter-current aortography, Rev. Cubana Cardiol., pp. 187-205, July 1939-April 1940.

Robb, George P., and Steinberg, Israel: Visualization of the chambers of the heart, the pulmonary circulation, and the great blood vessels in man, Amer. J. Roentgen. 41:1-18, 1939.

1940 Dougherty, J., and Homans, J.: Venography—a clinical study, Surg. Gynec. Obstet. 71:697-702, 1940.

Farinas, P. L.: Una nueva técnica para el examen arteriográfico de la aorta y sus ramas, Rev. Med. Hosp. Mexico, October, 1940.

1941 Allen, E., and Camp, J.: Angiography. In Golden, Ross, editor: Diagnostic roentgenology, ed. 2, New York, 1941, Thomas Nelson & Sons.

Farinas, P. L.: New technique for the arteriographic examination of the abdominal aorta and its branches, Amer. J. Roentgen. 46:641-645, 1941.

Lindblom, Knut: Phlebographische Untersuchung des Unterschenkels bei Kontrastinjektion in eine subkutane Vene, Acta Radiol. 22:288-296, 1941.

Sussman, Marcy L., Steinberg, Morris F., and Grishman, Arthur: Multiple exposure technique in contrast visualization of the cardiac chambers and great vessels, Amer. J. Roentgen. 46:745-747, 1941.

1942 Nelson, O. A.: Arteriography of abdominal organs by aortic injection, Surg. Gynec. Obstet. 74:655-662, 1942.

Sussman, Marcy L., Steinberg, Morris F., and Grishman, A.: A rapid film changer for use in contrast angiocardiography, Radiology 38:232-233, 1942.

1943 Lough, Thomas W.: Abdominal arteriography, Xray Techn. 14:235-237, 1943.

Mahorner, Howard: A method for obtaining venograms of the veins of extremities, Surg. Gynec. Obstet. 76:41-42, 1943.

Taylor, Henry K., and McGovern, Theresa: Evaluation of angiocardiography, J.A.M.A. 121:1270-1275, 1943.

1944 Baker, E. C., and Miller, F. A.: Further experiences with venography, Radiology 43:129-134, 1944.

Stoltz, Sister Mary F.: The technique of angiography, Xray Techn. 15:219-222, 1944.

Taylor, Henry K., and McGovern, Theresa: Angiocardiography; anatomy of the heart in health and disease, Radiology 43:364-372, 1944.

1945 Baker, Edgar C.: Venography of the lower extremities, Ohio Med. J. 41:330-332, 1945.

Farinas, P. L.: Retrograde arteriography in study of abdominal aorta and iliac arteries, Surgery 18:244-249, 1945.

Nelson, O. A.: Arteriography in renal and abdominal conditions, J. Urol. 53:521-533, 1945.

1946 Farinas, P. L.: Retrograde abdominal aortography, Amer. J. Roentgen. 55:448-451, 1946.

1947 Baker, Edgar C.: Clinical and roentgenologic evaluation of venography, Amer. J. Roentgen. 58:603-613, 1947.

Farinas, Pedro L.: Abdominal venography, Amer. J. Roentgen. 58:559-602, 1947.

O'Loughlin, J. B.: Roentgen visualization of the inferior vena cava, Amer. J. Roentgen. 58:617-619, 1947.

Wagner, F. B., Price, A. H., and Swenson, P. C.: Abdominal arteriography; technique and diagnostic application, Amer. J. Roentgen. 58:591-598, 1947.

1948 Brocklebank, J. A.: Angiocardiography applied to congenital heart disease; observations on radiology and technique, Brit. J. Radiol. 21:393-397, 1948.

1950 Castellanos, A., and Pereiras, R.: Retrograde or countercurrent aortography, Amer. J. Roentgen. 63:559-563, 1950.

Dos Santos, R.: Arteriography in bone tumors, J. Bone Joint Surg. 32-B:17-29, 1950.

Goodwin, W. E., and others: Translumbar aortic puncture and retrograde catheterization of aorta in aortography and renal arteriography, Ann. Surg. 132:944-958, 1950.

McEnerney, P. E.: Technical aspects of arterial visualization of the placenta, Xray Techn. 21:189-195, 1950.

Moore, G. E., and Bridenbaugh, R. B.: Portal venography, Surgery 28:827-831, 1950.

Sutton, George C., and others: Circulation times for angiocardiography, Amer. J. Roentgen. 63:186-190, 1950.

1951 Abeatici, S., and Campi, L.: Sur les possibilités de l'angiographie hépatique—la visualisation du système portal, Acta Radiol. 36:383-392, 1951.

Child, C. G., O'Sullivan, W. D., Payne, M. A., and McClure, R. D.: Portal venography, Radiology 57:691-701, 1951.

Dotter, C. T., and Steinberg, I.: Angiocardiography; series of monographic atlases, New York, 1951, Paul B. Hoeber.

Dotter, C. T., and Steinberg, I.: Rapid serial contrast angiography, Angiology 2:173-183, 1951.

Goyette, E. M., and Keirns, M. M.: Angiocardiography in the localization of foreign bodies in the heart, Amer. Heart J. 42:362-369, 1951.

Jönsson, G., and others: Thoracic aortography with special reference to its value in patent ductus arteriosus and coarctation of aorta, Acta Radiol. 89(supp.): 1-176, 1951.

Leger, L., and others: La portographie (technique et indications), J. Radiol. Electr. 32:633-636, 1951.

Leger, L., and others: La phlébographie portale dans l'exploration des affections hépato-spléniques, Presse Méd. 59:1230-1231, 1951.

Moore, G. E., and Bridenbaugh, R. B.: Roentgen demonstration of the venous circulation in the liver; portal venography, Radiology 57:685-690, 1951.

Scott, W. G.: The development of angiocardiography and aortography, Radiology **56:**485-518, 1951.

1952 Deterling, R. A., Jr.: Direct and retrograde aortography, Surgery **31:**88-114, 1952.

Smith, P. G., and others: Translumbar arteriography, Amer. J. Roentgen. **67:**183-196, 1952.

1953 Astle, W. E. C., and Wallace-Jones, D.: A simple radiographic technique for femoral angiography, Brit. J. Radiol. **26:**658-659, 1953.

Bahnson, H. T., and others: Splenic-portal venography; a technique utilizing percutaneous injection of radiopaque material into the spleen, Bull. Hopkins Hosp. **92:**331-345, 1953.

Gvozdanović, V., and others: Percutaneous splenic venography, Acta Radiol. **40:**17-26, 1953.

Ott, T. T.: Venography of the upper and lower extremities, Xray Techn. **25:**9-13, 1953.

Pierce, E. C., and Ramey, W. P.: Renal arteriography; report of a percutaneous method using the femoral artery approach and a disposable catheter, J. Urol. **69:**578-585, 1953.

Rousselot, L. M., Ruzicka, F. F., and Doehner, G. A.: Portal venography via the portal and percutaneous splenic routes, Surgery **34:**557-569, 1953.

Seldinger, S. I.: Catheter replacement of needle in percutaneous arteriography; new technique, Acta Radiol. **39:**368-376, 1953.

1954 Dotter, Charles T.: The technic of angiocardiography, Med. Radiogr. Photogr. **30:**68-79, 1954.

Evans, Arthur T.: Renal arteriography, Amer. J. Roentgen. **72:**574-585, 1954.

Evans, J. A., Dubilier, W., Jr., and Monteith, J. C.: Nephrotomography; a preliminary report, Amer. J. Roentgen. **71:**213-223, 1954.

Felson, B.: Translumbar arteriography in intrinsic disease of the abdominal aorta and its branches, Amer. J. Roentgen. **72:**597-608, 1954.

Greitz, T.: Technique of ascending phlebography of the lower extremity, Acta Radiol. **42:**421-441, 1954.

Rigler, L. G., and Olfelt, P. C.: Abdominal aortography for the roentgen demonstration of the liver and spleen, Amer. J. Roentgen. **72:**586-596, 1954.

1955 Evans, J. A., and O'Sullivan, W. D.: Percutaneous splenoportal venography, Med. Radiogr. Photogr. **31:**98-107, 1955.

Evans, J. A., and others: Nephrotomography, Radiology **64:**655-663, 1955.

Figley, M. M., and others: Percutaneous splenoportography, Gastroenterology **28:**153-162, 1955.

Greitz, T.: Ascending phlebography in venous insufficiency, Acta Radiol. **44:**145-162, 1955.

O'Sullivan, W. D., and Evans, J. A.: Splenoportal venography, Surg. Gynec. Obstet. **101:**235-241, 1955.

Steinberg, I., Dubilier, W., and Evans, J. A.: New twelve by twelve-inch roll-film magazine for rapid serial roentgenography, Radiology **65:**276-280, 1955.

1956 Dimtza, A.: Die Arteriographie der Hand, Radiol. Clin. **25:**305-320, 1956.

Figley, M. M.: The expanding scope of cardiovascular radiology, Amer. J. Roentgen. **76:**721-729, 1956.

Menendez, C. V., and Linton, R. R.: A technique of abdominal aortography and femoral arteriography, Surgery **40:**718-736, 1956.

Ödman, Paul: Percutaneous selective angiography of the main branches of the aorta (preliminary report), Acta Radiol. **45:**1-14, 1956.

Ödman, Paul: Thoracic aortography by means of radiopaque polythene catheter inserted percutaneously, Acta Radiol. **45:**117-124, 1956.

Rogoff, Stanley M.: Technique of serial long film angiography in arteriosclerosis obliterans, Amer. J. Roentgen. **76:**787-800, 1956.

1957 Evans, John A.: Nephrotomography in the investigation of renal masses, Radiology **69:**684-689, 1957.

Evans, J. A., and O'Sullivan, W. D.: Percutaneous splenoportal venography utilizing rapid serial roentgenography, Amer. J. Roentgen. **77:**312-323, 1957.

Morton, S. A., and Byrne, R. W.: Scanographic methods in visualization of the blood vessels and skeleton, Radiology **69:**63-69, 1957.

Paul, R. E., and others: Intravenous carbon dioxide for intracardiac gas contrast in roentgen diagnosis of pericardial effusion and thickening, Amer. J. Roentgen. **78:**224-225, 1957.

Steinberg, I., and Ryan, B. K.: Corner positioning for visualization of the branchiocephalic vessels, Radiology **68:**242-244, 1957.

1958 Bernstein, E. F., and others: Intravenous abdominal aortography; preliminary report, Surgery **44:**529-535, 1958.

Kincaid, O. W., and Davis, G. D.: Abdominal aortography, New Eng. J. Med. **259:**1017-1024, 1958.

Nelson, S. W., and others: Aortic valvulography and ascending aortography, Radiology **70:**697-712, 1958.

Van Velzer, D. A., and Lanier, R. R.: A simplified technic for nephrotomography, Radiology **70:**77-81, 1958.

1959 Bobbio, A., and others: Pelvic angiography in diseases of the prostatic gland, Amer. J. Roentgen. **82:**784-792, 1959.

De Weese, J. A., and Rogoff, S. M.: Functional ascending phlebography of the lower extremity by serial long film technique, Amer. J. Roentgen. **81:**841-854, 1959.

Jones, D. R.: Nephrotomography, Xray Techn. **30:**487-490, 1959.

Linton, R. R.: Peripheral vascular disease, New Eng. J. Med. **260:**322-328, 1959.

Sammons, B. P., and others: Simplified phlebography of the inferior vena cava in urologic diagnosis, Radiology **72:**222-226, 1959.

Scatliff, J. H., and others: Diagnosis of pericardial effusion with intracardiac carbon dioxide, Radiology **73:**871-883, 1959.

Steinberg, I., Finby, N., and Evans, J. A.: A safe and practical intravenous method for abdominal aortography, peripheral arteriography, and cerebral angiography, Amer. J. Roentgen. **82:**758-772, 1959.

1960 Cullinan, J. E.: The role of the x-ray technician in the cardiopulmonary laboratory, Xray Techn. **31:**623-627, 1960.

Detrie, P., and others: Cavographie par voie transsomatique, Presse Méd. **31:**1223-1226, 1960.

Dotter, Charles T.: Left ventricular and systemic arterial catheterization; simple percutaneous method using spring guide, Amer. J. Roentgen. **83:**969-984, 1960.

Gregg, D. McC., and others: Thoracic aortography; a symposium, Brit. J. Radiol. **33:**531-576, 1960.

Haimovici, H., and others: Serial femoral arteriography in occlusive disease; clinical-roentgenologic considerations with new classification of occlusive patterns, Amer. J. Roentgen. **83:**1042-1062, 1960.

Steinberg, I.: Localization of bullets and metallic fragments in the cardiovascular system; role of angiocardiography in 7 cases, Amer. J. Roentgen. **83:**998-1010, 1960.

1961 Bréhant, J., and others: La phlébographie mammaire interne trans-sternale, Presse Méd. **69:**140-143, 1961.

De Weese, J. A., and others: Deep venous thrombosis. Postgrad. Med. **29:**614-618, 1961.

Halpern, M., and others: Percutaneous transfemoral renal arteriography in hypertension, Radiology **77:**25-34, 1961.

Hemley, S. D., Arida, E. J., and Ring, E. M.: The renal arteries; an evaluation of roentgen methods of opacification, Radiology **76:**402-406, 1961.

Rogoff, S. M.: Lumbar aortography; background technique and indications. In Abrams, H. L., editor: Angiography, Boston, 1961, Little, Brown & Co., pp. 475-484.

Roy, P., and others: Extra large field angiography technique and results, J. Canad. Ass. Radiol. **12:**27-35, 1961.

Schobinger, R. A., and others: Comparison of intraosseous vertebral venography and Pantopaque myelography in diagnosis of surgical conditions of the lumbar spine and nerve roots, Radiology **77:**376-398, 1961.

Steinberg, I., and Marshall, V.: Intravenous abdominal aortography in urologic diagnosis, J. Urol. **86:**456, 1961.

Zerbi-Ortez, A., and Weldon, W. V.: Aortography by catheterization of the right atrium; a safe and reliable method, New Eng. J. Med. **264**:19-23, 1961.

1962 Alang, D.: The aortoarteriogram, Xray Techn. **34**:70-72, 1962.

Bucht, H.: Percutaneous catheterization of the left adrenal vein in man, Scand. J. Clin. Lab. Invest. **14**:27, 1962.

Honey, M., and others: Cardiac catheterisation and angiocardiography, Radiography **28**:69-74, 1962.

Isherwood, I.: Spinal intra-osseous venography, Clin. Radiol. **13**:73-82, 1962.

Lagergren, C., and Lindblom, A.: Angiography of peripheral tumors, Radiology **79**:371-377, 1962.

Lockery, R. M.: Pelvic phlebography, Xray Techn. **34**:11-12, 1962.

Steinberg, I.: Bilateral simultaneous intravenous angiocardiography, Amer. J. Roentgen. **88**:38-48, 1962.

Steinberg, I., and others: Experience with an automatic table for serial peripheral vascular arteriography, Amer. J. Roentgen. **88**:1175-1181, 1962.

Viamonte, M. J.: CO_2 angiocardiography, Amer. J. Roentgen. **88**:31-37, 1962.

1963 Beal, A. C., Jr., and others: Translumbar aortography; a simple, safe technic, Ann. Surg. **157**:882, 1963.

Grainger, R. G.: Aortography; its technique, indications and interpretation, Radiology **29**:45-60, 1963.

Gullmo, A.: The phlebographic Trendelenburg test, Brit. J. Radiol. **36**:812-821, 1963.

Hanafee, W.: Axillary artery approach to carotid, vertebral, abdominal aorta, and coronary angiography, Radiology **81**:559-567, 1963.

Karras, B. G., and others: Percutaneous left brachial aortography, Amer. J. Roentgen. **90**:564-570, 1963.

Olsson, O.: Angiographic diagnosis of islet cell tumor of the pancreas, Acta Chir. Scand. **126**:346-351, 1963.

Roy, P.: Le catheterisme percutané de l'artère axillaire; nouvelle voie d'approche pour l'artériographie carotidienne et vertébrale, Roentgen. Europ. **6-7**:122-147, 1963.

Schobinger, R. A., and Krueger, E. G.: Intraosseous epidural venography in the diagnosis of surgical diseases of the lumbar spine, Acta Radiol. [Diagn.] **1**:763-776, 1963.

Steinberg, I., and Evans, J. A.: Intravenous abdominal aortotomography, Amer. J. Roentgen. **89**:284-294, 1963.

1964 Ainsworth, J., and Gilman, P. W.: Diagnosis of placenta previa by aortography, Proc. Roy. Soc. Med. **57**:697-700, 1964.

Almeén, T., and Nylander, G.: False signs of thrombosis in lower leg phlebography, Acta Radiol. [Diagn.] **2**:345-352, 1964.

Bookstein, J. J., and Stewart, B. H.: The current status of renal arteriography, Radiol. Clin. N. Amer. **2**:461-482, 1964.

Bookstein, J. J., and Whitehouse, W. M.: Splenoportography, Radiol. Clin. N. Amer. **2**:447-460, 1964.

Bucht, H., and others: Catheterization of the left adrenal vein for contrast injection and steroid analysis in a case of Conn's syndrome, Acta Med. Scand. **176**:233-241, 1964.

Finney, L. A., and others: Interosseous vertebral venography in the diagnosis of lumbar disk disease, Amer. J. Roentgen. **92**:1282-1292, 1964.

Glenn, F., and others: Selective celiac and superior mesenteric arteriography, Surg. Gynec. Obstet. **118**:93-100, 1964.

Guibert, G. E.: Aortography in a small general hospital, Radiol. Techn. **36**:172-175, 1964.

Keats, T. E.: Trends in peripheral arteriography, Radiol. Clin. N. Amer. **2**:483-498, 1964.

Marshall, T. R., and Ling, J. T.: Percutaneous noncatheter left brachial renal arteriography, Amer. J. Roentgen. **92**:315-320, 1964.

Steinberg; I.: Method of intravenous abdominal aortography; report on present status and value in diagnosis of peripheral vascular diseases, Vasc. Dis. **1**:233-241, 1964.

Steinberg, I., and Stein, H.: Intravenous angiocardiog-

1965 raphy, abdominal aortography, and peripheral arteriography with single arm pressure injection, Amer. J. Roentgen. **92**:893-906, 1964.

Eiken, M., and others: Intra-osseous costal venography, Amer. J. Roentgen. **94**:172-181, 1965.

Friedenberg, M. J., and Carlsson, E.: Bilateral aortoilio-femoral arteriography via unilateral common femoral artery needle, Acta Radiol. [Diagn.] **3**:1-8, 1965.

Halpern, M., and Freiberger, R. H.: Arteriography in orthopedics, Amer. J. Roentgen. **94**:194-206, 1965.

Hendrick, C. K., and Schreiber, M. H.: Intravenous placentography, Amer. J. Roentgen. **93**:948-954, 1965.

Riley, J. M.: The Valsalva maneuver in renal angiography, J. Urol. **93**:631-634, 1965.

Riley, J. M., and others: Left axillary approach to the abdominal aorta, Radiology **84**:96-99, 1965.

Rösch, J., and Bret, J.: Arteriography of the pancreas, Amer. J. Roentgen. **94**:182-193, 1965.

Roy, Paul: Percutaneous catheterization via the axillary artery, Amer. J. Roentgen. **94**:1-18, 1965.

Sewell, W. H.: Coronary arteriography by the Sones technique—technical considerations, Amer. J. Roentgen. **95**:673-683, 1965.

Skinner, G. B.: The use of cinefluorography in peripheral arteriography, Amer. J. Roentgen. **95**:745-750, 1965.

Starer, F.: Percutaneous suprarenal venography, Brit. J. Radiol. **38**:675-681, 1965.

Steinberg, I., and Stein, H. L.: Visualization of abdominal aortic aneurysms, Amer. J. Roentgen. **95**:684-695, 1965.

Steinberg, I., and others: Thoracic aortography; intravenous and selective techniques, Amer. J. Roentgen. **94**:129-144, 1965.

Templeton, A. W.: Renal aortography; advantages and technique using the Valsalva maneuver, Amer. J. Roentgen. **95**:383-388, 1965.

Viamonte, M., Jr., and Stevens, R. C.: Guided angiography, Amer. J. Roentgen. **94**:30-39, 1965.

Viamonte, M., Jr., and others: Guided catheterization of the bronchial arteries, Radiology **85**:205-230, 1965.

Weidner, W., and others: Percutaneous transaxillary selective coronary angiography, Radiology **85**:652-657, 1965.

Wholey, M. II., and others: Fundamentals of angiographic techniques, Surg. Gynec. Obstet. **121**:517-527, 1965.

1966 Boijsen, E., and Reuter, S. R.: Subclavian and internal mammary angiography in the evaluation of anterior mediastinal masses, Amer. J. Roentgen. **98**:447-450, 1966.

Hyat, D. B.: Upright inferior vena cavography, Radiology **86**:865-870, 1966.

Janover, M. L., and others: Azygography and lung cancer, New Eng. J. Med. **275**:803-808, 1966.

Laubenberger, T., and Berghaus, H.: The roentgenographic exploration of the prostate and the urinary bladder floor veins; periprostatic phlebography; a new method, Amer. J. Roentgen. **98**:208-211, 1966.

Marshall, T. R., and others: Hand arteriography, Radiology **86**:299-304, 1966.

Nebesar, R. A., and Pollard, J. J.: Portal venography by selective arterial catherization, Amer. J. Roentgen. **97**:477-487, 1966.

Porstmann, W., and others: Die selektive Nebennierenangiographie [selective adrenal angiography], Fortschr. Roentgenstr. **104**:150-157, 1966. Abst.: Amer. J. Roentgen. **98**:262, 1966.

Puyau, F. A., and Burko, H.: The tilted left anterior oblique position in the study of congenital cardiac anomalies, Radiology **87**:1069-1073, 1966.

Shuford, W. H., and others: A comparison of carbon dioxide and radiopaque angiocardiographic methods in the diagnosis of pericardial effusion, Radiology **86**:1064-1069, 1966.

Sutton, D.: Arterial placentography and placenta previa, Brit. J. Radiol. **39**:47-51, 1966.

Turner, A. F., and others; Carbon dioxide cineangiocardiography in the diagnosis of pericardial disease, Amer. J. Roentgen. **97**:342-349, 1966.

1025

1967 Amsler, F. R., and Wilber, M. C.: Intraosseous vertebral venography as a diagnostic aid in evaluating disease of the lumbar spine, J. Bone Joint Surg. **49-A**:703-712, 1967.

Aronson, K. F., and Nylander, G.: Use of direct portography in diagnosis of liver diseases, Radiology **88**:40-47, 1967.

Bannister, R. J.: Arteriography, Radiol. Techn. **38**:328-345, 1967.

Bayindir, S., and Fabbender, C. W.: Die Bedeutung der selektiven Angiographie von A. coeliaca und A. mesenterica sup. für die Diagnostik von chirurgischen Oberbaucherkrankungen, Fortschr. Roentgenstr. **106**:13-23, 1967.

Chiandussi, L., and others: Hepatic portography by direct catheterization of the portal vein through the round ligament of the liver (ligamentum teres), Amer. J. Roentgen. **99**:625-628, 1967.

Deutsch, V.: Cholecystoangiography; visualization of the gallbladder by selective celiac and mesenteric angiography, Amer. J. Roentgen. **101**:608-616, 1967.

Düx, A., Winkler, C., Eber, G., and Bücheler, E.: Vergleichende vasographische und szintigraphische Untersuchungen bei Lebertumoren, Fortschr. Roentgenstr. **106**:502-524, 1967.

Feldman, F., Habif, D. V., Fleming, R. J., and others: Arteriography of the breast, Radiology **89**:1053-1061, 1967.

Hanafee, W., and Weiner, M.: Transjugular percutaneous cholangiography, Radiology **88**:35-39, 1967.

Hemley, S. D., Kanick, V., Kittredge, R. D., and Finby, N.: Intravenous aortography, Med. Radiogr. Photogr. **43**:1-31, 1967.

Kahn, P. C., and Nickrosz, L. V.: Selective angiography of the adrenal glands, Amer. J. Roentgen. **101**:739-749, 1967.

Lang, Erich K.: Arteriography in gynecology, Radiol. Clin. N. Amer. **5**:133-149, 1967.

Nordenström, B.: Selective catheterization and angiography of bronchial and mediastinal arteries in man, Acta Radiol. [Diagn.] **6**:13-24, 1967.

Wholey, M. H.: Evaluation of arteriography in obstetrics, Radiol. Clin. N. Amer. **5**:121-131, 1967.

Wickbom, I., Zachrisson, B. F., and Heinmann, P.: Thyroid angiography, Acta Radiol. [Diagn.] **6**:497-512, 1967.

1968 Frick, P. C.: Translumbar aortography, Radiol. Techn. **39**:261-266, 1968.

Herlinger, H.: Single film inclined angioplacentography in the diagnosis of placenta praevia, Clin. Radiol. **19**:59-64, 1968.

Lecky, J. W., Bashore, R. A., Tobin, P. A., and Hanafee, W. N.: Percutaneous intrauterine fetal transfusion; roentgenologic aspects and results, Amer. J. Roentgen. **103**:186-194, 1968.

McNulty, J. G.: High dose percutaneous transplenic portal venography, Brit. J. Radiol. **41**:55-58, 1968.

Moskowitz, H., Chait, A., Margulies, M., and Mellins, H. Z.: Prone splenoportography, Radiology **90**:1132-1135, 1968.

1969 Agee, O. F., and Kaude, J.: Angiography of the pelvis and lower extremities with moving table techniques, Amer. J. Roentgen. **107**:860-865, 1969.

Hynes, D. M., Verel, D., Moore, R. D., and Bates, P. F.: Assessment of a technique for coronary arteriography using 70 mm films, Brit. J. Radiol. **42**:736-743, 1969.

Morettin, L. B., and Wilson, McC.: A device for simplified femoral arteriography, Amer. J. Roentgen. **107**:866-868, 1969.

Ogden, J. A., Wade, M. E., and Davis, C. D.: Radiological aspects of fetal intrauterine transfusion, Radiology **93**:1315-1321, 1969.

Takahashi, M., Ishibashi, T., and Kawanami, H.: Angiographic diagnosis of benign and malignant tumors of the thyroid, Radiology **92**:520-526, 1969.

1970 Horner, R. W.: Angled bilateral cervical arteriography in the investigation of ischemia, Radiol. Techn. **42**:125-132, 1970.

Kattan, K. R.: Angled view in pulmonary angiography, Radiology **94**:79-82, 1970.

1971 Eisenman, J. I., and O'Loughlin, B. J.: Value of lateral abdominal aortography, Amer. J. Roentgen. **112**:586-592, 1971.

Di Rienzo, A.: Persistent portohepatography, Rev. Interamer. Radiol. **6**:40-60, 1971. (In Spanish.) Abst.: Radiology **100**:724, 1971.

1972 Damascelli, B., Cascinelli, N., Terno, G., and others: Second thoughts on the value of selective thyroid angiography, Amer. J. Roentgen. **114**:822-829, 1972.

Lea, Thomas M., and Andress, M. R.: Value of oblique projections in translumbar aortography, Amer. J. Roentgen. **116**:187-193, 1972.

1973 Bussat, P., Rossier, A. B., Djindjian, R., and others: Spinal cord angiography in dorsolumbar vertebral fractures with neurological involvement, Radiology **109**:617-620, 1973.

Lymphography

1901 Cunéo, B., and Marcille, M.: Topographie des ganglions ilio-pelviens, Bull. Soc. Anat. **3**:653-663, 1901.

1932 Pfahler, G. E.: A demonstration of the lymphatic drainage from the maxillary sinuses, Amer. J. Roentgen. **27**:352-356, 1932.

Rouvière, H.: Anatomie des lymphatiques de l'homme, Paris, 1932, Masson & Cie.

1933 Hudak, S. S., and McMaster, P. D.: Lymphatic participation in human cutaneous phenomena, J. Exp. Med. **57**:751-774, 1933.

1938 Rouvière, H.: Anatomy of the human lymphatic system, Ann Arbor, Mich., 1938, Edwards Bros.

1952 Kinmonth, J. B.: Lymphangiography in man; method of outlining lymphatic trunks at operation, Clin. Sci. **11**:13-20, 1952.

1954 Kinmonth, J. B., and Taylor, G. W.: Lymphatic circulation in lymphedema, Ann. Surg. **139**:129-136, 1954.

1955 Kinmonth, J. B., Harper, R. A. K., and Taylor, G. W.: Lymphangiography by radiological methods, J. Fac. Radiologists **6**:217-223, 1955.

Kinmonth, J. B., Taylor, G. W., and Harper, R. A. K.: Lymphangiography; technique for its clinical use in lower limb, Brit. Med. J. **1**:940-942, 1955.

1958 Collette, J. M.: Envahissements ganglionnaires inguino-ilio-pelviens par lymphographie, Acta Radiol. **39**:154-165, 1958.

Gergely, R.: The roentgen examination of the lymphatics in man, Radiology **71**:59-68, 1958.

1959 Fischer, H. W.: Lymphangiography and lymphadenography with various contrast agents, Ann. N. Y. Acad. Sci. **78**:799-808, 1959.

Jacobsson, S., and Johansson, S.: Normal roentgen anatomy of the lymph vessels of the upper and lower extremities, Acta Radiol. **51**:321-328, 1959.

1961 Fuchs, W. A., and Böök-Hederström, G.: Inguinal and pelvic lymphography, Acta Radiol. **55**:340-354, 1961.

Moulonguet-Doleris, P., and others: La lymphographie; technique, indications et resultats (conclusions portant sur 230 explorations), J. Radiol. Electr. **42**:281-296, 1961.

Sheehan, R., Herschyshyn, M., Lin, R. K., and Lessmann, F. P.: The use of lymphangiography as a diagnostic method, Radiology **76**:47-53, 1961.

Wallace, S., Jackson, L., Schaffer, B., Gould, J., Greening, R. R., Weiss, A., and Kramer, S.: Lymphangiograms: their diagnostic and therapeutic potential, Radiology **76**:179-199, 1961.

1962 Ditchek, T., and others: Lymphadenography in normal subjects, Radiology **80**:175-181, 1962.

Dolan, P. A., and Moore, E. B.: Improved technique for lymphangiography, Amer. J. Roentgen. **88**:110-111, 1962.

1963 De Roo, T.: Technick van de lymphografie, J. Belg. Radiol. **46**:462-480, 1963.

Greening, R. R., and Wallace, S.: Further observations in lymphangiography, Radiol. Clin. N. Amer. **1**:157-174, 1963.

Herman, P. G., Benninghoff, D. L., Nelson, J. H., and Mellins, H. Z.: Roentgen anatomy of the ilio-pelvic-aortic lymphatic system, Radiology **80**:182-193, 1963.

1964 Benninghoff, D. L., and Herman, P. G.: Ilio-pelvic abdomino-aortic lymphatic structures; a chart. Med. Radiogr. Photogr. **40**:35-37, 1964.

Brody, H. S., and others: Lymphangiography; an aid in urological surgery, J. Urol. **91**:606-607, 1964.

Clouse, M. E., and others: Lymphangiographic criteria for diagnosis of retroperitoneal fibrosis, Radiology **83**:1-5, 1964.

Herman, P. G., Benninghoff, D. L., and Schwartz, S.: A physiologic approach to lymph flow in lymphography, Amer. J. Roentgen. **91**:1207-1215, 1964.

Koehler, P. R., and others: Lymphangiography; a survey of its current status, Amer. J. Roentgen. **91**:1216-1221, 1964.

Lachapèle, A. P., and others: De l'étude anatomo-radiologique du canal thoracique d'après 60 opacifications sur l'être humain vivant, J. Radiol. Electr. **45**:1-10, 1964. Abst.: Amer. J. Roentgen. **92**:723, 1964.

1965 Buonocore, E., and Young, J. R.: Lymphangiographic evaluation of lymphedema and lymphatic flow, Amer. J. Roentgen. **95**:751-765, 1965.

De Roo, T.: Une nouvelle technique simple pour la lymphographie, Ann. Radiol. **8**:97-100, 1965.

De Roo, T., Thomas, P., and Kropholler, R. W.: The importance of tomography for the interpretation of the lymphographic picture of lymph node metastases, Amer. J. Roentgen. **94**:924-934, 1965.

O'Leary, J. A., and Friedman, P. J.: Lymphography and pelvic carcinoma, Amer. J. Obstet. Gynec. **92**:777-791, 1965.

Van Rensburg, L. C. J.: Lymphography—its technique and value, S. Afr. Med. J. **39**:271-277, 1965.

1966 Dolan, P. A.: Lymphography; complications encountered in 522 examinations, Radiology **86**:876-880, 1966.

Jackson, R. J. A.: Complications of lymphography, Brit. Med. J. **1**:1203-1205, 1966.

Jing, Bao-Shan: Improved technique of lymphangiography, Amer. J. Roentgen. **98**:952-956, 1966.

Love, R. W., and Takaro, T.: Lymphangiography with direct roentgenographic magnification, Radiology **87**:123-127, 1966.

1967 Ditchek, T., and Scanlon, G. T.: Direct magnification lymphography, J.A.M.A. **199**:654-656, 1967.

Kuisk, H., and Panning, W. P.: A simple, practical technic of lymphography, Radiology **88**:576-583, 1967.

Maddison, F. E.: Lymphatic cannulation without dye, Radiology **88**:362-363, 1967.

Miller, W. E.: A simplified cannulation technique for lymphangiography, Amer. J. Roentgen. **101**:978-980, 1967.

1968 O'Brien, P. H., Sherman, J. O., Brand, W. N., and Scarff, J. E.: Lymphangiography, Surg., Gynec. Obstet. **126**:131-143, 1968.

1969 Burgener, F., and Fuchs, W. A.: The importance of lymphography in the diagnosis and treatment of malignant testicular tumors, Schweiz. Med. Wschr. **99**:764-774, 1969. (In German.) Abst.: Radiology **94**:477, 1970.

1971 Lee, K. F., Hodes, P. J., and Lin, S. R.: The value of the inlet and outlet views of the pelvis in lymphography, Amer. J. Roentgen. **111**:297-300, 1971.

1972 Howland, W. J.: A cannula method of lymphangiography, Amer. J. Roentgen. **114**:830-831, 1972.

1973 Bergstrom, J. F.: A simplified and reliable cannulation technique for lymphography, Amer. J. Roentgen. **117**:701-703, 1973.

Bruna, J.: Suprailiac lymphography, Acta Radiol. [Diagn.] **14**:157-160, 1973.

PARARADIOLOGIC IMAGING MODALITIES
Ultrasonography

1952 Howry, D. H., and Bliss, W. R.: Ultrasonic visualization of soft tissue structures of the body, J. Lab. Clin. Med. **40**:579-592, 1952.

1959 De Vlieger, M. D., and Ridder, H. J.: Use of echoencephalography, Neurology **9**:216-223, 1959.

1961 Lithander, B.: Echoencephalography in children, Acta Psychiat. Scand. **36**(supp. 159):37-50, 1961.

1963 Ford, Robert, and Ambrose, J.: Echoencephalography—the measurement of the position of midline structures in the skull with high frequency pulsed ultrasound, Brain **86**:189-196, 1963.

1964 Willocks, J., Donald, I., Duggan, T. C., and Day, N.: Foetal cephalometry by ultrasound, J. Obstet. Gynaec. Brit. Comm. **71**:11-20, 1964.

1966 Bernstine, R. L., and Callagan, D. A.: Ultrasonic Doppler inspection of fetal heart, Amer. J. Obstet. Gynec. **95**:1001-1003, 1966.

Goldberg, B. B., Ostrum, B. J., Isard, H. J.: Ultrasonic aortography, J.A.M.A. **198**:353-358, 1966.

Gottesfeld, K. R., Thompson, H. E., Holmes, J. H., and Taylor, E. S.: Ultrasound placentography—a new method for placental localization, Amer. J. Obstet. Gynec. **96**:538-547, 1966.

Grossman, C. C.: A and B scan sonoencephalography (SEG)—a new dimension in neurology. In Grossman, C. C., and others, editors: Diagnostic ultrasound, New York, 1966, Plenum Press, pp. 130-141.

Lehman, J. S.: Ultrasound in the diagnosis of hepatobiliary disease, Radiol. Clin. N. Amer. **4**:605-623, 1966.

1967 Donald, I., and Abdulla, U.: Ultrasound in obstetrics and gynaecology, Brit. J. Radiol. **40**:604-611, 1967.

Ostrum, B. J., Goldberg, B. B., and Isard, H. J.: A-mode ultrasound differentiation of soft tissue masses, Radiology **88**:745-749, 1967.

Strandness, D. E., Jr., Schultz, R. D., Sumner, D. S., and Rushmer, R. F.: Ultrasonic flow detection; a useful technique in the evaluation of peripheral vascular disease, Amer. J. Surg. **113**:311-320, 1967.

1968 Brown, R. E.: Detection of intrauterine death, Amer. J. Obstet. Gynec. **102**:965-968, 1968.

Brown, R. E.: Diagnostic ultrasound associated with departments of radiology, J. Canad. Ass. Radiol. **19**:83-89, 1968.

Feuerlein, W., and Dilling, H.: The echoencephalogram of the third ventricle in different age groups. In Proceedings in echoencephalography, New York, 1968, Springer-Verlag, pp. 143-145.

Goldberg, B. B., Ostrum, B. J., and Isard, H. J.: Nephrosonography: ultrasound differentiation of renal masses, Radiology **90**:1113-1118, 1968.

Goldberg, B. B., Sklaroff, D. M., and Isard, H. J.: Echoencephalography in the management of patients receiving radiation therapy, Radiology **91**:363-366, 1968.

Sigel, B., Popky, G. L., Wagner, D. K., Boland, J. P., Mapp, E. McD., and Feigl, P.: Comparison of clinical and Doppler ultrasound evaluation of confirmed lower extremity venous disease, Surgery **64**:332-338, 1968.

Thiery, M.: Diagnostic uses of the fetal pulse detector, Bull. Soc. Roy. Belg. Gynec. Obstet. **38**:71-79, 1968.

1969 DeLand, F. H.: A modified technique of ultrasonography for the detection and differential diagnosis of breast lesions, Amer. J. Roentgen. **105**:446-452, 1969.

Kohorn, E. I., Morrison, J., Ashford, C., and Blackwell, R. J.: Ultrasonic scanning in obstetrics and gynecology, Obstet. Gynec. **34**:515-522, 1969.

1970 Engelhart, G., Blaunstein, U. H.: Ultrasound in the diagnosis of malignant pancreatic tumors, Gut **11**:443-449, 1970.

Eycleshymer, A. C., and Schoemaker, D. M.: A cross-section anatomy, ed. 2, New York, 1970, Appleton-Century-Crofts.

Freimanis, A. K.: Echographic exploration of abdominal structures, CRC Crit. Rev. Radiol. Sci. **1**:207, 1970.

Gottesfeld, K. R.: Ultrasonic diagnosis of fetal death, Amer. J. Obstet. Gynec. **108**:623-634, 1970.

1971 Brown, R. E.: Doppler ultrasound in obstetrics, J.A.M.A. **218**:1395-1399, 1971.

Thompson, H. E., and Makowski, E. L.: Estimation of birth weight and gestational age, Obstet. Gynec. **37**:44-47, 1971.

1972 Barnett, B.: Ultrasound in abdominal conditions, Radiography **38**:233-241, 1972.

Falus, M., Koranyi, G., and Sobel, M.: Follow-up studies on infants examined by ultrasound during fetal age, Orv. Hetil. **113**:2119-2121, 1972. (In Hungarian.)

Noah, B. A., and Igal, G.: Diagnosis of placenta praevia; use of the ultrasonic method compared with the radioisotope method, J. Gynec. Obstet. Biol. Reprod. 1:361-364, 1972.

Schupbach, M.: Ultrasonic diagnosis of retinal detachment, Mod. Probl. Ophthalmol. 10:443-448, 1972. (In German.)

Winsberg, F., and Mercer, E. N.: Echocardiography in combined valve disease, Radiology 105:405-411, 1972.

1973   Mason, D. T.: Non-invasive methods for the assessment of cardiac function, Calif. Med. 119:53-55, 1973.

Reed, M. F.: Ultrasonic placentography, Brit. J. Radiol. 46:255-258, 1973.

Watmough, D.: A critical assessment of ultrasonic fetal cephalometry, Brit. J. Radiol. 46:566-567, 1973.

Thermography

1840   Herschel, J. R. W.: Account of a process for rendering visible the caloric spectrum by its effects on paper properly prepared, and some further results obtained respecting the distribution of heat therein, Philos. Trans. Roy. Soc. 90:225-283, 1840.

1871   Wunderlick, C. H.: On the temperature in diseases: a manual of medical thermometry, London, 1871, The New Sydenham Society.

1876   Seguin, E.: Medical thermometry and human temperature, New York, 1876, William Wood & Co.

1916   Woodhead, G. S., and Varrier-Jones, P. C.: Investigations on clinical thermometry, Lancet 1:173-180; 338-340; 495-502, 1916.

1934   Hardy, J. D.: Radiation of heat from the human body: an instrument for measuring the radiation and surface temperature of the skin, J. Clin. Invest. 13:593-604, 1934.

1936   Hardy, J. D., and Muschenheim, C.: The emission, reflection and transmission of infrared radiation by the human skin, J. Clin. Invest. 15:1-9, 1936.

1937   McGuignan, H. A.: Medical thermometry, Ann. Med. Hist. 9:148-154, 1937.

1948   DuBois, E. F.: Fever and the regulation of body temperature, Springfield, Ill., 1948, Charles C Thomas, Publisher.

1949   Urbach, F., Nail, N. R., and Perlman, D.: The observations of temperature distributions and of thermal radiations by means of nonlinear phosphors, J. Opt. Soc. Amer. 59:1011-1019, 1949.

1954   Hardy, J. D.: Summary review of the influence of thermal radiation on human skin, Report N. NADC-MA-5415, U.S. Naval Air Development Center, Johnsville, Pa., 1954.

Hardy, J. D., and Stoll, A. M.: Radiometric methods for measurement of skin temperature, Methods Med. Res. 6:85-100, 1954.

1956   Lawson, R. N.: Implications of surface temperatures in the diagnosis of breast cancer, Canad. Med. Ass. J. 75:309-310, 1956.

1963   Barnes, R. B.: Thermography of the human body, Science 140:870-877, 1963.

1964   Albert, S. M., Glickman, M., and Kallish, M.: Thermography in orthopedics, Ann. N. Y. Acad. Sci. 121:157-170, 1964.

Atkins, E.: Body temperature elevation in disease, Ann. N. Y. Acad. Sci. 121:26-29, 1964.

Brueschke, E. E., Haberman, J. D., and Gershon-Cohen, J.: Relative densitometric analysis of thermograms for more precise temperature determinations, Ann. N. Y. Acad. Sci. 121:80-89, 1964.

Gershon-Cohen, J.: A short history of medical thermometry, Ann. N. Y. Acad. Sci. 121:4-11, 1964.

Gershon-Cohen, J., Berger, S. N., Haberman, J. D., and Barnes, R. B.: Thermography of the breast, Amer. J. Roentgen. 91:919-926, 1964.

Minard, D., Copman, L., and Dasler, A. R.: Elevation of body temperature in health, Ann. N. Y. Acad. Sci. 121:12-25, 1964.

Stoll, A. M.: Techniques and uses of skin temperature measurements, Ann. N. Y. Acad. Sci. 121:49-56, 1964.

Wolfe, William L.: Infrared imaging devices in infrared medical radiography. Ann. N. Y. Acad. Sci. 121:57-70, 1964.

1965   Birnbaum, S. J., and Kliot, D.: Thermoplacentography: placental localization by infrared sensing techniques, Obstet. Gynec. 25:515-519, 1965.

Gershon-Cohen, J., and Barnes, R. G.: Thermography, Gevaert X-ray Bulletin, No. 1, pp. 12-16, 1965.

Gershon-Cohen, J., and Haberman, J. D.: Medical thermography, Amer. J. Roentgen. 94:735-740, 1965.

Gershon-Cohen, J., and Haberman, J. D.: Obstetric and gynecologic thermography, Obstet. Gynec. 26:842-847, 1965.

Gershon-Cohen, J., Haberman, J. D., and Brueschke, E.: Medical thermography: summary of current status, Radiol. Clin. N. Amer. 3:403-431, 1965.

Lawson, R. N., and Alt, L. L.: Skin temperature recording with phosphers; a new technique, Canad. Med. Ass. J. 92:255-260, 1965.

Smessaert, A., Befeler, D., and Hicks, R. G.: Use of thermography for evaluation of sympathetic blocks, Amer. J. Surg. 109:594-598, 1965.

Wood, E. H.: Thermography in the diagnosis of cerebrovascular disease, Radiology 85:270-283, 1965.

Wright, M. M., and Korr, L. M.: Neural and spinal components of disease: progress in the application of thermography, J. Amer. Osteopath. Ass. 64:918-921, 1965.

1966   Crandell, Clifton E., and Hill, H.: Thermography in dentistry, Oral Med. Oral Path. 21:316-320, 1966.

Goldberg, H. I., Heinz, E. R., and Taveras, J. M.: Thermography in neurological patients, Acta Radiol. [Diagn.] 5:786-795, 1966.

Johnson, P. M., Siarra, J. G., and Brogg, D. G.: Placental localization; a comparison of radiopharmaceutic and thermographic methods, Amer. J. Roentgen. 96:681-689, 1966.

1967   Bjork, N. A.: AGA Thermovision, a high speed infrared camera with instantaneous picture display, J. Radiol. Electr. 48:30-33, 1967.

Gershon-Cohen, J.: Medical thermography, Sci. Amer. 216:94-102, 1967.

Lane, Warren Z.: Infrared mapping of peripheral vascular disorders, Hosp. Prac. 2:36-39, 1967.

1968   Barnes, B. R.: Diagnostic thermography, Appl. Optics 7:1673-1685, 1968.

Branemark, P., and Johansson, B. W.: Thermography as an aid in hibernation research, Acta Physiol. Scand. 73:300-304, 1968.

Edeiken, J., Wallace, J. D., Curley, R. E., and Lee, S.: Thermography and herniated lumbar discs, Amer. J. Roentgen. 102:790-796, 1968.

Freundlich, I., Wallace, J., and Dodd, G.: Thermography of the venous diameter rates in the detection of non-palpable breast carcinoma, Amer. J. Roentgen. 102:927-932, 1968.

Haberman, J. D.: The present status of mammary thermography, CA 18:314-321, 1968.

Haberman, J. D., Ehrlich, G. E., and Levinson, C.: Thermography in rheumatic diseases, Arch. Phys. Med. Rehab. 49:187-192, 1968.

Hitchcock, C. R., Hitkok, D. F., and Soucherey, R.: Thermography in mass screening for occult breast cancer, J.A.M.A. 204:419-422, 1968.

Mawdsley, C., Samuel, E., and Sumerling, M. D.: Thermography in occlusive cerebrovascular diseases, Brit. Med. J. 3:521-524, 1968.

1969   Dodd, G. D., Zermeno, A., Marsh, L., and Boyd, D.: New developments in breast thermography, Cancer 24:1212-1221, 1969.

Isard, H. J., Ostrum, B. J., and Shilo, R.: Thermography in breast carcinoma, Surg. Gynec. Obstet. 128:1289-1293, 1969.

Lilienfeld, A., Barnes, G. M., Barnes, R. B., and Brasfield, R.: An evaluation of thermography in the detection of breast cancer; a cooperative pilot study, Cancer 24:1206-1211, 1969.

Parker, J. E., and Bradham, G. B.: Thermographic demonstration of nicotine-induced vasoconstriction, J. S. Carolina Med. Ass. 65:423-425, 1969.

Thorne, F. L., Georgiado, N., and Mladick, R.: Use of thermography in determining viability of pedicle flaps, Arch. Surg. 99:97-99, 1969.

Weill, F., Colette, C., Zurlinden, B., and others: Radiology without x-rays: placenta localization by thermography and tomoechoradiography, Ann. Radiol. **12**:797-810, 1969. (In French.) Abst.: Radiology **96**:235, 1970.

1970 Feasey, C. M., James, W. B., and Davison, M.: A technique for breast thermography, Brit. J. Radiol. **43**:462-465, 1970.

Gershon-Cohen, J., Hermel, M. B., and Murdock, M. G.: Thermography in the detection of early breast cancer, Cancer **26**:1153-1156, 1970.

Guibor, P., and Kenney, A. H.: Ophthalmologic thermography, Trans. Amer. Acad. Ophthal. Otolaryng. **74**:1032-1043, 1970.

Ryan, J.: Thermography in the diagnosis of breast cancer, Australas. Radiol. **14**:70-78, 1970.

1971 Curcio, B., and Haberman, J.: Infrared thermography: a review of current medical application, instrumentation and technique, Radiol. Techn. **42**:233-247, 1971.

Farrell, C., Wallace, J. D., and Mansfield, C. M.: The use of thermography in the detection of metastatic breast cancer, Amer. J. Roentgen. **111**:148-152, 1971.

Haberman, J.: Image analysis of medical infrared thermograms, CRC Crit. Rev. Radiol. Sci. **2**:427-465, 1971.

1972 Haberman, J., Francis, J., and Love, T. J.: Thermographic responses to local external heat sources, Radiology **102**:341-348, 1972.

NUCLEAR MEDICINE AND NUCLEAR MEDICINE TECHNOLOGY

1960 Overman, R. T., and Clark, H. M.: Radioisotope techniques, New York, 1960, McGraw-Hill Book Co.

1964 Price, W. J.: Nuclear radiation detection, ed. 2, New York, 1964, McGraw-Hill Book Co.

1967 Chase, G., and Rabinowitz, J.: Principles of radioisotope methodology, ed. 3, Minneapolis, Minn., 1967, Burgess Publishing Co.

Hine, G., editor: Instrumentation in nuclear medicine, vol. 1, New York, 1967, Academic Press, Inc.

1968 Silver, S.: Radioactive nuclides in medicine and biology, Medicine **3**:1968.

Wagner, H. N., editor: Principles of nuclear medicine, Philadelphia, 1968, W. B. Saunders Co.

1969 Freeman, L., and Johnson, P., editors: Clinical scintillation scanning, New York, 1969, Harper & Row, Publishers.

Maynard, C. D.: Clinical nuclear medicine, Philadelphia, 1969, Lea & Febiger.

Sodee, D. B., Early, P. J., and Razzak, M. A.: Textbook of nuclear medicine technology, St. Louis, 1969, The C. V. Mosby Co.

1970 Quimby, E. H., Feitelberg, S., and Gross, W.: Radioactive nuclides in medicine and biology, Basic Physics Instrumentation **3**:1970.

Simmons, G.: Training manual for nuclear medicine technologists, Rockville, Md., 1970, U. S. Dept. of Health, Education and Welfare, Bureau of Radiologic Health.

1971 Arena, V.: Ionizing radiation and life, St. Louis, 1971, The C. V. Mosby Co.

Beierwaltes, W., Keyes, J., and Carey, J.: Manual of nuclear medicine procedures, Cleveland, 1971, Chemical Rubber Press Co.

Hoffer, P., Beck, R., and Gottschalk, A.: Semiconductor detectors in the future of nuclear medicine, New York, 1971, The Society of Nuclear Medicine, Inc.

Powsner, E. R., and Raeside, D. E.: Diagnostic nuclear medicine, New York, 1971, Grune & Stratton, Inc.

1972 Sodee, D. B., and Early, P. J.: Technology and interpretations of nuclear medicine procedures, St. Louis, 1972, The C. V. Mosby Co.

1973 Byers, B. J., Dielman, R. W., and Mueller, M. I.: Essentials of nuclear medicine technology, Glenview, Ill., 1973, The Society of Nuclear Medical Technologists, Inc.

Lange, R. C.: Nuclear medicine for technologists, Chicago, 1973, Year Book Medical Publishers, Inc.

Quinn, J. L., III, editor: Year book of nuclear medicine, Chicago, 1973, Year Book Medical Publishers, Inc.

Periodicals

Journal of Nuclear Medicine, New York, 1955-
Vignettes in Nuclear Medicine, St. Louis, 1966-
Seminars in Nuclear Medicine, New York, 1971-
Abbott Laboratories Radio-Pharmaceutical Bulletins, North Chicago, Ill., 1973-
Journal of Nuclear Medicine Technology, New York, 1973-

RADIATION THERAPY

1932 Thoraeus, R.: A study of the conization method for measuring the intensity and absorption of x-rays and of different filters used in therapy, Acta Radiol., supplement 15, 1932.

1955 Tsien, K. D.: The application of automatic computing machines to radiation therapy treatment planning, Brit. J. Radiol. **28**:543, 1955.

1957 Alexander, P.: Atomic radiation and life, Baltimore, 1957, Penguin Books.

1963 American Cancer Society, Inc.: A cancer source book for nurses, 1963.

American Cancer Society, Inc.: Essentials of cancer nursing, 1963.

National Bureau of Standards (NBS): Clinical dosimetry, Handbook 88, August, 1963.

National Bureau of Standards (NBS): Radiological dosimetry, Handbook 87, April, 1963.

Paterson, R.: The treatment of malignant disease by radiotherapy, ed. 2, London, 1963, Edward Arnold, Ltd.

1965 Grigg, E. R.N.: Trail of the invisible light, Springfield, Ill., 1965, Charles C Thomas, Publisher.

1966 Kaplan, H. S., and Rosenberg, S. A.: Treatment of Hodgkin's disease, Med. Clin. N. Amer. **50**:1591-1610, 1966.

Schwartz, E. E.: The biological basis of radiation therapy, Philadelphia, 1966, J. B. Lippincott Co.

1967 Elkind, M. D., and Whitmore, G. F.: The radiobiology of cultured mammalian cells, New York, 1967, Gordon & Breach.

1968 Fenner, M. L.: Elementary clinical radiotherapy, London, 1968, Butterworth & Co.

International Commission on Radiation Units and Measurements (ICRU): Radiation quantities and units, No. 11, September, 1968.

1969 Bogardus, C. R., Jr.: Clinical applications of physics of radiology and nuclear medicine, St. Louis, 1969, Warren H. Green, Inc.

International Commission on Radiation Units and Measurements (ICRU): Radiation dosimetry, 0.6-50 MeV, No. 14, September, 1969.

Johns, H. E., and Cunningham, J. R.: The physics of radiology, ed. 2, Springfield, Ill., 1969, Charles C Thomas, Publisher.

Stanton, L.: Basic medical radiation physics, New York, 1969, Appleton-Century-Crofts.

Walter, J., and Miller, H.: A short textbook of radiotherapy for technicians and students, ed. 3, Boston, 1969, Little, Brown & Co.

1970 Ackerman, L. V. and Del Regato, J. A.: Cancer diagnosis, treatment and prognosis, ed. 4, St. Louis, 1970, The C. V. Mosby Co.

American Cancer Society, Inc.: Clinical oncology for medical students and physicians, a multidisciplinary approach, ed. 3, 1970-1971.

Burch, R. J.: New approach to cancer, Nature **225**:512, 1970.

Grant, R. N., and Silverberg, E.: Cancer statistics, 1970, New York, 1970, American Cancer Society, Inc.

Florey, H.: General pathology, Philadelphia, 1970, W. B. Saunders Co.

National Council Radiation Protection and Measurements (NCRP): Basic radiation protection criteria, No. 39, 1971.

1972 Barnes, P. A., and Rees, D. J.: A concise textbook of

radiotherapy, Philadelphia, 1972, J. B. Lippincott Co.

Pizzarello, D. J., and Witcofski, R.: Medical radiation biology, Philadelphia, 1972, Lea & Febiger.

Vaeth, J. M.: Frontiers of radiation therapy and oncology. Volume 7, The interrelationship of the immune response and cancer, Baltimore, 1972, University Park Press.

1973 Dalrymple, G. V., and others: Medical radiation biology, Philadelphia, 1973, W. B. Saunders Co.

Fletcher, G. H.: Textbook of radiotherapy, ed. 2, Philadelphia, 1973, Lea & Febiger.

Moss, W. T., Brand, W. N., and Battifora, H.: Radiation oncology: rationale, technique, results, ed. 4, St. Louis, 1973, The C. V. Mosby Co.

Index

1

7